STOCHASTIC PROCESSES IN EPIDEMIOLOGY

STOCHASTIC PROCESSES IN EPIDEMIOLOGY

HIV/AIDS, Other Infectious Diseases and Computers

Charles J Mode
Candace K Sleeman

Drexel University, USA

World Scientific
Singapore • New Jersey • London • Hong Kong

Published by

World Scientific Publishing Co. Pte. Ltd.

P O Box 128, Farrer Road, Singapore 912805

USA office: Suite 1B, 1060 Main Street, River Edge, NJ 07661

UK office: 57 Shelton Street, Covent Garden, London WC2H 9HE

British Library Cataloguing-in-Publication Data
A catalogue record for this book is available from the British Library.

STOCHASTIC PROCESSES IN EPIDEMIOLOGY

ISBN 981-02-4097-X

This book is printed on acid and chlorine free paper.

Printed in Singapore by World Scientific Printers

Dedication

To the idea that stochastic models, coupled with computer intensive methods, will in future play a significant role in man's quest to understand and control epidemics of infectious diseases.

Preface

AIDS, acquired immune deficiency syndromes, is a devastating disease caused by HIV, human immunodeficiency virus, which may be transmitted by either sexual or other contacts in which body fluids are exchanged. Following a few recognized cases among homosexual men in the United States in the early 1980's, cases of AIDS were subsequently reported in a majority of countries throughout the world among heterosexuals, intravenous drugs users and others, indicating that HIV/AIDS was a global pandemic. It is indeed a pandemic of such proportions that it ranks as one of the most destructive microbial scourges in human history and has posed formidable challenges to the biomedical research and public health communities of the world. In response to these challenges, a voluminous biomedical literature on HIV/AIDS has been generated during the last two decades, including mathematical papers in numerous journals of applied mathematics, applied probability, biomathematics and biostatistics. When this book was first conceived, the original intention was to confine attention to those mathematical and statistical techniques underlying the models used to understand the dynamics of epidemics of HIV/AIDS as they developed in populations, with an emphasis of computer intensive methods. But as the development of ideas progressed, it became apparent that many of the techniques would be applicable to the populations dynamics of other infectious diseases. Consequently, the scope of the book was broadened to include other infectious diseases, although the main focus of the book has remained that of HIV/AIDS and other sexually transmitted diseases.

Mathematical models of epidemics of infectious diseases may be classified into two broad classes, deterministic and stochastic. Ordinary non-linear differential equations are among the principal tools used in the formulation of most deterministic models of epidemics, but when ages of individuals are accommodated in models, some authors have based their formulations on first order non-linear partial differential equations, belonging to the McKendrick-von Foerster class. Even though there is an extensive literature on deteministic models of epidemics, all deterministic models are incomplete in the sense that the variation and uncertainty that characterizes the development of most epidemics in populations cannot be accommodated in purely deteministic formulations. A widely recognized need to accommodate this variation and uncertainty has given rise to a rather large literature on stochastic models of epidemics, which takes into account variability in the development of epidemics and quantifies the uncertainties as to what course an epidemic may take in terms of probabilities. Because, for the most part, the mathematics underlying stochastic formulations is more difficult to penetrate than that used in deteministic formulations, this difficulty has in the past proven to be a barrier to applying stochastic models in practical situations. But, with the help of computer intensive methods designed to compute sample realizations of an epidemic, practical illustrations of the variability inherent in the evolution of a stochastic process are provided, and the barriers to practical application may, in part, be removed.

Computer intensive methods, whose aim is to compute random samples from probability distributions or stochastic processes, are often referred to collectively as Monte Carlo simulation. Contained within the literature of epidemiology published during the last three decades, as well as other fields of the biological sciences, are numerous papers devoted to reporting the results of Monte Carlo simulation experiments designed to gain some understanding of the intrinsic variability and uncertainty inherent in the evolution of most biological phenomena. Although the intent of these papers is impeccable, most of them are unsatisfactory to the mathematical scientist because they usually lack a formal account of the mathematical structures underlying their computer experiments. This lack of any formal account of mathematical structures on which their simulations are based is a serious impediment to understanding and interpreting the results of their computer experiments, for it can be demonstrated by examples that the results one obtains in Monte Carlo simulation experiments can depend significantly on the assumptions going into the design of the stochastic process from which the sample of realizations was supposed to have come. In short, this lack of formal documentation of the stochastic model underlying some Monte Carlo simulation models is analogous to asking a chemist or experimental biologist to evaluate the credibility of a laboratory experiment in which only the final results are reported, but the techniques used to obtain the results are withheld from his or her scrutiny so that any attempt to duplicate the results would be very difficult and time consuming.

One of the distinguishing features of this book is that a concerted attempt has been made to make clear the assumptions going into the design of the stochastic processes underlying all reported computer simulation experiments. No attempt has been made, however, to include listings of the computer code used in the implementations of the stochastic processes developed in this book. The reasons for this omission are two fold. Firstly, because it is a succinct and powerful medium in which to develop experimental code for not only computing Monte Carlo samples of realizations of stochastic processes, but also for computing informative summary statistics of these samples, such as the trajectories of order statistics, the programming language APL has been used to write the code for all the implementations of stochastic processes presented in this book. But, unfortunately, even though the authors have had over a decade of experience programming in this language, and there is a sizeable international community devoted to it, most readers would be unfamiliar with the succinct, but powerful notation that characterizes this language. Consequently, a second reason for not listing the computer code is that relatively few people would be able read it without a specialized knowledge of the symbols peculiar to APL. In principle, however, because an attempt has been made to carefully outline all computational procedures, the experimental results could be duplicated, using such widely used programming languages as C++, FORTRAN, or even MATLAB, a computer software package with numerous capabilities that is being used by an increasing number of engineers and scientists.

Another distinguishing feature of this book is that deterministic and stochastic models are not discussed in isolation, but are presented in a framework that synthesizes the two approaches in formulating models of epidemics. This synthesis is accomplished by systematically using a scheme of embedding deterministic models in a stochastic process by taking conditional expectations of present values of the sample functions, given the past, and using other approximation schemes borrowed from theories of statistical estimation. An advantage of this embedding scheme is that it allows for comparison of the trajectory of some feature of an epidemic based on the embedded deterministic model with the corresponding trajectories of statistical summaries of a sample of Monte Carlo realizations of the process. Included in these summaries are the trajectories of chosen quantiles and the mean trajectory of a Monte Carlo sample. By inspecting graphs of these summary trajectories, it becomes possible to assess to what degree a projection of an epidemic made solely on the basis of a deterministic model would be misleading or under what circumstances a deterministic projection may be adequate. Background and motivational material for developing deterministic and stochastic models within a unified formulation amenable to using computer intensive methods is considered in Chapters 1 through to 9, but, for the most part, computer intensive methods were used extensively only in Chapters 10, 11 and 12. Consequently, an overview of the themes used in the development of these chapters will be provided.

Four themes underlie the development of the new non-linear stochastic models of epidemics of HIV/AIDS and other sexually transmitted diseases presented in Chapters 10, 11, and 12, which accommodate one or more risk groups or behavioral classes and states of disease in definitions of the types of individuals. The same themes will underlie the age dependent models outlined in Chapter 13, which are extensions of the model developed in Chapter 12. As yet, however, the rather difficult task of developing software for these more complex models has not been undertaken. The first of these themes is to define state spaces for semi-Markovian life cycle models, which include types of individuals, along with matrices of competing latent risks, governing transitions among states. For the case of the one-sex model presented in Chapter 10, the life cycle model pertains to the evolution of individuals in the population, but, for models accommodating marital partnership or couples in Chapters 11 and 12, life cycle models for singles and couples are included. Among the latent risks in all life cycle models are those governing the infection of susceptibles due to sexual contacts with infected individuals.

Whether a susceptible individual becomes infected during any time interval depends upon his or her choices of sexual partners among the types of individuals present in the population at any time. Consequently, a second theme that underlies the models presented in Chapters 10, 11 and 12 is that of the use of an acceptance probability, which is a parametric function expressing the probability that a person of one type finds another acceptable as a sexual partner. In order for a sexual contact to occur, both partners must find each other acceptable, and by using set of probability arguments, including the law of total probability and Bayes' theorem, it is possible to express the latent risk that a susceptible person becomes infected during any time interval as non-linear functions of the sample functions of the process at any time, as well as functions of the parameters of the acceptance probabilities. By varying these parameters, it is possible to consider random and highly assortative mixing patterns in choosing sexual partners. For the partnership models of Chapters 11 and 12, the idea of acceptance probabilities is also used to model couple formation.

A third theme common to Chapters 10, 11, and 12 is the use of matrices of competing latent risks in the life cycle models to systematically compute vectors of conditional probabilities for chains of multinomial distributions that are used in the recursive computation of Monte Carlo realizations of the sample functions of the process on a time lattice of equally spaced points. Such computational schemes are sometimes referred to as chain multinomial models. According to these models, given values of the sample functions at some time point on the lattice, the conditional distribution of the sample functions at the next point in time is a multinomial distribution whose probabilities depend on the values of the sample functions of the preceding point in time. By taking conditional expectations of these vectors of multinomial random variables, given the past, along with other operations, it becomes possible to systematize procedures for embedding non-linear difference equations in the stochastic epidemic models on the discrete time lattice. Given a numerical specification of any point in the parameter space of the model and a set of initial conditions, it is then possible to compute trajectories describing various aspects of the evolution of an epidemic as it would develop in time according to the embedded deterministic model. Furthermore, by using computer generated graphs, the trajectories determined by the embedded difference equations may be compared visually with various statistical trajectories, such as selected quantiles, summarizing a Monte Carlo sample computed according to a chain multinomial model.

Unlike many stochastic models of epidemics, branching process approximations cannot be used to derive threshold conditions of the non-linear models of Chapter 10, 11, and 12, particularly in those cases where the parameters in the acceptance probabilities are chosen such that the selection of sexual partners is highly assortative. Consequently, it became necessary to find other approaches to finding threshold conditions for the stochastic models. Let $h > 0$ denote the distance between any two points in a discrete time lattice. Then, by letting $h \downarrow 0$, it can be shown, under rather general conditions, that the embedded non-linear difference equations give rise to a system of ordinary non-linear differential equations. Thus, a fourth theme common to Chapters 10, 11, and 12 is that of finding threshold conditions by deriving formulas for the partial derivatives that arise as elements in the Jacobian matrix for the embedded differential equations, and testing whether this matrix is stable or unstable when evaluated at a stationary population state vector for the case where the population is free of infected individuals. The stability or non-stability of this Jacobian matrix provides a useful indicator as to whether an epidemic will or will not develop according to a stochastic model, following the introduction of a few infectives into a population of susceptibles, and this is demonstrated empirically in the computer experiments reported in these chapters. Because many types of individuals in a population give rise to large Jacobian matrices, and the parameter spaces of the models are of high dimensions, it was not practically feasible to derive stability conditions symbolically. Consequently, software was written to compute Jacobian matrices and their eigenvalues numerically at any parameter point so that it could be numerically determined whether all real parts of the eigenvalues were negative. Furthermore, search engines were written to explore what regions in a parameter space would yield stable or unstable Jacobian matrices.

Among the countless numbers of numerical examples that could be have been chosen to illustrate biologically interesting realizations of the stochastic models, only a select sample of experiments was chosen for presentation, due to space limitations. It seems appropriate, therefore, to offer an explanation as to why these computer experiments were chosen for presentation. A theme common to most of the reported computer experiments was that the evolution of an epidemic was started by either the invasion of a few initial infectives into a population of susceptibles in demographic equilibrium, or by a recurrent stream of infective recruits that could enter the population during any time interval with low probability. In such experiments, it was observed that trajectories of the epidemic determined by the embedded deterministic model were often representative of only the worst cases of the epidemic that would occur in a Monte Carlo sample, especially in those cases where there was a positive probability of extinction or infective recruits entered the population with low probability during any time interval. Thus, if investigators confined their attention to using only deterministic models to forecast an epidemic, they could be seriously misled as to the severity of an epidemic. Epidemics of HIV/AIDS develop slowly in populations, and it seems reasonable to suppose that in many parts of the world, the pandemic is still in its early stages. This supposition motivated the selection of most of the computer experiments that have been presented in an attempt to highlight the importance of taking stochastic fluctuations into account in forecasting the future course of an epidemic still in its early stages.

Mention should also be made of the results of some computer experiments that were not reported due to space limitations. Among these experiments were those in which it was assumed that an epidemic had reached maturity in a population and that strategies of prevention to rid the population of infectives over time had been implemented. The effectiveness of a set of such strategies could be expressed by assigning values to parameters and testing whether the Jacobian matrix of the embedded differential equations was stable at a parameter point in question, when evaluated at a stationary vector for a population containing only susceptibles. By adjusting such parameters as the probability that a susceptible was infected per sexual contact with an infective, as well as those in acceptance probabilities so that a susceptible finds an infective acceptable as a sexual partner with low probability, one could attain stability of the Jacobian matrix, which would suggest that eventually the epidemic would become extinct. However, it was found in a number of experiments that if an investigator relied solely on the embedded deterministic model to forecast the evolution of an epidemic or its path to extinction, he or she could be seriously misled if the stochastic fluctuations exhibited in a sample of Monte Carlo projections were ignored. In conclusion, based on the evidence collected from the large number of computer experiments conducted so far, significant stochastic fluctuations will occur when a population undergoes a transition from one point of equilibrium to another. Indeed, it is this transient behavior with its stochastic fluctuations, rather than the existence of points equilibria, that produces the phenomena of most interest in computer experiments designed to study the development and control of epidemics of infectious diseases.

Acknowledgments

A number of people have provided help, encouragement and inspiration while the authors were working on this book. Among them is Guenther Hasibeder, who in 1994 and 1996 invited the senior author, C.J.M., to give a series lectures on Stochastic Processes in Epidemiology in the Institute of Algebra and Computational Mathematics of the Technical University of Vienna. Words of thanks are also due Dietmar Dornenger, Head of the Department of Algebra, and his colleagues, who with customary Viennese hospitality and camaraderie, made the author's visits to Austria most rewarding and pleasant. It was during these visits that most of the material presented in Chapters 6 and 7 was developed.

Three professional colleagues have read initial drafts of Chapters 6 and 7 and have offered constructive criticisms. John Jacquez, a late Professor Emeritus of the University of Michigan Medical School, read a draft of Chapter 6 and made a number of valuable suggestions. Frank Ball, Department of Mathematics, University of Nottingham, United Kingdom, read drafts of Chapters 6 and 7 and offered a number of valuable technical and historical comments that improved the presentation. Finally, Ingemar Nasell, Department of Mathematics, The Royal Institute of Technology, Stockholm, Sweden, read Chapter 7 and made a number of insightful comments that were included in the final version of the chapter.

Words of thanks are due also to Ms. Sook Chen Lim of World Scientific Publishing Company, who read preliminary drafts of the book and made many useful annotations, pointing out grammatical and typographical errors that were subsequently corrected.

The senior author, C.J.M., also wishes to extend a special word of thanks to his wife Eleanore, who with patience and forbearance agreed to postpone recreational travel until work on the book was completed.

The junior author, C.K.S., wishes to thank her father Richard Sleeman, Professor Emeritus of the Massachusetts College of Liberal Arts, for all his support and counsel, as well as her husband Ralph Fife for all his love and encouragement.

Acknowledgments

Contents

Chapter 1
BIOLOGY AND EPIDEMIOLOGY OF HIV/AIDS

1.1 Introduction

Mathematical models of any natural phenomenon should rest on some basic knowledge of the phenomenon in question and the data collected to track and understand it. Accordingly, the purpose of this chapter is to provide a brief outline of the basic biology underlying what has become known as the international HIV/AIDS epidemic and the diseases associated with it. Just as a biologist might find it difficult to penetrate the terminology and concepts used by a mathematical scientist, so it is with a mathematical scientist who attempts to penetrate the specialized biological literature. Consequently, the literature chosen for review in this chapter has been taken, for the most part, from interdisciplinary journals whose aim is to communicate with a wide audience. Even though such literature may lack the details required for a specialist in biology, the material presented in what follows seems adequate as a starting point for construction and analysis of mathematical models designed to understand the population dynamics underlying the possibilities for controlling the epidemic.

1.2 Emergence of a New Disease

When first encountered, the causative factors or agents underlying some reported human ailment may not be well understood. This was certainly the case for what has become known as AIDS (acquired immunodeficiency syndromes), when, during the early eighties, young homosexual men in the USA appeared at clinics with diseases not common to their age group. Among the reported cases were five young homosexual men who were treated for *Pneumosystis carinii* pneumonia, a disease associated with depression of the immune system, at hospitals in the city of Los Angeles between October 1980 and May 1981. At about the same time, a type of cancer, *Kaposi's sarcoma,* was being diagnosed with increasing frequency among young homosexual men in the cities of New York and San Francisco. By early 1982, workers in public health began to suspect that some causal agent, transmitted through semen in sexual contacts, may be a common link among these reported cases involving young homosexual men.

By the fall of 1981, the United States Public Health Service had taken initiatives aimed at trying to understand and define this new disease, and during 1982 cases of AIDS were being reported among people suffering from hemophilia, persons receiving blood transfusions, intravenous drug users (IVDU's), and children born to mothers at high risk of contracting AIDS. These latter cases clearly implicated blood as a medium of transmission and confirmed the suspicion that some causal infectious agent was involved. For technical and scientific references on the history of the early development of the AIDS epidemic the well-known book by Anderson and May[2] may be consulted. An interesting and informative account of the politics and people involved in the early stages of the epidemic in the United States and elsewhere, particularly among homosexual men as they became aware of the presence of some unknown causal agent of a collection of diseases that were devastating their communities, has been given by the late journalist Shilts,[32] a casualty of AIDS.

1.3 A New Virus as a Causal Agent

As recently as the early eighties, it was widely believed by public health workers that infectious diseases were no longer much of a threat in the developed world, for it was thought that the remaining challenges to public health stemmed from noninfectious conditions such as cancer, heart disease, and degenerative diseases. The advent of AIDS in the early eighties shattered these beliefs, but, thanks to rapid progress in basic molecular biology during the preceding three decades, science responded quickly and much light was shed on the nature of the epidemic in the short time period mid-1982 to mid-1984. During this period, a new retrovirus – the human immunodeficiency virus (HIV) – was isolated and shown to be the cause of the disease; a blood test was formulated to detect the virus in a person, and the virus's targets in the body were established. An account of this work for the scientific layman has been given by two investigators credited with the discovery of HIV, Gallo and Montagnier.[12] Even though it is not universally accepted that HIV is a causative agent of AIDS, these authors may also be consulted for a discussion of the evidence that HIV is indeed now firmly established as the causal agent of AIDS, a view that is accepted by a vast majority of investigators.

As AIDS emerged, the fact that retroviruses were not new to science contributed greatly to the basic understanding of the epidemic by narrowing the search for a causative agent. By the beginning of the twentieth century, a number of investigators had identified transmissible agents in animals that were capable of causing solid-tissue tumors as well as leukemias, cancers of blood cells. During the subsequent decades, retroviruses were identified in many animal species. However, the life cycles of retroviruses remained obscure until 1970, when H. M. Temin of the University of Wisconsin, Madison, and D. Baltimore of the Massachusetts Institute of Technology independently discovered an enzyme, reverse transcriptase. A property that characterizes retroviruses is their capacity to reverse the flow of genetic information from DNA to RNA to proteins, the structural and functional molecules of cells. For in retroviruses RNA is the genetic material and the reverse transcriptase carried by the virus uses RNA as a template for making DNA, which, in turn, integrates itself into the genome (chromosome complement) of the host. After making itself at home among the host's genes, the viral DNA remains latent until it is activated to make new virus particles. Tumor formation may also result from a process initiated by the latent DNA in the host.

The process just described takes place at the cellular level and, like many biological phenomena, is complex in nature. When entering the blood stream, a particle of HIV has two main targets among white blood cells, the lymphocyte and the macrophage. In particular, a subset of lymphocytes called T4 cells are infected and subsequently killed by HIV. In fact, a clinical hallmark of AIDS is the depletion of the T4 cell population, which helped establish HIV as the causal agent of AIDS. Unlike T4 cells, macrophage cells are not killed by HIV and may serve as a reservoir for the virus and thus can be transported in the circulatory system to various parts of the body, such as the brain, where some AIDS defining disease may develop. Among the key findings in the understanding of HIV infection was that infection begins when a virus particle binds to a molecule called $CD4^+$ on a target cell membrane, and the ensuing events have been described in detail by Weber and Weiss.[35] Once the virus enters a cell, subsequent events are controlled by an array of regulatory genes, making up the genetically complex HIV genome (see Haseltine and Wong-Staal[14] and also Fauci[11]) for details. An interesting and informative review of retroviruses has been given by Varmus.[34]

1.4 On the Evolutionary Origins of HIV

Another avenue to explore in attempting to understand and control the AIDS epidemic is to seek answers to questions regarding the evolutionary origin of the virus causing AIDS by studying related pathogens. Such an opportunity arose when many blood samples were tested from people who had lived in Guinea-Bissau, a former Portuguese colony in West Africa. Although many of these people had been diagnosed by Portuguese clinicians and investigators as having AIDS, their blood showed no signs of HIV infection. In October 1985, samples of blood from such people were tested for HIV by Montagnier and his coworkers (see Gallo and Montagnier[12]). It turned out that these people were infected with a new AIDS virus, which was designated as HIV-2 to distinguish it from the virus HIV-1 that was first discovered and which is responsible for the main AIDS epidemic in the USA and other developed countries. A comparative structural analysis revealed that HIV-1 and HIV-2 were similar in their overall structure and both can cause AIDS, suggesting they are related from an evolutionary point of view. The existence of two viruses that can cause AIDS suggested that other HIV's may exist as part of a spectrum of related pathogens.

As reported by Essex and Kanki,[9] a prior knowledge of related

T lymphotrophic retroviruses in monkeys and humans led investigators to search for a virus related to HIV in other primates. A serologic examination of a large number of primates was undertaken in 1984 to detect antibodies to HIV in monkey blood, a search that soon yielded evidence of a virus in blood samples from Asian macaques housed at the New England primate center. At about the same time, veterinary pathologists at several primate research centers in the USA were reporting outbreaks of AIDS-like disease in captive macaques called simian AIDS or SAIDS. The virus causing SAIDS was isolated, characterized, and designated simian immunodeficiency virus, SIV. Just as with HIV, this virus infected the same $CD4^+$ subset of lymphocytes, and the biochemical and biophysical properties of SIV proteins were very similar to those of HIV proteins. Genetic studies subsequently showed that SIV was approximately 50% related to HIV at the nucleotide-sequence level. Although the organization of structural and regulatory genes of SIV and HIV was virtually identical in many respects, SIV contained genes not found in HIV.

As the study of SIV continued in 1985, investigators began to wonder whether a knowledge of the geographic distribution of SIV found in Asian macaques might provide clues to the origin of the virus causing human AIDS. Extensive seroepidemiological studies of wild and captive Asian monkeys, including macaques, failed to find evidence for a SIV- or an HIV-like agent, suggesting that SIV did not naturally infect Asian monkeys in the wild and that primate center macaques had been infected with SIV while in captivity. These results led to a seroepidemiological survey of African primates, including chimpanzees, African green monkeys, baboons, and patas monkeys. No evidence of SIV infection was found in chimpanzees, baboons, or patas monkeys, but, in an initial survey, 50% of wild African green monkeys showed signs of SIV infection. Later surveys, conducted by taking blood samples from various regions of sub-Saharan Africa and others housed in research facilities throughout the world, showed that 30% to 70% of green monkeys tested positive for SIV, but, unlike the Asian macaques, these monkeys showed no signs of immunodepression and disease. The fact that various green monkey subspecies are among the most ecologically successful African primates suggested that such high rates of infection had not been exerting adverse selection pressure on the species.

Like other intracellular parasites, retroviruses tend to coexist with their natural host species in such a way that both the pathogen and host survive. For some retroviruses of rodents and chickens, for example, there has been mutual adaptation so that the viral genome has been integrated into the host genome and is regularly inherited by all members of the species. In such cases, the virus becomes endogenous to the host and is no longer pathogenic. Indeed, such observations in nature of interspecies transfer of genetic material has led to the concept of genetically engineering a species by transferring desirable genes from one species to another of economic value. But, SIV and HIV are exogenous in the sense that they may be transmitted horizontally among individuals of a species. Just as with other infectious agents, it seems plausible that retroviruses may be most pathogenic when they first enter a new host, but, subsequently natural selection may modify the genomes of both the host and parasite so that they may coexist. In this connection, it is of interest to note the existence of complementary genetic systems of an obligate rust fungus that attacks flax, a plant of economic importance as a source of fiber for linens and linseed oil. Even though the fungus may not be completely fatal to the host, a mathematical analysis suggested that their complementary genetic systems have evolved so as to permit the coexistence of both species (see Mode[27] for details).

Because SIV was the closest known animal-virus related to HIV, Essex and Kanki[9] investigated the possibility of finding a human virus that may be an intermediate between SIV and HIV, by acting on the idea that various HIV's and/or SIV's might exist as a spectrum of viruses in different monkey and human populations. To investigate this possibility, high-risk people from those diverse parts of Africa, where SIV-infected monkey populations had been found earlier, were examined. Female prostitutes were included in these studies, because in these parts of the world, they were at an elevated risk for being infected with sexually transmitted viruses. Moreover, unlike many industrialized countries, male homosexuals, IVDU's, and hemophiliacs are either rare or are difficult to identify in these parts of Africa. Early in 1985, evidence for such a SIV-related virus was found in Senegal,

West Africa, where about 10% of blood samples from prostitutes contained antibodies that reacted with both SIV and HIV. It turned out that the antibodies reacted much better with SIV antigens than with those of HIV; furthermore, the reactivity of the prostitutes' antibodies to SIV was indistinguishable from that of the antibodies in the blood of SIV-infected macaques and African green monkeys.

At about the same time, F. Clavel and L. Montagnier of the Pasteur Institute also showed that West African people were infected with a virus very similar to SIV. Their studies, as well as those of Essex and Kanki, showed that people infected with HIV-2 have antibodies entirely cross-reactive with SIV antigens. Indeed, on the basis of serological criteria, it was impossible to distinguish between SIV and HIV-2. An examination of the nucleotide sequences of the two viruses also revealed that they were closely related. Such evidence suggests that the primate and human viruses share evolutionary roots and thus raise the possibility that there may have been interspecies infection, i.e., SIV-infected monkeys may have transmitted the virus to humans and vice versa. The fact that HIV-2 seemed to be less pathogenic than HIV-1 also suggested that this difference may provide clues to the biological control of HIV-1 infections.

1.5 AIDS Therapies and Vaccines

As soon as HIV-1 was identified as the causal agent of AIDS, intensive research to find therapies and vaccines was undertaken by a number of investigators. Yarchoan et al.[36] reviewed results in progress as of 1988 and reported on evidence that one drug, AZT, which was already in clinical use, relieved HIV-induced dementia and other AIDS defining diseases. A common thread running throughout the search for therapies was that from a basic knowledge of the viral life cycle it might be possible to design drugs that interrupted specific phases of the cycle and thus slow down the growth of the virus population in an infected individual. Researchers are not, however, optimistic about finding therapies that would clear an infected person of all virus particles.

In principle, the best way to combat any disease is to prevent it, and, historically, vaccination has been the simplest, safest, and most effective form of prevention. Furthermore, vaccines have achieved legendary success against viruses. Matthews and Bolognesi[26] reported on the development of AIDS vaccines and reviewed a number of candidates currently being tested and others in development at a number of universities, government laboratories, and international pharmaceutical companies. An example of the types of vaccines being tested was a killed virus tested by the Salk Institute for Biological Studies, University of California at Davis, in which a whole inactivated HIV, with genetic material removed, was an immunogen tested in people. But, success in these ventures is far from assured, for the life cycle of the virus and the logistics of testing any AIDS vaccine make HIV-1 a challenge without precedent.

An alternative approach to the development of a vaccine is to use one type of HIV to protect against another type. In the 18th century, Edward Jenner, a British country doctor, observed that milkmaids who developed the mild cowpox disease rarely suffered the ravages of smallpox. This observation led to the development of vaccines for smallpox, which was caused by a type of cowpox virus. Marlink, Kanki, Essex et al.[25] found that, although persons infected with HIV-2 can develop an AIDS defining disease, this form of HIV takes on average a much longer time to cripple the immune system. Current evidence suggests that the average time from infection to crippling of the immune system could be about 25 years, which is much longer than that for HIV-1. A team of researchers led by P. Kanki (see Travers et al.[33]) followed the status and health of 756 women registered as prostitutes in Dakar, Senegal for 9 years. Of the 618 women who were not initially infected with either form of HIV, 61 became infected with HIV-1 during the study. But, of the 187 women who became infected with HIV-2, either before or during the study, only 7 became infected with HIV-1 as well, a result that suggests HIV-2 confers some protection from HIV-1.

Thus, there may exist some parallelism between HIV-2 and HIV-1 and the cowpox-smallpox case and other so-called "heterologous virus" systems, in which a weak cousin protects against its aggressive relative by stimulating immune molecules that recognize both strains. To further investigate this point, Kanki et al.[25] used a risk assessment analysis to estimate that in the study population, HIV-2 infection reduced the risk of HIV-1 infection by about 70%. A vaccine against HIV-1 with 70% efficacy would be a significant advance; yet, work with animal models suggests that people infected with HIV-1 need to be very cautious about being infected with HIV-2 to slow the degradation of the immune system. Daniel et al.[8] reported protective effects of a live attenuated SIV vaccine with a deletion of the nef gene, which appeared to confer immunity on adult Rhesus monkeys challenged by the intravenous inoculation of live, pathogenic SIV. Subsequently, Baba et al.[4] reported similar experiences with adult macaques, but, unfortunately, the attenuated virus caused SAIDS in newborns. Evidently, the long latent periods of retroviruses and their high levels of mutability make it very hard to predict the behavior of any attenuated form of HIV-2, but the epidemiological experience with HIV-2 and HIV-1 in West Africa offers some hope for the development of an AIDS vaccine. Recently, Letvin[19] has provided a review of the progress in the development of an HIV-1 vaccine.

Among the most dramatic developments of HIV therapies during the last few years has been the use of protease inhibitors and other combinations of drugs designed to eradicate or control HIV infection. Ho,[17] who is one of the leading researchers in this field, has provided an overview of the mechanisms underlying these therapies and the tasks that lie ahead in achieving a durable control of HIV-1 replication in vivo. Among the problems of attaining such control is the evolution of strains of HIV-1 in the bodies of patients under treatment. Perrin and Telenti[29] have discussed HIV treatment failure as well as testing for HIV resistance in clinical practice. Among the drawbacks to these aggressive therapies are that not all patients respond to them favorably and they are very expensive, so that they are practical only in the more developed countries of the world. Unfortunately, at this juncture, it does not appear practical to apply aggressive treatments of HIV in much of the underdeveloped world, where in some countries the incidence of HIV infections is increasing. In this regard, Fauci[10] has recently put forward the thesis that global efforts aimed at preventing HIV infection must be intensified, because effective treatment becomes less and less of an option for controlling the disease on a worldwide scale. Moreover, he stated that "Unless methods of prevention, with or without a vaccine, are successful, the worst of the global pandemic will occur in the 21st century."

1.6 Clinical Effects of HIV Infection

Brookmeyer and Gail,[5] along with the references cited therein, provide an informative picture of the clinical effects of HIV infection; two other interesting papers on this subject are those of Redfield and Burke[31] and Greene.[13] To understand some basic biology underlying the clinical effects of HIV infection, it is of interest to provide a brief and overly simplified view of some aspects of the body's immunologic defense system. For further details on the workings of the immune system in general, the September 1993 issue of *Scientific American* may be consulted. Immunologic defense is provided by cells that are generated in the bone marrow and thymus and are found in lymphoid tissue throughout the body in widely distributed lymph nodes and also the spleen. A lymphatic circulatory system, which communicates with peripheral blood, provides a medium of communication among these tissues.

The peripheral blood contains various types of white cells, in characteristic proportions per μl, that are involved in immunologic defense. Included among these types of cells are lymphocytes, and, even though all these types of cells and others are thought to play a role in immune defense, specificity of response to foreign antigen is determined by lymphocytes. Among the lymphocytes in peripheral blood are T and B lymphocytes, which constitute, respectively, about 75% and 12% of the population of these types of cells. Two broad classes of immune defense, humoral response and cell-mediated response, involve lymphocytes. Humoral response refers to the production of antibodies to foreign antigens, which can bind to virus particle or bacteria and, in conjunction with other elements of the immune system, clear these foreign invaders from the host's circulatory system. The role played by B lymphocytes is to produce antibodies, but a special type of lymphocyte, called T-helper cell or $CD4^+$ T cell, is essential to the B cell humoral response, because the $CD4^+$ T cell recognizes foreign antigen and causes previously challenged B cells to proliferate and produce appropriate antibodies.

Cell-mediated response, the second major type of immune defense, is important in ridding the body of those host cells that have been infected by some intracellular pathogen, such as viruses, fungi, protozoa, and some bacteria. In recognizing a foreign antigen, the $CD4^+$ T cell plays a major role in stimulating other cells, such as the macrophages, to ingest and destroy infected cells. However, a "suppressor T lymphocyte" or "$CD8^+$ T cell" can suppress cell-mediated response and limit damage to host tissue. Furthermore, $CD8^+$ T cells can also attack cells infected with a virus directly, by a process called "cell-mediated cytotoxicity". Because $CD4^+$ T cells not only have direct cytotoxic activity but also secrete factors that stimulate the proliferation of $CD8^+$ cytotoxic T cells, they are also important in promoting cell-mediated cytotoxicity. Thus, the $CD4^+$ T cell plays a central role in both humoral and cell-mediated defenses.

Following infection with HIV-1, the clinical response is complex, progressive, and varies among individuals. Typically, within a few days, an individual develops an acute mononucleosis-like syndrome with fever, malaise, and lymphadenopathy, the swelling of the lymph glands, but symptoms abate as HIV-1 bonds to cells with $CD4^+$ receptor. More particularly, HIV-1 attacks $CD4^+$ T cells, because they contain the $CD4^+$ receptors, and, through a process that is not completely understood, kills $CD4^+$ T lymphocytes and progressively destroys the immunocompetence of the host. In the first few months following infection, the $CD4^+$ T lymphocyte levels drop rapidly from a pre-infection normal level of about 1125 $CD4^+$ T cells per μl to about 800 cells per μl, but, thereafter, the decline proceeds at a slower pace. For further technical details, the foregoing references may be consulted.

Like many biological phenomena, longitudinal studies of patients infected with HIV-1 reveal long and variable incubation periods between infection and the development of AIDS. Nowak et al.[28] reported data from a small number of infected patients which showed temporal changes in the number of genetically distinct strains of virus throughout the incubation period, with a slow but increasing rise in genetic diversity during the progression to disease. These authors suggested the existence of an antigen diversity threshold, below which the immune system is able to regulate the virus population growth, but above which the virus population induces the collapse of the $CD4^+$ T lymphocyte population. On the basis of a mathematical model, these authors also suggested that antigenic diversity is the cause, not a consequence, of immunodeficiency disease. Based on observations of other host-pathogen systems, it is, perhaps, not too implausible to suggest that variability in resistance to HIV-1, as reflected in the length of the incubation period, may also be partially controlled by the genotype of the host.

At least two sets of stages of HIV-disease have been defined, based on blood tests for seropositivity to HIV-1 and symptomatic criteria. In one set, there are four stages: in stage 1, an individual is infected with HIV-1 but not seropositive; in stage 2, an individual is seropositive but exhibits no visible symptoms of AIDS defining disease; in stage 3, an individual is said to be in the ARC phase or AIDS related complex; and finally in stage 4, an individual has full-blown AIDS. Redfield and Burke[31] have proposed a classification system based on six stages of HIV-disease of the Walter Reed system; among the criteria defining these stages are the $CD4^+$ T cell counts per cubic millimeter. Longini et al.[20,21,22,23] have studied Markov models for the variability among patients in the durations of stay in the stages of HIV-disease. In a later chapter, the models of Longini et al., and those of others, will be discussed more extensively.

1.7 An International Perspective of the AIDS Epidemic

Piot et al.[30] and Mann et al.,[24] who provided international perspectives on the AIDS epidemic, described three types of patterns of HIV-1 infection in various geographical regions of the world. In pattern 1, homosexual/bisexual men and intravenous drug users (IVDU's) are the major risk groups affected. In this pattern, infected females are usually IVDU's or sexual partners of male IVDU's or other high risk males. Also included in this pattern are those who were infected by blood transfusion or the use of blood products contaminated with HIV-1, during the early stages of the epidemic; but, since 1985, such contamination has been brought under control. The geographical areas that fit this pattern are North America, Western Europe, some areas of South

America, Australia, and New Zealand.

In pattern 2 regions, HIV-1 is transmitted mainly through heterosexual contacts so that heterosexuals are the principal population group that develop AIDS, but homosexual transmission of the virus, although it may occur, is not a major factor in the development of the epidemic. In some areas with this pattern, up to 90% of prostitutes have tested positive for HIV-1. Transfusion with HIV-1 infected blood may be a public health problem, particularly in some areas, and the use of non-sterile needles and syringes may also account for some infections. In areas where 5% to 15% of women are seropositive for HIV-1, perinatal transmission, mothers infecting their infants, can also be a problem. Geographical regions of the world falling into this pattern are Africa, the Caribbean, and some areas of South America. As mentioned previously, there is also a region in West Africa where HIV-1 and HIV-2 occur simultaneously.

Pattern 3 occurs in some regions of Asia, the Pacific (excluding Australia and New Zealand), Eastern Europe, and some rural areas of South America. In these regions, both homosexual and heterosexual transmission of HIV-1 has been documented, but the seroprevalence of the virus is low even among prostitutes. Cases of infection among recipients of imported blood and blood products have occurred and have received considerable attention in the media. Unlike the pattern 1 and 2 regions of the world, where infections with HIV-1 were thought to have begun sometime in the early 1970's to 80's, infections in pattern 3 regions were thought to have occurred during the early to mid-1980's.

Curran et al.[7] and Heyward and Curran[16] presented overviews of the epidemiology of HIV and AIDS in the United States as of 1988, but, for the most part, the patterns they presented persist to this day. Even within a country, such as the US, there can exist sub-patterns by race and sex (see CDC report[15]). Presented in Table 1.7.1 are the percentages of the cumulative number of AIDS cases diagnosed among males living in the United States up to December 1994 by race and risk category. In this table, the acronym HOMO/BI-NIVDU stands for homosexual-bisexual males who are not intravenous drug users, while the acronym HOMO/BI-IVDU stands for such males who are intravenous drug users. Among White (non-Hispanic) males, the vast majority of the cases, 77%, belong to the risk category HOMO/BI-NIVDU; the other major risk categories, IVDU and HOMO/BI-IVDU, amount to 16%. For Black (non-Hispanic) and Hispanic males, however, these latter two categories amount to 45% of the reported AIDS cases, the other major risk category being HOMO/BI-NIVDU, accounting for 40% and 45%, respectively, for these two racial classifications.

Table 1.7.1. Percentages of AIDS Cases Diagnosed among USA Males up to December 1994 by Race and Risk Category.

Risk Category	White	Black	Hispanic
HOMO/BI-NIVDU	77	40	45
IVDU	8	37	38
HOMO/BI-IVDU	8	8	7
Hemophilia/Coagulation Disorder	1	>0, rare	>0, rare
Heterosexual	1	5	4
Recipient of Blood Transfusion, Blood Components, or Tissue	1	1	1
Risk not Reported or Identified	3	9	6
Total Number	198882	12016	62934

Presented in Table 1.7.2 are the percentages of the reported cumulative number of AIDS cases diagnosed among females in the US up to December 1994 by race and risk category. Unlike that for males, the risk group IVDU constitutes the majority of cases in all three risk categories, White (non-Hispanic), Black (non-Hispanic), and Hispanic, with 43%, 50%, and 46%, respectively. The next highest percentages for these racial classifications were in the heterosexual risk category, with 37%, 33%, and 43% for Whites, Blacks, and Hispanics, respectively. It is also of interest to note that the percentages of cases in which the risk category was neither reported nor identified was significant for both males and females (see second row from the bottom in each table). Another observation of interest in Table 1.7.2 is that the total number of reported AIDS cases for Blacks exceeds that for Whites, even though they make up a smaller percentage of the total US population. Among the total number of AIDS cases reported among women in the US, the percentage of AIDS cases among Hispanic women also exceeds their percentage in the total population of US women as of December 1994.

Table 1.7.2. Percentages of AIDS Cases Diagnosed among USA Females up to December 1994 by Race and Risk Category.

Risk Category	White	Black	Hispanic
IVDU	43	50	46
Hemophilia/Coagulation Disorder	>0, rare	>0, rare	>0, rare
Heterosexual	37	33	43
Recipient of Blood Transfusion, Blood Components, or Tissue	11	2	3
Risk not Reported or Identified	8	14	7
Total Number	14166	31821	11909

Data such as that summarized in the foregoing tables suggest that a knowledge of sexual preferences of a population, as well as the number of sexual partners individuals have during some time interval, would be of great value in projecting the number of people infected with HIV in a population. By using such projections, it would also be possible to obtain estimates of the costs of caring for people with HIV disease. In the USA, however, obtaining funds from government agencies for conducting such behavioral surveys has met with stiff political opposition. Nevertheless, Laumann et al.,[18] using funds from private sources, have conducted a national survey on the social organization of sexuality and sexual practices in the United States, which will be a source of valuable information for years to come.

1.8 Evolution of Antibiotic Resistance

Mention has already been made of increases in genetic diversity of HIV, following an infection in an individual, but evolutionary changes in other disease causing organisms have also been documented in recent years. These changes have an impact on the HIV/AIDS epidemic by not only increasing the risk of contracting some fatal disease, which can have a severe impact on a person with a depressed immune system, but by also causing lesions expediting the entrance of HIV into the blood stream. Since the period following the end of World War II in 1945, the three classical venereal diseases, gonorrhea, syphilis, and chancroid, have nearly disappeared in almost all the industrialized countries. Throughout Europe, Australia, New Zealand, and Japan the incidence of gonorrhea, for example, has declined in the past two decades. In Sweden, between 1970 and 1989, the incidence of gonorrhea dropped by more than 95%. It is thought that these improvements reflect the effectiveness of public health measures taken in these countries.

There are some urban minority sub-populations in the USA, on the other hand, where these three sexually transmitted diseases (STD's) have actually been increasing at rates that are a cause for concern. In such sub-populations, urban poverty, social disintegration, prostitution, and the relatively new phenomenon of sex in exchange for drugs seem to be among the underlying social causes of this epidemic. The rise of drug resistant strains of sexually transmitted bacterial infections and the rapid spread of incurable viral infections have further compounded the STD problems in the USA. To an increasing extent, the situation in urban underclasses in the USA resembles that seen in the slums of the least developed countries, where HIV/AIDS has been spreading at epidemic rates among heterosexuals. Aral and Holmes[3] have reviewed the available data on the incidence of STD's, along with the social, economic, and political factors that seem to be underlying the epidemic and have recommended public health measures that should be taken to prevent an HIV/AIDS epidemic among heterosexuals in the urban USA underclass.

Evolution of strains in disease causing organisms has not been confined to STD's. For, in recent years, increasing attention has been focused on the resurgence of tuberculosis, a disease that had almost disappeared in industrialized countries thanks to the use of antibiotics in patients identified by massive drug screening efforts. These efforts had been so successful that no new drugs for tuberculosis had been introduced for the last 30 years. But, now multi-drug resistant strains of tuberculosis are being isolated with increasing frequency. The evolution of drug-resistant strains of tuberculosis was not new; in fact, as early as the late 1940's, only a few years after streptomycin proved to be the first effective anti-tuberculosis drug, resistant strains emerged. Shortly thereafter, clinicians observed that tuberculosis could easily develop resistance to a single drug (and often two), but three drugs seemed invincible.

Based on these observations, the Centers for Disease Control (CDC) and the Food and Drug Administration (FDA) approved a combination drug containing rifampin, isoniazid, and pyrazinamide for treatment of tuberculosis; however, not even a three-drug regime has proved sufficient to control recently emerged strains of the bacterium causing the disease. Moreover, strains of the bacterium have evolved that are resistant to every available tuberculosis drug, resulting in the reintroduction of isolated tuberculosis wards in hospitals to help control the spread of the disease. A factor associated with the rise of resistant strains is the failure of patients to complete a full course of drug therapy, but, in isolation wards, this factor can be controlled.

After starting treatment, patients begin to feel well within 2 to 3 months, but it can take up to 18 months before all of the tuberculosis causing organisms are killed. In the past, patients were routinely kept in hospitals throughout the treatment period. Recently, however, the move to outpatient treatment care and self-administered drugs, which often leads to patients not completing a prescribed regimen and a relapse of the disease, has increased the rise of strains resistant to more than three drugs. Evidently, such circumstances create conditions for the selection of drug-resistant strains of organisms. In New York City, for example, from 1982 to 1984, about 9.8% of *Mycobacterium tuberculosis* cells isolated from untreated patients were resistant to one or more drugs, but, in relapsed patients, 52% of such isolates were resistant. These observations also suggest that communities, with many people suffering from HIV disease and depressed immune systems, might provide fertile environments for the evolution of not only strains of drug resistant tuberculosis but also resistant strains of organisms causing STD's. Further details may be found in Amábile-Cuevas et al.[1]

1.9 Mathematical Models of the HIV/AIDS Epidemic

Because biological phenomena are, for the most part, characterized by diversity and variability, and, moreover, the data collected in attempts to monitor and understand them involve uncertainties, stochastic models, with roots in stochastic processes, will be the primary focus of this book. Although the list in not complete, the foregoing overview of the biological literature suggests that the following classes of models should be given attention.

- *Models of the Latent Period:* The waiting time from the infection of a disease causing agent to the development of symptoms or death from disease of the infected individual is often called the latent period. For the case of HIV disease, as well as other diseases, this period exhibits considerable variability among individuals. A basic component of any mathematical model of the population dynamics underlying the HIV/AIDS epidemic should, therefore, contain a component dealing with the latent period of a HIV infection. In constructing such models, there are at least two possibilities, namely, the latent period may be viewed as evolving without stages or in stages.

- *Models Describing the Evolution of Genetic Diversity in HIV for Infected Individuals:* Compared to most organisms, HIV is known to undergo relatively high rates of genetic mutations. It has also been suggested that an infected individual succumbs to an AIDS defining disease when the genetic diversity of the HIV in the body goes beyond a certain threshold. Models describing the evolution of this genetic diversity and its impact on the length of the incubation period would, therefore, be of interest.

- *Models Accommodating Behavioral Heterogeneity in the Population:* Data collected by departments of public health bear witness to the existence of population behavioral heterogeneity, as described by such risk categories as male homo-bisexual non-IVDU's, male homo-bisexual IVDU's, and female and male heterosexuals. Mathematical models should, therefore, accommodate such population heterogeneity.

- *Contact Structures in Populations with Behavioral Heterogeneity:* The existence of population behavioral heterogeneity suggests that there are contacts among risk categories that may lead to the transmission of a disease causing agent. For the case of HIV, these contacts are primarily of two types, sexual and the sharing of needles, and perhaps a mixture of the two. Models of such contacts structures are a necessary component of any mathematical model describing the population dynamics underlying the evolution of an HIV/AIDS epidemic.

- *Models Accommodating Formation and Dissolution of Partnerships and Other Assemblies of People:* Contacts among individuals in a population may be modeled in a number of ways. In one approach, it can be assumed that sexual contacts and needle sharing occur among individuals in random or semi-random ways, ignoring the existence of partnerships, consisting of a female and a male, or, in the case of homosexuals, two males. An alternative approach is to take into explicit account the formation and dissolution of partnerships consisting of a female and male. Alternatively, assemblages of three people consisting of, for example, of two males and a female or one male and two females could also be considered. Such models seem to be worthy of consideration when studying the spread of HIV infections in a heterosexual component of a population.

- *Age Dependent Models:* Even though it leads to structures of high dimensionality, age is a basic component of any mathematical model describing the dynamics of a human population, particularly when demographic considerations are important. Consequently, these types of models play a fundamental role not only in demography but also stochastic models in epidemiology.

- *Models for the Evolution of Resistance to Antibiotics:* When more than one biological organism is considered in models of population dynamics, the co-evolution of their genetic structure should be taken into account. Such basic problems underlie the evolution of resistance to antibiotics and such models accommodating such co-evolution will, in all probability, receive increasing attention in the future.

1.10 References

1. C. F. Amábile-Cuevas, M. Cárdenas-García and M. Ludgar, Antibiotic Resistance, *Scientific American* **83**: 320-329, 1995.
2. R. M. Anderson and R. M. May, *Infectious Diseases of Humans - Dynamics and Control,* Oxford University Press, Oxford, New York, Tokyo, 1992.
3. S. O. Aral and K. K. Holmes, Sexually Transmitted Diseases in the AIDS Era, *Scientific American* **264:** 62-69, 1991.
4. T. W. Baba, Y. S. Jeong, D. Penninck, R. Bronson, M. F. Greene and R. M. Ruprecht, Pathogenicity of Live, Attenuated SIV After Mucosal Infection of Neonatal Macaques, *Science* **267:** 1820-1825, 1995.
5. R. Bookmeyer and M. H. Gail, *AIDS Epidemiology: A Quantitative Approach,* Oxford University Press, Oxford, New York, Tokyo, 1994.
6. W. Cavert and A. T. Hasse, A National Tissue Bank to Track HIV Eradication and Immune Reconstruction, *Science* **280:** 1865-1866, 1998.
7. J. W. Curran and H. W. Jaffe et al., Epidemiology of HIV Infection and AIDS in the United States, *Science* **239:** 610-616, 1988.

8. M. D. Daniel, F. Kirchoff, S. C. Czajak, P. K. Sehga and R. C. Desrosiers, Protective Effects of a Live Attenuated SIV Vaccine with a Deletion of the nef Gene, *Science* **258:** 1938-1941, 1992.

9. M. Essex and P. J. Kanki, The Origins of the AIDS Virus, *Scientific American* **259:** 64-71, 1988.

10. A. S. Fauci, The AIDS Epidemic - Considerations for the 21-st. Century, *The New England Journal of Medicine* **341:** 1046-1049, 1999.

11. A. S. Fauci, The Human Immunodeficiency Virus: Infectivity and Mechanisms of Pathogenesis, *Science* **238:** 617-622, 1988.

12. R. C. Gallo and L. Montagnier, AIDS in 1988, *Scientific American* **259:** 41-48, 1988.

13. W. C. Greene, AIDS and the Immune System, *Scientific American* **269:** 98-105, 1993.

14. W. A. Haseltine and F. Wong-Staal, The Molecular Biology of the AIDS Virus, *Scientific American* **259:** 52-62, 1988.

15. *HIV/AIDS Surveillance Report*, Centers for Disease Control and Prevention, Atlanta, Georgia, December, 1994

16. W. L. Heyward and J. W. Curran, The Epidemiology of AIDS in the US, *Scientific American* **259:** 72-81, 1988.

17. D. D. Ho, Toward HIV Eradication or Remission: The Tasks Ahead, *Science* **280:** 1866-1867, 1998.

18. E. O. Laumann, J. H. Gagnon, R. T. Michael and S. Michaels, *The Social Organization of Sexuality - Sexual Practices in the United States*, The University of Chicago Press, Chicago and London, 1994.

19. N. L. Letvin, Progress in the Development of an HIV-1 Vaccine, *Science* **280:** 1875-1880, 1998.

20. I. M. Longini, Jr., Modeling the Decline of CD4+ T-Lymphocyte Counts in HIV-Infected Individuals, *Journal of Acquired Immune Deficiency Syndromes* **3:** 930-931, 1990.

21. I. M. Longini, Jr., B. H. Byers, N. A. Hessol and W. Y. Tan, Estimating Stage-Specific Numbers of HIV Infection Using a Markov Model and Back Calculation, *Statistics in Medicine* **11:** 831-843, 1992.

22. I. M. Longini, Jr., W. S. Clark, and R. H. Byers et al., Statistical Analysis of the Stages of HIV Infection Using a Markov Model, *Statistics in Medicine* **8:** 831-843, 1989.

23. I. M. Longini, Jr., W. S. Clark, L. M. Haber and R. Horsburgh, Jr., The Stages of HIV Infection: Waiting Times and Infection Transmis-

sion Probabilities, *Lecture Notes in Biomathematics* **83:** 111-137, C. Castillo-Chavez (ed.), *Mathematical and Statistical Approaches in AIDS Epidemiology,* Springer-Verlag, Berlin, New York, Tokyo, 1989.

24. J. Mann, J. Chin, P. Piot and T. Quinn, The International Epidemiology of AIDS, *Scientific American* **259:** 82-89, 1988.
25. R. Marlink and P. Kanki et al., Reduced Rate of Disease Development After HIV-2 Infection as Compared to HIV-1, *Science* **265:** 1587-1590, 1994.
26. T. J. Matthews and D. P. Bolognesi, AIDS Vaccines, *Scientific American* **259:** 120-127,1988.
27. C. J. Mode, A Mathematical Model for the Coevolution of Obligate Parasites and Their Hosts, *Evolution* **12:** 158-165, 1958.
28. M. A. Nowak and R. M. Anderson et al., Antigenic Diversity Thresholds and the Development of AIDS, *Science* **254:** 963-969, 1991.
29. L. Perrin and A. Telenti, HIV Treatment Failure: Testing for HIV Resistance in Clinical Practice, *Science* **280:** 1871-1873, 1998.
30. P. Piot and F. A. Plummer et al., AIDS: An International Perspective, *Science* **239:** 573-579, 1988.
31. R. R. Redfield and D. S. Burke, HIV Infection: The Clinical Picture, *Scientific American* **259:** 90-98, 1988.
32. R. Shilts, *And The Band Played On - Politics, People, and the AIDS Epidemic,* St. Martin's Press, New York, 1987.
33. K. Travers, S. Mboup and R. Marlink et al., Natural Protection Against HIV-1 Infection Provided by HIV-2, *Science* **268:** 1612-1615, 1995.
34. H. Varmus, Retroviruses, *Science* **240:** 1427-1435, 1988.
35. J. N. Weber and R. A. Weiss, HIV Infection: The Cellular Picture, *Scientific American* **259:** 100-109, 1988.
36. R. Yarchoan, H. Mitsuya and S. Broder, AIDS Therapies, *Scientific American* **259:** 110-119, 1988.

Chapter 2
MODELS OF INCUBATION AND INFECTIOUS PERIODS

2.1 Introduction

Following an infection by some disease causing organism, there will usually be a waiting time before symptoms defining the disease develop. The time span elapsing from the time of infection to the development of symptoms is referred to as the incubation period. During the period an individual is infected with some disease causing organism, he or she may be able to pass the disease causing agent to others in a population by various forms of contact. The span of time in which an infected individual can pass a disease causing agent to others will be referred to as the infectious period. Both the incubation and infectious periods may vary among individuals in a population and the purpose of this chapter is to explore methods that have been used to choose distributions describing this variation and to provide some examples in which parameters of the distributions have been estimated from data. Even though the principles governing these choices apply to many types of waiting time phenomena, such as incubation, infectious and other periods of interest in the study of infectious diseases, particular attention will be paid to HIV disease.

2.2 Distribution Function of the Incubation Period

By definition, the length of time taken to develop some AIDS-defining disease following infection with HIV is called the incubation period, and this period will vary considerably among infected individuals. Although HIV disease will be the primary focus of attention, the remarks that follow will apply, in principle, to the incubation period of any disease caused by some biological or other agent. Let the continuous type random variable T represent the variability in the incubation period among infected individuals in a population, and suppose the range of this random variable is $R_T = [0, \infty) = [t : 0 \leq t < \infty]$, the set of non-negative real numbers representing time. Then, for $t \in R_T$, the probability,

$$\mathbb{P}[T \leq t] = F(t) , \tag{2.2.1}$$

that the incubation period is less than or equal to t is called the distribution function (*d.f.*) of the random variable T. The survival function $S(t) = \mathbb{P}[T > t] = 1 - F(t)$ is the probability the duration of the incubation period is greater than $t \in R_T$. Throughout this section and subsequent sections it will be assumed that $F(0) = 0$ so that $S(0) = 1$, unless otherwise stated. A problem to be considered in this section is that of general methods for choosing a parametric form of the *d.f.* $F(t)$. Another function that is useful in finding solutions to this problem is that of the probability density function (*p.d.f.*), which is defined by:

$$f(t) = \frac{dF(t)}{dt} \tag{2.2.2}$$

for those points $t \in R_T$ for which the derivative exists.

A concept that is widely used in biostatistics, demography, and reliability theory in engineering is that of a risk or hazard function. Some authors also refer to this function as the failure rate. Given that $T > t$, the conditional probability that $T \in (t, t + h]$ for $h > 0$ is:

$$\mathbb{P}[t < T \leq t + h \mid T > t] = \frac{F(t+h) - F(t)}{S(t)} . \tag{2.2.3}$$

The risk function of the random variable T is defined as:

$$\theta(t) = \lim_{h \downarrow 0} \frac{\mathbb{P}[t < T \leq t + h]}{h} = \frac{f(t)}{S(t)} \tag{2.2.4}$$

for those $t \in R_T$ for which the limit exists. An equivalent form of Eq. (2.2.4) is the differential equation

$$-\frac{d \ln S(t)}{dt} = \theta(t) , \tag{2.2.5}$$

with the initial condition $S(0) = 1$. If it is assumed that the risk function may be integrated, then an equivalent form of this equation is

$$S(t) = \exp\left[-\int_0^t \theta(s)ds\right] \qquad (2.2.6)$$

for $t \in R_T$. It thus follows that in terms of the risk function, the distribution function has the formula

$$F(t) = 1 - \exp\left[-\int_0^t \theta(s)ds\right], \qquad (2.2.7)$$

and the *p.d.f.* takes the form,

$$f(t) = \theta(t)S(t) \qquad (2.2.8)$$

for $t \in R_T$. From the general theory just outlined, it can be seen that in choosing a parametric form for the incubation period of HIV, or indeed any incubation period of a disease caused by some agent, one may proceed in at least three ways by specifying the *d.f.*, the *p.d.f.*, or the risk function.

2.3 The Weibull and Gamma Distributions

Where the approach to the problem involves choosing a parametric form for the distribution function of the incubation period, an appropriate starting point would be that of investigating some properties of distributions widely used in probability and mathematical statistics. Among these distributions is the Weibull, which, in the standard case, has the one-parameter risk function,

$$\theta(t) = \alpha t^{\alpha-1} \qquad (2.3.1)$$

where α is a positive parameter. As can be seen from this formula, the properties of the risk function are determined by the shape parameter α. If, for example, $0 < \alpha < 1$, then the risk function is well defined only for $t > 0$ and is a decreasing function of t. But, if $\alpha > 1$, then the risk function is well defined for all $t \geq 0$ and is an increasing function of t. If, however, $\alpha = 1$, then the risk function is constant for all $t \geq 0$.

If a random variable T_0 has the risk function in Eq. (2.3.1), then the corresponding survival function for any value of $\alpha > 0$ is:

$$S_0(t) = \exp\left[-\int_0^t \theta(s)ds\right] = e^{-t^\alpha} , \tag{2.3.2}$$

for all $t \geq 0$. An alternative to the standard form of this distribution is to introduce a positive scale parameter β and define a random variable T by $T = \beta T_0$. It then follows that the survival function for this random variable takes the form,

$$S(t) = \mathbb{P}\left[T > t\right] = \mathbb{P}\left[T_0 > \frac{t}{\beta}\right] = \exp\left[-\left(\frac{t}{\beta}\right)^\alpha\right] , \tag{2.3.3}$$

for $t \geq 0$. Quite frequently another form of this survival function is used in the literature. This form may be derived from Eq. (2.3.3) by introducing the parameter $\gamma = 1/\beta^\alpha$, so that the survival function takes the form,

$$S(t) = e^{-\gamma t^\alpha} . \tag{2.3.4}$$

Whether one chooses to use the Weibull distribution as a model of an incubation period depends on existing empirical evidence or a rational belief that the risk function is either a decreasing or an increasing function of t, for all $t > 0$.

It is of interest to note that if $\alpha = 1$, then the survival function in Eq. (2.3.4) reduces to that for the famous exponential distribution with positive parameter γ. As is well known, this distribution has the so-called memoryless property characterized by the conditional probability,

$$\mathbb{P}\left[T > t_0 + t \mid T > t_0\right] = \frac{S(t_0 + t)}{S(t_0)} = e^{-\gamma t} , \tag{2.3.5}$$

which holds for every $t_0 \geq 0$ and $t > 0$. The distribution is memoryless in the sense that given that an object has survived to time $t_0 \geq 0$, the conditional probability of survival for an additional $t > 0$ time units does not depend on t_0. This memoryless or non-aging property seems to make the exponential distribution an implausible model for variation in incubation times among infected individuals for many diseases, since it seems plausible that the longer an individual is infected, the greater the conditional probability that symptoms of a disease will develop. Similarly, if one is considering aging, it is reasonable to expect that the longer one lives, the greater one's conditional probability of dying. Even though the exponential distribution seems to be an appropriate model for many waiting time problems in the physical world, its applicability as a model of waiting times for biological phenomena seems limited, because of this memoryless property.

Since the risk function of the Weibull distribution either decreases or increases as a function of $t > 0$ when $\alpha \neq 1$, investigators have been led to consider other distributions from mathematical probability and statistics as models for the incubation periods of diseases. Among these models is the two-parameter gamma whose *p.d.f.* has the form,

$$f(t) = \frac{\beta^\alpha}{\Gamma(\alpha)} t^{\alpha-1} e^{-\beta t} , \tag{2.3.6}$$

where α and β are positive parameters, $t > 0$, and $\Gamma(\alpha)$ is the gamma function defined for $\alpha > 0$. In this case, the *d.f.* may be expressed in the integral form,

$$F(t) = \frac{\beta^\alpha}{\Gamma(\alpha)} \int_0^t s^{\alpha-1} e^{-\beta s} ds , \tag{2.3.7}$$

for $t > 0$. The parameter α is sometimes referred to as the shape parameter, and β is a scale parameter. Much is known about this widely used distribution; for example, if $\alpha = 1$, then the *p.d.f.* reduces to that of the exponential distribution with constant risk function $\theta(t) = \beta$. If $0 < \alpha < 1$, then the risk function is a decreasing function of t; while if $\alpha > 1$, then $\theta(t)$ increases as t increases. In both these cases, the risk function converges to the asymptote $\beta > 0$ as $t \to \infty$. Thus, for large waiting times, the risk function is essentially constant, a property that resembles the exponential distribution. Because of the monotonicity properties of the risk functions for both the Weibull and gamma distributions, one would also be led to consider distributions with risk functions that are not necessarily monotone.

Brookmeyer and Gail[4] may be consulted for many references on applying the Weibull and gamma distributions as models of the incubation period of HIV based on various sets of data, including individuals infected with HIV through blood transfusions and the use of blood products, male homosexuals, and heterosexuals. An informative theoretical development of properties of the risk function for the gamma distribution may be found in Barlow and Proschan.[2] By way of illustrating some parameter estimates reported in the late eighties, it is of interest to consider maximum likelihood estimates of the parameters in the Weibull distribution, based on a cohort study of the incubation period in homosexual men and in adults who contracted AIDS through blood transfusions as reported by Lui et al.[14] According to these authors, for male homosexuals, the estimates of the parameters α and γ were $\widehat{\alpha} = 2.571000$ and $\widehat{\gamma} = 0.003807$; while for the transfusion associated AIDS cohort, these estimates were $\widehat{\alpha} = 2.396000$ and $\widehat{\gamma} = 0.004799$.

From these estimates, it is of interest to note that the values of α suggest the risk function is strictly increasing in t. Furthermore, for these estimates, the estimated mean incubation period for male homosexuals was estimated at 7.8 years with a 90% confidence interval ranging form 4.2 to 15.0 years, which was close to the estimated mean of 8.2 years for adults developing transfusion associated AIDS. One important point to keep in mind when interpreting these estimates, is that the incubation period of HIV may not have a standard definition in the literature. Sometimes, for example, it refers to the time of infection to the time at which an AIDS-defining disease is diagnosed; while in other cases, it may be the time from infection to the time a person becomes seropositive for HIV.

It should also be kept in mind that these estimates are based on small samples, because data on larger cohort sets was not available. A limitation of such small samples is that persons with naturally long incubation periods may have inadvertently been excluded in the samples, because they would have no apparent need to come to a clinic, and thus the reported mean incubation periods may be underestimated. There is also the question of whether the Weibull and gamma distributions have sufficiently long right-hand tails to accommodate naturally occurring variability that can encompass the possibility of long incubation periods for HIV.

2.4 The Log-Normal, Log-Logistic and Log-Cauchy Distributions

From time to time one hears of reports in the press that a patient has been infected with HIV for an apparently long period of time, but, as yet, has not developed symptoms of an AIDS-defining disease. From the point of view of choosing a model for the incubation period of HIV, there are at least two ways to interpret such observations; namely, the patient could be a sample of size one from a distribution such as the Weibull or gamma, or he/she could be an observation from some other distribution that would naturally encompass such "outliers" better than either of these distributions. From an historical point of view, such outliers have been the subject of some debate as to whether they represent errors in measurement or they are actually a sample from a distribution whose natural variation would encompass such outliers. Stigler[16] may be consulted for a very interesting history of statistics and the measurement of uncertainty before 1900, where, among many other things, the problem of interpreting outliers in the 19th century is discussed. Apart from the problem of outliers, it is also of interest to consider distributions of the latent period of a disease other than the Weibull and gamma, because HIV-2 seems to have a longer incubation period than HIV-1, the virus for which most data is available. There is also a need to consider the possibility that a treatment intervention, including diet and drugs, may alter the form of the distribution of the latent period.

In this age of computers, it is important to construct distributions in terms of procedures that make it apparent how samples may be simulated from these distributions by Monte Carlo methods. With this goal in mind, a useful way of deriving distributions is that of considering random variables that are a function of a random variable with a known distribution. Suppose, for example, the random variable (*r.v.*) Z has a standard normal distribution with a mean of 0 and a variance of 1. In symbols, $Z \sim N(0,1)$. Then, as is well-known, if $\mu \in R$, the set of real numbers, and $\sigma \in (0,\infty)$, the set of positive real numbers, then the random variable $X = \mu + \sigma Z$ has a normal distribution with a mean or expectation μ and variance σ^2. In symbols, $X \sim N(\mu, \sigma^2)$. The *d.f.* of a standard normal random variable is given by the well-known formula,

$$\Phi(z) = \mathbb{P}\left[Z \le z\right] = \frac{1}{\sqrt{2\pi}} \int_{-\infty}^{z} e^{-\frac{s^2}{2}} ds \text{ for } z \in R \,. \tag{2.4.1}$$

Hence, by elementary manipulations, it follows that the *d.f.* of X is:

$$F(x) = \mathbb{P}\left[X \le x\right] = \Phi\left(\frac{x-\mu}{\sigma}\right) \text{ for } x \in R \,. \tag{2.4.2}$$

A useful way of introducing the log-normal distribution is to consider a *r.v.* T with range $R_T = (0, \infty)$ defined by:

$$T = e^X \,. \tag{2.4.3}$$

Then, as the name suggests, $\ln T = X \sim N(\mu, \sigma^2)$ and the *d.f.* of T is:

$$G(t) = \mathbb{P}\left[T \le t\right] = \mathbb{P}\left[\ln T \le \ln t\right] = \Phi\left(\frac{\ln t - \mu}{\sigma}\right) \,, \tag{2.4.4}$$

for $t \in R_T$. It thus follows that the *p.d.f.* of T is:

$$g(t) = \frac{dG(t)}{dt} = \frac{1}{\sqrt{2\pi}\sigma t} \exp\left[\frac{(\ln t - \mu)^2}{2\sigma^2}\right] \,, \tag{2.4.5}$$

for $t \in R_T$.

A random variable Z_0 with range $R_{Z_0} = R$, is said to have a logistic distribution with *d.f.*,

$$H_0(z) = \mathbb{P}\left[Z_0 \le z\right] = \left(1 + e^{-z}\right)^{-1} \text{ for } z \in R \,. \tag{2.4.6}$$

Evidently, the name of the distribution is derived from the form of the *p.d.f.*,

$$h_0(z) = \frac{dH_0(z)}{dz} = H_0(z)\left(1 - H_0(z)\right) \text{ for } z \in R \,, \tag{2.4.7}$$

which resembles the logistic differential equation for density dependent deterministic population growth. It can be shown that $h_0(z) = h_0(-z)$ for all $z \ge 0$, so that the *p.d.f.* is an even function; moreover, the distribution has a finite expectation, $E[Z_0] = 0$, and variance, $var[Z_0] = \pi^2/3$.

The $r.v.Z = (\sqrt{3}/\pi)Z_0$ thus has expectation 0 and variance 1, and we let $H(z) = H_0(z/c)$, where $c = \sqrt{3}/\pi$, be its distribution function. Just as in the case of the standard normal distribution, the random variable $X = \mu + \sigma Z$, $\mu \in R$ and $\sigma \in (0, \infty)$, has the expectation $E[X] = \mu$ and variance $var[X] = \sigma^2$.

A $r.v.T$ is said to have a log-logistic distribution if it has the form $T = \exp[X]$. Like the log-normal distribution, T is a function of a random variable X, with expectation μ and variance σ^2, which will expedite making comparisons between the log-normal and log-logistic distributions as choices for models of a latent period. The *d.f.* of the $r.v.T$, with range $R_T = (0, \infty)$, in this case is:

$$G(t) = \mathbb{P}[T \leq t] = H\left(\frac{\ln t - \mu}{\sigma}\right) = \left(1 + \exp\left[-\frac{(\ln t - \mu)}{c\sigma}\right]\right)^{-1} \tag{2.4.8}$$

for $t \in (0, \infty)$.

From a theoretical point of view, an understanding of the properties of a set of distributions, which may be candidates for models of a latent period, can be enhanced through comparison with a distribution with distinctly different properties. A $r.v.Z$ is said to follow a Cauchy distribution if its *p.d.f.* is:

$$f(z) = \frac{1}{\pi(1 + z^2)} \text{ for } z \in R\,, \tag{2.4.9}$$

with *d.f.*,

$$F(z) = \mathbb{P}[X \leq z] = \int_{-\infty}^{z} f(s)ds = \frac{1}{\pi}\tan^{(-1)}(z) + \frac{1}{2}\,, \tag{2.4.10}$$

where $z \in R$ and the function on the right is the inverse tangent. It is known that the Cauchy distribution has neither a finite expectation nor a finite variance, because the integrals defining these expectations do not converge. Distributions with these properties are said to have heavy tails and if one has samples from these distributions, then outliers would be expected. Again if $\mu \in R$ and $\sigma \in (0, \infty)$, then $X = \mu + \sigma Z$ is a well-defined random variable but it does not have a finite expectation or variance. However, μ may be interpreted as a location parameter and σ a scale parameter. Actually, μ is the median of the distribution of X. Just as for the log-normal and log-logistic distributions, a $r.v.\,T$ defined by $T = \exp[X]$ will be said to have a log-Cauchy distribution with location parameter μ and scale parameter σ.

It should be mentioned in passing that there is a family of distributions that will include the log-Cauchy and log-normal as special cases and is worthy of consideration. As is well-known, the density of the student's T-distribution is symmetric about $t = 0$ and depends on a single parameter ν, the degrees of freedom. Let the random variable T_ν have a T-distribution with ν degrees of freedom. For $\nu = 1$, the T-distribution reduces to the Cauchy and for $\nu = 2$, this distribution does not have a finite variance. Thus, the distribution of a random variable of the form $\exp[\mu + \sigma T_\nu]$ will have heavy right-hand tails. For $\nu > 2$, the variance of this distribution is $\nu/(\nu - 2)$ so that the random variable $Z = T_\nu/\sqrt{\nu/(\nu - 2)}$ has expectation 0 and variance 1. Thus, one may proceed as above to construct a family of distributions with support $(0, \infty)$, whose right-hand tail behavior depends on the parameter ν. For the range $2 < \nu < 30$, the heaviness of the right-hand tail diminishes as ν increases and for $\nu \geq 30$, the distribution will be virtually indistinguishable from the log-normal.

Most of the material in this section may be found in introductory books to mathematical probability and statistics. Included among these books are the very readable accounts by Mood et al.[15] and Bain and Engelhardt.[1] Many examples of applications of well-known probability distributions have been given in the interesting book by Derman et al.[7] Brookmeyer and Gail[4] cite applications of the log-logistic distribution to the incubation period of HIV in a different but equivalent form than that introduced above.

2.5 Quantiles of a Distribution

When searching for or trying to invent a distribution to describe the variation in the measurement of some phenomenon, it is of interest to compare a proposed distribution with others. One way of comparing parametric distributions is to derive formulas for their expectations and variances as functions of unknown parameters. Then, by adjusting values of parameters to attain equal expectations and variances for two distributions, one could investigate random samples from these distributions and compare them statistically, using Monte Carlo simulation. But, for some distributions of interest it may not be possible to express the expectation and variance as simple functions of parameters, and, moreover, some distributions may not have an expectation. Every distribution, however, has quantiles, which can be very helpful in comparing properties of samples from distributions; but in what follows, attention will be confined to continuous-type random variables.

In particular, consider the class of continuous-type random variables Z with range $R_Z \subset R$, the set of real numbers, that has a continuous and strictly increasing $d.f.\, F(z)$. Mathematically, this function is a mapping from its domain R_Z into the set $(0,1) = \{x \in R \mid 0 < x < 1\}$. For any $q \in (0,1)$, a number $z_q \in R_Z$ is called the qth quantile of the distribution if

$$\mathbb{P}\left[Z \leq z_q\right] = F(z_q) = q \,. \tag{2.5.1}$$

Because the function $F(z)$ is strictly increasing on R_Z, it has an inverse $F^{(-1)}(y)$ mapping each $y \in (0,1)$ to a point $z \in R_Z$, which may be found by formally solving the equation $y = F(z)$ for z. Hence, the formal solution of Eq. (2.5.1) is:

$$z_q = F^{(-1)}(q) \,. \tag{2.5.2}$$

If $q = 1/2$, then z_q is called the median of the distribution.

In the foregoing section, $r.v.$'s X that were functions of a $r.v.\, Z$ were considered. It is, therefore, of interest to compute the quantiles of a $r.v.\, X$ in terms of those for Z. For example, for a $r.v.\, X = \mu + \sigma Z$, with $\mu \in R$, $\sigma \in (0,\infty)$ and $q \in (0,1)$, the qth quantile of X is:

$$G(x_q) = \mathbb{P}\left[X \leq x_q\right] = F\left(\frac{x_q - \mu}{\sigma}\right) = F\left(z_z\right) = q \,, \tag{2.5.3}$$

which implies $x_q = \mu + \sigma z_q$. Similarly, if a $r.v.\, T$ is defined by $T = \exp\left[X\right]$, then

$$G(t_q) = \mathbb{P}\left[T \leq t_q\right] = F\left(\frac{\ln t_q - \mu}{\sigma}\right) = F(z_q) = q \,, \tag{2.5.4}$$

so that $t_q = \exp[\mu + \sigma z_q]$. From these simple formulas, it is clear that once the quantile z_q is computed, x_q and t_q may be easily determined.

For such well-known distributions as the standard normal and gamma, it is not possible to solve the equation $y = F(x)$ for x as an elementary function of $y \in (0,1)$, but there are numerical methods for accomplishing such calculations and many software packages contain programs implementing them. The books Kennedy and Gentle[8] and Thisted[18] may be consulted for a discussion of widely used methods for the numerical computation of inverses of distribution functions. For many distributions, however, their quantiles may be evaluated in terms of elementary functions. In the case of the standard Weibull distribution with shape parameter $\alpha > 0$, the equation,

$$F(z_q) = 1 - e^{-z_q^{\alpha}} = q \tag{2.5.5}$$

may be easily solved for z_q to yield:

$$z_q = (-\ln(1-q))^{\frac{1}{\alpha}} \tag{2.5.6}$$

for $q \in (0,1)$, and if a *r.v.* $T = \beta Z$, then its qth quantile is $t_q = \beta z_q$.

The logistic and Cauchy distributions are other examples whose quantiles may be expressed in terms of elementary functions. When a *r.v.* Z has a standard logistic distribution, i.e., Z has expectation zero and variance one, the qth quantile of Z is given by:

$$z_q = \frac{\sqrt{3}}{\pi} \ln\left(\frac{q}{1-q}\right) \tag{2.5.7}$$

for $q \in (0,1)$. If a *r.v.* Z has a Cauchy distribution with *d.f.*,

$$F(z) = \frac{1}{\pi} \tan^{(-1)}(z) + \frac{1}{2} \tag{2.5.8}$$

for $z \in R$, then for $q \in (0,1)$, the qth quantile of Z is given by:

$$z_q = \tan\left(\pi(q - \frac{1}{2})\right) . \tag{2.5.9}$$

Among the widely used distributions in statistics is the Chi-square, which is a special case of the gamma with shape parameter

$\alpha = n/2$ and scale parameter $\beta = 1/2$, where the positive integer n is the degrees of freedom. Many computer packages contain programs for computing the inverse of the Chi-square distribution function; in some programs, for example, if one enters the degrees of freedom n and $q \in (0,1)$, then a numerical value of the qth quantile is returned. Let a *r.v.* Z have a Chi-square distribution with n degrees of freedom and let z_q be the qth quantile of the distribution. If a *r.v.* X has a gamma distribution with shape parameter α and scale parameter β, then it is of interest to find the qth quantile x_q as a function of z_q. If $n = 2\alpha$, then the transformation $X = Z/2\beta$ transforms a Chi-square random variable with n degrees of freedom into a gamma *r.v.* with shape parameter α and scale parameter β. Thus, for $q \in (0,1)$:

$$G(x_q) = P\left[X \le x_q\right] = F(2\beta x_q) = F(z_q) = q\ , \tag{2.5.10}$$

which implies $x_q = z_q/2\beta$.

To illustrate the use of quantiles in comparing distributions, consider the estimates $\widehat{\alpha} = 2.57100$ and $\widehat{\gamma} = 0.00387$ of the parameters of the Weibull distribution as reported for a cohort of male homosexuals by Lui et al.[14] Given these estimates of the parameters, it can be shown that the expected value of the distribution is 7.752. For purposes of illustration, the scale parameter in the exponential distribution was chosen such that its expectation was 7.752 years. Similarly, if one chooses the scale parameter in the gamma distribution as one and shape parameter equal to 7.752, then this distribution also has the expectation 7.772. Table 2.5.1 contains a set of selected quantiles for these three distributions. It is of interest to observe that the quantiles of the Weibull and gamma distributions computed in this way are very similar. Indeed, it would be difficult to distinguish samples from these distributions, which suggests that variability in the incubation for HIV in this cohort of homosexual males could have also been described by a one parameter gamma distribution. When, however, one inspects the quantiles in Table 2.5.1 for the exponential distribution, it can be seen that they are larger for $q \geq 0.90$ than those for the Weibull and gamma. In the samples from this distribution, 5% of the values would exceed 23.223 years.

Table 2.5.1. Selected Quantiles in Years of Exponential, Weibull, and Gamma Distributions with Same Expectations.

q	Exponential	Weibull	Gamma
0.25	2.230	5.362	5.738
0.50	5.373	7.549	7.423
0.75	10.747	9.885	9.410
0.90	17.850	12.041	11.469
0.95	23.223	13.339	12.824
0.999	53.549	18.461	19.380

The log-normal, log-logistic, and log-Cauchy distributions are of particular interest in comparing candidates as possible models of the incubation period, because the latter two distributions can accommodate outliers, i.e., those individuals with particularly long incubation periods. To gain some insight into the properties of samples from these distributions, it is of interest to investigate quantiles comparable to those in Table 2.5.1. All these distributions depend on a location parameter μ and a scale parameter σ. By way of an illustrative example, the parameter μ was chosen such that all three distributions had the same median $\exp[\mu] = 7.549$ years, the median of the Weibull distribution in Table 2.5.1. Values of σ were chosen such that all distributions had the same 0.75th quantile as for the Weibull distribution in Table 2.5.1. Table 2.5.2 contains selected values of the quantiles for the three distributions with these choices of parameter values.

Table 2.5.2. Selected Quantiles in Years of Log-Normal, Log-Logistic, and Log-Cauchy Distributions with Same Medians.

q	Log-Normal	Log-Logistic	Log-Cauchy
0.25	5.782	5.782	5.782
0.50	7.549	7.549	7.549
0.75	9.913	9.913	9.913
0.90	12.639	12.981	17.357
0.95	14.617	15.593	41.532
0.999	26.053	41.232	1.409×10^{38}

From this table it can be seen that the quantiles of the log-normal and log-logistic are of comparable magnitudes for the values $0.25 \leq q \leq 0.95$, but for $q = 0.999$, the quantile of the log-logistic, 41.232, is larger than that for the log-normal, 26.053. Therefore, given these parameter values, if variability in incubation periods followed a log-logistic distribution, then one would expect larger outliers than if the periods followed a log-normal distribution. On the other hand, if the log-Cauchy distribution governed variability in incubation periods, then, with these parameter values, it can be seen from Table 2.5.2 that 5% of these periods would exceed 41.532 years and one out of a thousand would exceed 1.409×10^{38} years, which, in view of the expected human life spans, makes this distribution implausible as a model for incubation periods. Nevertheless, the log-Cauchy distribution is a model of theoretical interest. Because these three distributions are very sensitive to parameter values, it should be emphasized that the parameter values used in this section were meant only for illustrative comparisons.

2.6 Some Principles and Results of Monte Carlo Simulation

Among the many uses of computer simulation is that of computing random samples from some given distribution to gain some insights into what to expect when sampling from this distribution. Although Monte Carlo samples may be computed from discrete distributions, in this section attention will be confined to a continuous-type *r.v.* X, with a strictly increasing *d.f.* $F(x)$ for $x \in R_X$, the range of X. Typical examples of such distributions are those for the incubation period described in the previous section, which will be given special attention along with simulations of outliers. A random variable that plays a central theoretical role in Monte Carlo simulation is a continuous-type *r.v.* U, with a uniform distribution on the interval $(0, 1)$. The *d.f.* of this *r.v.* is:

$$F_U(u) = u \text{ for } u \in (0, 1) , \tag{2.6.1}$$

so that its *p.d.f.* is $F_U'(u) = f_U(u) = 1$, for all $u \in (0, 1)$.

As in the previous section, let the function $F^{(-1)}(y)$, with domain $y \in (0, 1)$ and range R_X , be the inverse of the *d.f.* $F(x)$ of the *r.v.* X. Then, if $y = F(x)$, $F^{(-1)}(y) = x$ and $F(F^{(-1)}(y)) = y$. In what follows, it will be necessary to use the property that $F^{(-1)}(y)$ on $(0,1)$ is a non-decreasing function. It is perhaps obvious that the non-decreasing property of the *d.f.* $F(x)$ on $x \in R_X$ implies this property, but, nevertheless, the following simple proof is of interest. Because $F(x)$ is non-decreasing $x_1 \leq x_2$ implies $y_1 = F(x_1) \leq F(x_2) \leq y_2$, and it follows that $F^{(-1)}(y_1) = x_1 \leq x_2 = F^{(-1)}(y_2)$. Hence, the function $F^{(-1)}(y)$ is non-decreasing in $y \in (0,1)$.

A rather remarkable mathematical fact is that there is a transformation such that any continuous-type *r.v.* X of the class under consideration may be transformed to a *r.v.* U with a uniform distribution on the interval $(0,1)$. Suppose the *r.v.* X has *d.f.* $F(x)$ and consider the *r.v.* Y defined by $Y = F(X)$, with range $R_Y = (0,1)$. Then, because $F^{(-1)}(y)$ is non-decreasing in $y \in (0,1)$, the *d.f.* of Y is:

$$G(y) = \mathbb{P}\left[F(X) \leq y\right] = \mathbb{P}\left[X \leq F^{(-1)}(y)\right] = F\left(F^{(-1)}(y)\right) = y\ , \tag{2.6.2}$$

for $y \in (0,1)$. Thus (see Eq. (2.6.1)), the *r.v.* Y has a uniform distribution on the interval $(0,1)$.

Computers may be programmed to compute realizations of a uniform *r.v.* U that are approximately independent and identically distributed (*i.i.d*). A mapping that transforms a uniform *r.v.* U into a *r.v.* X with *d.f.* $F(x)$, $x \in R_X$, is, therefore, of interest in constructing algorithms for computing *i.i.d* realizations of a *r.v.* X. To this end, consider a *r.v.* Z defined by $Z = F^{(-1)}(U)$, with range $R_Z = R_X$. Then, it follows from Eq. (2.6.1) that the *d.f.* of Z is:

$$H(z) = \mathbb{P}\left[F^{(-1)}(U) \leq z\right] = \mathbb{P}\left[U \leq F(z)\right] = F(z) \tag{2.6.3}$$

for all $z \in R_X$. Therefore, the *r.v.* Z has *d.f.* $F(z)$ and the *r.v.*'s X and Z are equal in distribution. In symbols, $X \cong Z$. From this result, it can be seen that if one has an algorithm for computing the inverse of a *d.f.* $F(x)$, $x \in R_X$ and *i.i.d.* realizations of a uniform *r.v.* U on $(0,1)$, then approximate *i.i.d* realizations of a *r.v.* X may be computed by using the formula $X = F^{(-1)}(U)$.

Actually, a computer may be programmed to compute approximate *i.i.d.* realizations of a discrete *r.v.* Z_N with a uniform distribution on the set of positive integers $S_N = \{z \mid z = 1, 2, \cdots, N\}$, where N is a large positive integer, and with *p.d.f.* $f_{Z_N} = 1/N$ for $z \in S_N$. The approximation to a continuous-type *r.v.* U used in computer simulations is a discrete type *r.v.* of the form,

$$U_N = \frac{Z_N}{N} \,. \tag{2.6.4}$$

It can be shown that this *r.v.* has expectation,

$$E\left[U_N\right] = \frac{1}{2} + \frac{1}{2N} \tag{2.6.5}$$

and variance,

$$var\left[U_N\right] = \frac{1}{12} - \frac{1}{12N^2} \tag{2.6.6}$$

When N is large, this expectation and variance are very good approximations to $E\left[U\right] = 1/2$ and $var\left[U\right] = 1/12$ for a uniform *r.v.* U on $(0, 1)$.

There is a large and growing literature on random number generators used in computer simulation. The book Knuth[9] is a classic; the books, Deák[6] and Kennedy and Gentle,[8] and the references cited therein, may be consulted for details. Before any random number generator is used for simulation, it is wise to investigate whether it passes a number of statistical tests for *i.i.d.* realizations of a uniform random variable U on $(0, 1)$. Over the years, the authors and their associates have tested the random number generator implemented in the programming language APL*PLUS III, a language that operates under Microsoft Windows, using a variety of statistical tests, including the estimation of an auto-correlation function. Because this generator has passed many tests for *i.i.d.* realizations of uniform *r.v.*'s, it has been used widely in the computer simulations reported in this book.

Devising numerical algorithms for computing the inverse of a *d.f.* that are very accurate numerically, can pose difficult problems. Methods for transforming *i.i.d.* realizations of uniform *r.v.*'s directly into random variables of interest without finding the inverses of distribution functions have, therefore, been given much attention. A case in point is the distribution function of the standard normal distribution.

Fortunately, if $Z \sim N(0,1)$, then there are several methods for transforming *i.i.d.* realizations of uniform *r.v.*'s into *i.i.d.* realizations of Z. Among these methods are the Box-Muller algorithm. A *r.v.* R is said to have a Rayleigh distribution if its *d.f.* is:

$$\mathbb{P}[R \leq r] = F(r) = 1 - e^{-\frac{r^2}{2}}, \; r \in (0, \infty) \; . \tag{2.6.7}$$

If U_1 and U_2 are *i.i.d.* uniform *r.v.*'s on $(0,1)$, then $\Theta = 2\pi U_1$ has a uniform distribution on $(0, 2\pi)$. Moreover, it is the case that the independent *r.v.* $R = F^{(-1)}(U_2)$ has a Rayleigh distribution, where from Eq. (2.6.7) the inverse can be expressed in an elementary form. The Box-Muller algorithm consists of observing that:

$$Z_1 = R\cos\Theta \text{ and } Z_2 = R\sin\Theta \tag{2.6.8}$$

are two *i.i.d* realizations of $Z \sim N(0,1)$. Note the result in Eq. (2.6.8) may be proved easily by considering the joint *p.d.f.* of Z_1 and Z_2 in $R^{(2)} = \{(z_1, z_2) \mid z_1 \in R, z_2 \in R\}$ and transforming to polar coordinates.

To investigate the behavior of outliers in random samples from the Weibull, log-normal, and log-logistic distributions, the following Monte Carlo simulation exercise was carried out. Suppose one has m random samples of size n from some distribution and let the *r.v.* X_{ij} represent the jth observation in the ith sample, where $i = 1, 2, \cdots, m$ and $j = 1, 2, \cdots, n$. Then, the *r.v.*,

$$Y_i = \max_{1 \leq j \leq n} X_{ij} \tag{2.6.9}$$

is the maximum value in the ith sample, which may be viewed as a possible outlier. The sampling properties of these maximum values were investigated by computing the mean, standard deviation, minimum, and maximum of the m values Y_i, $i = 1, 2, \cdots, m$, for the three distributions in question and for the same parameter values as those used to compute Tables 2.5.1 and 2.5.2. The number of samples was $m = 100$ and for each sample the size was $n = 101$. Table 2.6.1 contains the results of these simulation experiments.

Table 2.6.1. Simulation of Outliers in Weibull, Log-Normal, and Log-Logistic Distributions.

Dist.	Mean	Std. Dev.	Min.	Max.
Weibull	16.304	1.479	13.076	21.143
Log-Normal	21.345	4.169	14.747	33.812
Log-Logistic	28.827	22.943	16.012	241.017

As can be seen from Table 2.6.1, for the parameter values used in the Weibull distribution, the variability in the maximum value statistic is relatively small, which suggests that if the variability in the incubation period of HIV was, in fact, governed by this distribution, one would not encounter many "large" outliers. For example, the maximum of the maximum sample value for the Weibull distribution was about 21.143 years. Even though the log-normal and log-logistic normal distributions have the same median and the same 0.75th quantile as the Weibull in the numerical examples in Table 2.6.1, samples from these three distributions can, nevertheless, have significantly different properties. By inspecting this table, it can be seen that the variability about the mean of the maximum value statistic, as measured by the standard deviations, is much greater for the log-normal and log-logistic distributions than for the Weibull. Moreover, this simulation exercise clearly differentiates between the log-normal and log-logistic distributions, for although these distributions had the same parameter values in the simulation exercise, the standard deviation, 22.943, for the log-logistic is over five times that for the log-normal, 4.169. In passing, it should be mentioned that the log-Cauchy distribution was not included in the simulation exercise, because simulated values from the Cauchy distribution were sometimes outside the permissible domain of the exponential function $\exp[\cdot]$ on the computer used in the simulation.

Thus, if a log-logistic distribution governed the variability in lengths of incubation periods of HIV, one would expect, as can be seen by inspecting the maximum of the maximum value statistics in Table 2.6.1, that there would be more outliers in the population than if this period were governed by a log-normal distribution. These observations, comparing the three distributions, could be significant in choosing a model for the variability in the incubation period of HIV. For, suppose a distribution such as the log-logistic actually governed the incubation period of HIV in a population and, as in the United States, there was no massive screening for seropositivity to HIV, then only those with relatively short incubation periods would be diagnosed with an AIDS-defining disease. Furthermore, if the data for testing a model of an incubation period were chosen from a sample whose infection times were known, then the sample could be biased against outliers and thus not be representative of the population of infected people as a whole. Simulation exercises, such as that described in this section, can be very useful in assessing the existence and consequences of such biases.

2.7 Compound Distributions

Choosing a parametric form for distributions other than the incubation period of HIV, or that of some other disease causing agent, can often be of interest in attempting to estimate HIV prevalence in a population and to project future AIDS cases. Among these distributions is one investigated by Tan and Byers,[17] which is defined as follows. Consider a susceptible male in a homosexual population at some time t_0. Let the $r.v.\, T_1$ be the waiting time to the first infection with HIV. Then, the $r.v.\, T_2 = T_1 - t_0$ is referred to as the infection time for this person and its distribution is then called the infection distribution. Similarly, if the $r.v.\, T_3$ denotes the waiting time to the first appearance of HIV antibodies in the blood of this infected person, then the distribution of the $r.v.\, T_4 = T_3 - t_0$ is referred to as the seroconversion time distribution. In applying the method of back-calculation to estimating the prevalence of HIV and for projecting future cases of AIDS, the infection time distribution plays a basic role (see Brookmeyer and Gail[4]) for details.

Upon reflection, one may conclude that the infection time distribution is actually determined by a number of factors governing the development of a HIV/AIDS epidemic in a population of male homosexuals. Among these factors are the distribution of the number of sexual partners per unit time and the probability of infection per sexual contact, which may in turn be a function of the stage of HIV disease of the infected partner. The main focus of the interesting paper of Tan and Byers[17] was to derive formulas for this distribution as determined by a stochastic model of a HIV/AIDS epidemic in a population of male homosexuals. As expected, this distribution can be quite complicated and can only be computed in terms of algorithms rather than by the relatively simple formulas for well-known parametric distributions. However, as these authors demonstrated by computer simulations, it is sometimes possible to approximate these complex distributions in terms of relatively simple parametric distributions. Among the distributions considered was a so-called three-parameter generalized log-logistic distribution, which gave the best fits to the simulated data. The purpose of this section is to provide a brief overview of the structure of this class of generalized distributions.

In what follows, all random variables and their distribution functions will be continuous. Suppose a *r.v.* X has range $R_X = (0,1)$ and *d.f.* $F(x)$ for $x \in R_X$, and suppose the *r.v.* Y has range R_Y and *d.f.* $G(y)$ for $y \in R_Y$. Then, consider a *r.v.* Z with range $R_Z = R_Y$ and suppose the *d.f.* of Z is:

$$H(z) = F(G(z)) \text{ for } z \in R_Z \, . \tag{2.7.1}$$

If the *p.d.f.*'s of the *d.f.*'s $F(x)$ and $G(y)$ are $f(x)$ and $g(y)$, then $H(z)$ has the *p.d.f.*,

$$h(z) = f(G(z))g(z) \text{ for } z \in R_Z \, . \tag{2.7.2}$$

Because the construction of generalized distributions involves functional composition, it seems appropriate to call such structures compound distributions.

By way of illustration, suppose the *r.v.* X has a beta distribution with *d.f.*,

$$F(x) = \frac{\Gamma(\alpha+\beta)}{\Gamma(\alpha)\Gamma(\beta)} \int_0^x s^{\alpha-1}(1-s)^{\beta-1} ds \, , \tag{2.7.3}$$

where $x \in (0,1)$, α and β are positive parameters, and $\Gamma(\cdot)$ is the gamma function. Now suppose the *r.v.* Y has a standard normal distribution function,

$$G(y) = \Phi(y) = \frac{1}{\sqrt{2\pi}} \int_{-\infty}^{y} e^{-\frac{s^2}{2}} ds \text{ for } y \in R \, . \tag{2.7.4}$$

Then, the general structure outlined above applies so that the *d.f.* of a *r.v.* Z could be defined by applying Eq. (2.7.1). From this simple illustration, it can be seen that the functions $F(x)$ and $G(y)$ may be chosen in a multitude of ways and it is natural to seek criteria for choosing particular forms of these functions.

A method that is often informative for interpreting a random variable with some distribution is to think of it as a transformation of a random variable with a known distribution. For example, the inverse of the *d.f.* in Eq. (2.7.1) is:

$$H^{(-1)}(y) = G^{(-1)}(F^{(-1)}(y)) \tag{2.7.5}$$

with domain $y \in (0,1)$ and range R_Z. Hence, from the general principles of computer simulation outlined in the previous section, it follows that if the *r.v.* U has a uniform distribution on the interval $(0,1)$, then the *r.v.*,

$$Z = G^{(-1)}(F^{(-1)}(U)) \tag{2.7.6}$$

has *d.f.* $H(z)$ for $z \in R_Z$.

This result is not only of interest in simulating realizations of a *r.v.* Z, but also suggests that a random variable with a compound distribution has a double sampling interpretation. For, if U has a uniform distribution on $(0,1)$, then the random variable,

$$X = F^{(-1)}(U) \tag{2.7.7}$$

with range $R_X = (0,1)$ has *d.f.* $F(x)$ for $x \in R_X$, and from Eq. (2.7.6) it follows that the *r.v.*,

$$Z = G^{(-1)}(X) \tag{2.7.8}$$

has range R_Z and *d.f.* $H(z)$. A random variable with a compound distribution may, therefore, be thought of as arising from a sampling process that produces a realization of the *r.v.* X with range $(0,1)$ and *d.f.* $F(x)$, then, given a realization of X, the transformation appearing in Eq. (2.7.8) yields a realization of a *r.v.* Z with the compound distribution function in Eq. (2.7.1). Observe that the assumption that X may not have a uniform distribution on $(0,1)$ plays a key role, for, if $X = U$ has a uniform distribution on the interval $(0,1)$, then the *r.v.*,

$$Y = G^{(-1)}(U) \tag{2.7.9}$$

has $d.f.\, G(y)$ for $y \in R_Y = R_Z$.

Even though they exist, it may not be possible to express expectations of random variables with compound distributions in simple forms. Because many computer packages contain programs for computing inverses of distribution functions, it will often be useful to compute quantiles of a random variable with a compound distribution so as to gain insights into its pattern of variation. For $q \in (0,1)$, the corresponding quantile $z_q \in R_Z$ is determined by the formula,

$$z_q = G^{(-1)}(F^{(-1)}(q)) = G^{(-1)}(x_q) \,, \tag{2.7.10}$$

where $x_q = F^{(-1)}(q)$, the qth quantile of the $r.v.\, X$. Thus, whenever there are computer programs available for computing the inverses of the distribution functions $F(x)$ and $G(y)$, then the quantiles of a random variable with a compound distribution may be easily computed.

The particular compound distribution used by Tan and Byers[17] in their study of the HIV infection distribution was that of choosing a two-parameter beta distribution as Eq. (2.7.3) and selecting the $d.f.\, G(t)$ of a $r.v.\, T$ as a form of the log-logistic distribution with the formula,

$$G(t) = \left(1 + \exp\left[-\frac{(\ln t - \mu)}{\sigma}\right]\right)^{-1} \,, \tag{2.7.11}$$

where $t \in R_T = (0, \infty)$, $\mu \in R$, and $\sigma > 0$. For this choice of distribution functions $F(\cdot)$ and $G(\cdot)$, the general form of the $p.d.f.$ in Eq. (2.7.2) takes the four-parameter special form,

$$h(t) = \frac{\Gamma(\alpha+\beta)}{\Gamma(\alpha)\Gamma(\beta)t\sigma} \left(G(t)\right)^{\alpha} \left(1 - G(t)\right)^{\beta} \,, \tag{2.7.12}$$

for $t \in R_T$. When $\beta = 1$, this distribution reduces to a three-parameter model, which was found to give the best fits to simulated data on the HIV infection distribution. The references cited in Tan and Byers[17] may also be consulted for examples in which this distribution gave the best fits to cancer survival data.

Although the well-known and extensively used beta distribution has many nice properties, such as all moments may be expressed as elementary functions of the parameters, it is natural to ask whether some other distribution with support $(0,1)$ might be equally well-suited as a choice for the distribution function $F(\cdot)$. One approach to constructing a large class of distribution functions whose support is the interval $(0,1)$ is to let $F_V(v)$ for $v \in R_V \subset R$ be the *d.f.* of some *r.v.* V. If W is some other *r.v.* with range R_W and *d.f.* $F_W(w)$ for $w \in R_W$, then the *r.v.* X defined by:

$$X = F_V(W) \tag{2.7.13}$$

has range $R_X = (0,1)$. Observe that if the *r.v.* W is replaced by the *r.v.* V, then X has a uniform distribution on $(0,1)$, but, in general, the distribution of X is not uniform on $(0,1)$ and is determined by the distribution of the *r.v.* W and the function F_V. Unlike that of the inverse of a *d.f.* in Eq. (2.7.8) in constructing compound distributions, it is a distribution function that plays a crucial role in determining the distribution of the *r.v.* X in Eq. (2.7.13).

Even in this age of powerful desktop computers, mathematical tractability is still an important consideration in choosing the distribution functions $F_V(\cdot)$ and $F_W(\cdot)$. A very computationally tractable distribution arises if $F_V(\cdot)$ is chosen as the logistic distribution function and it is assumed that the *r.v.* $W \sim N(\mu, \sigma^2)$. With these assumptions, the transformation in Eq. (2.7.13) takes the form,

$$X = \frac{e^W}{1+e^W} \tag{2.7.14}$$

and it follows by straightforward manipulations that the distribution function of X has the form:

$$\mathbb{P}\left[X \le x\right] = F(x) = \Phi\left(\frac{\ln\frac{x}{1-x} - \mu}{\sigma}\right), \tag{2.7.15}$$

where $\Phi(\cdot)$ is the standard normal distribution function and $x \in (0,1)$. In this case, the *p.d.f.* takes the form,

$$f(x) = \frac{1}{\sqrt{2\pi}\sigma x(1-x)} \exp\left[-\frac{\left(\ln\frac{x}{1-x} - \mu\right)^2}{2\sigma^2}\right], \tag{2.7.16}$$

for $x \in (0,1)$. As the parameters $\mu \in R$ and $\sigma \in (0,\infty)$ vary over pairs of values, a family of $p.d.f,$'s is generated whose graphs resemble those of the beta density.

Because the logistic and normal distributions were used in the derivation of this family, it seems appropriate to call this distribution the logistic-normal. Like many distributions of the form under consideration, expectations cannot be expressed as elementary functions of the parameters μ and σ. However, from Eq. (2.7.14), it follows that the quantiles of the distribution may be expressed in the computationally tractable form,

$$x_q = \frac{\exp\left[\mu + \sigma z_q\right]}{1 + \exp\left[\mu + \sigma z_q\right]} , \tag{2.7.17}$$

where z_q is the qth quantile of the standard normal distribution.

From the computational point of view, there are some advantages to considering the logistic-normal as an alternative to the beta distribution. For example, if a good algorithm is available for simulating realizations of the random variable $W \sim N(\mu, \sigma^2)$, then the simple formula in Eq. (2.7.14) may be applied to compute realizations of the $r.v.\, X$. This formula holds for all $\mu \in R$ and $\sigma \in (0,\infty)$; whereas in the case of a beta random variable, rather complicated algorithms are needed to simulate realizations of X when either $0 < \alpha < 1$ or $0 < \beta < 1$. Another advantage of the logistic-normal distribution is that its extension to the multidimensional case is straightforward, because Eq. (2.7.14) holds for each component of a random vector $\mathbf{W} = (W_1, \cdots, W_n)$ with a $n \geq 2$ dimensional normal distribution. Furthermore, the formula for the density in Eq. (2.7.16) may be easily generalized to the multidimensional case.

2.8 Models Based on Symptomatic Stages of HIV Disease

At the clinical level, individuals infected with HIV have been observed to pass through a series of stages from infected but antibody negative to a diagnosis of AIDS, as defined by one or more AIDS-defining diseases. In modeling the incubation period of HIV, it is, therefore, natural to consider models of the incubation period that accommodate transitions through various stages or states of some stochastic process. Among the classes of stochastic processes that have a state space and provide for probabilistic transitions among states are Markov processes in continuous time; for example, Chiang[5] may be consulted for a development of the theory of such processes and their applications in biostatistics. In a subsequent chapter, the general structure of this class of processes, as well as related processes, will be described in more detail. Even though Markov processes had been used in biological applications for at least three decades, among the first investigators to consider such a process in connection with HIV disease were Longini et al.,[11] who worked with the stages or states of HIV disease described in Table 2.8.1.

Table 2.8.1. Symptomatic Stages of HIV Disease.

State of HIV	Symptoms
E_1	Infected but Antibody Negative
E_2	Antibody Positive but Asymptomatic
E_3	AIDS-Related Complex (ARC)
E_4	Full Blown AIDS
E_5	Death due to AIDS

When formulating a stochastic model as a Markov process in continuous time with some defined state space, an essential step is to specify the patterns of transition among the states of the process. For the state space described in Table 2.8.1, it was assumed that transitions among these states were unidirectional as depicted in the diagram:

$$E_1 \to E_2 \to E_3 \to E_4 \to E_5 \,. \tag{2.8.1}$$

According to this diagram, after being infected with HIV, a person spends some random length of time T_1 in E_1 before moving to state E_2, when antibodies to HIV may be detected in his/her blood. After a random length of time T_2 in state E_2, there is a transition to state E_3, when some AIDS-related disease or diseases become apparent. Then, after a random length of time T_3 in state E_3, a patient is diagnosed with full-blown AIDS and is said to be in state E_4. Finally, after a random time T_4 in state E_4, a patient succumbs to some AIDS-defining disease and enters state E_5, where the process terminates.

To complete the formulation of the model, it was necessary to specify the distribution of each of the random variables, T_i for $i = 1, 2, 3, 4$, as well as their joint distribution. As is well-known and will also be discussed in a subsequent chapter, if one assumes that each $r.v. T_i$ has an exponential distribution with parameter $\beta_i > 0$ and all random variables are independent, then a Markov process in continuous time arises. An advantage of assuming a process is Markov in continuous time is that it then becomes possible to write down likelihood functions for data sets and estimate parameters even though the data may be heavily censored. But, because the assumption that each of these random variables has an exponential distribution seems too restrictive, some formulas for current state probabilities will be derived for the case where all random variables are independent but the $r.v. T_i$ has the arbitrary $p.d.f.\ f_i(t)$ with distribution and survival functions $F_i(t)$ and $S_i(t)$ for $i = 1, 2, 3, 4$.

It should also be observed that, due to the assumption the $p.d.f.$'s $f_i(t)$ do not change in calendar time, the process is said to have time homogeneous laws of evolution. Thus, given that the process is in some state E_i at time $t_1 \geq 0$, the conditional probability it is in state E_j at time $t_2 > t_1$ depends only on the difference $t_2 - t_1$. Without loss of generality, we may take $t_1 = 0$ in the discussion that follows. From now on, to simplify the notation, states will be denoted by the symbols i, j. Mention should also be made that the formulation under consideration does not take into account population heterogeneity in the sense that the model is assumed to apply to all members of a population who become infected with HIV.

Current state probabilities are defined as the following set of conditional probabilities that are essential for estimating the unknown parameters from data, and understanding some basic properties of the process. Given that the process enters state i at $t = 0$, let $P_{ij}(t)$ be the conditional probability that the process is in state j at time $t > 0$. Because transitions through states are unidirectional, $P_{ij}(t) = 0$ for all $t \geq 0$ when $j < i$, the task of deriving the required formulas reduces to considering the cases $j \geq i$. When $i = j$, the formula for a current state probability takes a simple form. For, if at time $t = 0$ the process enters state i, then $1 - F_i(t) = S_i(t)$ is the conditional probability it is in state i at time $t > 0$. Therefore,

$$P_{ii}(t) = S_i(t) \tag{2.8.2}$$

for all $i = 1, 2, 3, 4$.

Due to the assumption that transitions through states are unidirectional, it is also possible to set down a general formula for all cases such that $4 \geq j > i \geq 1$. If at $t = 0$, the process is in state 1, then the waiting times to first entrance into state 2, 3, or 4 are given, respectively, by the random variables T_1, $T_1 + T_2$, and $T_1 + T_2 + T_3$. In general, if at time $t = 0$ the process enters state i, then the waiting time to first entrance into state j is given by the random variable,

$$T_i + \cdots + T_{j-1} \ , \tag{2.8.3}$$

with the proviso that $T_{j-1} = 0$ if $j = i+1$. Let $g_{12}(t)$ be the conditional $p.d.f.$ of the waiting time to first entrance into state 2, given that the process entered state 1 at $t = 0$. Then, by definition, $g_{12}(t) = f_1(t)$. Because the random variables T_1 and T_2 are assumed to be independent, for $t > 0$ the convolution,

$$g_{13}(t) = f_1 * f_2(t) = \int_0^t f_1(s) f_2(t-s) ds \tag{2.8.4}$$

is the conditional $p.d.f.$ of the waiting time for first entrance into state 3, given that at $t = 0$ the process entered state 1.

Similarly, in the general case, if at $t = 0$ the process enters state i, then from Eq. (2.8.3) it follows that:

$$g_{ij}(t) = f_1 * f_2 * \cdots * f_{j-1}(t) \tag{2.8.5}$$

is the conditional $p.d.f.$ of the waiting time to first entrance into state j. Given these definitions, the current state probability $P_{ij}(t)$ may be derived by a so-called renewal argument. If at $t = 0$ the process enters state i and at $t > 0$ the process is in state j, then at some time $u \in (0, t]$ the process entered state j with probability $g_{ij}(u)du$ and has remained there for $t - u$ time units with probability $S_j(t - u)$. An integration "summation" over all $u \in (0, t]$ yields the formula:

$$P_{ij}(t) = \int_0^t g_{ij}(u) S_j(t-u) du \tag{2.8.6}$$

for the desired current state probability. According to the notation in Eq. (2.8.5), the *p.d.f.* of the incubation period is $g_{14}(t)$; while the *p.d.f.* of the waiting time from infection with HIV to death from an AIDS-defining disease is $g_{15}(t)$ for $t > 0$.

As mentioned above, Longini et al.[11] used formulas of the above type when all *p.d.f.*'s had the simple exponential form

$$f_i(t) = \beta_i \exp\left[-\beta_i t\right] \text{ for } i = 1, 2, 3, 4 \tag{2.8.7}$$

where β_i is a positive parameter, to estimate the four unknown parameters by the method of maximum likelihood, under the assumption that the underlying process was Markovian in continuous time. It is important to also take note that the data used by these investigators came from two types of sources. All data on individuals whose infection times were known consisted of patients who had been infected with HIV by either a blood transfusion or by the use of blood products contaminated with HIV. There were 105 such individuals in the sample who accounted for observed transition of the type $E_1 \to E_1$, $E_1 \to E_2$, $E_1 \to E_3$, and $E_1 \to E_4$ in the likelihood function. The remaining 650 individuals in the sample consisted of San Francisco cohorts of homosexual-bisexual men, who accounted for transitions out of states E_i for $i = 2, 3, 4$. Again, Longini et al.[11] should be consulted for details. Presented in Table 2.8.2 are the maximum likelihood estimates of the scale parameters in the exponential distributions for the Markov model for stages of HIV disease along with estimated mean and median waiting times expressed in months for each stage as reported by Longini et al.[11]

Table 2.8.2. Maximum Likelihood Estimates of Scale Parameters in Exponential Distributions for a Markov Model of Stages of HIV Disease Along with Estimated Mean and Median Waiting Times in Each Stage Expressed in Months.

Stage i	$\widehat{\beta}_i$ months^{-1}	Mean	Median
1	0.4571	2.1877	1.5164
2	0.0190	52.632	36.481
3	0.0159	62.893	43.594
4	0.0424	23.585	16.348

where the mean is:

$$\widehat{E\left[T_i\right]} = \frac{1}{\widehat{\beta}_i}\,, \tag{2.8.8}$$

and the median is:

$$\widehat{t}_{\frac{1}{2}} = \frac{\ln 2}{\widehat{\beta}_i}\,. \tag{2.8.9}$$

According to these estimates, the mean waiting time in stage E_1 is 2.1877 months or $2.1877/12 = 0.1823$ years; while, the mean waiting time in E_3, the ARC stage of the disease, is 62.8930 months or $62.8930/12 = 5.2411$ years. Because $E\left[T_i\right] = 1/\beta_i$ for $i = 1, 2, 3, 4$, it follows that, according to the Markov model, the estimated mean length of the incubation period of HIV is:

$$\frac{1}{\widehat{\beta}_1} + \frac{1}{\widehat{\beta}_2} + \frac{1}{\widehat{\beta}_3} = 2.1877 + 52.6320 + 62.8930 = 117.7127 \tag{2.8.10}$$

months or $117.7127/12 = 9.8094$ years. By a similar calculation, the estimated mean waiting time from infection with HIV to death from an AIDS-defining disease is 141.2977 months or $141.2977/12 = 11.7750$ years. In principle, one could use the distribution function of the incubation period:

$$G_{14}(t) = \int_0^t g_{14}(s)ds \text{ for } t > 0 \tag{2.8.11}$$

to compute the quantiles of this distribution as well as $G_{15}(t)$, the distribution function of the waiting time from infection to death, but exercises of this type will be postponed until the next section.

2.9 CD4$^+$ T Lymphocyte Decline

The symptomatic stages of HIV disease used in the preceding section were among the first attempts to model the progression of the disease by stages. Even though different systems of staging the disease have evolved since this work appeared, it remains of interest, because some of the later stages may become apparent to an infected individual and thus affect his or her ability to attract sexual partners. As mentioned in Chapter 1, however, one of the primary targets of HIV in the host is CD4$^+$ T lymphocytes (T4 cells); consequently, T4 cell decline is often used as a leading indicator of HIV disease progression. Longini et al.[12] have used a Markov process similar to that described in the previous section to model the progression of HIV by stages based on the T4 cell count per mm^3. Presented in Table 2.9.1 are the definitions of six stages of HIV disease, based on the Walter Reed System, as used by these authors.

Table 2.9.1. Stages of HIV Disease Based on T4 Cell Counts.

Stage	T4 Count per mm^3
1	> 899
2	700 – 899
3	500 – 699
4	350 – 499
5	200 – 349
6	0 – 199

When considering the stages defined in this table, it should be kept in mind that T4 cell counts in an individual can exhibit considerable variation due to measurement error and even with diurnal changes in physiological conditions. In an earlier stage of infection, an abnormally low T4 cell count could place an individual in a more advanced stage of HIV disease than is actually the case. To control these types of errors, the authors used the fairly large intervals displayed in the table with lengths of 200 units, and to determine the initial stage of a patient the higher of the first two T4 cell counts were used. Longini et al.[12] may be consulted for further details on the control procedures used in analyzing the data. From the point of view of the population as a whole, in addition to those in Table 2.9.1, three other stages are needed. Stage 0 represents a non-infected individual; stage 7 represents a diagnosis of full-blown AIDS as defined by some opportunistic infection resulting from the degradation of the immune system by HIV; while stage 8 represents a deceased individual.

Just as with the model discussed in Section 2.8, it is assumed that transitions through these states are unidirectional. Consequently, if no cofactors are taken into account, then six scale parameters β_j for $j = 1, 2, \cdots, 6$, in exponential distributions need to be estimated from data providing information on transitions among the states in Table 2.9.1. If each individual is also classified by three levels $i = 1, 2, 3$, of a cofactor such as age, then 18 parameters β_{ij}, for $i = 1, 2, 3$, and $j = 1, 2, \cdots, 6$, need to be estimated. The data used by Longini et al.[12] came from individuals in the US Army, who had been infected with HIV-1. Virtually all personnel of the US Army have been screened at least once and those testing positive for HIV-1 have been carefully followed. During the period June 1985 to April 1990, 1796 HIV infected individuals had at least two seropositive exams, and, in this sample, 1533 were seropositive at their first exam and 263 seroconverted. The patients were seen periodically with an average waiting time among exams of 6.9 ± 4.5 months and an average of 4.2 ± 2.0 exams per person. All patients were classified by age, where $i = 1, 2, 3$ stand for the age groups ≤ 25, $26 - 30$, and > 30. The method of maximum likelihood was again used to estimate the 18 parameters.

Presented in Table 2.9.2 are the estimates of the scale parameters and the mean durations of stay in each stage of HIV disease by age grouping of patients as determined by T4 cell counts. The mean values in this table have been calculated from the estimated mean values μ_{ij} expressed in years, as reported by Longini et al.[12] in their Table 4 and adjusted to a monthly time scale. To make the estimates comparable to those in the previous section, the relationship $\beta_{ij} = 1/\mu_{ij}$ was then used to compute values of the scale parameters rounded to four places. It is interesting to observe that the estimated mean durations of stay in stages 1, 2, and 3 of HIV disease, for which the T4 cell counts were ≥ 500, did not seem to differ significantly among the age groups ≤ 25, $26 - 30$, and > 30. However, significant differences among these age groups seemed to appear when the T4 cell count was < 500 in stages 4, 5, and 6.

According to the Markov model under consideration, the mean length of the incubation period of HIV for individuals in age group i is:

$$\nu_i = \sum_{j=1}^{6} \mu_{ij} \ . \tag{2.9.1}$$

According to the estimates in Table 2.9.2, it then follows that the means $\widehat{\nu}_1 = 133.2$, $\widehat{\nu}_2 = 120$, and $\widehat{\nu}_3 = 106.8$ months, or, equivalently that $133.2/12 = 11.1$, $120/12 = 10.0$ and $106.8/12 = 8.9$ years. From these estimates, one reaches the tentative conclusion that age at infection with HIV may significantly affect the length of the incubation period.

Table 2.9.2. Estimates of Scale Parameters in Exponential Distributions and Mean Durations of Stay in Stages Expressed in Months, Classified by Age, and Based on T4 Cell Count Data.

Stage j	$\widehat{\beta}_{1j}$	$\widehat{\mu}_{1j}$	$\widehat{\beta}_{2j}$	$\widehat{\mu}_{2j}$	$\widehat{\beta}_{3j}$	$\widehat{\mu}_{3j}$
1	0.0758	13.2	0.0641	15.6	0.0758	13.2
2	0.0595	16.8	0.0694	14.4	0.0694	14.4
3	0.0521	19.2	0.0521	19.2	0.0490	20.4
4	0.0347	28.8	0.0439	22.8	0.0490	20.4
5	0.0321	31.2	0.0417	24.0	0.0439	22.8
6	0.0417	24.0	0.0417	24.0	0.0641	15.6
Means		133.2		120		106.8

Estimates of mean lengths of the latent period by age groups are of interest, but to gain further insights into the effects of age on the latent period of HIV, it is also of interest to compute some quantiles of the distributions determined by the estimates of the β-parameters in Table 2.9.2. Because the distribution function of the latent period is determined by a six-fold convolution of exponential distributions in this case, finding numerical values of selected quantiles by root extraction methods is not a straight-forward task, if one wishes to strive for high numerical accuracy. On the other hand, if one is interested in getting approximate values of some selected quantiles, then Monte Carlo methods may be used in an elementary way to obtain estimates of quantiles. Table 2.9.3 contains Monte Carlo estimates of selected quantiles based on the estimates of the β parameters in Table 2.9.2 and samples of size 10000.

Table 2.9.3. Monte Carlo Estimates of Selected Quantiles in Months of Distributions of Latent Period by Age Group.

Quantile	≤ 25	$26-30$	>30
0.25	91.74	83.58	74.27
0.50	123.49	112.81	100.57
0.75	163.94	148.28	132.79
0.95	235.61	211.33	190.05

The basic principles underlying the Monte Carlo estimations of quantiles are simple. Let X_{ij} be independent exponential random variables with scale parameters β_{ij} for $i = 1, 2, 3$, and $j = 1, 2, \cdots, 6$, and let the random variable Y_i represent the latent period for the ith age group. Then, the distribution of Y_i is that of the sum

$$Y_i = \sum_{j=1}^{6} X_{ij} \ . \tag{2.9.2}$$

Briefly, the quantiles were estimated by computing the order statistics in samples of 10000 realizations of Y_i and then choosing the smallest order statistic, say y_q, such that some fraction q of the sample was less than or equal to that value. It is of interest to observe that for all age groups, the estimated medians were less than the mean, suggesting that graphs of the *p.d.f.*'s would be skewed to the left. For example, for the age group ≤ 25, the estimated mean was 133.20 and the median was 123.49 months (see Tables 2.9.2 and 2.9.3). These estimates also suggest that persons of age > 30, when first infected with HIV, would progress more rapidly to an AIDS-defining disease than those in the age group ≤ 25. As can be seen from Table 2.9.3, among those in the age group > 30, by 190.05 months 95% of cohorts of infectives would have progressed to full-blown AIDS; whereas for the age group ≤ 25, 95% of cohorts would have progressed to AIDS by 235.61 months, a difference of $235.61 - 190.05 = 45.56$ months or $45.56/12 = 3.7967$ years.

2.10 Concluding Remarks

Various waiting time distributions play important roles in developing stochastic models of epidemics, and as will be demonstrated in subsequent chapters, projections of an epidemic in a population are very sensitive to assumptions made about the distribution of the incubation period of the disease. Assumptions as to the form of the distribution also play an important role in estimating the number of persons infected with HIV in a population (see, for example, Longini et al.[10] on applying the method of back calculation to estimate stage specific numbers of persons infected with HIV). Another important component going into stochastic models of a HIV/AIDS epidemic is information on the probability that a susceptible person becomes infected per sexual contact with a partner infected with HIV. Longini et al.[13] have addressed this problem and have obtained valuable results. There are also other approaches to modeling the incubation period of HIV that do not entail the concept of stages. An example of this alternative approach is the paper by Berman,[3] where the incubation period is modeled as a stochastic process in continuous time. But, before this and other approaches to modeling the incubation period and other waiting time phenomena can be considered, it will be necessary to delve more deeply into the widely ranging field of stochastic processes, the subject of the next chapter.

2.11 References

1. L. J. Bain and M. Engelhardt, *Introduction to Probability and Mathematical Statistics,* Duxbury Press, Boston, 1987.
2. R. E. Barlow and F. Proschan, *Statistical Theory of Reliability and Life Testing Probability Models,* Holt, Rinehart, and Winston, Inc., New York, Chicago, 1975.
3. S. M. Berman, A Stochastic Model for the Distribution of HIV Latency Time Based on T4 Counts, *Biometrika* **77:** 733-741, 1990.
4. R. Brookmeyer and M. H. Gail, *AIDS Epidemiology: A Quantitative Approach,* Oxford University Press, Oxford, New York, Tokyo, 1994.
5. C. L. Chiang, *An Introduction to Stochastic Processes in Biostatistics,* 2nd ed., Krieger, New York, 1980.
6. I. Deák, *Random Number Generators and Simulation,* Akadémiai Kiadó, Budapest, 1990.
7. C. Derman, L. J. Gleser and I. Olkin, *A Guide to Probability Theory and Application,* Holt, Rinehart and Winston, Inc., New York, Chicago, 1973.
8. W. J. Kennedy, Jr. and J. E. Gentle, *Statistical Computing,* Marcel Dekker, Inc., New York and Basel, 1980.
9. D. E. Knuth, *Seminumerical Algorithms - The Art of Computer Programming, II,* Addison-Wesley, Reading Mass., London, Sydney, 1969.
10. I. M. Longini, Jr., B. H. Byers, N. A. Hessol and W. Y. Tan, Estimating Stage-Specific Numbers of HIV Infection Using a Markov Model and Back Calculation, *Statistics in Medicine* **11:** 831-843, 1992.
11. I. M. Longini, Jr., W. S. Clark and R. H. Byers et al., Statistical Analysis of the Stages of HIV Infection Using a Markov Model, *Statistics in Medicine* **8:** 831-843, 1989.
12. I. M. Longini, Jr., W. S. Clark, L. I. Gardner and J. F. Brundage, Modeling the Decline of CD4+ T-Lymphocyte Counts in HIV-Infected Individuals: A Markov Modeling Approach, *Journal of Acquired Immune Deficiency Syndromes* **4:** 1141-1147, 1991.
13. I. M. Longini, Jr., W. S. Clark, L. M. Haber and R. Horsburgh, Jr., The Stages of HIV Infection: Waiting Times and Infection Transmission Probabilities, *Lecture Notes in Biomathematics* **83:** 111-137, C. Castillo-Chavez (ed.), *Mathematical and Statistical Approaches in AIDS Epidemiology,* Springer-Verlag, Berlin, New York, Tokyo, 1989.

14. K.-J. Lui, W. W. Darrow and G. W. Rutherford, III, A Model-Based Estimate of the Mean Incubation Period for AIDS in Homosexual Men, *Science* **240:** 1333-1335, 1988.

15. A. M. Mood, F. A. Graybill and D. C. Boes, *An Introduction to the Theory of Statistics,* McGraw-Hill, New York, 1963.

16. S. M. Stigler, *The History of Statistics - The Measurement of Uncertainty Before 1900,* The Belknap Press of Harvard University Press, Cambridge, Mass. and London, England, 1986.

17. W. Y. Tan and R. H. Byers, Jr., A Stochastic Model of the HIV Epidemic and HIV Infection Distribution in a Homosexual Population, *Mathematical Biosciences* **113:** 115-143, 1993.

18. R. A. Thisted, *Elements of Statistical Computing - Numerical Computation,* Chapman and Hall, New York and London, 1988.

Chapter 3
CONTINUOUS TIME MARKOV AND SEMI-MARKOV JUMP PROCESSES

3.1 Introduction

A number of classes of stochastic processes have been used to model the incubation period of HIV as well as other aspects of HIV/AIDS epidemiology. Accordingly, the purpose of this chapter is to give an overview of several classes of stochastic processes that have been used in the construction of stochastic models in epidemiology. When attempting to construct a stochastic model of some phenomenon of interest, it is natural for an investigator to focus on the substantive aspects of the problem without paying attention to the mathematical foundations underlying the class of stochastic process that has been chosen. Unfortunately, by not paying attention to mathematical foundations, one may be led into intractable analytic problems which can obscure the underlying conceptual simplicity of the model and reduce its practical usefulness as a tool for understanding the phenomenon being considered. One may find that by choosing another class of stochastic process as the framework for modeling the phenomenon, analytic difficulties disappear. Moreover, by focusing on some limited aspect of the process, the construction of algorithms for computing Monte Carlo realizations of the process may not be apparent. In this computer age, the computation of Monte Carlo realizations of a process can be very helpful in understanding the implications of a model from both the theoretical and practical points of view. Consequently, throughout this chapter the advantages and disadvantages of each class of stochastic processes will be considered, and whenever classes of stochastic processes are introduced, attention will be given to the problem of developing algorithms for computing Monte Carlo realizations of the process.

In addition to the references cited in Chapter 2, some further background in probability and stochastic processes will be useful but not absolutely essential to an understanding of the material of this chapter. An excellent reference is the classic book, Feller.[7] The textbooks, Breiman,[3] Hoel et al.[9] and Cinlar[5] also contain readable and useful background material. A more comprehensive treatment of stochastic processes is contained in the well-known textbook, Karlin.[11] Finally, two more advanced and classic books on stochastic processes, Doob[6] and Gikhman and Skorokhod,[8] may also be consulted for background material. At times it will be helpful in clarifying concepts to introduce the concept of a probability space $(\mathbf{\Omega}, \mathfrak{A}, \mathbb{P})$ in what follows, where $\mathbf{\Omega}$ is the sample space of the process, $\mathfrak{A}$ is a σ-algebra of events, i.e., subset of $\mathbf{\Omega}$, and $\mathbb{P}$ is a probability measure on $\mathfrak{A}$. If a reader feels compelled to delve more deeply into these concepts, the latter two references are excellent sources. Another excellent textbook that gives a comprehensive treatment of these concepts is that of Billingsley.[2]

3.2 Stationary Markov Jump Processes

Among the classes of stochastic processes that have been widely applied in epidemiology is that of continuous time parameter Markov jump processes with stationary transition probabilities. In the construction of a model within this class of stochastic processes, a first step is to define some set $\mathfrak{S}$ of states among which the process moves at random points in time. If, for example, one is considering HIV disease by stages as discussed the Chapter 2, then the elements of $\mathfrak{S}$ would be the stages of HIV disease. In what follows, time will be chosen as the set of non-negative real numbers $\mathbb{T}= [t \mid 0 \leq t < \infty] = [0, \infty)$. Let $(\mathbf{\Omega}, \mathfrak{A}, \mathbb{P})$ be a probability space underlying the process, and for $(\omega, t) \in \mathbf{\Omega} \times \mathbb{T}$ (the Cartesian product of the sets $\mathbf{\Omega}$ and $\mathbb{T}$), let $X(\omega, t)$ be a random function with range $\mathfrak{S}$, representing the state of the system at time $t \in \mathbb{T}$. As an aid to understanding the stochastic nature of the structure under consideration, observe that for each $\omega \in \mathbf{\Omega}$, $X(\omega, t)$ is a sample function or realization of the process as t varies over the time set $\mathbb{T}$. Intuitively, the process moves by jumps, i.e., it starts in some state i_0

and stays there for some length of time, then moves to another state i_1 and stays there for a time, and so the process continues. As ω varies over $\mathbf{\Omega}$, the length of stays in states becomes "random". This notion of randomness or stochasticity is basic to the understanding of stochastic processes, but to lighten the notation, the symbol ω will often be dropped so that the state of the process at time t will be represented by $X(t)$.

A basic property characterizing Markov processes in continuous time is the so-called Markov property; namely, the present state of the process depends only on the past state and all previous history is forgotten. More precisely, for any integer $n \geq 1$, let $i_0, i_1, \cdots, i_n$ be states in $\mathfrak{S}$, let $0 \leq t_0 \leq t_1 \leq \cdots \leq t_n$ points in $\mathbb{T}$, let:

$$\mathfrak{B}(n-1) = \{X(t_k) = i_k \mid k = 0, 1, 2, \cdots, n-1\} \ , \tag{3.2.1}$$

and suppose the probability measure $\mathbb{P}$ on $\mathfrak{A}$ has the property,

$$\mathbb{P}\left[X(t_n) = i_n \mid \mathfrak{B}(n-1)\right] = \mathbb{P}\left[X(t_n) = i_n \mid X(t_{n-1}) = i_{n-1}\right] \ . \tag{3.2.2}$$

Because the process is assumed to have the Markov property as characterized by Eq. (3.2.2), it is natural to introduce a function $P(s,t)$ defined on $\mathbb{T}\times\mathbb{T}$, called a transition probability, such that for $s < t$ and any states i and j in $\mathfrak{S}$:

$$\mathbb{P}\left[X(t) = j \mid X(s) = i\right] = P_{i,j}(s,t) \ . \tag{3.2.3}$$

Conversely, if we are given a transition probability $P_{ij}(s,t)$, then as is well-known, a probability measure $\mathbb{P}$ on $\mathfrak{A}$ with the Markov property may be determined, up to an initial distribution, by defining the finite dimensional distribution of the process as:

$$\begin{aligned} &\mathbb{P}\left[X(t_k) = i_k, k = 1, 2, \cdots, n \mid X(t_0) = i_0\right] \\ &\qquad = \prod_{k=1}^{n} P_{i_{k-1},i_k}(t_{k-1}, t_k) \ , \end{aligned} \tag{3.2.4}$$

for ordered points t_ν in $\mathbb{T}$ and states i_k, $k = 0, 1, 2, \cdots, n$, in $\mathfrak{S}$ for every positive integer $n \geq 1$. A Markov process is said to have stationary transition probabilities if there is a function $P_{ij}(\cdot)$ defined on $\mathbb{T}$ for every pair of states i and j in $\mathfrak{S}$, such that:

$$P_{i,j}(s,t) = P_{ij}(t-s), \tag{3.2.5}$$

when $s < t$. Thus, for a process with stationary transition probabilities, if at some time $s < t$, the process is in state i, then the conditional probability that the process is in state j at time t depends only on the time difference $t - s$.

Because the transition probability function $P_{ij}(t)$ determines the probability measure $\mathbf{P}$ underlying the process, it seems natural to attempt to find some formula for this function of i, j and t. At the outset, it is clear that this function must satisfy at least three conditions. Since it is a probability, the condition,

$$0 \leq P_{ij}(t) \leq 1 , \tag{3.2.6}$$

must be satisfied for all $t \in \mathbb{T}$ and states i and j in $\mathfrak{S}$. A second condition that must be satisfied is:

$$\sum_{j \in \mathfrak{S}} P_{ij}(t) = 1 \tag{3.2.7}$$

for all $i \in \mathfrak{S}$ and $t \in \mathbb{T}$. Intuitively, this condition states that if the process is in any state i at time $t = 0$, then it must be in some state $j \in \mathfrak{S}$ at time $t > 0$ with probability one. Lastly, if one rules out instantaneous jumps, then the initial condition,

$$P_{ij}(0) = \delta_{ij} , \tag{3.2.8}$$

where δ_{ij} is the Kronecker delta, i.e., $\delta_{ii} = 1$ and $\delta_{ij} = 0$ if $i \neq j$, must also be satisfied.

Since the process whose underlying probability measure is to have the Markov property, it turns out that the function $P_{ij}(t)$ must also satisfy another condition known as the Chapman-Kolmogorov equation. To derive this equation, let the symbol $[X(t) = j]$ for $j \in \mathfrak{S}$ stand for the ω set,

$$[X(t) = j] = [\omega \in \boldsymbol{\Omega} \mid X(\omega, t) = j] \tag{3.2.9}$$

Then, because

$$\boldsymbol{\Omega} = \bigcup_{k \in \mathfrak{S}} [X(s) = k] \tag{3.2.10}$$

for any $s, t \in \mathbb{T}$, it follows that:

$$[X(s+t) = j] = \bigcup_{k \in \mathfrak{S}} [X(s) = k, X(s+t) = j] \ , \tag{3.2.11}$$

where the symbol in the disjoint union stands for the intersection of the sets $[X(s) = k]$ and $[X(s+t) = j]$. Therefore, by the Markov property, it can be seen that:

$$\mathbb{P}[X(s+t) = j \mid X(0)] = \sum_{k \in \mathfrak{S}} \mathbb{P}[X(s) = k, X(s+t) = j \mid X(0) = i]$$

$$= \sum_{k \in \mathfrak{S}} \mathbb{P}[X(s) = k \mid X(0) = i] \, \mathbb{P}[X(s+t) = j \mid X(s) = k, \ X(0) = i]$$

$$= \sum_{k \in \mathfrak{S}} \mathbb{P}[X(s) = k \mid X(0) = i] \, \mathbb{P}[X(s+t) = j \mid X(s) = k] \ . \tag{3.2.12}$$

Equivalently, for the case of stationary transition probabilities $P_{ij}(t)$, this result becomes the Chapman-Kolmogorov equation,

$$P_{ij}(s+t) = \sum_{k \in \mathfrak{S}} P_{ik}(s) P_{kj}(t) \ . \tag{3.2.13}$$

In summary, if a transition function $P_{ij}(t)$ is to be that of a continuous time Markov jump process with stationary transition probabilities, then the conditions in Eqs. (3.2.5), (3.2.6), (3.2.7), (3.2.8) and (3.2.13) must be satisfied for all $i, \, j \in \mathfrak{S}$ and $s, \, t \in \mathbb{T}$.

3.3 The Kolmogorov Differential Equations

An approach that has been used extensively to obtain formulas for the transition probabilities is to assume that the functions $P_{ij}(t)$ are differentiable for all $t \in \mathbb{T}$ and then set down a set of differential equations which may be solved to obtain the desired formulas. Accordingly, let $P'_{ij}(t)$ be the continuous derivative of the function $P_{ij}(t)$ at $t \in \mathbb{T}$. The values of these derivatives at $t = 0$ and their probabilistic interpretation will play an important role in deriving the desired set of differential equations. If the process is in state i at time $t = 0$, then $P_{ii}(t)$ is the conditional probability the process is in state i at time $t > 0$, and $1 - P_{ii}(t)$ is the conditional probability that at least one jump has occurred during the time interval $(0, t]$. A useful set of differential equations may be derived by supposing that during any small time interval $(0, h]$, at most one jump can occur if h is sufficiently small. More precisely, assume that for every $i \in \mathfrak{S}$ there is a finite positive constant q_i such that:

$$\lim_{h \downarrow 0} \frac{1 - P_{ii}(h)}{h} = q_i \ . \tag{3.3.1}$$

Equivalently, $1 - P_{ii}(h) = q_i h + o(h)$ is the conditional probability of at least one jump during $(0, h]$, where $o(h)/h \to 0$ as $h \downarrow 0$. Also observe that because $P_{ii}(0) = \delta_{ii} = 1$,

$$q_{ii} = \lim_{h \downarrow 0} \frac{P_{ii}(h) - 1}{h} = P'_{ii}(0) = -q_i \tag{3.3.2}$$

for all $i \in \mathfrak{S}$. It will also be supposed that if $i \neq j$, then the derivatives:

$$q_{ij} = P'_{ij}(0) = \lim_{h \downarrow 0} \frac{P_{ij}(h) - \delta_{ij}}{h} = \lim_{h \downarrow 0} \frac{P_{ij}(h)}{h} \geq 0 \tag{3.3.3}$$

at $t = 0$ are finite for all $i, j \in \mathfrak{S}$.

For the sake of simplicity, it will assumed in what follows that the state space $\mathfrak{S}$ is finite in deriving the desired set of differential equations so that the operations of summation and differentiation can be interchanged with impunity. The references cited previously may be consulted for the derivation of these equations in the more complicated case where $\mathfrak{S}$ is countably infinite. If t in the Chapman-Kolmogorov Eq. (3.2.13) is fixed and one differentiates the equation with respect to s, the equation,

$$P'_{ij}(s + t) = \sum_{k \in \mathfrak{S}} P'_{ik}(s) P_{kj}(t) \tag{3.3.4}$$

arises. Similarly, if one fixes s in this equation and differentiates with respect to t, one obtains the equation,

$$P'_{ij}(s + t) = \sum_{k \in \mathfrak{S}} P_{ik}(s) P'_{kj}(t) \ . \tag{3.3.5}$$

By letting $s \downarrow 0$ in Eq. (3.3.4), $t \downarrow 0$ in Eq. (3.3.5), and by substituting t for s in the resulting expression, the pair,

$$P'_{ij}(t) = \sum_{k \in \mathfrak{S}} q_{ik} P_{kj}(t) \tag{3.3.6}$$

$$P'_{ij}(t) = \sum_{k \in \mathfrak{S}} P_{ik}(t) q_{kj} \ , \tag{3.3.7}$$

which are known as the Kolmogorov differential equations, arise.

Further, Eqs. (3.3.6) are known as the backward equations and Eqs. (3.3.7) as the forward equations. This terminology seems justified, for if one imagines taking derivatives with respect to s from the left in the Chapman-Kolmogorov equation (3.2.13), i.e., backwards in time, then equations Eqs. (3.3.6) would arise. Similarly, if one imagines taking derivatives in this equation with respect to t from the right, i.e., forwards in time, the process just described would yield the forward equations. Thc problcm of finding solutions to these differential equations can be stated much more succinctly if it is cast in matrix form. To this end, let $\mathbf{P}(t) = (P_{ij}(t))$, $\mathbf{P}'(t) = (P'_{ij}(t))$, and $\mathbf{Q} = (q_{ij}) = \mathbf{P}'(0)$ be finite square matrices. Then, for $t \in \mathbb{T}$, the Kolmogorov differential equations take the form,

$$\mathbf{P}'(t) = \mathbf{Q}\mathbf{P}(t) \tag{3.3.8}$$

$$\mathbf{P}'(t) = \mathbf{P}(t)\mathbf{Q} \tag{3.3.9}$$

with the initial condition

$$\mathbf{P}(0) = \mathbf{I} \ , \tag{3.3.10}$$

where $\mathbf{I}$ is an identity matrix. Furthermore, in matrix notation, for $s, t \in \mathbb{T}$ the Chapman-Kolmogorov equation takes the form,

$$\mathbf{P}(s+t) = \mathbf{P}(s)\mathbf{P}(t) \ . \tag{3.3.11}$$

Let $\mathbf{1}$ be column vector of $1's$. Then, in matrix form the condition that all sums over columns in $\mathbf{P}(t)$ should be one (see Eq. (3.2.7)), becomes

$$\mathbf{P}(t)\mathbf{1} = \mathbf{1} \tag{3.3.12}$$

for all $t \in \mathbb{T}$. Finally, by differentiating this equation with respect to t and letting $t \downarrow 0$, it follows that:

$$\mathbf{Q1} = \mathbf{0} , \tag{3.3.13}$$

a column vector containing all zeros. The matrix $\mathbf{Q}$ is sometimes called the infinitesimal generator of the process; it is also known as the intensity matrix of the process.

Fortunately, it is easy to formally find the solution of the Kolmogorov differential equations, satisfying Eqs. (3.3.10) and (3.3.11) for all $s, t \in \mathbb{T}$. For, let

$$\mathbf{P}(t) = \exp\left[\mathbf{Q}t\right] = \mathbf{I} + \mathbf{Q}t + \frac{\mathbf{Q}^2 t^2}{2!} + \frac{\mathbf{Q}^3 t^3}{3!} + \cdots \tag{3.3.14}$$

be the exponential matrix function defined by the series on the right, which converges for all $t \in \mathbf{T}$. Then, by differentiating this series term by term with respect to t, it is easy to see that the matrix exponential defined in Eq. (3.3.14) is a solution of differential equations Eq. (3.3.8) and Eq. (3.3.9). It can also be seen from Eq. (3.3.14) that Eq. (3.3.13) implies that condition Eq. (3.3.12) is satisfied for all $t \in \mathbf{T}$. That the exponential matrix satisfies the Chapman-Kolmogorov equation can also be seen from the equation,

$$\begin{aligned} \mathbf{P}(s+t) &= \sum_{n=0}^{\infty} \frac{\mathbf{Q}^n (s+t)^n}{n!} \\ &= \sum_{n=0}^{\infty} \sum_{i=0}^{n} \frac{\mathbf{Q}^i s^i \mathbf{Q}^{n-i} t^{n-i}}{i!(n-i)!} \\ &= \left(\sum_{i=0}^{\infty} \frac{\mathbf{Q}^i s^i}{i!} \right) \left(\sum_{j=0}^{\infty} \frac{\mathbf{Q}^j t^j}{j!} \right) \\ &= \mathbf{P}(s)\mathbf{P}(t) , \end{aligned} \tag{3.3.15}$$

which is valid for all $s, t \in \mathbb{T}$. In deriving this equation, the condition that the matrix series in Eq. (3.3.14) converges absolutely element by element has been tacitly used to justify rearrangement of terms in the infinite series.

The method just outlined for solving the Kolmogorov differential equations has been known for several decades for the case where the state space $\mathfrak{S}$ is a finite set, but it has not been used extensively in applications because of numerical and algebraic difficulties in finding values of the exponential matrix. However, from a theoretical standpoint, much is known about the exponential matrix; for example, the classic book on differential equations, Bellman,[1] may be consulted for technical details. Briefly, when the eigenvalues of $\mathbf{Q}$ are simple, the elements of the exponential matrix may be represented as linear combinations of exponential functions of t with the eigenvalues of the matrix $\mathbf{Q}$ appearing as constants in the exponents. If $\mathbf{Q}$ has multiple eigenvalues, then for some elements of the matrix, the exponentials may have polynomials in t as coefficients. As computers become more powerful and user-friendly, however, software packages often include the implementation of accurate algorithms for finding symbolic as well as numerical values of the exponential matrix. For example, the word processor that is being used for this manuscript is linked to a computer algebra software package called MAPLE, which not only does symbolic manipulations, but also numerical computations. The book Char et al.[4] may be consulted for details on the MAPLE programming language.

By way of illustration, suppose the intensity matrix $\mathbf{Q}$ of a three-state process has the simple form,

$$\mathbf{Q} = \begin{bmatrix} -2 & 1 & 1 \\ 0 & -3 & 3 \\ 2 & 2 & -4 \end{bmatrix} . \tag{3.3.16}$$

Then, the symbolic form of the matrix $\mathbf{P}(t)$ for $t \in \mathbb{T}$ is:

$$\begin{bmatrix} \frac{1}{3} + \frac{2}{3}e^{-3t} & -\frac{1}{3}e^{-3t} + \frac{1}{3} & -\frac{1}{3}e^{-3t} + \frac{1}{3} \\ \frac{1}{3}e^{-6t} - \frac{2}{3}e^{-3t} + \frac{1}{3} & \frac{1}{3}e^{-3t} + \frac{1}{3}e^{-6t} + \frac{1}{3} & -\frac{2}{3}e^{-6t} + \frac{1}{3}e^{-3t} + \frac{1}{3} \\ \frac{1}{3} - \frac{1}{3}e^{-6t} & \frac{1}{3} - \frac{1}{3}e^{-6t} & \frac{1}{3} + \frac{2}{3}e^{-6t} \end{bmatrix} . \tag{3.3.17}$$

It is of interest to observe that if one sums each row of this matrix over the columns, the sum is one for all $t \in \mathbb{T}$, as it should be, in accordance with the condition in Eq. (3.3.13). In this case, the matrix $\mathbf{Q}$ has three simple eigenvalues; namely, $-6, -3$, and 0 which appear in the exponents. At $t = 1$, the transition matrix has the numerical value

$$\mathbf{P}(1) = \begin{bmatrix} 0.36652 & 0.31674 & 0.31674 \\ 0.30097 & 0.35076 & 0.34828 \\ 0.33251 & 0.33251 & 0.33499 \end{bmatrix} . \tag{3.3.18}$$

Other software packages contain implementations of algorithms making it possible to compute numerical values of the exponential matrix for finitely many values of $t \in \mathbb{T}$ with relative ease, but even with good packages, the computations may become unwieldy if the intensity matrix $\mathbf{Q}$ is too large. Having a capability for computing numerical values of the exponential matrix also makes it feasible to do statistical inference for models based on Markov jump processes with stationary transition probabilities, particularly for those models in which the state space $\mathfrak{S}$ is not too large. For example, suppose the intensity matrix $\mathbf{Q}(\boldsymbol{\theta})$ depends on a vector parameters $\boldsymbol{\theta} \in \boldsymbol{\Theta}$, a finite dimensional parameter space, and let $\mathbf{P}(t) = \exp[\mathbf{Q}(\boldsymbol{\theta})t] = (P_{ij}(\boldsymbol{\theta};t))$ be a symbolic form of the matrix of transition probabilities, depending on $t \in \mathbb{T}$ and $\boldsymbol{\theta} \in \boldsymbol{\Theta}$. Next suppose an investigator has the following observations on $n \geq 1$ individuals. At times $t_{jk,}$ where for each $j = 1, 2, \cdots, n$, and $k = 0, 1, 2, \cdots, n_j$, $0 \leq t_{j0} < t_{j1} < \cdots < t_{jn_j}$, the states $i_{jk} \in \mathfrak{S}$ occupied by these individuals are known at time t_{jk}. Then, by using the Markov property in continuous time, it follows that the likelihood function of the data has the form,

$$L(\boldsymbol{\theta}) = \prod_{j=1}^{n} \prod_{k=1}^{n_j} P_{i_{j,k-1}, i_{j,k}}(\boldsymbol{\theta}; t_{jk} - t_{j,k-1}) \tag{3.3.19}$$

Given a capability for finding numerical values of the transition matrix for these time points, states, and any value $\boldsymbol{\theta} \in \boldsymbol{\Theta}$, it becomes possible to conduct numerical searches of the parameter space to find a maximum likelihood estimator of the parameter vector $\boldsymbol{\theta}$. Among the authors that have used these ideas to estimate the parameters for staged models of HIV disease are Longini et al.[13] It should be noted that the Markov property in continuous time (see Eq. (3.2.2)), and the assumption of stationary transition probabilities are essential to the mathematical validity of the likelihood function in Eq. (3.3.19).

3.4 The Sample Path Perspective of Markov Processes

As stated previously, when thinking about continuous time Markov jump processes, one usually has in mind the following simple picture. At time $t = 0$, the process is in some state $i \in \mathfrak{S}$. After a random length of time, it jumps to some state $j \in \mathfrak{S}$ and remains there for a random length of time until it jumps to another state, and so the process continues. Given an intensity matrix $\mathbf{Q} = (q_{ij})$ of a Markov jump process with stationary transition probabilities, it is natural to ask: What is the distribution of the sojourn time, length of stay in some state $i \in \mathfrak{S}$, and, given that a jump from i occurs, what is the conditional probability of the jump to state j? Because the matrix $\mathbf{Q}$ completely determines the process, answers to these questions can be expressed in terms of the elements of this matrix.

Among others, Doob[6] has shown that from the Markov property, as expressed in Eq. (3.2.4), one may deduce that

$$P\left[X(u) = i, \text{ for all } u \in (s, s+t] \mid X(s) = i\right] = \exp\left[-q_i t\right] \tag{3.4.1}$$

for every $s, t \in \mathbb{T}$ and state $i \in \mathfrak{S}$, where, by definition, $q_i = -q_{ii} \geq 0$. By letting $s = 0$, it can be seen that the sojourn time in some initial state i is exponentially distributed with parameter q_i. Furthermore, Eq. (3.4.1) implies that whatever the length of the stay in state i, if the process is in state i at time $s \geq 0$, then the conditional probability that it is still in state i at time $s + t$ is $\exp[-q_i t]$. Observe that the memoryless property of the exponential distribution plays an essential role in the mathematical validity of this statement.

Let π_{ij} for $i \neq j$ be the conditional probability of a jump to state j, given that a jump from state i has occurred. Doob and others have shown how this probability is determined. Eq. (3.3.13) implies that:

$$q_i = \sum_{j \neq i} q_{ij} \tag{3.4.2}$$

for all $i \in \mathfrak{S}$, and from this equation, it can be shown that the probability in question is given by $\pi_{ij} = q_{ij}/q_i$, provided that $q_i \neq 0$. Hence, for $q_i \neq 0$ equation Eq. (3.4.2) implies:

$$\sum_{j \neq i} \pi_{ij} = 1 \, , \tag{3.4.3}$$

so that the matrix $\mathbf{\Pi} = (\pi_{ij})$, where $\pi_{ii} = 0$, may be interpreted as a one step transition matrix of a Markov chain with stationary transition probabilities.

From the analysis just described, a very simple picture for the evolution of the process from the perspective of the sample paths emerges. Suppose the process starts in state i_0, let $i_k, k = 1, 2, \cdots, n$, be the states visited for the first $n \geq 1$ jumps, and let the random variable T_{i_k} represent the sojourn time in state i_k, for $k = 0, 1, 2, \cdots, n-1$. Then, each of these random variables has an exponential distribution with *p.d.f.*,

$$f_{i_k}(t) = q_{i_k} \exp\left[-q_{i_k} t\right] , \; t \in \mathbb{T}, \tag{3.4.4}$$

and, given the sample path, $i_0, i_1, \cdots, i_{n-1}, i_n$, the random variables:

$$T_{i_0}, T_{i_1}, \cdots, T_{i_{n-1}} \tag{3.4.5}$$

are conditionally independent. As we saw in the Chapter 2, the exponential distribution, with its memoryless property, is a very special case and may not be sufficiently realistic as a waiting model for many biological phenomena. A question that arises, therefore, is whether it is possible to construct jump processes such that the random variables representing sojourn times in states have arbitrary distributions on $\mathbb{T}$, but are conditionally independent, given a sample path. As we shall see in a subsequent section, the question may be answered in the affirmative and gives rise to a class of stochastic processes known as semi-Markov processes.

At this point, it will be instructive to recast the Kolmogorov differential equations in a form that provides some insight into the process from the sample path perspective. In the notation of this section, the forward Kolmogorov differential equations may be represented in the form

$$P'_{ij}(t) = -P_{ij}(t) q_j + \sum_{k \neq j} P_{ik}(t) q_k \pi_{kj} \tag{3.4.6}$$

and the backwards equations take the form,

$$P'_{ij}(t) = -q_i P_{ij}(t) + \sum_{k \neq i} q_i \pi_{ik} P_{kj}(t) \ . \tag{3.4.7}$$

By multiplying the first equation by $\exp[q_j t]$ and the second by $\exp[q_i t]$, these equations may be cast in the form:

$$\frac{d}{dt}\left(e^{q_j t} P_{ij}(t)\right) = \sum_{k \neq j} P_{ik}(t) q_k \pi_{kj} e^{q_j t} \tag{3.4.8}$$

and

$$\frac{d}{dt}\left(e^{q_i t} P_{ij}(t)\right) = \sum_{k \neq i} q_i e^{q_i t} \pi_{ik} P_{kj}(t) \ . \tag{3.4.9}$$

Then, by using the initial condition $P_{ij}(0) = \delta_{ij}$ and doing some rearranging after integration, the pair,

$$P_{ij}(t) = \delta_{ij} e^{-q_j t} + \sum_{k \neq j} \int_0^t P_{ik}(s) q_k \pi_{kj} e^{-q_j (t-s)} ds \tag{3.4.10}$$

and

$$P_{ij}(t) = \delta_{ij} e^{-q_i t} + \sum_{k \neq i} \int_0^t q_i e^{-q_i s} \pi_{ik} P_{kj}(t-s) ds \ , \tag{3.4.11}$$

of renewal type integral equations arise, which hold for all $t \in \mathbb{T}$ and states $i, j \in \mathfrak{S}$.

For the most part, in choosing a continuous time Markov jump process as a model of some phenomenon, attention is usually focused on the forward differential equations to find the probabilities $P_{ij}(t)$. But, when modeling a phenomenon from the perspective of a semi-Markov process, attention is focused on a "backward" renewal type integral equation of form (3.4.11) to find the probabilities $P_{ij}(t)$ for $t \in \mathbb{T}$ and $i, j \in \mathfrak{S}$. To derive such renewal type integral equations, a so-called first step decomposition and renewal argument is used. To illustrate these ideas, suppose the process starts in state i at $t = 0$. Then, at time $t > 0$ the event that the process is still in state i has probability $\exp[-q_t t]$. On the other hand, if the first event is a jump at $s \in (0, t]$ with probability $q_i \exp[-q_i s]ds$, and a jump to state k with probability π_{ik}, then the process begins anew or renews and is in state j with probability $P_{kj}(t - s)$ at time t. Because these events are disjoint, an integration over $s \in (0, t]$ and a summation over $k \neq i$ leads to Eq. (3.4.11). For the sake of brevity, the intuitive statements just made are often referred to as the derivation of an integral equation by a renewal argument.

Viewing a continuous time Markov jump process from the sample path perspective also leads to a simple algorithm for computing Monte Carlo realizations of the process. To simplify the writing, an expression of the form $T \sim EXP(\beta)$ will indicate that the random variable T has an exponential distribution with positive parameter β. Suppose the process is in state i_0 at time $t = 0$. Then, the first step in the evolution of the process may be represented by the pair (i_0, t_{i_0}), where the sojourn time t_{i_0} in state i_0 is a realization of the random variable $T \sim EXP(q_{i_0})$. Given that a jump occurs, the next state i_1 visited by the process is a realization of a sample of size one from a multinomial distribution with probabilities $\{\pi_{i_0,j} \mid j \neq i_0\}$ and the sojourn time in this state t_{i_1} is a realization of the random variable $T \sim EXP(q_{i_1})$. By continuing in this way, a realization of the process up to the time of the $(n + 1)$st jump may be represented by the collection of pairs,

$$\{(i_0, t_{i_0}), (i_1, t_{i_1}), \cdots, (i_n, t_{i_n})\} \ , \tag{3.4.12}$$

which may also be called a sample path. By repeating this process $m \geq 1$ times, a statistical analysis could be performed on a sample realization to provide some insights into the behavior of the process.

Depending on the objectives of the simulation study, the experiments could proceed in at least two ways. If, for example, one was interested in studying the time taken for the process to undergo $n + 1$ jumps, then computing realizations of the process as just described would be appropriate. On the other hand, if one were interested in studying the evolution of the process during some fixed time interval $(0, t]$, $t > 0$, then a jump would be counted only if a cumulative sum of sojourn times in states were in this interval. For example, the $(n+1)$st jump would be counted only if

$$t_{i_0} + t_{i_1} + \cdots + t_{i_n} \leq t \,. \tag{3.4.13}$$

Observe that for t fixed, the number of jumps the process makes during time interval $(0, t]$ would be a random variable.

3.5 Non-Stationary Markov Processes

It is easy to conceive of situations in which the laws of evolution of a stochastic process chosen to model some phenomenon may not be time homogeneous. An example of this kind of situation in HIV/AIDS epidemiology occurs when patients are administered drugs to control HIV. During the course of treatment, new and improved drugs may be developed, which affect the rates of progression from infection with HIV to full-blown AIDS. Under such circumstances, one would expect that any stochastic process chosen to model the progression of patients through the various stages of HIV disease would not have time homogeneous laws of evolution. If the model were formulated as a continuous time Markov jump process, then the transition probabilities would not be stationary, and thus the structure discussed in the foregoing sections would not be applicable. When a transition probability $P_{ij}(s,t)$, defined for $s \leq t$, of a continuous time Markov process does not depend only on the difference $t-s$, then the process becomes more complicated mathematically.

Just as for processes with stationary transition probabilities, it is possible to derive the forward and backward Kolmogorov differential equations under certain assumptions. As before, it will be assumed that the state space $\mathfrak{S}$ of the process is finite and the transition probabilities satisfy the condition $P_{ij}(t,t) = \delta_{ij}$ for all $t \in \mathbb{T}$. It will also be supposed that for every $i \in \mathfrak{S}$, there is a continuous non-negative function $q_i(t)$ defined for all $t > 0$, such that:

$$\lim_{h \downarrow 0} \frac{1 - P_{ii}(t-h,t)}{h} = \lim_{h \downarrow 0} \frac{1 - P_{ii}(t,t+h)}{h} = q_i(t) \,. \tag{3.5.1}$$

Observe that the first limit is "backwards" in time, but the second is "forwards" in time. It will also be assumed that to every pair of states

i and j in $\mathfrak{S}$, $i \neq j$, there are continuous functions $\pi_{ij}(t)$ on $t \in \mathbb{T}$ such that $0 \leq \pi_{ij}(t) \leq 1$,

$$\lim_{h\downarrow 0} \frac{P_{ij}(t-h,t)}{h} = \lim_{h\downarrow 0} \frac{P_{ij}(t,t+h)}{h} = q_i(t)\pi_{ij}(t) \ , \tag{3.5.2}$$

and

$$\sum_{j\neq i} \pi_{ij}(t) = 1 \tag{3.5.3}$$

for all $t > 0$.

As a first step in deriving the forward differential equations, observe that for $s \leq t$ and $h > 0$ the Chapman-Kolmogorov equation may be represented in the form,

$$P_{ij}(s,t+h) = P_{ij}(s,t)P_{jj}(t+h) + \sum_{k\neq j} P_{ik}(s,t)P_{kj}(t+h) \ . \tag{3.5.4}$$

Similarly, if one looks backwards in time, this equation takes the form:

$$P_{ij}(s-h,t) = P_{ii}(s-h,s)P_{ij}(s,t) + \sum_{k\neq i} P_{ik}(s-h,s)P_{kj}(s,t) \ . \tag{3.5.5}$$

For h small, Eq. (3.5.1) implies $P_{jj}(t,t+h) = 1 - q_j(t)h + o(h)$ and $P_{ii}(s-h,s) = 1 - q_i(s)h + o(h)$, where $o(h)/h \to 0$ as $h \downarrow 0$. Upon substituting these equations into Eqs. (3.5.4) and (3.5.5), it can be seen that:

$$\begin{aligned}\frac{P_{ij}(s,t+h) - P_{ij}(s,t)}{h} &= -q_j(t)P_{ij}(s,t) \\ &\quad + \sum_{k\neq j} P_{ik}(s,t)\frac{P_{kj}(t,t+h)}{h} + \frac{o(h)}{h}\end{aligned} \tag{3.5.6}$$

and

$$\begin{aligned}\frac{P_{ij}(s-h,t) - P_{ij}(s,t)}{h} &= -q_i(s)P_{ij}(s,t) \\ &\quad + \sum_{k\neq i} \frac{P_{ik}(s-h,s)}{h}P_{kj}(s,t) + \frac{o(h)}{h} \ .\end{aligned} \tag{3.5.7}$$

Then, by letting $h \downarrow 0$ and using Eq. (3.5.2), it follows from these equations that the forward differential equations take the form

$$\frac{\partial P_{ij}(s,t)}{\partial t} = -q_j(t)P_{ij}(s,t) + \sum_{k \neq j} P_{ik}(s,t)q_k(t)\pi_{kj}(t) \ ; \tag{3.5.8}$$

while the backward differential equations have the form

$$\frac{\partial P_{ij}(s,t)}{\partial s} = q_i(s)P_{ij}(s,t) - \sum_{k \neq i} q_i(s)\pi_{ik}(s)P_{kj}(s,t) \ , \tag{3.5.9}$$

for all pairs of states $i, j \in \mathfrak{S}$. It will be noted that the signs on the right in Eq. (3.5.8) and Eq. (3.5.9) differ because as $h \downarrow 0$, the limit of the ratio on the left in Eq. (3.5.7) is $-\partial P(s,t)/\partial s$. The assumption that the state space $\mathfrak{S}$ is finite has been tacitly used throughout these derivations through free interchange of the operations of summation and limits. But, if it had been assumed that the state space was infinite, then these operations could not have been interchanged with impunity and the derivation of the Kolmogorov differential equations would have been much more complicated (see Feller[7] and other authors, who have extensively studied the case where the state space is infinite).

Gikhman and Skorokhod,[8] among other authors, have shown that for a Markov jump process $X(t)$, $t \in \mathbb{T}$, whose underlying probability measure $\mathbb{P}$ is determined by a transition function $P_{ij}(s,t)$ with the above properties, the conditional probability that $X(\tau) = i$ for all $\tau \in (s,t]$, given that $X(s) = i$, has the form,

$$\mathbb{P}\left[X(\tau) = i \text{ for all } \tau \in (s,t] \mid X(s) = i\right] = \exp\left[-\int_s^t q_i(\tau)d\tau\right] . \tag{3.5.10}$$

This result reminds one of a survival function determined by a risk function $q_i(\tau)$ as discussed in Chapter 2, Section 2.1. Indeed, one may interpret $q_i(t)$ for $t > 0$, as the risk function for the distribution of a sojourn time in state $i \in \mathfrak{S}$. Moreover, once entered, the process will eventually leave state i with probability one if, and only if, for every $s \in \mathbb{T}$:

$$\lim_{t \uparrow \infty} \int_s^t q_i(\tau)d\tau = \infty \tag{3.5.11}$$

so that the conditional probability in Eq. (3.5.10) converges to 0 as $t \uparrow \infty$ for all $s \in \mathbb{T}$. Henceforth, it will be assumed that condition Eq. (3.5.11) is satisfied for all $i \in \mathfrak{S}$ unless stated otherwise for a particular state.

Just as in the derivation of integral Eqs. (3.4.10) and (3.4.11), if one introduces integrating factors of the form,

$$\exp\left[\int_s^t q_i(\tau)d\tau\right] \tag{3.5.12}$$

and uses the boundary condition $P_{ij}(t,t) = \delta_{ij}$ for all $t \in \mathbb{T}$, it can be shown that the forward differential equations are equivalent to the integral equations,

$$P_{ij}(s,t) = \delta_{ij}\exp\left[-\int_s^t q_j(\tau)d\tau\right]$$

$$+\sum_{k\neq j}\int_s^t P_{ik}(s,\tau)q_k(\tau)\pi_{kj}(\tau)\exp\left[-\int_\tau^t q_j(\eta)d\eta\right]d\tau\ ; \tag{3.5.13}$$

while the integral equations corresponding to the backward equations have the form,

$$P_{ij}(s,t) = \delta_{ij}\exp\left[-\int_s^t q_i(\tau)d\tau\right]$$

$$+\sum_{k\neq i}\int_s^t q_i(\tau)\exp\left[-\int_s^\tau q_i(\eta)d\eta\right]\pi_{ik}(\tau)P_{kj}(\tau,t)d\tau\ . \tag{3.5.14}$$

As they should, when the q's and π's are constants, all transition probabilities $P_{ij}(s,t)$ depend only on $t-s$, and $s=0$, these integral equations reduce to Eqs. (3.4.10) and (3.4.11).

Though the forward differential equations are most frequently the focus of attention when a Markov jump process is chosen as a model for some phenomenon, the backward differential equations and their equivalent integral equation representation in Eq. (3.5.14) are, in many ways, the easiest with which to work. Among other things, these equations suggest avenues of generalization and emphasize the step-like nature of the process when attention is focused on the sample paths. To illustrate these notions and to lighten the notation, define a one-step transition density by:

$$a_{ij}(s,t) = q_i(t) \exp\left[-\int_s^t q_i(\eta)d\eta\right] \pi_{ik}(t) \tag{3.5.15}$$

for a transition from state i at time s to state j at time t, $s \leq t$. Then, Eq. (3.5.14) may be written in the more compact form,

$$P_{ij}(s,t) = \delta_{ij} \exp\left[-\int_s^t q_i(\tau)d\tau\right] + \sum_{k\neq i}\int_s^t a_{ik}(s,\tau)P_{kj}(\tau,t)d\tau \ . \tag{3.5.16}$$

To emphasize the jump or step-like nature of the process, let

$$P_{ij}^{(0)}(s,t) = \delta_{ij} \exp\left[-\int_s^t q_i(\tau)d\tau\right] \tag{3.5.17}$$

and define $P_{ij}^{(n)}(s,t)$ as the conditional probability that at time s the process is in state i, and at time $t > s$ it is in state j after $n \geq 1$ jumps have occurred. Then, for $n \geq 1$, these probabilities may be determined recursively by:

$$P_{ij}^{(n)}(s,t) = \sum_{k\neq i}\int_s^t a_{ik}(s,\tau)P_{kj}^{(n-1)}(\tau,t)d\tau \ . \tag{3.5.18}$$

It then follow that

$$P_{ij}(s,t) = \sum_{n=0}^{\infty} P_{ij}^{(n)}(s,t) \tag{3.5.19}$$

is the conditional probability that if the process is in state i at time s, it is state j at time $t > s$ after finitely many jumps. By summing over $n = 1, 2, \cdots$, and adding Eq. (3.5.17) to each side of the resulting equation, it can be seen that the series defined by Eq. (3.5.19) is a solution of integral Eq. (3.5.16). Moreover, if it is required that $P_{ij}^{(n)}(t,t) = 0$ for all $n \geq 1$, i, j, and $t \in \mathbb{T}$, then the probabilities in Eq. (3.5.19) satisfy the condition $P_{ij}(t,t) = \delta_{ij}$ for all states i and j. With regard to mathematical rigor, it may be mentioned in passing that showing

Eq. (3.5.19) is a solution of Eq. (3.5.16) involves an interchange of integration and summation in Eq. (3.5.18). Because all the terms in this series are non-negative, this interchange may be justified by appealing to the monotone convergence theorem.

The procedure just described can, in principle, be used to construct solutions of the forward and backward Kolmogorov differential equations such that the condition,

$$\sum_{j \in \mathfrak{S}} P_{ij}(s,t) = 1 \tag{3.5.20}$$

for all $i \in \mathfrak{S}$, $s, t \in \mathbb{T}$, with $s \leq t$, and the Chapman-Kolmogorov equations are satisfied, but no further details will be pursued here (see Feller[7] and other authors for details). For models with a small number of states, the method of finding solutions to the Kolmogorov differential equations just described may actually be an interesting and practical way of computing numerical solutions of these equations on powerful and user-friendly desktop computers, particularly if the probabilities $P_{ij}^{(n)}(s,t)$ are of some interest for chosen values of $n \geq 1$.

Even though for some models, it may be very difficult to find solutions of the Kolmogorov differential equations, it will, nevertheless, be useful to simulate realizations of the sample paths of a Markov jump process with time inhomogeneous laws of evolution. Suppose, for example, that for every $t > 0$ and state $i \in \mathfrak{S}$, a risk function $q_i(t)$ and the conditional jump probabilities $\pi_{ij}(t)$, $i \neq j$, have been specified. Then, if the process starts in state i_0 at time $t = 0$, the time t_{i_0} spent in this state is a realization of a random variable T_{i_0} with distribution function,

$$F_{i_0}(t) = 1 - \exp\left[-\int_0^t q_{i_0}(\tau)d\tau\right], \quad t > 0\,. \tag{3.5.21}$$

And, i_1, the next state visited by the process, is a sample of size one from a multinomial distribution with the probability vector

$$\{\pi_{i_0,j}(t_{i_0}) \mid j \neq i_0\}\ . \tag{3.5.22}$$

Then the time t_{i_1} spent in state i_1 is a realization of a random variable

T_{i_1} with distribution function,

$$F_{i_1}(t_{i_0}, t) = 1 - \exp\left[\int_{t_{i_0}}^{t} q_{i_1}(\tau)d\tau\right], \quad t > 0\ . \tag{3.5.23}$$

Similarly, the next state i_2 visited by the process is a sample of size one from a multinomial distribution with the probability vector

$$\{\pi_{i_1,j}(t_{i_1}) \mid j \neq i_1\} \tag{3.5.24}$$

and so the simulation continues.

3.6 Models for the Evolution of HIV Disease

Having outlined the theory of Markov jump processes with finite state spaces and either time homogeneous or inhomogeneous laws of evolution, it is appropriate to pause and give some concrete examples of applications of these processes as models for the evolution of HIV disease in cohorts of infected persons. Let $\mathcal{S} = \{E_i \mid i = 1, 2, \cdots, 6\}$ be the six stages of HIV disease as designated by the Walter Reed system and defined in Table 2.9.1 by disjoint intervals of $CD4^+$ counts. Unlike the simpler models discussed in Chapter 2, evolution among these stages may not be linear. That is, because $CD4^+$ cell counts may fluctuate in time, a patient observed at time t_1 in stage E_i may be in either stage E_{i-1} or E_{i+1} at some time $t_2 > t_1$. If one also wishes to consider those cases in which a patient would be diagnosed with full-blown AIDS, then it would be useful to append a state E_7 to the set $\mathcal{S}$, indicating that a patient has developed one or more AIDS-defining diseases. Over time, the symptoms defining AIDS have been changed officially by the United States Centers for Disease Control so that at the clinical level a one-step transition of the form, $E_i \to E_7$, corresponding to a diagnosis of AIDS, may occur for a person last observed in state E_i for some indcx $i > 1$. As will be demonstrated in the examples that follow, the possibility of such transition, as well as other types of transitions, can easily be accommodated by choosing forms of the intensity matrix $\mathbf{Q}$, when the model is formulated as a Markov jump process with time homogeneous laws of evolution.

Example 3.6.1. A Model for the Incubation Period of HIV.

Suppose a continuous time Markov jump process with time homogeneous laws of evolution and a state space $\mathfrak{S} = \{E_7\} \cup \mathcal{S}$ consisting of seven states is considered. Since attention is being focused on the incubation period, the process terminates at first entrance into state E_7, signalling a patient has reached a state of full-blown AIDS. A mathematical device for stopping a process is to introduce the idea of an absorbing state when considering a state space. A state will be called absorbing if, after entering this state, the process remains there with probability one, or equivalently, transitions out of this state have probability zero. Thus, to make a state absorbing, it suffices to assign a zero to all the elements in the row of the matrix $\mathbf{Q}$ corresponding to transitions from this state. By convention, to conform to a more general treatment of jump processes to be outlined in subsequent sections of this chapter, the set of absorbing states will be listed first, followed by a set of transient states among which the process may move prior to termination in an absorbing state. In this example, the states will therefore be ordered as:

$$\mathfrak{S} = \{E_7, E_1, E_2, \cdots, E_6\} \tag{3.6.1}$$

so that $\mathfrak{S}_1 = \{E_7\}$ is a set of one absorbing state, and the set of transient states is $\mathfrak{S}_2 = \{E_i \mid i = 1, 2, \cdots, 6\} = \mathcal{S}$. From now on, to comply with this ordering and to simplify the notation, let the symbol $i = 1$ stand for the absorbing state E_7 and the symbols $i = 2, 3, \cdots, 7$, stand for the transient states in the set $\mathfrak{S}_2$.

For this state space, the 7×7 intensity matrix may be represented in the partitioned form,

$$\mathbf{Q} = \begin{bmatrix} 0 & \mathbf{0}_{12} \\ \mathbf{Q}_{21} & \mathbf{Q}_{22} \end{bmatrix} . \tag{3.6.2}$$

In this matrix, $\mathbf{0}_{12}$ is a 1×6 matrix of zeros, indicating transitions from state E_7 do not occur, $\mathbf{Q}_{21}$ is a 6×1 matrix governing transitions from the set of transient states $\mathfrak{S}_2$ into the absorbing state, and $\mathbf{Q}_{22}$ is a 6×6 matrix governing transitions among transient states prior to termination of the process. The forms of these sub-matrices depend on the assumptions made about transitions among states. For example, if it is assumed that transitions to full-blown AIDS can occur only from the last three intervals of CD4$^+$ counts, then the 6×1 matrix $\mathbf{Q}_{21}$ takes the form,

$$\mathbf{Q}_{21} = \begin{bmatrix} 0 \\ 0 \\ 0 \\ q_{51} \\ q_{61} \\ q_{71} \end{bmatrix} . \tag{3.6.3}$$

Similarly, the form of the 6×6 matrix governing transitions among transient states may be chosen as:

$$\mathbf{Q}_{22} = \begin{bmatrix} -q_2 & q_{23} & 0 & 0 & 0 & 0 \\ q_{32} & -q_3 & q_{34} & 0 & 0 & 0 \\ 0 & q_{43} & -q_4 & q_{45} & 0 & 0 \\ 0 & 0 & q_{54} & -q_5 & q_{56} & 0 \\ 0 & 0 & 0 & q_{65} & -q_6 & q_{67} \\ 0 & 0 & 0 & 0 & q_{76} & -q_7 \end{bmatrix} . \tag{3.6.4}$$

Observe that the positions of positive off-diagonal elements in this matrix conform to the assumption that for $i = 3, 4, 5$, only transitions of the form $i \to i-1$ or $i \to i+1$ are possible among transient states; whereas, for states $i = 2$ or 7, the only possible transitions to another transient state have, respectively, the forms $2 \to 3$ and $7 \to 6$. It will also be recalled that for $i = 2, 3, \cdots, 7$, the elements on the principal diagonal of this matrix are defined by:

$$q_i = \sum_{j \neq i} q_{ij} , \tag{3.6.5}$$

in compliance with the general treatment of Markov jump processes with time homogeneous laws of evolution.

Given the 7×7 intensity matrix $\mathbf{Q}$, if one is interested in the matrix $\mathbf{P}(t)$ of transition probabilities, then numerical values of these functions may, in principle, be found by evaluating the exponential matrix,

$$\mathbf{P}(t) = \exp\left[\mathbf{Q}t\right] \text{ for } t \in \mathbb{T} . \tag{3.6.6}$$

As explained in a foregoing section, a capability for computing values of the exponential matrix can make it possible to find maximum likelihood estimates of the elements of the intensity matrix. But, once these estimates are available, in other applications of the theory, it is of interest to find the distribution function of the latent period of HIV disease based on a model of the type under consideration. More precisely, suppose an individual is infected with HIV at time $t = 0$ and let the random variable T_{21} represent the time the process reaches the absorbing state $i = 1$. Formally, within this framework, the distribution function of the latent period of HIV is that of the random variable T_{21}. Thus, one is led to consider the problem of finding the conditional distribution function,

$$\mathbb{P}\left[T_{21} \le t \mid X(0) = 1\right] = F_{21}(t) \text{ for } t \in \mathbb{T} \tag{3.6.7}$$

as a function of the elements of the matrix $\mathbf{Q}$. As we shall see, this problem may be approached in several ways, which will be developed in subsequent sections of this chapter.

Example 3.6.2. On Including Mortality in Models for the Evolution of HIV Disease.

As will be shown in subsequent chapters, when developing models for projecting the number of individuals with HIV disease in a population, it becomes necessary to design structures that include deaths as absorbing states. After a person has been infected with HIV, his or her death may be classified as either due to an AIDS-defining disease or due to some other cause. Accordingly, it is of interest to incorporate two absorbing states into any model formulated as a Markov jump process in continuous time. Let the symbol S_1 stand for a death not attributable to an AIDS-defining disease, and let the symbol S_2 stand for a death attributable to AIDS. Then, the set of absorbing states is $\mathfrak{S}_1 = \{S_1, S_2\}$, and the set $\mathfrak{S}_2$ of transient states will be defined as the seven states:

$$\mathfrak{S}_2 = \{S_i \mid i = 3, 4, \cdots, 9\} , \tag{3.6.8}$$

where the symbols S_i, $i = 3, 4, \cdots, 8$, represent the six stages of HIV described above and the symbol S_9 stands for a person with full-blown AIDS.

For the state space $\mathfrak{S} = \mathfrak{S}_1 \cup \mathfrak{S}_2$, the 9×9 intensity matrix may be represented in the partitioned form:

$$\mathbf{Q} = \begin{bmatrix} \mathbf{0}_{11} & \mathbf{0}_{12} \\ \mathbf{Q}_{21} & \mathbf{Q}_{22} \end{bmatrix} . \tag{3.6.9}$$

In this matrix, $\mathbf{0}_{11}$ is a 2×2 matrix of zeros, $\mathbf{0}_{12}$ is a 2×7 matrix of zeros, $\mathbf{Q}_{21}$ is a 7×2 governing transitions from transient states to absorbing states, and $\mathbf{Q}_{22}$ is a 7×7 matrix governing transitions among transient states. If it is assumed that deaths due to AIDS will be classified as such only for persons in state S_9, then the 7×2 matrix $\mathbf{Q}_{21}$ would take the form,

$$\mathbf{Q}_{21} = \begin{bmatrix} q_{31} & 0 \\ q_{41} & 0 \\ q_{51} & 0 \\ q_{61} & 0 \\ q_{71} & 0 \\ q_{81} & 0 \\ q_{91} & q_{92} \end{bmatrix} . \tag{3.6.10}$$

When all the q's in the first column of this matrix are positive, then a person in any of the transient states in $\mathfrak{S}_2$ may die due to causes other than AIDS. Moreover, when the q's in the last row of this matrix are positive, then a person with AIDS may die from causes other than AIDS. The structure of the 7×7 matrix $\mathbf{Q}_{22}$ in Eq. (3.6.9) will be similar to that in Eq. (3.6.4), but a detailed enumeration of this matrix will be left as an exercise for the reader.

Just as for the model of the incubation period of HIV, the conditional distribution functions of the waiting time for termination of the process in some absorbing state are of interest. Given that the process starts in state 3 at $t = 0$, let the random variable T_{3j}, $j = 1, 2$, be the waiting time to absorption in state j. Then, the conditional distribution function of the random variable T_{3j} is defined by:

$$\mathbb{P}\left[T_{3j} \le t \mid X(0) = 3\right] = F_{3j}(t) \text{ for } t \in \mathbb{T} . \tag{3.6.11}$$

Unlike the simpler model for the incubation period of HIV, in this case a need arises for calculating two distribution functions determined by the 9×9 matrix $\mathbf{Q}$. In a subsequent section of this chapter, general methods for calculating such functions will be developed.

Example 3.6.3. Processes with Time Inhomogeneous Laws of Evolution.

To formulate either of the models just discussed as Markov jump processes with time inhomogeneous laws of evolution, it would be assumed that all elements in the intensity matrix $\mathbf{Q}(t)$ were continuous functions of $t \in \mathbb{T}$. Choosing explicit forms of the elements of the intensity matrix is not always a straightforward task. To overcome these difficulties, several authors have partitioned the set of time points $\mathbb{T} = [0, \infty)$ into disjoint intervals $[t_{u-1}, t_u)$, where $u = 1, 2, 3, \cdots$, and $0 = t_0 < t_1 < t_2 < \cdots$, and then assumed that there are constant matrices $\mathbf{Q}_u$ such that $\mathbf{Q}(t) = \mathbf{Q}_u$ for all $t \in [t_{u-1}, t_u)$. Under this assumption, the matrix $\mathbf{P}(t) = (P_{ij}(t))$ of transition probabilities may be represented in terms of the exponential matrix by using the Chapman-Kolmogorov equation repeatedly. For processes with time inhomogeneous laws of evolution for any time points $s < v < t$, the matrix form of this equation is:

$$\mathbf{P}(s,t) = \mathbf{P}(s,v)\mathbf{P}(v,t) \ . \tag{3.6.12}$$

Now suppose the interval $[t_{u-1}, t_u)$ is partitioned into n subintervals $[s_{k-1}, s_k)$ determined by the points $t_{u-1} = s_0 < s_1 < \cdots < s_n = t_u$ and let $h_k = s_k - s_{k-1}$ for $k = 1, 2, \cdots, n$. Then, if the state space $\mathfrak{S}$ of the process contains $N \geq 2$ states, h_k small conditions in Eqs. (3.5.1) and (3.5.2) may be represented in the matrix form:

$$\mathbf{P}(s_{k-1}, s_k) = \mathbf{I}_N + \mathbf{Q}_u h_k + \mathbf{o}(h_k) \ , \tag{3.6.13}$$

where $\mathbf{o}(h_k)/h_k \to \mathbf{0}$, a zero matrix as $h_k \downarrow 0$. It will supposed that $\max_k h_k \to 0$ as $n \to \infty$. But, by applying Eq. (3.6.12) repeatedly, it then can be shown that:

$$\mathbf{P}(t_{u-1}, t_u) = \lim_{n \to \infty} \prod_{k=1}^{n} \mathbf{P}(s_{k-1}, s_k)$$

$$= \lim_{n\to\infty} \prod_{k-1}^{n} [\mathbf{I}_n + \mathbf{Q}_u h_k + \mathrm{o}(h_k)]$$

$$= \exp[\mathbf{Q}_u(t_u - t_{u-1})] \ . \tag{3.6.14}$$

Tan[15] used these kind of ideas to develop models of the incubation period for HIV under treatment, and the references cited in this paper may be consulted for the technical details underlying this derivation.

Models of this type have also been used extensively in multidimensional mathematical demography (see Hoem and Jensen[10] as well as other papers in this conference volume). Although algorithms for computing values of the exponential matrix have been implemented in many software packages, finding estimates of the intensity matrix $\mathbf{Q}_u$ for selected time intervals can be problematic even if this matrix is of moderate size. For large but finite intensity matrices, however, specifying values of this matrix and computing values of the exponential matrix can become unwieldy. A question that arises, therefore, is whether it is possible to find alternative methods for the numerical analysis of models formulated as Markov jump processes with time inhomogeneous laws of evolution. In a subsequent section of this chapter, questions of this type will be addressed.

3.7 Time Homogeneous Semi-Markov Processes

Historically, Markov jump processes evolved by focusing attention on the transition functions $P_{ij}(s,t)$ for points $0 \le s \le t$ in $\mathbb{T}$, and letting these functions determine a probability measure $\mathbb{P}$ underlying the process as outlined in the preceding sections. An alternative approach is to focus attention on the sample paths of the process, and then construct a probability measure $\mathbb{P}$ underlying the process by making assumptions about the joint distribution of the random variables whose realizations constitute the sample paths. For example, consider a jump process with finite state space $\mathfrak{S}$ and let the random variables X_n, $n = 0, 1, 2, \cdots$ represent the state in $\mathfrak{S}$ entered at the nth jump. If $X_n = i_n \in \mathfrak{S}$, then let the random variable T_n be the sojourn time or length of stay in state i_n, and let $T_n = t_{i_n} \in \mathbb{T}$ be a realization of this random variable.

A sample path consisting of $n \geq 1$ jumps may be represented as the set of ordered pairs $\{(i_k, t_{i_k}) \mid k = 0, 1, 2, \cdots, n\}$. By constructing the joint distribution of these sample paths for all $n \geq 1$, it is possible to construct a probability measure $\mathbb{P}$ underlying the process. Unlike Markov jump processes with time homogeneous laws of evolution, in which the sojourn times in states necessarily follow an exponential distribution, it becomes possible to construct the measure $\mathbb{P}$ such that these times have arbitrary distributions. Such processes have become known as semi-Markov processes and the purpose of this section is to outline some basic principles underlying this class of processes for the case of time homogeneous laws of evolution.

To formulate models within this class of stochastic processes, one needs to specify a state space $\mathfrak{S}$ with $r \geq 2$ elements and a $r \times r$ matrix $\mathbf{a}(t) = (a_{ij}(t))$ of continuous non-negative transition densities. Furthermore, suppose the state space $\mathfrak{S}$ may be partitioned into two disjoint sets $\mathfrak{S}_1$ and $\mathfrak{S}_2$, where $\mathfrak{S}_1$ is a set of $r_1 \geq 1$ absorbing states and $\mathfrak{S}_2$ is a set of $r_2 \geq 1$ non-absorbing or transient states. Once the process reaches an absorbing state, no transition out of this state is possible. Thus, for every $i \in \mathfrak{S}_1$, $a_{ij}(t) = 0$ for all $j \in \mathfrak{S}$ and $t \geq 0$. In a continuous time formulation, only transitions out of a state are taken into account; hence, $a_{ii}(t) = 0$ for all $i \in \mathfrak{S}$ and $t \geq 0$.

Once the density matrix $\mathbf{a}(t)$ is chosen, the construction of the probability measure $\mathbb{P}$ underlying the process may proceed as follows. With a view towards defining conditional probabilities, let the symbol $\mathfrak{B}(n-1)$ stand for any set of realizations of the sample path random variables prior to the nth jump. Then, the fundamental assumption underlying a semi-Markov process with stationary transition probabilities may be expressed as:

$$\mathbb{P}\left[X_n = j, T_{n-1} \leq t \mid \mathfrak{B}(n-1)\right]$$

$$= \mathbb{P}\left[X_n = j, T_{n-1} \leq t \mid X_{n-1} = i\right] = \int_0^t a_{ij}(s)ds \qquad (3.7.1)$$

for all $n \geq 1$ and $t \in \mathbb{T}$. It will be noted that in this formulation, the future probabilistic evolution of the process depends not only on the state $i \in \mathfrak{S}$ last visited, but that the time to the next state $j \neq i$ visited by the process also depends on i. Unlike continuous time Markov jump processes, this is an assumption about the evolution of the sample paths rather than an assumption about the probabilities the process is in for a specified set of states at fixed points in time (see Eq. (3.2.2)). From Eq. (3.7.1) it follows that, given $X_0 = i_0$, the finite dimensional distributions of the process are determined by the joint conditional densities,

$$f_n(i_k, t_{k-1},\ 1 \leq k \leq n \mid X_0 = i_0)$$

$$= \prod_{k=1}^{n} a_{i_{k-1},i_k}(t_{k-1}) \tag{3.7.2}$$

of the collection of random variables $\{X_k, T_{k-1} \mid k = 1, 2, \cdots, n\}$, which hold for all integers $n \geq 1$, the states $i_0, i_1, \cdots, i_n$ in $\mathfrak{S}$ and the points $t_0, t_1, \cdots, t_{n-1}$ in $\mathbb{T}$.

Just as for Markov jump processes, the conceptual picture underlying this class of processes is a simple one. By way of illustration, suppose the process starts in some transient state $i \in \mathfrak{S}_2$ at $t = 0$. After a random length of time, it jumps to state j. If j is an absorbing state, the process terminates; but, if j is another transient state, then it remains there for a random length of time until the next jump and so the process continues until some absorbing state is reached. Due to stationarity assumptions, i.e., the assumption of time homogeneous laws of evolution, once the process enters some transient state, a probabilistic renewal occurs and the laws of evolution henceforth are as if this state were the initial one.

To every semi-Markov process in this class, there corresponds an absorbing Markov chain with a $r \times r$ matrix $\mathbf{P} = (p_{ij})$ of transition probabilities determined as follows. If the process is in some transient state $i \in \mathfrak{S}_2$ at $t = 0$, then the conditional probability of a jump to state j by time $t > 0$ is given by:

$$A_{ij}(t) = \int_0^t a_{ij}(s)ds\ . \tag{3.7.3}$$

The distribution function of the sojourn time in state i is given by

$$A_i(t) = \sum_j A_{ij}(t) \tag{3.7.4}$$

for $j \in \mathfrak{S}$. If i and j are not equal, then the conditional probability of an eventual jump to j is

$$p_{ij} = \lim_{t \to \infty} A_{ij}(t) \ . \tag{3.7.5}$$

But if $i = j$, then the process is still in state i at time $t > 0$, with probability $1 - A_i(t)$. Hence, the probability of never leaving state i is:

$$p_{ii} = \lim_{t \to \infty} (1 - A_i(t)) \ . \tag{3.7.6}$$

For all the models under consideration, if i is a transient state, then $p_{ii} = 0$; but if i is an absorbing state, then $p_{ii} = 1$. For ease of reference, let $Z(t)$ be a random function representing the state of the semi-Markov process at $t \geq 0$.

Thanks to the pioneering work of Kemeny and Snell[12] much is known about absorbing Markov chains with a finite state space; moreover, the results are expressed in a form amenable to computer implementation. To facilitate the analysis and computer implementation of this class of discrete time stochastic processes, these authors arranged the $r \times r$ matrix $\mathbf{P}$ in the partitioned form:

$$\mathbf{P} = \begin{bmatrix} \mathbf{I} & \mathbf{0} \\ \mathbf{R} & \mathbf{Q} \end{bmatrix} , \tag{3.7.7}$$

where $\mathbf{I}$ is a $r_1 \times r_1$ identity matrix corresponding to the absorbing states; $\mathbf{R}$ is a $r_2 \times r_1$ matrix governing transitions from transient to absorbing states; and $\mathbf{Q}$ is a $r_2 \times r_2$ matrix governing transitions among transient states.

A random function for absorbing semi-Markov processes that is of interest is $N_j(t)$, the number of entrances into transient state j during the time interval $[0, t]$, for $t > 0$, prior to the time the process terminates in some absorbing state. To gain insight into the random function $N_j(t)$, it will be useful to represent it in terms of indicator functions. Let $\delta_j(n, t) = 1$ if transient state j is entered at some point during the time interval $[0, t]$, and let $\delta_j(n, t) = 0$ otherwise. If i is the initial transient state at $t = 0$, then, because the state at $t = 0$ is counted in $N_j(t)$, it follows that:

$$N_j(t) = \delta_{ij} + \sum_{n=1}^{\infty} \delta_j(n,t) \ , \tag{3.7.8}$$

where δ_{ij} is the Kronecker delta. Conditional expectations of this random function may be computed in terms of matrix convolutions of the functions in the $r_2 \times r_2$ density matrix $\mathbf{Q}(t) = (a_{ij}(t))$, corresponding to the transient states.

For all i and j in $\mathfrak{S}_2$, let $a_{ij}^{(1)}(t) = a_{ij}(t)$ and define the sequence $(a_{ij}^{(n)}(t))$ recursively by:

$$a_{ij}^{(n)}(t) = \sum_{\nu \in \mathfrak{S}_2} \int_0^t a_{i\nu}(s) a_{\nu j}^{(n-1)}(t-s) ds \tag{3.7.9}$$

for $n \geq 2$. Now let

$$A_{ij}^{(n)}(t) = \int_0^t a_{ij}^{(n)}(s) ds \ . \tag{3.7.10}$$

Then, because

$$E\left[\delta_j(n,t) \mid Z(0) = i\right] = A_{ij}^{(n)}(t) \ , \tag{3.7.11}$$

it follows that

$$m_{ij}(t) = E\left[N_j(t) \mid Z(0) = i\right] = \delta_{ij} + \sum_{n=1}^{\infty} A_{ij}^{(n)}(t) \tag{3.7.12}$$

for $t \geq 0$.

With probability one, the random step function $N_j(t)$ is nondecreasing in t by construction. Therefore, the limit $N_j = \lim_{t\to\infty} N_j(t)$, finite or infinite, exists with probability one when $Z(0) = i$ for any $i \in \mathfrak{S}_2$. To show that under rather general conditions the random variable N_j is finite with probability one, whenever the process starts in some transient state, it will be useful to define a $r_2 \times r_2$ matrix $\mathbf{Q}^{(n)}(t) = (A_{ij}^{(n)}(t))$, where i and j are transient states in $\mathfrak{S}_2$. Then, from well-known properties of matrix convolutions, it may be shown that:

$$\lim_{t\to\infty} \mathbf{Q}^{(n)}(t) = \mathbf{Q}^n \ , \tag{3.7.13}$$

the nth power of the matrix $\mathbf{Q}$ for $n \geq 1$. By applying the monotone convergence theorem, it also follows that:

$$m_{ij} = E\left[N_j \mid Z(0) = i\right] = \lim_{t \to \infty} E\left[N_j(t) \mid Z(0) = i\right] . \tag{3.7.14}$$

Moreover, the random variable N_j will be finite with probability one, when i is the initial state, if the conditional expectation m_{ij} is finite. Let $\mathbf{M} = (m_{ij})$ be a $r_2 \times r_2$ matrix of these conditional expectations and let $\mathbf{I}$ be a $r_2 \times r_2$ identity matrix. Then, by letting $t \to \infty$ in Eq. (3.7.12), it follows that:

$$\mathbf{M} = \mathbf{I} + \mathbf{Q} + \mathbf{Q}^2 + \cdots . \tag{3.7.15}$$

If $\mathbf{Q}^n \to 0$, a zero matrix, as $n \to \infty$, the matrix series converges to the matrix inverse $(\mathbf{I} - \mathbf{Q})^{-1}$, so that:

$$\mathbf{M} = (\mathbf{I} - \mathbf{Q})^{-1} . \tag{3.7.16}$$

For state spaces of moderate size, this inverse matrix may be computed with relative ease on many computer platforms. A sufficient condition for the matrix $\mathbf{Q}^n$ to converge to the zero matrix may be given in terms of a matrix norm:

$$\|\mathbf{A}\| = \max_i \sum_j |a_{ij}| , \tag{3.7.17}$$

defined for any rectangular matrix $\mathbf{A} = (a_{ij})$. If for some $m \geq 1$, $\|\mathbf{Q}^m\| < 1$, a condition that is often easy to check, then it can be shown that the matrix series in Eq. (3.7.15) converges.

When using the structure under consideration in the formulation of a model, attention focuses on constructing the transition densities rather than on solving the Kolmogorov differential equations as was the case for Markov jump processes. Accordingly, in applications of the general theory just outlined, it is desirable to express the functions of the density matrix $\mathbf{a}(t)$ in parametric form. A useful way of accomplishing this parameterization is to apply the classical theory of competing risks (see Mode[14] for a review of the literature). To apply this theory to semi-Markov processes, each pair of states i and j has associated with it a non-negative and continuous latent risk function $\theta_{ij}(t)$, governing transitions from state i to state j in the absence of other competing risks. The total risk function governing transitions out of state i is:

$$\theta_i(t) = \sum_{j \neq i} \theta_{ij}(t) \tag{3.7.18}$$

so that the survival function for state i is:

$$S_i(t) = \exp\left[-\int_0^t \theta_i(s)ds\right] . \tag{3.7.19}$$

Thus, when the classical theory of competing risks is in force, it can be shown that the function $A_{ij}(t)$ takes the form,

$$A_{ij}(t) = \int_0^t S_i(u)\theta_{ij}(u)du . \tag{3.7.20}$$

In principle, the integrals in Eq. (3.7.20) may be evaluated numerically for many choices of the latent risk functions, provided good software packages are available on the computer platform being used. However, when all latent risk functions are assumed to be constant, these integrals take an elementary form.

When all latent risk functions are constants, i.e., $\theta_{ij}(t) = \theta_{ij}$ for all $t \in \mathbb{T}$, then all latent distributions are simple exponentials. In this case, when θ_i is not zero, the integral in Eq. (3.7.20) takes the simple form,

$$A_{ij}(t) = \frac{\theta_{ij}}{\theta_i}(1 - \exp[-\theta_i t]), \ t \in \mathbb{T} \tag{3.7.21}$$

and the corresponding density function has the form,

$$a_{ij}(t) = \theta_{ij} \exp[-\theta_i t] \tag{3.7.22}$$

for $t \in \mathbb{T}$ and $i \neq j$. By letting $t \to \infty$ in Eq. (3.7.21), it follows that for $i \neq j$, the transition probabilities of the embedded Markov chain have the form,

$$p_{ij} = \frac{\theta_{ij}}{\theta_i} \tag{3.7.23}$$

for $\theta_i > 0$. According to the theory just outlined, to parameterize a semi-Markov process under the foregoing assumptions, it suffices to specify a $r \times r$ matrix of $\mathbf{\Theta} = (\theta_{ij})$ of constant latent risk functions. As is well-known, when a semi-Markov process is constructed in this way, it is equivalent to a Markov jump process in continuous time with stationary transition probabilities.

For some models, the matrix $\mathbf{I} - \mathbf{Q}$ can be quite large, which may raise some questions as to the stability of the numerical procedures used to compute its inverse. A measure that is widely used to judge whether a non-singular square matrix $\mathbf{A}$ may be inverted with some degree of confidence as to its numerical validity is the condition number, which is defined by:

$$\kappa(\mathbf{A}) = \|\mathbf{A}\| \cdot \left\|\mathbf{A}^{-1}\right\| , \tag{3.7.24}$$

where the matrix norm $\|\cdot\|$ may be computed as in Eq. (3.7.17). A large value for the condition number indicates that the matrix is nearly singular, signalling the possibility of numerical problems.

It should be mentioned that the formula in Eq. (3.7.20), which was derived by appealing to the theory of competing risks, is merely one of several methods for constructing matrices of transition densities. An alternative approach is to specify a matrix (p_{ij}) of transition probabilities for the embedded Markov chain, and let $f_{ij}(t)$ be a conditional probability density of the time taken for the transition $i \rightarrow j$, given that the process is in state i and jumps to state $j \neq i$ eventually. Then, a transition density would have the form,

$$a_{ij}(t) = p_{ij} f_{ij}(t) \text{ for } t \in \mathbb{T} . \tag{3.7.25}$$

If $F_{ij}(t)$ is the distribution function corresponding to the *p.d.f.* $f_{ij}(t)$, then the distribution function of the sojourn time in state i is the mixture,

$$A_i(t) = \sum_{j \neq i} p_{ij} F_{ij}(t) \text{ for } t \in \mathbb{T} . \tag{3.7.26}$$

This approach can be useful when risk functions are not of a simple form such as those for the gamma and log-normal families, but in this case modelling parametric forms of the matrix (p_{ij}) of transition probabilities for the embedded Markov chain can be problematic.

One interesting approach to modelling the transition matrix (p_{ij}) is to generalize Eq. (3.7.23), which was based on the assumption that the latent distributions are simple exponentials. If a random variable has an exponential distribution with parameter $\theta_{ij} > 0$, then its expectation is $\mu_{ij} = 1/\theta_{ij}$ so that $\theta_{ij} = 1/\mu_{ij}$. With this observation in mind, it seems plausible to assume that in the absence of other competing risks, the longer the process stays in state i before a jump to state j, the smaller the probability p_{ij} of an eventual jump to state j. One is thus led to consider transition probabilities of the form,

$$p_{ij} = \frac{c_i}{\mu_{ij}} \,, \tag{3.7.27}$$

where the constant c_i is chosen such that $\sum_{j \neq i} p_{ij} = 1$. If the densities $f_{ij}(t)$ have been specified, then the expectation μ_{ij} would be determined by:

$$\mu_{ij} = \int_0^\infty t f_{ij}(t) dt \,. \tag{3.7.28}$$

Observe that, in general, these expectations will be a function of the parameters of the densities, so that it will not be necessary to introduce additional parameters to specify the matrix (p_{ij}).

An advantage of utilizing the theory of competing risks to specify the matrix of transition densities is that the transition matrix (p_{ij}) for the embedded Markov chain is completely determined by the latent risk functions, as illustrated in the following example.

Example 3.7.1. On Constructing a Density Matrix Based on Weibull Type Risk Functions.

Suppose the state space for a semi-Markov process contains three elements 1, 2, and 3, and suppose the latent risk function for the transition $1 \to 2$ is $\theta_{12}(t) = 2t$, and that for $1 \to 3$ is $\theta_{13}(t) = 3t^2$ for $t \in \mathbb{T}$. Then,

$$A_{12}(t) = 2 \int_0^t s e^{-s^2 - s^3} ds \tag{3.7.29}$$

and

$$A_{13}(t) = 3 \int_0^t s^2 e^{-s^2 - s^3} ds \tag{3.7.30}$$

for $t \in \mathbb{T}$. Therefore,

$$p_{12} = \lim_{t \uparrow \infty} A_{12}(t) = 2 \int_0^\infty s e^{-s^2 - s^3} ds = 0.52719 \tag{3.7.31}$$

and

$$p_{13} = \lim_{t \uparrow \infty} A_{13}(t) = 3 \int_0^\infty s^2 e^{-s^2 - s^3} ds = 0.47281 \ . \tag{3.7.32}$$

As they should, these probabilities satisfy the condition $p_{12} + p_{13} = 1$. Computer implementations of algorithms for evaluating the above integrals numerically are available on many computer platforms. In fact, the integrals in Eqs. (3.7.31) and (3.7.32) were evaluated by MAPLE linked to the word processor used for this book.

3.8 Absorption and Other Transition Probabilities

As indicated in Section 3.6, when considering models for the evolution of HIV disease, it is of interest to compute the distribution function of the waiting time from infection with HIV to a diagnosis of AIDS. Within the framework of a semi-Markov process, such distribution functions are referred to as first passage time distributions. More precisely, suppose the process begins in state i at time $t = 0$ and let the random variable Υ_j be the time of first entrance into state $j \neq i$. One approach for computing such distribution functions is to reconstruct the density matrix so that j becomes an absorbing state and i is a transient state. Then let the random variable Υ_j represent time of absorption into state $j \neq i$, given that the process starts in state i at $t = 0$. Thus, one may consider a semi-Markov process with a set $\mathfrak{S}_1$ of $r_1 \geq 1$ absorbing states, and a set of $\mathfrak{S}_2$ of $r_2 \geq 1$ transient states, and let $f_{ij}(t)$ be the conditional density of the time of first entrance into an absorbing state $j \in \mathfrak{S}_1$, given that the process starts in transient state $i \in \mathfrak{S}_2$ at time $t = 0$. Given this density, the conditional distribution function of the random variable T is:

$$\mathbb{P}\left[\Upsilon_j \leq t \mid X_0 = i\right] = F_{ij}(t) = \int_0^t f_{ij}(s) ds \text{ for } t \in \mathbb{T} \ . \tag{3.8.1}$$

Like many functions of interest, when considering models based on semi-Markov processes with a matrix $\mathbf{a}(t) = (a_{ij}(t))$ of continuous transition densities, formulas for a first passage density $f_{ij}(t)$ may be derived by using a first step decomposition and a renewal argument. For example, if the process starts in transient state $i \in \mathfrak{S}_2$ at time $t = 0$, then the process may enter the absorbing state $j \in \mathfrak{S}_1$ on the first step or it may jump to another transient state $k \neq i$ on the first step at some time $s \in (0, t]$. Upon entrance into state k, a probabilistic renewal occurs and future evolution of the process behaves as if k were the initial state. Hence, it follows that the $r_2 \times r_1$ matrix of densities $\mathbf{f}(t) = \{f_{ij}(t) \mid i \in \mathfrak{S}_2, j \in \mathfrak{S}_1\}$ satisfies the system of renewal type integral equations:

$$f_{ij}(t) = a_{ij}(t) + \sum_{k \neq i} \int_0^t a_{ik}(s) f_{kj}(t-s) ds \text{ for } t \in \mathbb{T} . \tag{3.8.2}$$

To further analyze this system of integral equations, it will be convenient to cast them in matrix form. For the class of semi-Markov processes under consideration, the matrix of one-step transition densities may be represented in the partitioned form:

$$\mathbf{a}(t) = \begin{bmatrix} \mathbf{0}_{r_1,r_1} & \mathbf{0}_{r_1,r_2} \\ \mathbf{r}(t) & \mathbf{q}(t) \end{bmatrix} , \ t \in \mathbb{T} , \tag{3.8.3}$$

where $\mathbf{r}(t)$ is a $r_2 \times r_1$ matrix governing one-step transitions from transient states to absorbing states, and $\mathbf{q}(t)$ is a $r_2 \times r_2$ matrix governing one-step transitions among transient states. In matrix notation, the system of renewal type integral equations may be represented in the succinct form

$$\mathbf{f}(t) = \mathbf{r}(t) + \int_0^t \mathbf{q}(s) \mathbf{f}(t-s) ds \text{ for } t \in \mathbb{T} . \tag{3.8.4}$$

Methods for finding numerical solutions of integral equations of this form are essential in this computer age, and in the next chapter, methods for numerically solving such equations will be discussed. But, before proceeding to a discussion of these methods, it will be informative to derive formulas for calculating the conditional probability F_{ij}

that the process terminates in absorbing state $j \in \mathfrak{S}_1$, given that it starts in transient state $i \in \mathfrak{S}_2$. In terms of the distribution function in Eq. (3.8.1), this probability is:

$$F_{ij} = \lim_{t\uparrow\infty} F_{ij}(t) = \int_0^\infty f_{ij}(s)ds \ . \tag{3.8.5}$$

A useful way of computing this probability is to pass to matrices of Laplace transforms in Eq. (3.8.4). Let

$$\widehat{\mathbf{a}}(\lambda) = \int_0^\infty e^{-\lambda t}\mathbf{a}(s)ds \text{ for } \lambda > 0 \tag{3.8.6}$$

be the matrix of Laplace transforms of the one-step transition densities $\mathbf{a}(t)$. In what follows, a symbol of the form $\widehat{\mathbf{f}}$ will stand for a matrix of Laplace transforms of any matrix $\mathbf{f}$ of functions. Then, in terms of Laplace transforms, the integral equations in Eq.(3.8.4) become

$$\widehat{\mathbf{f}}(\lambda) = \widehat{\mathbf{r}}(\lambda) + \widehat{\mathbf{q}}(\lambda)\widehat{\mathbf{f}}(\lambda) \text{ for } \lambda > 0 \ . \tag{3.8.7}$$

Hence, if $\mathbf{I}_{r_2}$ is a $r_2 \times r_2$ identity matrix, then the solution of Eq. (3.8.7) is:

$$\widehat{\mathbf{f}}(\lambda) = (\mathbf{I}_{r_2} - \widehat{\mathbf{q}}(\lambda))^{-1}\widehat{\mathbf{r}}(\boldsymbol{\lambda}) \text{ for } \lambda > 0 \ . \tag{3.8.8}$$

On computer platforms where implementations of algorithms for computing numerical inverses of Laplace transforms are available, this formula may be useful for finding numerical values of the matrix $\mathbf{f}(t)$ at chosen values of $t \in \mathbb{T}$. It may also be useful for those cases in which the matrix of Laplace transforms $\widehat{\mathbf{a}}(\lambda)$ has elementary forms as, for example, when all sojourn time distributions for transient states have simple exponential distributions so that the matrix $\widehat{\mathbf{f}}(\lambda)$ may be represented in a usable symbolic form. In any case, Eq. (3.8.8) is very useful for deducing a general formula for the $r_2 \times r_1$ matrix $\mathbf{F} = (F_{ij})$ of absorption probabilities. For, from Eqs. (3.8.5) and (3.8.8), it can be seen that:

$$\mathbf{F} = \lim_{\lambda\downarrow 0} \widehat{\mathbf{f}}(\lambda) = (\mathbf{I}_{r_2} - \mathbf{Q})^{-1}\mathbf{R} = \mathbf{MR} \ , \tag{3.8.9}$$

where $\mathbf{Q}$ and $\mathbf{R}$ are sub-matrices of the transition matrix $\mathbf{P}$ for the embedded Markov chain (see Eq. (3.7.7)) and it is assumed $\mathbf{Q}^n \to \mathbf{0}$, a zero matrix, as $n \uparrow \infty$. It will be noted that Eq. (3.8.9) holds, because for every state $i \in \mathfrak{S}_2$, the transition probability p_{ij} for the embedded Markov chain is given by:

$$p_{ij} = \lim_{t\uparrow\infty} A_{ij}(t) = \lim_{\lambda\downarrow 0} \widehat{a}_{ij}(\lambda) \text{ for } j \in \mathfrak{S}\ . \tag{3.8.10}$$

A question that naturally arises is whether one can guarantee that:

$$\sum_{j\in\mathfrak{S}_1} f_{ij} = 1 \tag{3.8.11}$$

for all $i \in \mathfrak{S}_2$ so that, given that the process starts in some transient state i at time $t = 0$, it will terminate eventually in some absorbing state $j \in \mathfrak{S}_1$ with probability one. For the case that the state space is finite, it is easy to answer this question in the affirmative. By an induction argument, it can be shown that the nth power of the transition matrix $\mathbf{P}$ for the embedded Markov chain may be represented in the partitioned form:

$$\mathbf{P}^n = (p_{ij}^{(n)}) = \begin{bmatrix} \mathbf{I}_{r_1} & \mathbf{0} \\ \left(\sum_{k=0}^{n-1} \mathbf{Q}^k\right)\mathbf{R} & \mathbf{Q}^n \end{bmatrix}. \tag{3.8.12}$$

But, for every $n \geq 1$ and $i \in \mathfrak{S}$,

$$\sum_{j\in\mathfrak{S}} p_{ij}^{(n)} = 1\ . \tag{3.8.13}$$

Therefore, because the state space is finite, it follows that:

$$\lim_{n\uparrow\infty} \sum_{j\in\mathfrak{S}} p_{ij}^{(n)} = \sum_{j\in\mathfrak{S}} \lim_{n\uparrow\infty} p_{ij}^{(n)} = 1\ . \tag{3.8.14}$$

But, from Eq. (3.8.12) it is clear that:

$$\lim_{n\uparrow\infty} \mathbf{P}^n = \begin{bmatrix} \mathbf{I}_{r_1} & \mathbf{0} \\ \mathbf{MR} & \mathbf{0} \end{bmatrix} \tag{3.8.15}$$

which proves Eq. (3.8.11) holds.

Another random function of interest in the applications of models based on semi-Markov processes is $Z(t)$, indicating the state occupied by the process at time $t > 0$. Some authors refer to this random function as a semi-Markov process. If the process starts in state $X_0 = i$ at time $t = 0$ and $t < T_1$, the time of the first jump from i, then $Z(t) = i$. To define $Z(t)$ more generally, let the random variable,

$$U_n = T_1 + T_2 + \cdots + T_n \tag{3.8.16}$$

be the time of the nth jump, $n \geq 1$. Then, in general for $t \geq T_1$, $Z(t) = j$, if, and only if, $X_n = j$ and

$$U_n \leq t < U_{n+1} \tag{3.8.17}$$

for some $n \geq 1$. Just as for Markov jump processes in continuous time, a set of functions of basic interest in the analysis of absorbing semi-Markov processes consists of the conditional probabilities,

$$\mathbb{P}\left[Z(t) = j \mid X_0 = i\right] = P_{ij}(t) \ , \tag{3.8.18}$$

defined for all states i, j in $\mathfrak{S}$ and $t \in \mathbb{T}$ and satisfying the initial conditions $P_{ij}(0) = \delta_{ij}$.

If $i \in \mathfrak{S}_2$ and $j \in \mathfrak{S}_1$, then $P_{ij}(t) = F_{ij}(t)$, the distribution function defined in Eq. (3.8.1). When i and j are transient states in $\mathfrak{S}_2$, these probabilities also satisfy a system of renewal type integral equations. For if the process starts in some transient state $i \in \mathfrak{S}_2$ at $t = 0$, then it is still in state i at time $t > 0$ with probability $1 - A_i(t)$. On the other hand, if there is a jump to another transient state $k \neq i$ at some time $s \in (0, t]$, then $P_{kj}(t - s)$ is the probability the process is in some transient state j at time $t > 0$. Again by a renewal type argument, it can be seen that the matrix $\mathbf{P}(t) = (P_{ij}(t) \mid i, j \in \mathfrak{S}_2)$ of functions satisfies the integral equations,

$$P_{ij}(t) = \delta_{ij}(1 - A_i(t)) + \sum_{k \neq i} \int_0^t a_{ik}(s) P_{kj}(t - s) \text{ for } t \in \mathbb{T} \ . \tag{3.8.19}$$

By letting $\mathbf{D}(t) = (\delta_{ij}(1 - A_i(t)))$ be a diagonal matrix, it can be seen that these equations may also be represented in the more compact matrix form:

$$\mathbf{P}(t) = \mathbf{D}(t) + \int_0^t \mathbf{q}(s)\mathbf{P}(t-s)ds, \ t \in \mathbb{T} \ . \tag{3.8.20}$$

Just as for the case of absorption probabilities, it is possible to pass to Laplace transforms in this equation to derive useful formulas for $\widehat{\mathbf{P}}(\lambda)$, the transform of the matrix $\mathbf{P}(t)$, but the details will be omitted.

3.9 References

1. R. Bellman, *Stability Theory of Differential Equations,* McGraw-Hill, New York, Toronto, London, 1953.
2. P. Billingsley, *Probability and Measure,* John Wiley and Sons, Inc., New York, London, 1979.
3. L. Breiman, *Probability and Stochastic Processes: With a View Toward Applications,* Houghton Mifflin Company, Boston, New York, Atlanta, 1969.
4. B. W. Char, K. O. Geddes, G. H. Gonnet, B. Leong, M. B. Monagan and S. M. Watt, *MAPLE V Language Reference Manual,* Springer-Verlag, Berlin, 1991.
5. E. Cinlar, *Introduction to Stochastic Processes,* Prentice-Hall, Inc., Englewood Cliffs, New Jersey, 1975.
6. J. L. Doob, *Stochastic Processes,* John Wiley and Sons, Inc., New York, London, 1953.
7. W. Feller, *An Introduction to Probability Theory and Its Applications, I,* 3rd ed., John Wiley and Sons, Inc., New York, London, 1968.
8. I. I. Gikhman and A. V. Skorokhod, *Introduction to the Theory of Random Processes,* W. B. Saunders Company, Philadelphia, London, Toronto, 1969.
9. P. C. Hoel, S. C. Port and C. J. Stone, *Introduction to Stochastic Processes,* Houghton Mifflin Company, Boston, New York, Atlanta, 1972.
10. J. M. Hoem and U. F. Jensen, Multistate Life Table Methodology: A Probabilistic Critique, K. C. Land and A. Rogers (eds.), *Multidimensional Mathematical Demography,* Academic Press, New York and London, 1982, pp. 155-264.
11. S. Karlin, *A First Course in Stochastic Processes,* Academic Press, New York, London, 1966.

12. J. G. Kemeny and J. L. Snell, *Finite Markov Chains,* Springer-Verlag, Berlin, New York, 1976.

13. I. M. Longini, Jr., W. S. Clark, L. I. Gardner and J. F. Brundage, Modeling the Decline of CD4+ T-Lymphocyte Counts in HIV-Infected Individuals: A Markov Modeling Approach, *Journal of Acquired Immune Deficiency Syndromes* **4:** 1141-1147, 1991.

14. C. J. Mode, *Stochastic Processes in Demography and Their Computer Implementation,* Springer-Verlag, Berlin, Heidelberg, New York, Tokyo, 1985.

15. W. Y. Tan, First Passage Probability Distributions in Markov Models and the HIV Incubation Period Under Treatment, *Mathematical and Computer Modelling* **19:** 53-66, 1994.

Chapter 4
SEMI-MARKOV JUMP PROCESSES IN DISCRETE TIME

4.1 Introduction

As discussed in the preceding chapter, models based on continuous time Markov jump processes often center on finding solutions to some version of the Kolmogorov differential equations. These solutions, in turn, can be used to construct a probability measure $\mathbb{P}$ underlying the process such that for every $n \geq 1$, states $i_k \in \mathfrak{S}$, $k = 0, 1, 2, \cdots, n$, and time points $0 = t_0 < t_1 < \cdots < t_n$, the event $[X(t_k) = i_k \mid k = 1, 2, \cdots, n]$ can be assigned a conditional probability, given $X(t_0) = i_0$. For the case where the laws of evolution underlying the process are time homogeneous, it was shown that if a continuous time Markov process was viewed from the sample path perspective, then the structure could be generalized to a class of models called semi-Markov processes such that the condition that the sojourn time in any state must have an exponential distribution could be relaxed. But, as illustrated in the preceding chapter, models based on either continuous time Markov or semi-Markov processes may become mathematically intractable. If, however, attention is focused on models in discrete time, then many mathematical difficulties diminish and one may proceed to study a model using computer intensive methods. As we will see in this chapter, if attention is focused on discrete time models, then it becomes possible to consider models that are more general than those discussed in the previous chapter. Moreover, as the memory and computational power of desktop computers expand, it becomes increasingly feasible to work with such models using computer intensive methods.

4.2 Computational Methods

Because the computer implementation of any continuous time model must necessarily entail only finitely many computations, it is natural to consider discrete time approximations to a process in continuous time over finite time intervals. There are also situations in which it is natural to consider processes that may, for practical reasons, be observed at only discrete points in time. Such is the case, for example, in monitoring most HIV/AIDS epidemics, where AIDS cases are usually reported by departments of public health on a monthly time scale. One is thus led to consider an increasing sequence of equally spaced time points $0 = t_0 < t_1 < t_2 < \cdots$, where $t_k - t_{k-1} = h$, some unit of time, for all $k \geq 1$. To lighten the notation, it will be supposed that $h = 1$ so that one may consider the evolution of a stochastic process observed at the discrete time points $t = 0, 1, 2, \cdots$.

A discrete time semi-Markov process arises when the transition matrix $\mathbf{a}(t) = (a_{ij}(t))$ is specified at points $t = 0, 1, 2, \cdots$. All definitions set forth in the preceding chapter for continuous time processes continue to hold for a discrete time formulation except that all integrals are replaced by sums. For example, in the case of discrete time, the $r_2 \times r_1$ matrix $\mathbf{f}\,(t) = \{f_{ij}(t) \mid i \in \mathfrak{S}_2, j \in \mathfrak{S}_1\}$ of absorption densities satisfies the discrete type renewal equation:

$$\mathbf{f}(t) = \mathbf{r}(t) + \sum_{s=0}^{t} \mathbf{q}(s)\mathbf{f}(t-s) \text{ for } t = 0, 1, \cdots , \tag{4.2.1}$$

(see Eq. (3.8.4)). Similarly, the $r_2 \times r_2$ matrix $\mathbf{P}(t) = \{P_{ij}(t) \mid i, j \in \mathfrak{S}_2\}$ in Eq. (3.8.20) of probabilities for transitions among transient states satisfies the equation:

$$\mathbf{P}(t) = \mathbf{D}(t) + \sum_{s=0}^{t} \mathbf{q}(s)\mathbf{P}(t-s), \ t = 0, 1, \cdots . \tag{4.2.2}$$

In many applications of semi-Markov processes to problems in epidemiology, it becomes necessary to compute values of the matrices $\mathbf{f}(t)$ and $\mathbf{P}(t)$ at finitely many time points $t = 0, 1, 2, \cdots, N$.

There are at least two general methods for solving the matrix equations of Eqs. (4.2.1) and (4.2.2) numerically. If it is assumed that at least one time unit must transpire before any transition from a state can occur, then $\mathbf{a}(0) = \mathbf{0}$, a $r \times r$ zero matrix, so that all sub-matrices of $\mathbf{a}(0)$ are also zero matrices. Hence, $\mathbf{f}(0) = \mathbf{0}$, $\mathbf{f}(1) = \mathbf{r}(1)$ and it follows that for $t \geq 2$, Eq. (4.2.1) may be written in the form:

$$\mathbf{f}(t) = \mathbf{r}(t) + \sum_{s=1}^{t-1} \mathbf{q}(s)\mathbf{f}(t-s) \ . \tag{4.2.3}$$

From this equation, it is clear that if the matrices $\mathbf{f}(s)$ are known for $s = 1, 2, \cdots, t-1$, then Eq. (4.2.3) may be used to determine the matrix $\mathbf{f}(t)$ for $t \geq 2$. A similar recursive method may be used to solve Eq. (4.2.2). It can be seen, by observing the condition $\mathbf{q}(0) = \mathbf{0}$, that for $t \geq 1$ this equation takes the form:

$$\mathbf{P}(t) = \mathbf{D}(t) + \sum_{s=1}^{t} \mathbf{q}(s)\mathbf{P}(t-s) \ . \tag{4.2.4}$$

Therefore, by recalling $\mathbf{P}(0) = \mathbf{I}$, a $r_2 \times r_2$ identity matrix, it follows that $\mathbf{P}(1) = \mathbf{D}(1) + \mathbf{q}(1)$. Further, if $\mathbf{P}(s)$ has been computed for $s = 0, 1, 2, \cdots, t-1$, then Eq. (4.2.4) may be used to compute $\mathbf{P}(t)$ for $t \geq 2$.

Another approach to solving the renewal equations of Eqs. (4.2.1) and (4.2.2) is to consider a discrete time analogue of the $r_2 \times r_2$ matrix $\mathbf{M}(t) = (m_{ij}(t))$, whose ijth element is the conditional expectation:

$$E\left[N_j(t) \mid Z(0) = i\right] \tag{4.2.5}$$

defined in Eq. (3.7.12). Rather than working directly with this matrix as was the case in a continuous time formulation, in a discrete time formulation it is convenient to work with a renewal density matrix $\mathbf{u}(s) = (u_{ij}(s))$, which is defined such that:

$$\mathbf{M}(t) = \sum_{s=0}^{t} \mathbf{u}(s) \text{ for } t = 0, 1, \cdots \ . \tag{4.2.6}$$

Actually, if one was interested in computing the expected number of visits to transient state $j \in \mathfrak{S}_2$ up to time $t > 0$, given that the process was in state $i \in \mathfrak{S}_2$ at $t = 0$, then this matrix of expectations would be of importance in its own right. To determine this renewal density matrix, define a sequence $(\mathbf{q}^{(n)}(t))$ of matrices for $n = 1, 2, \cdots$, by letting $\mathbf{q}^{(1)}(t) = \mathbf{q}(t)$ and, for $n \geq 2$, let the sequence be determined recursively by the matrix convolutions:

$$\mathbf{q}^{(n)}(t) = \sum_{s=0}^{t} \mathbf{q}^{(n-1)}(s)\mathbf{q}(t-s) \text{ for } t = 0, 1, \cdots . \tag{4.2.7}$$

To complete the definition of the density matrix, it will be very helpful to define the algebraic notion of an identity for the operation of matrix convolution. Let the matrix-valued function $\mathbf{q}^{(0)}(t)$ be defined for all $t = 0, 1, 2, \cdots$, by letting $\mathbf{q}^{(0)}(0) = \mathbf{I}$, a $r_2 \times r_2$ identity matrix, and for $t \geq 1$ let $\mathbf{q}^{(0)}(t) = \mathbf{0}$, a $r_2 \times r_2$ zero matrix. Then, this function is an identity for the operation of matrix convolution in the sense that:

$$\mathbf{q}(t) = \sum_{s=0}^{t} \mathbf{q}^{(0)}(s)\mathbf{q}(t-s) = \sum_{s=0}^{t} \mathbf{q}(s)\mathbf{q}^{(0)}(t-s) \tag{4.2.8}$$

for $t = 0, 1, 2, \cdots$. Formally, the renewal density matrix $\mathbf{u}(t)$ is defined for each t by the infinite series:

$$\mathbf{u}(t) = \sum_{n=0}^{\infty} \mathbf{q}^{(n)}(t) . \tag{4.2.9}$$

It can be shown that the condition $\mathbf{q}(0) = \mathbf{0}$ implies that for any $t \geq 1$, the matrix series in Eq. (4.2.9) has only finitely many non-zero terms and thus converges element by element for any $t = 0, 1, 2, \cdots$. By inspection, it can also be seen that the density matrix $\mathbf{u}(t)$ satisfies the renewal equation:

$$\mathbf{u}(t) = \mathbf{q}^{(0)}(t) + \sum_{s=0}^{t} \mathbf{u}(s)\mathbf{q}(t-s) \tag{4.2.10}$$

for $t = 0, 1, 2, \cdots$. Therefore, because $\mathbf{u}(0) = \mathbf{I}$ and $\mathbf{q}(0) = \mathbf{0}$, the equation may be expressed in the form:

$$\mathbf{u}(t) = \sum_{s=0}^{t-1} \mathbf{u}(s)\mathbf{q}(t-s) \tag{4.2.11}$$

for $t = 1, 2, \cdots$. Hence, if $\mathbf{u}(s)$ has been computed for $s = 0, 1, 2, \cdots, t-1$, then $\mathbf{u}(t)$ may be determined from Eq. (4.2.11) for $t \geq 1$.

If the symbol t is dropped in Eqs. (4.2.3) and (4.2.4) and if we let the symbol $*$ stand for the operation of matrix convolution, then these equations may be represented in the forms:

$$(\mathbf{q}^{(0)} - \mathbf{q}) * \mathbf{f} = \mathbf{r} \tag{4.2.12}$$

and

$$(\mathbf{q}^{(0)} - \mathbf{q}) * \mathbf{P} = \mathbf{D} \, . \tag{4.2.13}$$

By writing Eq. (4.2.10) in the equivalent form:

$$\sum_{s=0}^{t} \mathbf{u}(s)(\mathbf{q}^{(0)}(t-s) - \mathbf{q}(t-s)) = \mathbf{q}^{(0)}(t) \, , \tag{4.2.14}$$

which holds for all $t = 0, 1, 2, \cdots$, it can be seen that the renewal density $\mathbf{u}(t)$ is actually the convolution inverse of $\mathbf{q}^{(0)}(t) - \mathbf{q}(t)$. Symbolically, $\mathbf{u} * (\mathbf{q}^{(0)} - \mathbf{q}) = \mathbf{q}^{(0)}$ and, because the operation $*$ is associative, numerical solutions of Eqs. (4.2.3) and (4.2.4) may also be computed using the formulas:

$$\mathbf{f}(t) = \sum_{s=0}^{t} \mathbf{u}(s)\mathbf{r}(t-s) \tag{4.2.15}$$

and

$$\mathbf{P}(t) = \sum_{s=0}^{t} \mathbf{u}(s)\mathbf{D}(t-s) \tag{4.2.16}$$

for $t = 0, 1, 2, \cdots$. These formulas will be particularly useful if the renewal density $\mathbf{u}(t)$ has already been computed so as to evaluate the matrix of expectations $\mathbf{M}(t)$ in Eq. (4.2.6).

The numerical procedures just outlined have been used extensively in applications of semi-Markov processes in models of biological phenomena as well as those of interest in the social sciences (see Mode[2] and Mode and Pickens[3] for further details and references). Experience with these procedures suggests they are very stable numerically and have performed well for state spaces of moderate size on several computer platforms. As computer memory expands, it will, in all likelihood, become feasible to apply these methods to models with state spaces larger than those considered previously. Sometimes, by taking advantage of the structure of the transition density matrix $\mathbf{a}(t)$, it is possible to derive special cases of the renewal type equations discussed, which results in reductions in the dimensionality of the problem. This will be illustrated in subsequent chapters.

A problem confronted by any investigator when constructing a model based on a semi-Markov process is that of modelling a discrete time version of the density matrix $\mathbf{a}(t) = (a_{ij}(t))$, $t = 0, 1, 2, \cdots$. In this connection, it is often fruitful to consider models based on risk functions in discrete time, when constructing models with time homogeneous laws of evolution. To this end, let T_i be a random variable representing the time of exit from state i and let the random variable C_i represent the state entered after leaving i. Then, the discrete risk function $q_{ij}(t)$ is defined as the conditional probability:

$$\mathbb{P}\left[C_i = j, T_i = t \mid T_i > t-1\right] = q_{ij}(t) \tag{4.2.17}$$

for $t = 1, 2, 3, \cdots$. The conditional probability that the process in state i at time $t-1$ leaves this state during the time interval $(t-1, t]$ is, therefore,

$$q_i(t) = \sum_{j \neq i} q_{ij}(t) = \mathbb{P}\left[T_i = t \mid T_i > t-1\right] \tag{4.2.18}$$

so that

$$p_i(t) = 1 - q_i(t) = \mathbb{P}\left[T_i > t \mid T_i > t-1\right] = \frac{\mathbb{P}\left[T_i > t\right]}{\mathbb{P}\left[T_i > t-1\right]} \tag{4.2.19}$$

is the conditional probability of remaining in state i during $(t-1, t]$. It will be observed that the conditional probability in the center of (4.2.19) is actually the ratio of two unconditional probabilities, because $T_i > t$ implies $T_i > t-1$. As with all discrete time processes considered in this section, by definition $q_i(0) = 0$ for all i so that $p_i(0) = \mathbb{P}\left[T_i > 0\right] = 1$.

From an inspection of the telescoping product:

$$\mathbb{P}\left[T_i > t\right] = \prod_{\nu=1}^{t} \frac{\mathbb{P}\left[T_i > \nu\right]}{\mathbb{P}\left[T_i > \nu-1\right]}\,, \tag{4.2.20}$$

it follows from Eq. (4.2.19) that the survival function for the sojourn time in state i may be expressed in the form

$$S_i(t) = \mathbb{P}[T_i > t] = \prod_{\nu=0}^{t} p_i(\nu) \tag{4.2.21}$$

for $t = 0, 1, 2, \cdots$. In the case of discrete time, $a_{ij}(t)$ is the conditional probability that if the process enters state i at time $t = 0$, there is a jump to state j by time $t \geq 1$. The probability the process is still in state i at time $t-1$ is $S_i(t-1)$ and, given it is in this state at $t-1$, $q_{ij}(t)$ is the conditional probability of a jump to $j \neq i$ during $(t-1, t]$. Therefore,

$$a_{ij}(t) = S_i(t-1)q_{ij}(t) \tag{4.2.22}$$

for $t = 1, 2, \cdots$. This density resembles the one derived in the case of continuous time by appealing to the theory of competing risks, and, in the demographic literature, the procedure for calculating it is referred to as a multiple decrement life table algorithm (see Mode[2] for details). The distribution of the function of the sojourn time in state i is:

$$A_i(t) = \sum_{s=0}^{t} \sum_{j \neq i} a_{ij}(s) \ . \tag{4.2.23}$$

The process leaves i eventually with probability one if, and only if, $A_i(t) \uparrow 1$ as $t \uparrow \infty$. But, this condition is satisfied if, and only if,

$$\lim_{t \uparrow \infty} (1 - A_i(t)) = \lim_{t \uparrow \infty} S_i(t) = \lim_{t \uparrow \infty} \prod_{\nu=0}^{t} p_i(\nu) = 0 \ . \tag{4.2.24}$$

When constructing models of the risk functions $q_{ij}(t)$ one needs to check whether this condition is indeed satisfied. In computer implementations of these ideas, the essential support of a sojourn time distribution in a state is actually a finite set so there is some integer t_0 such that $q_i(t_0) = 1$ so $p_i(t_0) = 0$. In such cases, the condition in Eq. (4.2.24) will automatically be satisfied.

A simple and useful case arises when all the risk functions $q_{ij}(t) = q_{ij}$ are constant for $t \geq 1$ so that q_i and $p_i = 1 - q_i$ are also constant. Under this constancy condition, the density in Eq. (4.2.22) takes the form:

$$a_{ij}(t) = p_i^{t-1} q_{ij} , \tag{4.2.25}$$

for $t \geq 1$, and the survival function for state i has the form:

$$S_i(t) = p_i^t \tag{4.2.26}$$

for $t = 0, 1, 2, \cdots$. In this case, $\lim_{t\uparrow\infty} S_i(t) = 0$ if, and only if, $0 \leq p_i < 1$. To avoid the trivial case, the process cannot remain in state i for more than one time unit, requiring that $0 < p_i < 1$. In this case, the transition probabilities for the embedded Markov chain are given by:

$$p_{ij} = \sum_{t=1}^{\infty} p_i^{t-1} q_{ij} = \frac{q_{ij}}{1 - p_i} = \frac{q_{ij}}{q_i} \text{ for } j \neq i. \tag{4.2.27}$$

The formula in Eq. (4.2.25) is actually a generalization of the geometric distribution, which, like its continuous analogue the exponential distribution, has the memoryless property. In fact, the structure just described may viewed as a Markov process of the lattice of time points $t = 0, 1, 2, 3, \cdots$.

Constructing models of the discrete risk functions $q_{ij}(t)$ can itself pose problems, so an alternative approach is to view these functions as an approximation to some continuous time model. Suppose, for example, it is possible to compute the functions $A_{ij}(t)$ for a continuous time model at selected points $t = 0, 1, 2, \cdots$ in $\mathbb{T}$. Then, if $S_i(t)$ is the survival function for state i, the discrete time risk functions could be chosen as:

$$q_{ij}(1, t) = \frac{A_{ij}(t) - A_{ij}(t-1)}{S_i(t-1)} \text{ for } t \geq 1. \tag{4.2.28}$$

With this approximation, the discrete density would have the form:

$$a_{ij}(1, t) = S_i(t-1)\, q_{ij}(1, t) = A_{ij}(t) - A_{ij}(t-1) . \tag{4.2.29}$$

It can be shown that this approximation has the property that if one uses a multiple decrement life table algorithm to compute the density and survival function as in Eqs. (4.2.21) and (4.2.22), using the risk functions in Eq. (4.2.28), then the resulting density agrees exactly with

Eq. (4.2.29) and the survival function at the points $t = 0, 1, 2, \cdots$. Tan[4] has used ideas similar to the ones outlined in this section to develop a non-Markovian discrete time model for the incubation period of HIV under treatment.

From the practical point of view, the length h of each time interval in a discrete approximation to a continuous model will depend on the size of the arrays that can be handled by the computer platform being used. The smaller the value of h, the greater the size of the arrays to be processed by the computer; in fact, if h is too small, their size may exceed the memory limitations of the computer. It is, nevertheless, of interest to consider the case $h \downarrow 0$. When $h > 0$ is small and $\theta_{ij}(t)$ is a risk function for a continuous time model for the transition $i \to j$, then the risk function in Eq. (4.2.28) may be expressed as:

$$q_{ij}(h,t) = \frac{A_{ij}(t+h) - A_{ij}(t)}{S_i(t)} = \theta_{ij}(t)h + o(h) , \tag{4.2.30}$$

Consequently,

$$\lim_{h \downarrow 0} \frac{a_{ij}(h,t)}{h} = \lim_{h \downarrow 0} \frac{S_i(t) q_{ij}(h,t)}{h} = S_i(t)\theta_{ij}$$

$$= \lim_{h \downarrow 0} \frac{A_{ij}(t+h) - A_{ij}(t)}{h} = a_{ij}(t) , \tag{4.2.31}$$

the density for the continuous time model. Thus, the discrete density is an approximation to the continuous time density in the sense that for $h > 0$ small:

$$a_{ij}(h,t) = a_{ij}(t)h + o(h) . \tag{4.2.32}$$

These observations could be used as a starting point in a study of discrete time processes as approximations to those in continuous time, but the details will not be pursued here.

4.3 Age Dependency with Stationary Laws of Evolution

A factor that has not been considered heretofore but needs to be reckoned with when constructing stochastic models of epidemiological phenomena is that of the age of an individual when entering a state. For, it seems reasonable to suppose that an individual's age when entering some state will affect his or her subsequent evolution among the states of the process. The need to accommodate this possibility has given rise to a class of stochastic processes called age-dependent semi-Markov processes. As before, let $\mathfrak{S}$ be a finite state space under consideration, and, with a view towards computer implementation, suppose time and age are measured on some discrete set of points $0, 1, 2, \cdots$. Just as in Section (3.7), the random variables X_n represent the state entered at the nth jump, but T_n is an integer-valued random variable representing the length of the stay in this state. A sample path consisting of $n \geq 1$ jumps will again be represented by the set of ordered pairs $\{(i_k, t_{i_k}) \mid k = 0, 1, 2, \cdots, n\}$, which is a particular realization of the pairs of random variables $\{(X_k, T_k) \mid k = 0, 1, 2, \cdots, n\}$. If an individual is of age x when entering the initial state $X_0 = i_0$ at time $t = 0$, then his or her age when entering state $X_n = i_n$ at the nth jump, $n \geq 1$, is given by the random variable $U_{n-1} = x + T_0 + \cdots + T_{n-1}$. In what follows, a realization of this random variable will be denoted by u_{n-1}.

A fundamental object underlying the theory of age-dependent semi-Markov processes is a density matrix $\mathbf{a}(x, t) = (a_{ij}(x, t))$ defined for all pairs of non-negative integers $x, t = 0, 1, 2, \cdots$ and pairs of states i, j in $\mathfrak{S}$. In a discrete time formulation, all elements in the density matrix are probabilities satisfying the inequalities $0 \leq a_{ij}(x, t) \leq 1$ for all pairs of non-negative integers $x, t = 0, 1, 2, \cdots$. Given the evolution of the process up to step $n - 1$, which as in Section 3.7 is symbolized by $\mathfrak{B}(n-1)$, the assumption that determines the probability measure $\mathbb{P}$ underlying an age-dependent semi-Markov process is:

$$\mathbb{P}\left[X_n = j, T_n = t \mid \mathfrak{B}(n-1)\right] =$$

$$\mathbb{P}\left[X_n = j, T_n = t \mid X_{n-1} = i\right] = a_{ij}(u_{n-1}, t) \tag{4.3.1}$$

From this assumption, it follows by using well-known properties of conditional probabilities that the finite dimensional densities of the process are given by:

$$\mathbb{P}[\, X_k = i_k, T_k = t_k, 1 \leq k \leq n \mid X_0 = i_0, T_0 = t_0 \,]$$

$$= \prod_{k=1}^{n} a_{i_{k-1}, i_k}(u_{k-1}, t_k) \tag{4.3.2}$$

for all states $i_0, i_1, \cdots, i_n$ in $\mathfrak{S}$ and non-negative integers $t_0, t_1, \cdots, t_n$ for $n \geq 1$. It will be noted from Eq. (4.3.1) that the laws governing the evolution of the process are stationary in the sense that the right-hand side of this equation depends on n only through the variable u_{n-1}.

As an aid to generalizing the renewal theory that yielded fruitful results for the case of semi-Markov processes, it will be useful to again consider the sequence of random variables:

$$U_n = x + T_0 + T_1 + \cdots + T_n \tag{4.3.3}$$

defined for $n = 0, 1, 2, \cdots$, for the case an individual is age x when entering the initial state at time $t = 0$. From this equation it can be seen that there is a one-to-one correspondence between the random variables $U_0, U_1, U_2, \cdots$ and the random variables $T_1, T_2, \cdots$. In fact,

$$T_n = U_n - U_{n-1} \tag{4.3.4}$$

for $n \geq 1$. Because of this one-to-one correspondence, it follows that the joint density of the pairs of random variables (X_k, U_k), $k = 1, 2, \cdots, n$, given $(X_0, T_0) = (i_0, t_0)$ is:

$$\mathbb{P}[X_k = i_k, U_k = u_k, k = 1, 2, \cdots, n|\ i_0, t_0]$$

$$= \prod_{k=1}^{n} a_{i_{k-1}, i_k}(u_{k-1}, u_k - u_{k-1}) \tag{4.3.5}$$

for all states $i_0, i_1, \cdots, i_n$ in $\mathfrak{S}$ and non-negative integers such that $u_0 \leq u_1 \leq \cdots \leq u_n$. But, from Eq.(4.3.5) it also follows that:

$$\mathbb{P}[X_n = i_n, U_n = u_n|\ X_k = i_k, U_k = u_k,\ k = 0, 1, 2, \cdots, n-1]$$

$$= a_{i_{n-1}, i_n}(u_{n-1}, u_n - u_{n-1}) \tag{4.3.6}$$

for all $n \geq 1$. Therefore, the sequence of pairs (X_k, U_k), $k = 1, 2, 3, \cdots$, has the Markov property with respect to jumps of the process. In other words, if the process enters a state at some jump, then the future evolution of the process depends only on the state last visited and the age of an individual when entering this state. As we shall see, this property plays an essential role in generalizing renewal theory for the age-dependent case. It should be noted that the conditioning just described applies only to sample paths of positive probability.

Before deriving age-dependent renewal equations for absorption and other transition probabilities, it will be necessary to briefly consider the concepts of absorbing and transient states in the structure under consideration. For all pairs of states $i, j \in \mathfrak{S}$ and non-negative integers $x, t = 0, 1, 2, \cdots$, let

$$A_{ij}(x,t) = \sum_{s=0}^{t} a_{ij}(x,s) \ , \tag{4.3.7}$$

and let

$$A_i(x,t) = \sum_{j \in \mathfrak{S}} A_{ij}(x,t) \ . \tag{4.3.8}$$

Because the sequence of pairs $(X_n, U_n), n \geq 0$, has the Markov property and the laws of evolution of the process are stationary, $A_i(x,t)$ is the conditional distribution function of the sojourn time in state i, given that an individual enters state i at age x.

Like the semi-Markov processes considered in the previous sections, it will be useful to introduce the concepts of absorbing and transient states. A state $i \in \mathfrak{S}$ will be called transient if, and only if,

$$\lim_{t \uparrow \infty} A_i(x,t) = 1 \tag{4.3.9}$$

for all $x \geq 0$. Thus, whatever the age x of an individual entering a transient state, departure from this state occurs eventually with probability one. A state i will be called absorbing if, and only if, $a_{ij}(x,t) = 0$ for all $j \in \mathfrak{S}$ and non-negative integers $x, t = 0, 1, 2, \cdots$. Once an absorbing state is entered, there are no transitions from this state.

Just as in previous discussions of semi-Markov processes, it will be useful to partition the state space into a set $\mathfrak{S}_1$ of $r_1 \geq 1$ absorbing states and a set $\mathfrak{S}_2$ of $r_2 \geq 1$ transient states for a total of $r = r_1 + r_2$ states. With these definitions, the $r \times r$ matrix of transition densities may be represented in the partitioned form:

$$\mathbf{a}(x,t) = \begin{bmatrix} \mathbf{0}_{r_1,r_1} & \mathbf{0}_{r_1,r_2} \\ \mathbf{r}(x,t) & \mathbf{q}(x,t) \end{bmatrix} \tag{4.3.10}$$

for all $x, t = 0, 1, 2, \cdots$, where $\mathbf{r}(x,t)$ is a $r_2 \times r_1$ matrix governing one-step transitions from transient states to absorbing states and $\mathbf{q}(x,t)$ is a $r_2 \times r_2$ matrix governing one-step transitions among transient states.

Given that an individual of age x enters a transient state $i \in \mathfrak{S}_2$ at time $t = 0$, let $f_{ij}(x,t)$ be the conditional probability absorbing state $j \in \mathfrak{S}_1$ is entered at time $t > 0$, and let $\mathbf{f}(x,t) = (f_{ij}(x,t))$ be a $r_2 \times r_1$ matrix of these functions. Then, in view of Eq. (4.3.10) and the condition that the future evolution of the process depends only on the age of an individual when entering a state, it can be seen, by using an age-dependent renewal argument, that this matrix satisfies the discrete time age-dependent renewal type equation:

$$\mathbf{f}(x,t) = \mathbf{r}(x,t) + \sum_{s=0}^{t} \mathbf{q}(x,s)\mathbf{f}(x+s, t-s) \tag{4.3.11}$$

for all $x, t = 0, 1, 2, \cdots$.

Another matrix of conditional probabilities concerns the probability of being in a transient state prior to entering some absorbing state. Given that an individual of age x enters transient state $i \in \mathfrak{S}_2$ at time $t = 0$, let $P_{ij}(x,t)$ be the conditional probability of being in transient state $j \in \mathfrak{S}_2$ at time $t > 0$, and let $\mathbf{P}(x,t) = (P_{ij}(x,t))$ be a $r_2 \times r_2$ matrix of these conditional probabilities. Next observe that if an individual of age x enters transient state i at time $t = 0$, then $1 - A_i(t)$ is the conditional probability that he is still in state i at time $t > 0$, and let $\mathbf{D}(x,t) = (\delta_{ij}(1 - A_i(x,t)))$ be a $r_2 \times r_2$ diagonal matrix containing these probabilities. Then, by using another age-dependent renewal type argument, it can be seen that this matrix satisfies the equation:

$$\mathbf{P}(x,t) = \mathbf{D}(x,t) + \sum_{s=0}^{t} \mathbf{q}(x,s)\mathbf{P}(x+s, t-s) \tag{4.3.12}$$

for all $x, t = 0, 1, 2, \cdots$.

Although Eqs. (4.3.11) and (4.3.12) may be solved by a recursive method in x and t, a more elegant approach is to compute a renewal density associated with the matrix-valued function $\mathbf{q}(x,t)$. A first step in developing a method to compute this density is to define an identity function for the operation of age-dependent matrix convolutions. Let $\mathbf{q}^{(0)}(x,t)$ be a $r_2 \times r_2$ matrix-valued function such that $\mathbf{q}^{(0)}(x,0) = \mathbf{I}_{r_2}$ and $\mathbf{q}^{(0)}(x,t) = \mathbf{0}_{r_2}$ for all $t \geq 1$, where $\mathbf{I}_{r_2}$ and $\mathbf{0}_{r_2}$ are, respectively, $r_2 \times r_2$ identity and zero matrices. Then, it can be shown that:

$$\begin{aligned}
&\sum_{s=0}^{t} \mathbf{q}^{(0)}(x,s)\mathbf{q}(x+s,t-s) \\
&= \sum_{s=0}^{t} \mathbf{q}(x,s)\mathbf{q}^{(0)}\mathbf{q}(x+s,t-s) \\
&= \mathbf{q}(x,t) \qquad (4.3.13)
\end{aligned}$$

for all non-negative integers $x, t = 0, 1, 2, \cdots$, so that $\mathbf{q}^{(0)}(x,t)$ is indeed an identity for the operation of age-dependent matrix convolutions.

Drop the symbols x and t in Eq. (4.3.12) and let the symbol $*$ stand for the operation of age-dependent matrix convolutions. Then, Eq. (4.3.12) may be written in the compact form:

$$(\mathbf{q}^{(0)} - \mathbf{q}) * \mathbf{P} = \mathbf{D}\ . \qquad (4.3.14)$$

To solve this equation, we must find a $r_2 \times r_2$ matrix-valued inverse function $\mathbf{m}(x,t) = (m_{ij}(x,t))$, the renewal density, such that:

$$\mathbf{m} * (\mathbf{q}^{(0)} - \mathbf{q}) = \mathbf{q}^{(0)}\ . \qquad (4.3.15)$$

An equivalent form of this equation expressed in the complete notation is:

$$\mathbf{m}(x,t) = \mathbf{q}^{(0)}(x,t) + \sum_{s=0}^{t} \mathbf{m}(x,s)\mathbf{q}(x+s,t-s)\ , \qquad (4.3.16)$$

which holds for all $x, t = 0, 1, 2, \cdots$. From this equation, it can be seen that $\mathbf{m}(x,0) = \mathbf{I}_{r_2}$ for all $x \geq 0$. If we further suppose that $\mathbf{q}(x,0) = \mathbf{0}_{r_2}$ for all $x \geq 0$ so that it takes at least one time unit for a transition to occur with positive probability, then Eq. (4.3.16) becomes:

$$\mathbf{m}(x,t) = \sum_{s=0}^{t-1} \mathbf{m}(x,s)\mathbf{q}(x+s,t-s) \qquad (4.3.17)$$

for $x \geq 1$ and $t \geq 1$. This equation is particularly useful, for if the values of the matrix $\mathbf{q}(x,t)$ are specified numerically on a finite lattice of (x,t)-points, then for each x the function $\mathbf{m}(x,t)$ may be computed recursively in $t = 0, 1, 2, \cdots$.

Having computed the renewal density $\mathbf{m}(x,t)$ on a finite lattice of (x,t)-points, it is easy, in principle, to find the numerical solutions of Eqs. (4.3.11) and (4.3.12). For example, the solution of Eq. (4.3.12) on a finite lattice of (x,t)-points is:

$$\mathbf{f}(x,t) = \sum_{s=0}^{t} \mathbf{m}(x,s)\mathbf{r}(x+s,t-s) . \tag{4.3.18}$$

A similar expression may be written down for the solution of Eq. (4.3.12) on a finite lattice of (x,t)-points, but the details will be omitted.

As the foregoing discussion illustrates, given a numerical specification of the density matrix $\mathbf{a}(x,t) = (a_{ij}(x,t))$ on a finite lattice of (x,t)-points, it becomes feasible to compute the matrix $\mathbf{f}(x,t)$ of absorption densities as well as the matrix $\mathbf{P}(x,t) = (P_{ij}(x,t))$ of transition probabilities on this lattice. But, up to now no mention has been made of the problems that arise in specifying the density matrix numerically. There are a number of methods that may be used to find numerical specification of the density matrix on a finite lattice of (x,t)-points.

One approach to numerically specifying the density matrix is to revert to a continuous time formulation and again appeal to the classical theory of competing risks. Suppose that for each state $i \in \mathfrak{S}$ there is a continuous latent risk function $\eta_{ij}(x,t)$ governing transitions to state $j \in \mathfrak{S}$ as a function of $t \geq 0$ for an individual entering state i at age x. Then, the latent distribution function corresponding to this risk function is:

$$F_{ij}(x,t) = 1 - \exp\left[-\int_0^t \eta_{ij}(x,s)ds\right] \tag{4.3.19}$$

for $t \geq 0$. And, the probability this individual is still in state i at time $t > 0$ is given by the survival function:

$$S_i(x,t) = \prod_{j=1}^{r} (1 - F_{ij}(x,t)) . \tag{4.3.20}$$

By appealing to the classical theory of competing risks, it follows that for $t > 0$:

$$A_{ij}(x,t) = \int_0^t S_i(x,u)\eta_{ij}(x,u)du \ . \tag{4.3.21}$$

If it is feasible to compute this function on a finite lattice of (x,t)-points, then the density matrix may be computed as:

$$a_{ij}(x,t) = A_{ij}(x,t) - A_{ij}(x,t-1) \ , \tag{4.3.22}$$

where $x, t = 0, 1, 2, \cdots$.

Choosing models for the latent risk functions $\eta_{ij}(x,t)$ can be problematic, since this function actually depends on four variables i, j, x and t. To reduce the dimensionality of the problem, it is useful to suppose that there are latent risk functions $\theta_{ij}(x)$ that govern transitions from any state i to any state j as a function of an individual's age x. Then, the latent risk functions going into Eq. (4.3.21) may be chosen as:

$$\eta_{ij}(x,t) = \theta_{ij}(x+t) \ . \tag{4.3.23}$$

This assumption seems plausible biologically, because there is reason to believe that transitions from some state to another will depend on the age of an individual. For example, suppose the state space of an age-dependent semi-Markov process contains the states i = "married" and j = "divorced". The longer a person is married, the less likely that the marriage will end in divorce, which suggests that the latent risk function for the transition $i \to j$ should be a decreasing function of age $x > 0$. Among the choices for the latent risk function in Eq. (4.3.23) for this transition is that of the Weibull distribution; namely,

$$\theta_{ij}(x) = \alpha_{ij} x^{\alpha_{ij}-1} \ , \tag{4.3.24}$$

where α_{ij} is a shape parameter such that $0 < \alpha_{ij} < 1$. If necessary, a scale parameter $\beta_{ij} > 0$ could be added to the risk function in Eq. (4.3.24) to gauge the timing of the transitions. When the state space contains relatively few states, as is frequently the case for many models discussed in this book, the methods just outlined become feasible for numerically specifying the $r \times r$ density matrix $\mathbf{a}(x,t)$, particularly when only a few transitions out of any state are possible.

Methods of the type just described, along with others, have been used extensively in Mode[2] and further discussion of these methods and their application to demography and other social sciences may by found in Mode.[1] These references, as well as the references cited therein, may be consulted for further details and examples of applications of age-dependent semi-Markov processes. Although this class of jump processes have not, as yet, been used extensively in HIV/AIDS epidemiology, they are worthy of consideration when age is a variable that should be accommodated in a model.

4.4 Discrete Time Non-Stationary Jump Processes

Apart from the discussion of Markov jump processes with non-stationary transition probabilities in Section 3.5, no attention has been given to processes with time inhomogeneous laws of evolution. Accordingly, the purpose of this section is explore two sub-classes of Markovian processes in discrete time, with laws of evolution that may change in time, from the sample path perspective. In one class, the age of an individual when entering a state will not be taken into account; while, in a second class, the age of an individual when entering a state will be accommodated in the model. As in previous sections, it will supposed that the state space $\mathfrak{S}$ of the process is partitioned into a set $\mathfrak{S}_1$ of $r_1 \geq 1$ absorbing states and a disjoint set $\mathfrak{S}_2$ of $r_2 \geq 1$ transient states with time represented by the set of non-negative integers $0, 1, 2, \cdots$.

When the laws governing the evolution of a jump process change with time, it will be convenient to refer to particular points in time as epochs to clearly distinguish between durations of time, such as the sojourn time in some state, and the time when a jump occurs or when we observe the state of the process at some time (epoch). In the non-age dependent case, a density matrix $\mathbf{a}(s,t) = (\, a_{ij}(s,t))$ of functions is again a basic ingredient underlying the process, given that the process enters state i at epoch s, $a_{ij}(s,t)$ is the conditional probability it jumps to state $j \neq i$ at epoch $t > s$. In this case, the sojourn time in state i is $t-s$. Let the sequence of random variable X_k, $k = 1, 2, \cdots$, represent the state entered at the kth jump and the random variable T_k represent the epoch at which the kth jump occurs. Then, because the time set under consideration is the non-negative integers and at least one unit of time must transpire before a jump is recorded, it follows that $T_0 < T_1 < T_2 < \cdots$ with probability one.

A sample path for the first $n \geq 1$ jumps is the set:

$$\{(i_k, t_k) \mid k = 0, 1, \cdots, n\} \tag{4.4.1}$$

of realizations of pairs of random variables (X_k, T_k), $k = 0, 1, 2 \cdots$. The probability measure $\mathbb{P}$ on the sample paths of the process is determined from the collection of conditional probabilities:

$$\mathbb{P}[A \mid B] = \prod_{k=1}^{n} a_{i_{k-1}, i_k}(t_{k-1}, t_k) \tag{4.4.2}$$

where $A = [X_k = i_k, T_k = t_k]$ and $B = [X_0 = i_0, T_0 = t_0]$, defined for $n \geq 1$, states $i_0, i_1, \cdots, i_n$ in $\mathfrak{S}$ and epochs $t_0 < t_1 < t_2 < \cdots$. From this assignment of the probability measure underlying the process, it is easy to see that the sequence of pairs of random variables (X_k, T_k), $k = 0, 1, 2, \cdots$ has the Markov property so that the future probabilistic evolution of the process depends only on the last state visited, the epoch at which this state was entered and the laws governing the evolution process beyond this epoch. As in the process discussed in the previous section, it is again useful to represent the density matrix in the partitioned form:

$$\mathbf{a}(s,t) = \begin{bmatrix} \mathbf{0}_{r_1, r_1} & \mathbf{0}_{r_1, r_2} \\ \mathbf{r}(s,t) & \mathbf{q}(s,t) \end{bmatrix}, \tag{4.4.3}$$

where the sub-matrices are defined similarly to those in Section 4.3. If we suppose that at least one unit of time must transpire before any jumps can occur with positive probability, then it follows that $\mathbf{a}(s,s) = \mathbf{0}$, a $r \times r$ zero matrix, for all $s \geq 0$.

Given that the process enters a transient state $i \in \mathfrak{S}_2$ at epoch s, let $f_{ij}(s,t)$ be the conditional probability the process enters the absorbing state $j \in \mathfrak{S}_1$ at epoch $t > s$, and let $\mathbf{f}(s,t) = (f_{ij}(s,t))$ be a $r_2 \times r_1$ matrix of these absorption probabilities. Then, because the sequence of pairs of random variables (X_k, T_k), $k \geq 0$, has the Markov property, it can be shown that this matrix satisfies the equation:

$$\mathbf{f}(s,t) = \mathbf{r}(s,t) + \sum_{u=s}^{t} \mathbf{q}(s,u)\mathbf{f}(u,t) \ . \tag{4.4.4}$$

With respect to evolution among transient states, let $P_{ij}(s,t)$ be the conditional probability the process is in transient state $j \in \mathfrak{S}_2$ at epoch t, given that it entered transient state $i \in \mathfrak{S}_2$ at epoch $s < t$, and let $\mathbf{P}(s,t) = (P_{ij}(s,t))$ be a $r_2 \times r_2$ matrix of these conditional probabilities. This matrix-valued function also satisfies an equation similar to Eq. (4.4.4), but to derive this equation further definitions will be needed.

For a process with time inhomogeneous laws of evolution, the density of a sojourn time in transient state i is given by:

$$a_i(s,t) = \sum_{j \in \mathfrak{S}} a_{ij}(s,t) \ , \tag{4.4.5}$$

when the process enters state i at epoch s, with corresponding distribution function:

$$A_i(s,t) = \sum_{u=s}^{t} a_i(s,t) \ . \tag{4.4.6}$$

Thus, $1 - A_i(s,t)$ is the conditional probability that the process is still in state t at epoch $t > s$, given that it entered state i at epoch s. It will be supposed that for all transient states i:

$$\lim_{t \uparrow \infty} A_i(s,t) = 1 \tag{4.4.7}$$

for all $s \geq 0$. Let $\mathbf{D}(s,t) = (\delta_{ij}(1 - A_i(s,t)))$ be a $r_2 \times r_2$ diagonal matrix. Then, it can be shown that the matrix $\mathbf{P}(s,t)$ satisfies the equation:

$$\mathbf{P}(s,t) = \mathbf{D}(s,t) + \sum_{u=s}^{t} \mathbf{q}(s,u)\mathbf{P}(u,t) \ . \tag{4.4.8}$$

Note that if this matrix equation was expressed in element-by-element form, then it would resemble equation Eq. (3.5.16), which was derived from the backward Kolmogorov differential equations for a continuous time Markov jump process with non-stationary transition probabilities.

Given a numerical specification of the density matrix $\mathbf{a}(s,t)$ on some finite triangular lattice of (s,t)-points, Eq. (4.4.4) for the matrix of absorption probabilities may be solved recursively for fixed values of $s < t$. Under the assumption that at least one unit of time must elapse before a jump is recorded, then it follows that $\mathbf{f}(t,t) = \mathbf{0}$, a $r_2 \times r_1$ zero matrix, for all $t \geq 0$. Therefore, if $s = t-1$, then from Eq. (4.4.4) it can be seen that:

$$\mathbf{f}(t-1,t) = \mathbf{r}(t-1,t) \ . \tag{4.4.9}$$

Similarly, if $s = t-2$, then

$$\begin{aligned}\mathbf{f}(t-2,t) &= \mathbf{r}(t-2,t) + \sum_{u=t-1}^{t-1} \mathbf{q}(t-2,u)\mathbf{f}(u,t) \\ &= \mathbf{r}(t-2,t) + \mathbf{q}(t-2,t-1)\mathbf{f}(t-1,t-2)\end{aligned} \tag{4.4.10}$$

More generally, suppose it is required to compute the triangular of matrices $\mathbf{f}(t-k,t)$ for $s < t$ and $k = 1, 2, \cdots, t-s$. If $s = t-k$, then

$$\mathbf{f}(t-k,t) = \mathbf{r}(t-k,t) + \sum_{u=t-(k-1)}^{t-1} \mathbf{q}(t-k,u)\mathbf{f}(u,t) \ . \tag{4.4.11}$$

Hence, if $\mathbf{f}(u,t)$ has been computed for $u = t-(k-1), \cdots, t-1$, then $\mathbf{f}(t-k,t)$ may be computed. It is thus clear that by executing this triangular procedure for $k = 1, 2, \cdots, t-s$, the desired array of matrices may be computed recursively.

Eq. (4.4.8) may also be solved by executing a triangular procedure recursively. In this case, the condition $\mathbf{P}(t,t) = \mathbf{I}_{r_2}$, a $r_2 \times r_2$ identity matrix, is satisfied for all $t \geq 0$. Therefore,

$$\begin{aligned}\mathbf{P}(t-1,t) &= \mathbf{D}(t-1,t) + \mathbf{q}(t-1,t)\mathbf{P}(t,t) \\ &= \mathbf{D}(t-1,t) + \mathbf{q}(t-1,t) \ .\end{aligned} \tag{4.4.12}$$

In general, for $k = 1, 2, \cdots, t-s$,

$$\mathbf{P}(t-k,t) = \mathbf{D}(t-k,t) + \sum_{u=t-(k-1)}^{t} \mathbf{q}(t-k,u)\mathbf{P}(u,t) \ . \tag{4.4.13}$$

Therefore, if $\mathbf{P}(u,t)$ has been computed for $u = t - (k-1), \cdots, t-1$, then $\mathbf{P}(t-k,t)$ may be determined.

Constructing models of Markovian processes with time inhomogeneous laws of evolution gives rise to the problem of constructing and computing the one-step transition densities. Unlike time homogeneous models, in which the basic ingredients of the model may be densities or distribution functions, in the time inhomogeneous case, a basic ingredient is a set of risk functions. To illustrate these ideas, attention will initially be focused on the non-age dependent case. For every transient state $i \in \mathfrak{S}_2$, let $q_{ij}(t)$ be the conditional probability that the process jumps to state $j \in \mathfrak{S}$ at epoch t, given it was in state i at epoch $t-1$. Observe that it is being assumed that the evolution of the process prior to epoch $t-1$ is being "forgotten" in the sense that $q_{ij}(t)$ depends only on the state the process was at epoch $t-1$.

Then, given that the process was in state i at epoch $t-1$,

$$q_i(t) = \sum_{j \in \mathfrak{S}} q_{ij}(t) \tag{4.4.14}$$

is the conditional probability of a jump to some other state by epoch t. The conditional probability that the process is still in state i at epoch t, given it was in state i at epoch $t-1$, is $p_i(t) = 1 - q_i(t)$. Therefore,

$$S_i(s,t) = \prod_{u=s+1}^{t} p_i(u) \tag{4.4.15}$$

is the conditional probability that the process is still in state i at epoch $t > s$, given that it was in state i at epoch s. Let $a_{ij}(s,t)$ be the conditional probability the process jumps to state $j \in \mathfrak{S}$ at epoch $t > s$, given that it was in state $i \in \mathfrak{S}_2$ at epoch s. Then,

$$a_{ij}(s,t) = S_i(s,t-1)q_{ij}(t) \,. \tag{4.4.16}$$

In principle, if the set $\{q_{ij}(t) \mid i \in \mathfrak{S}_2,\ j \in \mathfrak{S} \text{ and } t = 1,2,3,\cdots\}$ of finitely many risk functions has been determined, then the densities in Eq. (4.4.16) may be computed on a finite lattice of (s,t)-points such that $s < t$.

Various schemes may be used to specify finitely many risk functions and the following simple example illustrates an idea that may be useful. Suppose the risk functions have the form

$$q_{ij}(t) = q_i(t)\pi_{ij} \; , \tag{4.4.17}$$

where, for $j \neq i$, π_{ij} is the constant conditional probability of a jump to state j by epoch t, given that the process was in state i at epoch $t-1$. A question that natural arises is: What is a useful and understandable way of specifying the probabilities $q_i(t)$ for finitely many values of t? One approach to answering this question is to suppose that the value of $q_i(t)$ was in force indefinitely and let the random variable $U_i(t)$ be the sojourn time in state i when this constant prevails. Then, $U_i(t)$ would have a geometric distribution with density

$$P\left[U_i(t) = u\right] = p_i(t)(q_i(t))^{u-1} \tag{4.4.18}$$

for $u = 1, 2, 3, \cdots$, where $p_i(t) = 1 - q_i(t)$, and expectation

$$E\left[U_i(t)\right] = \frac{1}{p_i(t)} \; . \tag{4.4.19}$$

Thus, if one has some feeling for these expectations for finitely many values of t, then the conditional probabilities $p_i(t)$ and $q_i(t)$ could be determined. The procedure just suggested resembles constructing population projections for human populations when mortality is either decreasing or increasing, by specifying a sequence of period expectations of life at birth (see Mode[2] for details).

4.5 Age Dependency with Time Inhomogeneity

As was suggested in a foregoing section, there are situations in epidemiology in which it is desirable to take age into account when considering models describing the evolution of cohorts of individuals among a set of states in a Markovian type process. Previously, it was supposed that the laws of evolution underlying the process were time homogenous, but it is also of interest to consider the case where these laws may change in time. To this end, suppose that for every transient state

$i \in \mathfrak{S}_2$, densities have been specified such that $a_{ij}(x,s,t)$ is the conditional probability of a jump to state $j \in \mathfrak{S}$ at epoch t, given that state i was entered at epoch $s < t$ when an individual is of age x. Rather than going through the exercise of setting down the foundations of this class of processes, an exercise that will be left to the reader, we will proceed directly to the consideration of equations for the matrix $\mathbf{f}(x,s,t) = (f_{ij}(x,s,t) \mid i \in \mathfrak{S}_2, j \in \mathfrak{S}_1)$ of absorption probabilities and the matrix $\mathbf{P}(x,s,t) = (P_{ij}(x,s,t) \mid i \in \mathfrak{S}_2, j \in \mathfrak{S}_2)$ of transition probabilities for multiple jumps among transient states.

Like all equations considered thus far, equations for these matrices in the age-dependent case may be derived by using the Markov property underlying the process and a first step (jump) decomposition argument. With regard to the matrix of absorption probabilities, the matrix $\mathbf{r}(x,s,t)$ covers the case where there is a transition from some transient state to an absorbing state on the first jump at epoch $t > s$. But, if the first jump consists of a transition to another transient state at some epoch $u \geq s$, then the age of this individual when entering this transient state is $x+u-s$. Thus, by using the Markov property, it follows that the matrix of absorption probabilities satisfies the equation:

$$\mathbf{f}(x,s,t) = \mathbf{r}(x,s,t) + \sum_{u=s}^{t} \mathbf{q}(x,s,t)\mathbf{f}(x+u-s,u,t) \tag{4.5.1}$$

for all (x,s,t)-points such that $x \geq 0$ and $s \leq t$.

Let $1-A_i(x,s,t)$ be the conditional probability that the process is still in transient state i at epoch $t > s$, given that state i was entered at epoch s when an individual is age of x. Further, let it be the case that $\mathbf{D}(x,s,t) = (\delta_{ij}(1-A_i(x,s,t)))$ is a $r_2 \times r_2$ diagonal matrix. Then, by another first step decomposition argument, it can be shown, by using the Markov property, that the matrix $\mathbf{P}(x,s,t)$ satisfies the equation:

$$\mathbf{P}(x,s,t) = \mathbf{D}(x,s,t) + \sum_{u=s}^{t} \mathbf{q}(x,s,u)\mathbf{P}(x+u-s,u,t) \tag{4.5.2}$$

holds for all points (x,s,t) such that $x \geq 0$ and $s \leq t$. Even though the arrays of matrices arising in these equations are functions of three variables, it is still possible to solve these equations recursively by a triangular procedure.

Again, suppose that at least one unit of time has elapsed before a jump is recorded, so that $\mathbf{r}(x,s,s) = \mathbf{0}_{r_1,r_2}$ and $\mathbf{q}(x,s,s) = \mathbf{0}_{r_2,r_2}$ for all $x, s \geq 0$. Under this assumption

$$\mathbf{f}(x,t-1,t) = \mathbf{r}(x,t-1,t) \tag{4.5.3}$$

for all $x \geq 0$. If $s = t-2$, then

$$\mathbf{f}(x,t-2,t) = \mathbf{r}(x,t-2,t) + \mathbf{q}(x,t-2,t-1)\mathbf{f}(x+1,t-1,t)\ . \tag{4.5.4}$$

Thus, if $\mathbf{f}(x+1,t-1,t)$ has been computed for all $x+1$, then $\mathbf{f}(x,t-2,t)$ may be determined for all x. In general, for $k = 1,2,\cdots,t-s$,

$$\mathbf{f}(x,t-k,t) = \mathbf{r}(x,t-k,t) + \sum_{u=t-(k-1)}^{t-1} \mathbf{q}(x,s,u)\mathbf{f}(x+u-(t-k),u,t)\ . \tag{4.5.5}$$

In the sum on the right, the smallest age increment, say $\nu = u-(t-k)$, occurs when $u = t-(k-1)$, so that $\nu = 1$ and the largest occurs when $u = t-1$ so that $\nu = k-1$. Therefore, if $\mathbf{f}(x+\nu,u,t)$ has been computed for $\nu = 1,2,\cdots,k-1$ and $u = t-(k-1),\cdots,t-1$ for all x, then $\mathbf{f}(x,t-k,t)$ may be determined for all x under consideration.

Eq. (4.5.1) may also be solved by a similar procedure. For all x and t, let $\mathbf{P}(x,t,t) = \mathbf{I}_{r_2}$, be a $r_2 \times r_2$ identity matrix. Then, if $s = t-1$,

$$\mathbf{P}(x,t-1,t) = \mathbf{D}(x,t-1,t) + \mathbf{q}(x,t-1,t) \tag{4.5.6}$$

for all x. In general, for $k = 1,2,\cdots,t-s$,

$$\mathbf{P}(x,t-k,t) = \mathbf{D}(x,t-k,t) + \sum_{u=t-(k-1)}^{t} \mathbf{q}(x,t-k,u)\mathbf{P}(x+u-(t-k),u,t) \tag{4.5.7}$$

for all x and $t > s$. Hence, if $\mathbf{P}(x + \nu, u, t)$ has been computed for $\nu = 1, 2, \cdots, k - 1$ and $u = t - (k - 1), \cdots, t - 1$ for every x, then the matrix $\mathbf{P}(x, t - k, t)$ may be determined for all x. Rather large arrays may arise when finding numerical solutions to the triangular systems just discussed, but, as the amount of available memory in computers increases, the practical handling of such large arrays becomes more and more feasible, particularly when the state space $\mathfrak{S}$ is relatively small as is the case for stages of HIV disease.

Risk functions are also a basic ingredient in constructing an age-dependent Markovian process with time inhomogeneous laws of evolution. In this case, define $q_{ij}(x, t)$ as the conditional probability of a jump to state $j \neq i$ by epoch t, given an individual of age x was in transient state i at epoch $t - 1$. Like the time homogeneous case, it will be assumed that the past before epoch $t - 1$ is "forgotten". Then, given an individual of age x is in state i at epoch $t - 1$,

$$q_i(x, t) = \sum_{j \in \mathfrak{S}} q_{ij}(x, t) \tag{4.5.8}$$

is the conditional probability of a jump to another state by epoch t, and $p_i(x, t) = 1 - q_i(x, t)$ is the probability this individual is still in state i at epoch t. Given that an individual of age x is in state i at epoch s,

$$S_i(x, s, t) = \prod_{u=s+1}^{t} p_i(x + u - s, u) \tag{4.5.9}$$

is the conditional probability this individual is still in state i at epoch $t > s$. Let $a_{ij}(x, s, t)$ be the conditional probability that an individual makes a jump to state $j \neq i$ at epoch $t > s$, given the individual was of age x at epoch s and in state i. Then,

$$a_{ij}(x, s, t) = S_i(x, s, t - 1) q_{ij}(x + t - s, t) \tag{4.5.10}$$

for all x, s, and t such that $s < t$. Just as for the case of a time homogeneous model, a further discussion of methods for specifying models of the set $\{q_{ij}(x, t) \mid i \in \mathfrak{S}_2, j \in \mathfrak{S}\}$ of risk functions for finitely many pairs of points (x, t) is appropriate, but discussion of these details will be deferred to a subsequent chapter.

4.6 On Estimating Parameters From Data

Suppose one is considering a Markov process with the transition function $P_{ij}(s,t)$, which is a solution of the Kolmogorov differential equations, and let the random function $X(t)$ represent the state of the process at time t. If it is the case that the transition functions are stationary, then $P_{ij}(s,t) = P_{ij}(t-s)$, for $s < t$. Also suppose the transition function depends on some vector of parameters $\boldsymbol{\theta} \in \boldsymbol{\Theta}$, a parameter space. The time parameter may be either discrete or continuous. If in a sample of $n \geq 1$ individuals, the uth individual is observed to occupy states i_{uv}, $v = 0, 1, 2, \cdots, n_u$ at times $t_{u0} < t_{u1} < t_{u2} < \cdots < t_{un_u}$, then the likelihood function of the sample is:

$$L(\boldsymbol{\theta}) = \prod_{u=1}^{n} \prod_{v=1}^{n_u} P_{i_{u,v-1} i_{uv}}(t_{u,v-1}, t_{uv}) \,. \tag{4.6.1}$$

Whether it is practical to estimate the parameter vector $\boldsymbol{\theta}$ by the method of maximum likelihood will depend on the ease with which the transition function can be computed. For the case of a continuous time parameter model, the computation of the transition function can be very difficult except for very simple cases, but if a discrete time parameter model is under consideration, then, as we have seen in the previous sections, the computation of the transition function may be feasible. On the other hand, if the process does not have the Markov property on all sets of increasing time points, such as in a semi-Markov process, then the likelihood function in Eq. (4.6.1) would not be valid. In such circumstances, one would need to consider approaches to parameter estimation other than the method of maximum likelihood.

An alternative approach to parameter estimation would be that of the method of minimum Chi-square. By way of a simple illustration, suppose a random sample of $n \geq 1$ individuals enters some state i at time $t = 0$, but no further observations are taken until some time $t > 0$, when $O_{ij}(t)$ is the number observed to be in state j. Let $\mathfrak{S}$ be the state space of the process and suppose $E_{ij}(t; \boldsymbol{\theta})$ is the expected number of individuals in state j at time t, according to some model under consideration, which may be expressed as a function of $\boldsymbol{\theta} \in \boldsymbol{\Theta}$.

Then,

$$\sum_{j\in\mathfrak{S}} O_{ij}(t) = \sum_{j\in\mathfrak{S}} E_{ij}(t;\boldsymbol{\theta}) = n \tag{4.6.2}$$

and

$$\chi^2 = \sum_{j\in\mathfrak{S}} \frac{(O_{ij}(t) - E_{ij}(t;\boldsymbol{\theta}))^2}{E_{ij}(t;\boldsymbol{\theta})} \tag{4.6.3}$$

is the Chi-square criterion of goodness of fit of the model to data. The method of minimum Chi-square estimation consists of searching the parameter space $\boldsymbol{\Theta}$ to find a value of $\widehat{\boldsymbol{\theta}}_n \in \boldsymbol{\Theta}$ such that the criterion in Eq. (4.6.3) is minimized. Observe that this criterion could easily be extended to cover cases in which all individuals not only do not start in the same state at the same time, but also may be observed at different times subsequently.

If the model were such that transition probabilities $P_{ij}(t;\boldsymbol{\theta})$ could be calculated with relative ease as functions of t and $\boldsymbol{\theta}$, then the expected values would be given by $E_{ij}(t;\boldsymbol{\theta}) = nP_{ij}(t;\boldsymbol{\theta})$. As has been illustrated in the preceding sections of this chapter, it would be feasible to calculate these transition probabilities for discrete time models, provided that the state space was relatively small, for processes that do not have the Markov property on a set of increasing time points. But, even for discrete time processes, it may be difficult to compute transition probabilities as functions of some parameter vector $\boldsymbol{\theta}$. In such cases, it may be possible to compute Monte Carlo realizations of a stochastic process, for, even if it is difficult to compute a transition function, the structure of a process is often sufficiently simple so that Monte Carlo realizations of the process can be computed with relative ease on fast, high-powered computers. Let $\widehat{E}_{ij}(t;\boldsymbol{\theta})$ be a Monte Carlo estimate of the expectation $E_{ij}(t;\boldsymbol{\theta})$ at the parameter vector $\boldsymbol{\theta} \in \boldsymbol{\Theta}$. In principle, by doing repeated Monte Carlo simulations, it may be possible to search the parameter space to find a value of $\widehat{\boldsymbol{\theta}}_n \in \boldsymbol{\Theta}$ such that the Chi-square criterion is minimized.

Among the authors who have advocated and developed computer intensive methods of estimation similar to those just discussed, when dealing with models based on stochastic processes in which it is difficult to derive explicit formulas for the likelihood or other objective functions of the data used in classical methods of statistical estimation, are Thompson et al.[5] Further discussion of these methods, along with examples, may be found in Thompson et al.[6] There are also cases arising in theoretical physics, where the size of the arrays of transition probabilities needed to test some physical theory concerning the basic structure of matter becomes so large that not even super-computers can process them in sufficiently short periods of time to be of practical use. However, by computing realizations of the stochastic process underlying the physical theory of the structure of matter, the validity of the model could be checked within a reasonable degree of confidence (see Weingarten[7] for further details).

As models used in science become more and more complex, investigators can no longer rely on results that can be derived within the classical mathematical paradigm, using only pencil and paper. Much like the empirical scientist who conducts experiments to test hypotheses, the theoretical scientist is led to conduct experiments designed to explore the properties of a model using computer intensive methods. In physics, such activity gives rise to the oxymoron 'experimental theoretical physics', an expression that may be applied equally to other fields by exchanging the word "physics" with some other appropriate phrase or word.

4.7 References

1. C. J. Mode, Increment-Decrement Life Tables and Semi-Markovian Processes from a Sample Path Perspective, K. C. Land and A. Rogers (eds.), *Multidimensional Mathematical Demography,* Academic Press, New York and London, 1982, pp. 535-565.
2. C. J. Mode, *Stochastic Processes in Demography and Their Computer Implementation,* Springer-Verlag, Berlin, Heidelberg, New York, Tokyo, 1985.
3. C. J. Mode and G. T. Pickens, Computational Methods for Renewal Theory and Semi-Markov Processes with Illustrative Examples, *American Statistician* **42:** 143-152, 1988.
4. W. Y. Tan, On the HIV Incubation Period Under non-Markovian Models, *Statistics and Probability Letters* **21:** 49-57, 1994.
5. J. R. Thompson, E. N. Neely, and B. W. Brown, SIMTEST-An Algo-

rithm for Simulation-Based Estimation of Parameters Characterizing a Stochastic Process, J. R. Thompson and B. W. Brown (eds.), *Cancer Modeling,* Marcel Dekker Inc., New York, 1987, pp. 387-415.

6. J. R. Thompson, D. N. Stivers, and K. B. Ensor, SIMTEST-Technique for Model Aggregation with Considerations of Chaos, O. Arino, D. E. Axelrod, and M. Kimmel (eds.), *Mathematical Population Dynamics,* Marcel Dekker Inc., New York, 1991.
7. D. H. Weingarten, Quarks by Computer, *Scientific American* **274:** 116-120, 1996.

Chapter 5
MODELS OF HIV LATENCY BASED ON A LOG-GAUSSIAN PROCESS

5.1 Introduction

The outline of stochastic processes presented in the preceding two chapters does not exhaust the classes of processes that have been applied in HIV/AIDS epidemiology, among which are certain classes of stationary processes in discrete and continuous time. In order to provide some basis for making informed judgements as to the relative merits of alternative approaches to constructing models of potential use in studying the epidemic, it will be helpful to provide some background on and examples of stationary processes that have been used in the quest for models of the latency period of HIV. Accordingly, the purpose of this chapter is to present some background information on constructing stationary Gaussian processes as well as certain processes that may be derived from them. After the necessary background has been put into place, a specific model will be discussed in detail and applied to data on $CD4^+$ counts.

5.2 Stationary Gaussian Processes in Continuous Time

Before proceeding to a discussion of models of the incubation period of HIV other than those discussed in the preceding two chapters, it is appropriate to provide a brief overview of stationary processes in continuous time. Let $\mathbb{R} = (-\infty, \infty)$ be the set of real numbers and let the collection of random variables,

$$\{Z(t) \mid t \in \mathbb{R}\} \tag{5.2.1}$$

be a stochastic process taking values in $\mathbb{R}$. The variable t will be interpreted as time. This process is said to be stationary if for every integer $n \geq 1$ and points $t_1, t_2, \cdots, t_n$ in $\mathbb{R}$, the collection of random variables,

$$\{Z(t_1), \cdots, Z(t_n)\} \tag{5.2.2}$$

has the same distribution as the collection,

$$\{Z(t_1 + h), \cdots, Z(t_n + h)\} \tag{5.2.3}$$

for every $h \in \mathbb{R}$. In other words, a process is stationary if all its finite dimensional distributions are invariant under any time translation.

Assume that for every $t \in \mathbb{R}$ the random variable $Z(t)$ has a finite mean and variance. Then, because of the stationarity assumption, the mean and variance functions of the process are constant so that there are constants $\mu \in \mathbb{R}$ and $\sigma^2 \in (0, \infty)$ such that:

$$\begin{aligned} \mu &= E\left[Z(t)\right] \\ \sigma^2 &= var\left[Z(t)\right] = E\left[Z^2(t)\right] - \mu^2 \end{aligned} \tag{5.2.4}$$

for all $t \in \mathbb{R}$. The covariance function of the process is:

$$\begin{aligned} \Gamma(t_1, t_2) &= cov\left[Z(t_1), Z(t_2)\right] \\ &= E\left[Z(t_1)Z(t_2)\right] - \mu^2 . \end{aligned} \tag{5.2.5}$$

The assumption of stationarity requires that this function depend only on the difference $t_2 - t_1$. Therefore, to construct a stationary process, one must be able to find a function $\Gamma(\cdot)$ such that for every t and h in $\mathbb{R}$:

$$\begin{aligned} \Gamma(h) &= cov\left[Z(t), Z(t + h)\right] \\ &= cov\left[Z(t + h), Z(t)\right] = \Gamma(-h) . \end{aligned} \tag{5.2.6}$$

This function is often referred to as the auto-covariance function. Observe that $\Gamma(0) = \sigma^2$, and, from the Cauchy-Schwartz inequality,

$$|cov\left[Z(t), Z(t + h)\right]| \leq \left(var\left[Z(t)\right] var\left[Z(t + h)\right]\right)^{\frac{1}{2}} , \tag{5.2.7}$$

it also follows that $|\Gamma(h)| \leq \sigma^2$ for all $h \in \mathbb{R}$.

An approach to constructing a probability measure $\mathbb{P}$ underlying a stationary process is to assume that every finite collection of *r.v.*'s in Eq. (5.2.2) has a multi-dimensional normal distribution with n-dimensional mean vector $\boldsymbol{\mu} = (\mu, \mu, \cdots, \mu)$ and $n \times n$ covariance matrix:

$$\boldsymbol{\Gamma}_n = (\Gamma(t_j - t_i) \mid i, j = 1, 2, \cdots, n) \ . \tag{5.2.8}$$

Such a construction is known as a normal or Gaussian process and it is completely determined by the mean μ and the auto-covariance function $\Gamma(h)$. Thus, it can be seen that if a model of some phenomenon is chosen as a stationary Gaussian process, then a basic feature of the modeling process will be the construction or choice of the auto-covariance function.

For any $n \times n$ matrix $\boldsymbol{\Gamma}_n$ to be a candidate for a covariance matrix of a vector of random variables, it must be symmetric and positive definite. From now on, the superscript prime $'$ will stand for the transpose of a matrix or vector. A matrix $\boldsymbol{\Gamma}_n$ is symmetric if $\boldsymbol{\Gamma}_n' = \boldsymbol{\Gamma}_n$. From inspection, it can be seen that the matrix in Eq. (5.2.8) is symmetric. For example, if $n = 2$ and $t_2 = t_1 + h$, then this matrix becomes

$$\boldsymbol{\Gamma}_2 = \begin{bmatrix} \sigma^2 & \Gamma(h) \\ \Gamma(h) & \sigma^2 \end{bmatrix} . \tag{5.2.9}$$

Let $\mathbf{a}$ be any $n \times 1$ vector in $\mathbb{R}^n$, the set of all n-dimensional vectors of real numbers. Then, a symmetric matrix $\boldsymbol{\Gamma}_n$ is non-negative definite if, and only if,

$$\mathbf{a}' \boldsymbol{\Gamma}_n \mathbf{a} \geq 0 \tag{5.2.10}$$

for all $\mathbf{a} \in \mathbb{R}^n$. A function $\Gamma(h)$ with domain $\mathbb{R}$ and range $\mathbb{R}$ is said to be non-negative definite if for any $n \geq 2$ and finite set of points set of points $t_1, t_2, \cdots, t_n$ in $\mathbb{R}$, the matrix $\boldsymbol{\Gamma}_n$ in Eq. (5.2.8) is non-negative definite. Therefore, any choice of auto-covariance function must have the property of non-negative definiteness.

Before proceeding to discuss a range of choices for the auto-covariance function of a process, it will instructive to pause and see why the property of non-negative definiteness is necessary. To this end, let $\mathbf{Z}$ be a $n \times 1$ vector with elements $Z(t_i)$, $i = 1, 2, \cdots, n$, and let $\boldsymbol{\mu}$ be a $n \times 1$ vector with the constant value μ. Then, the covariance matrix of $\mathbf{Z}$ may be represented in the form:

$$\boldsymbol{\Gamma}_n = E\left[(\mathbf{Z} - \boldsymbol{\mu})(\mathbf{Z} - \boldsymbol{\mu})'\right]$$

$$= (cov\left[Z(t_i), Z(t_j)\right] \mid i, j = 1, 2, \cdots, n) \ . \tag{5.2.11}$$

For any vector $\mathbf{a}$ in $\mathbb{R}^n$, $Y = \mathbf{a}'(\mathbf{Z} - \boldsymbol{\mu})$ is a scalar random variable with variance:

$$var\left[Y\right] = E\left[\left(\mathbf{a}'\left(\mathbf{Z} - \boldsymbol{\mu}\right)\right)^2\right]$$

$$= E\left[\mathbf{a}'\left(\mathbf{Z} - \boldsymbol{\mu}\right)\left(\mathbf{Z} - \boldsymbol{\mu}\right)'\mathbf{a}\right]$$

$$= \mathbf{a}'\boldsymbol{\Gamma}_n\mathbf{a} \geq 0 \ , \tag{5.2.12}$$

for all $\mathbf{a} \in \mathbb{R}^n$. Hence, the covariance matrix $\boldsymbol{\Gamma}_n$ must be non-negative definite.

Among the choices for the auto-covariance function of a model based on a stationary Gaussian process is a member of the class of characteristic functions of symmetric distributions. A random variable X, taking values in $\mathbb{R}$, has a symmetric distribution if its continuous distribution function $F(x)$ has the property:

$$F(x) = \mathbb{P}\left[X \leq x\right] = \mathbb{P}\left[X \geq -x\right] = 1 - F(-x) \tag{5.2.13}$$

for all $x \in \mathbb{R}$. From this equation, it can be seen by differentiation that for all points x such that the distribution function has a density $f(x)$, the equation $f(x) = f(-x)$ holds so that the density is an even function. In the continuous case, the characteristic function of a random variable X is defined by:

$$g(u) = E\left[e^{iuX}\right] = \int_{-\infty}^{\infty} e^{iux} f(x)dx$$

$$= \int_{-\infty}^{\infty} \cos(ux)f(x)dx \ + \ i\int_{-\infty}^{\infty} \sin(ux)f(x)dx \tag{5.2.14}$$

for all $u \in \mathbb{R}$, where i is an imaginary element such that $i^2 = -1$. Because the integrand in the second integral on the right is an odd function, the integral vanishes so that the characteristic function is real and has the form:

$$g(u) = \int_{-\infty}^{\infty} \cos(ux) f(x) dx \tag{5.2.15}$$

for all $u \in \mathbb{R}$. For the case of discrete-valued random variables, the integral would be replaced by either finite sums or a convergent infinite series.

Characteristic functions are of interest as candidates for auto-covariance functions because, from Bochner's theorem (see Loève[16] page 207 for details), a complex-valued function $g(u)$ on $\mathbb{R}$, normed such that $g(0) = 1$, is continuous and non-negative definite if, and only if, it is a characteristic function. In particular, $g(u)$ may be real valued for all $u \in \mathbb{R}$ as is the case for symmetric distributions. Consequently, Eq. (5.2.15) may be used to generate candidates for auto-covariance functions.

A famous symmetric distribution is the standard normal and, in this case, Eq. (5.2.15) becomes:

$$g(u) = \frac{1}{\sqrt{2\pi}} \int_{-\infty}^{\infty} \cos(ux) e^{-\frac{x^2}{2}} dx = e^{-\frac{1}{2}u^2} \tag{5.2.16}$$

for $u \in \mathbb{R}$. This is a well-known formula and may be found in most books on probability theory, but if the formula is not available then MAPLE, which has been integrated into the word processor used for this book, may be used to derive it. Another famous symmetric distribution is the Cauchy, and in this case Eq. (5.2.15) takes the form:

$$g(u) = \frac{1}{\pi} \int_{-\infty}^{\infty} \frac{\cos(ux)}{1+x^2} dx = e^{-|u|} \tag{5.2.17}$$

for all $u \in \mathbb{R}$. For the case of the Laplace distribution, Eq. (5.2.15) becomes:

$$\begin{aligned} g(u) &= \frac{1}{2} \int_{-\infty}^{\infty} \cos(ux) e^{-|x|} dx \\ &= \int_{0}^{\infty} \cos(ux) e^{-x} dx = \frac{1}{1+u^2} \end{aligned} \tag{5.2.18}$$

for $u \in \mathbb{R}$.

All these examples may be used as candidates for the auto-covariance function $\Gamma(h)$ of a stationary Gaussian process by choosing a positive variance σ^2, a positive scale parameter $\theta > 0$, and letting $\Gamma(h) = \sigma^2 g(\theta h)$. It will be noted that for all these choices, $\Gamma(h) \to 0$ as $|h| \to \infty$, at rates depending on the choice of $g(\cdot)$ and the scale parameter θ, indicating that when the time difference $|t_2 - t_1|$ is large, the random variables $Z(t_1)$ and $Z(t_2)$ will be weakly correlated. A number of authors have shown that if a stationary process also has the Markov property, then the auto-covariance function must have the form

$$\Gamma(h) = \sigma^2 e^{-\theta|h|} , \tag{5.2.19}$$

for $h \in \mathbb{R}$ (see Feller[13] page 96 for details), where $\theta > 0$. It is of interest to note this formula, apart from the multiplier σ^2 and the scale parameter θ, is that of the characteristic function for the Cauchy distribution.

Many candidates for the auto-covariance function of a stationary process may be generated by the following symmetrization scheme. Let X_1 and X_2 be two identically distributed random variables with common characteristic function g, and define a random variable Y as $Y = X_1 - X_2$. Then, the characteristic function of Y is:

$$\begin{aligned} g_Y(u) &= E\left[e^{iuY}\right] = E\left[e^{iuX_1}\right] E\left[e^{-iuX_2}\right] \\ &= g(u)g(-u) = |g(u)|^2 \end{aligned} \tag{5.2.20}$$

because X_1 and X_2 are independent and $g(-u)$ is the complex conjugate of $g(u)$.

A large variety of candidates for an auto-covariance function may be generated from this formula. For example, if the common distribution of X_1 and X_2 is the uniform on $(0, 1)$, then their common characteristic function is:

$$g(u) = \int_0^1 e^{iux} dx = \frac{e^{iu} - 1}{iu} \tag{5.2.21}$$

and

$$g_Y(u) = \left(\frac{e^{iu} - 1}{iu}\right)\left(\frac{e^{-iu} - 1}{-iu}\right) = \frac{2(1 - \cos u)}{u^2} . \tag{5.2.22}$$

Observe this function vanishes at the points $k2\pi$, for $k = 0, \pm 1, \pm 2, \cdots$, which implies that the random variables $Z(t)$ and $Z(t+h)$ would be uncorrelated if $h = k2\pi$.

Another example of some interest arises when the common characteristic function is that for the discrete Poisson distribution with parameter $\lambda > 0$; namely

$$g(u) = \exp(\lambda(e^{iu} - 1)) . \tag{5.2.23}$$

Then,

$$g_Y(u) = g(u)g(-u) = \exp(2\lambda(\cos u - 1)) . \tag{5.2.24}$$

Curiously, this is a periodic function with period 2π such that $g_Y(u) = 1$ for $u = k2\pi$ and $k = 0, \pm 1, \pm 2, \cdots$. In this case, the random variables $Z(t)$ and $Z(t+h)$ are perfectly and positively correlated when $h = k2\pi$.

The auto-correlation function of a stationary process is defined by:

$$\rho(h) = \frac{\Gamma(h)}{\sigma^2} \tag{5.2.25}$$

for $h \in \mathbb{R}$, and if $\Gamma(h)$ is chosen as $\Gamma(h) = \sigma^2 g(\theta h)$, then $\rho(h) = g(\theta h)$, where $\theta > 0$ and $g(u)$ is a characteristic function. In all the examples considered so far involving symmetric distributions, the characteristic function has the property $g(u) \geq 0$ for all u so that $\rho(h) \geq 0$ for all h. It seems desirable, however, that the auto-covariance function should have the property that it may be negative for some values of $h \in \mathbb{R}$. Accordingly, it would be useful to have methods of choosing $\Gamma(h)$ such that this function may be negative for some values of h.

Another interpretation of Bochner's theorem is that if $\Gamma(h)$ is a real-valued auto-covariance function, then there is a non-negative and non-decreasing function $H(x)$ on $\mathbb{R}$ such that:

$$\Gamma(h) = \int_{-\infty}^{\infty} \cos(hx) H(dx) \tag{5.2.26}$$

for $h \in \mathbb{R}$. The function $H(x)$ is called the spectral distribution function corresponding to $\Gamma(h)$, where $\Gamma(0)$ is finite. Technically, the integral in Eq. (5.2.26) is of the Lebesgue-Stieltjes type so that it may be reduced to an infinite series when the jump points of $H(x)$ are a discrete set. This would be the case, for example, if $\Gamma(h) = \sigma^2 g_Y(\theta h)$ (see Eq. (5.2.13)), where the set of jump points is $\{x \mid x = 0, \pm 1, \pm 2, \cdots\}$. If $H(x)$ has a derivative $h(x)$ on some set of points in $\mathbb{R}$, then $h(x)$ is called the spectral density. Further, $H(dx) = h(x)dx$. In the foregoing examples, specific forms of this density have been specified to yield only a few illustrative examples.

An illustrative example, in which the auto-covariance function may assume negative and positive values, occurs when the spectral density has the form:

$$h(x) = \frac{3}{2}x^2 \text{ if } x \in [-1, 1]$$

and

$$= 0 \text{ if } x \notin [-1, 1] \,. \tag{5.2.27}$$

For this choice of $h(x)$, the auto-covariance function takes the form:

$$\Gamma(h) = \frac{3}{2}\int_{-1}^{1} \cos(hx)x^2 dx$$

$$= 3\frac{h^2 \sin h + 2h \cos h - 2\sin h}{h^3} \tag{5.2.28}$$

for $h \in \mathbb{R}$. If one plots this function, it may be seen that it assumes both positive and negative values. A simpler example arises when $h(x)$ is chosen as the uniform density on $[0, 1]$, giving rise to the auto-covariance function:

$$\Gamma(h) = \int_0^1 \cos(hx)dx = \frac{\sin(h)}{h} \,. \tag{5.2.29}$$

From these examples, it may be seen that judicious choices of the spectral density will yield a variety of candidates for the auto-covariance function of a stationary Gaussian process. Using MAPLE, or other software packages that do symbolic operations, a variety of examples may be derived with relative ease in exploratory experiments aimed at deciding which auto-covariance function may be appropriate for the model under consideration. An informative and elementary treatment of auto-covariance functions may be found in Prabhu[17] in discussions of covariance stationary processes; for an advanced treatment, the classic by Doob[11] may be consulted.

When attempting to judge the appropriateness of a model, a capability for simulating realizations of the process may be helpful. Suppose, for example, the constant μ and the auto-covariance function $\Gamma(h)$ have been specified and it is desired to simulate realizations of the *r.v.*'s $Z(t_i)$, where $i = 1, 2, \cdots, n$, and $t_1 < t_2 < \cdots < t_n$. Let $\mathbf{Z}_n$ be a $n \times 1$ vector of these random variables and let $\mathbf{\Gamma}_n$ be the $n \times n$ covariance matrix of this vector, $n \geq 2$, and suppose this matrix in non-singular. According to the Cholesky factorization of a real non-singular positive definite matrix (see Kennedy and Gentle[15]), there exists a lower triangular matrix $\mathbf{L}_n$ such that:

$$\mathbf{\Gamma}_n = \mathbf{L}_n \mathbf{L}_n' \ . \tag{5.2.30}$$

Let U_n be a $n \times 1$ vector of independent standard normal random variables with common mean 0 and variance 1. Then, as is well-known, the vector random variable,

$$\mathbf{Y}_n = \mathbf{L}_n \mathbf{U}_n \tag{5.2.31}$$

has a multivariate normal distribution with mean vector $E[\mathbf{Y}_n] = \mathbf{0}_n$ and covariance matrix,

$$\begin{aligned} E\left[\mathbf{Y}_n \mathbf{Y}_n'\right] &= E\left[\mathbf{L}_n \mathbf{U}_n \mathbf{U}_n' \mathbf{L}_n'\right] \\ &= \mathbf{L}_n E\left[\mathbf{U}_n \mathbf{U}_n'\right] \mathbf{L}_n' \\ &= \mathbf{L}_n \mathbf{I}_n \mathbf{L}_n' = \mathbf{\Gamma}_n \ . \end{aligned} \tag{5.2.32}$$

The vector $\mathbf{Y}_n$, therefore, has the same covariance matrix as the vector $\mathbf{Z}_n$. To simulate realizations of the random vector $\mathbf{Z}_n$, one computes:

$$\mathbf{Z}_n = \boldsymbol{\mu}_n + \mathbf{Y}_n \ , \tag{5.2.33}$$

where $\boldsymbol{\mu}_n$ is a $n \times 1$ vector with each element equal to μ. Because many software packages contain procedures for calculating the Cholesky factorization, the procedure just outlined should work well for moderate values of n. Moreover, if the covariance matrix is nearly singular, other procedures may be devised to simulate finitely many realizations of the vector random variable $\mathbf{Z}_n$.

5.3 Stationary Gaussian Processes in Discrete Time

Among the advantages of stationary processes in continuous time is that the joint distributions of the random functions of the process are specified for any finite set of time points in $\mathbb{R}$. However, when one is faced with the problem of finding useful computer implementations of the model or when dealing with actual data, which is often collected at equally spaced points in time, it is useful to consider models formulated in discrete time. Accordingly, in this section, the time set will be chosen as:

$$\mathbb{N} = \{t \mid t = 0, \pm 1, \pm 2, \cdots\} \ , \tag{5.3.1}$$

the set of all integers. Just as in a continuous time formulation, a collection of random variables,

$$\{Z(t) \mid t \in \mathbb{N}\} \ , \tag{5.3.2}$$

taking values in $\mathbb{R}$, will be called a stationary stochastic process if all its finite dimensional distributions are invariant under any translation of time points in $\mathbb{N}$.

As in the previous section, it will be assumed that the constant expectation $E[Z(t)] = \mu$ is finite and in the discussion that follows, the random function $Y(t)$ is defined by $Y(t) = Z(t) - \mu$ so that $E[Y(t)] = 0$ for all $t \in \mathbb{N}$. Up to now, a stationary process has been determined by specifying all finite dimensional distributions of the process, but it is also useful to define processes as functions of other random variables. For example, let

$$\{\epsilon(t) \mid t \in \mathbb{N}\} \tag{5.3.3}$$

be a collection of random variables where $E[\epsilon(t)] = 0$ and $E[\epsilon^2(t)] = \sigma_\epsilon^2$ for all $t \in \mathbb{N}$, and suppose they are uncorrelated, i.e., $E[\epsilon(t)\epsilon(t')] = 0$ when $t \neq t'$. For $n \geq 1$, let $\gamma_0, \gamma_1, \gamma_2, \cdots, \gamma_n$, be constants and consider a process defined by:

$$Y(t) = \gamma_0\epsilon(t) + \gamma_1\epsilon(t-1) + \cdots + \gamma_n\epsilon(t-n) \ . \tag{5.3.4}$$

This expression is often referred to as a moving average, a name that seems to stem from the case $\gamma_i = 1/\sqrt{n+1}$ for $i = 0, 1, 2, \cdots, n$.

By inspection, it can be seen the distribution of the random variable $Y(t)$ in Eq. (5.3.4) is invariant under translations of time, and, in particular, if it is also assumed that the collection of random variables in Eq. (5.3.3) is normally and independently distributed with a common mean of 0 and variance σ_ϵ^2, then it can be shown that Eq. (5.3.4) determines a stationary Gaussian process on $\mathbb{N}$ with constant mean $E[Y(t)] = 0$, variance

$$\Gamma(0) = \left(\sum_{l=0}^{n} \gamma_i^2\right) \sigma_\epsilon^2 \tag{5.3.5}$$

and auto-covariance function

$$\Gamma(h) = \left(\sum_{i=0}^{n} \gamma_i \gamma_{i+h}\right) \sigma_\epsilon^2 \,, \tag{5.3.6}$$

where $h \geq 0$ and $\gamma_{i+h} = 0$ if $i + h > n$. This function may assume either positive or negative values, depending the γ-parameters, and if $h \geq n + 1$, then $\Gamma(h) = 0$. Given specified values of the γ-parameters, Monte Carlo realizations of the random function $Y(t)$ may be easily computed for finitely many time points in $\mathbb{N}$. From now on, it will be assumed that the collection of random variables in Eq. (5.3.3) are normally and independently distributed with mean 0 and variance σ_ϵ^2, a property that is sometimes referred to as Gaussian noise. In much of what follows, however, these random variables need only be assumed uncorrelated.

A moving average process is conceptually simple, but the condition $\Gamma(h) = 0$ if $h \geq n+1$ may be an unnecessarily restrictive property of the auto-covariance function. It is of interest, therefore, to consider alternative methods for formulating stationary processes, depending on only a few parameters. One of the simplest cases is that of a process that satisfies the stochastic difference equation,

$$Y(t) = \beta Y(t-1) + \epsilon(t) \,, \tag{5.3.7}$$

where the parameter β is constant, the ϵ's belong to the class of random variables defined in Eq. (5.3.3) and $t \in \mathbb{N}$. This difference equation is also known as an auto-regressive model of order one. All solutions of this equation depend on the two parameters β and σ_ϵ^2, and it is natural to ask what conditions the parameter β must satisfy in order that the solution of Eq. (5.3.7) is a stationary Gaussian process.

By iterating equation Eq. (5.3.7), it can be shown that:

$$Y(t) - \sum_{\nu=0}^{n} \beta^\nu \epsilon(t-\nu) = \beta^{n+1} Y(t-(n+1)) \,, \tag{5.3.8}$$

and, by squaring and taking expectations, it follows that:

$$E\left[\left(Y(t) - \sum_{\nu=0}^{n} \beta^\nu \epsilon(t-\nu)\right)^2\right]$$
$$= \beta^{2(n+1)} E\left[Y^2(t-(n+1))\right] \,. \tag{5.3.9}$$

This result suggests that the solution of Eq. (5.3.7) has the form,

$$Y(t) = \sum_{\nu=0}^{\infty} \beta^\nu \epsilon(t-\nu) \tag{5.3.10}$$

for all $t \in \mathbb{N}$, where the random infinite series, or infinite moving average, must converge in some sense. In order that the Y-process be stationary and Gaussian, it is necessary that the expectation $E\left[Y^2(t)\right]$ be finite for all t. Because the ϵ's are uncorrelated, it can be seen by squaring and formally taking expectations in Eq. (5.3.10) that

$$E\left[Y^2(t)\right] = \sigma_\epsilon^2 \sum_{v=0}^{\infty} \beta^{2v} = \frac{\sigma_\epsilon^2}{1-\beta^2} \tag{5.3.11}$$

if, and only if, $|\beta| < 1$. Moreover, when this condition is satisfied, the right-hand side of (5.3.9) converges to 0 as $n \to \infty$ and the random infinite series in Eq. (5.3.10) is said to converge in quadratic mean to a solution of the auto-regressive equation in Eq. (5.3.7).

So far no mention has been made as to whether it is mathematically valid to take expectations term by term in an infinite random series so that the resulting infinite series converges to a valid formula.

However, it is well-known that for the case of convergence in quadratic mean, the operations of taking expectations and infinite sums can be interchanged with impunity. Thus, for $h \geq 0$, the auto-covariance function of the Y-process is given by:

$$\Gamma(h) = E\left[Y(t)Y(t+h)\right]$$

$$= E\left[\sum_{v_1=0}^{\infty}\sum_{v_2=0}^{\infty}\beta^{v_1+v_2}\epsilon(t-v_1)\epsilon(t+h-v_2)\right]$$

$$= \frac{\sigma_\epsilon^2\beta^h}{1-\beta^2}\,, \tag{5.3.12}$$

and for $h \geq 0$, the auto-correlation function is:

$$\rho(h) = \frac{\Gamma(h)}{\Gamma(0)} = \beta^h\,. \tag{5.3.13}$$

If $0 < \beta < 1$, then $\rho(h)$ is positive for all $h > 0$, but if $-1 < \beta < 0$, then $\rho(h)$ is positive or negative, depending on whether h is an even or odd positive integer. This property may render the formulation unrealistic as a model for some phenomena, making it necessary to search for alternative formulations. In passing, it should be mentioned that a stationary Gaussian process generated by a first-order auto-regressive model also has the Markov property.

A second-order auto-regressive model of the form

$$Y(t) = \beta_1 Y(t-1) + \beta_2 Y(t-2) + \epsilon(t) \tag{5.3.14}$$

is a straightforward extension of the first-order process, where β_1 and β_2 are parameters, the ϵ's are Gaussian noise, and $t \in \mathbb{N}$. For this model, one may place conditions on the β-parameters so that there exists a sequence (γ_v) such that the infinite series:

$$\sum_{v=0}^{\infty}\gamma_v^2 \tag{5.3.15}$$

converges and a solution of Eq. (5.3.14) has the form of an infinite moving average,

$$Y(t) = \sum_{v=0}^{\infty}\gamma_v\epsilon(t-v)\,. \tag{5.3.16}$$

It can be shown that the convergence of the series in Eq. (5.3.15) implies the random series in Eq. (5.3.16) converges in quadratic mean. In order for Eq. (5.3.15) to converge, it suffices to require that the series:

$$\sum_{v=0}^{\infty} |\gamma_v| \tag{5.3.17}$$

converge. For, if this series converges, then $|\gamma_n| \to 0$ as $n \to \infty$, and there is an n_0 such that $n \geq n_0$ implies $|\gamma_n|^2 \leq |\gamma_n|$.

From Eq. (5.3.15), it can be seen that:

$$E\left[\epsilon(t-v)Y(t)\right] = \gamma_v \sigma_\epsilon^2 \tag{5.3.18}$$

for all $v \geq 0$ and $t \in \mathbb{N}$. Therefore, by multiplying equation Eq. (5.3.14) and taking expectations, it can be seen that the sequence (γ_v) must satisfy the second-order difference equation,

$$\gamma_v = \beta_1 \gamma_{v-1} + \beta_2 \gamma_{v-2} \ . \tag{5.3.19}$$

We seek a solution of this equation such that $\gamma_v = 0$ if $v < 0$. Under this condition, if γ_0 and γ_1 are specified, then the sequence (γ_v) may be determined recursively for $v \geq 2$, but it will be necessary to find solutions such that the resulting infinite series converges. From now on, $\gamma_0 = 1$, and from Eq. (5.3.19), it can be seen that $\gamma_1 = \beta_1$, since $\gamma_{-1} = 0$.

Suppose one searches for solutions of Eq. (5.3.19) of the form $\gamma_v = r^v$, where r is a constant. Then, it can be shown that r is a root of the quadratic equation,

$$x^2 - \beta_1 x - \beta_2 = 0 \ . \tag{5.3.20}$$

The roots of this equation are:

$$r_1 = \frac{1}{2}\beta_1 + \frac{1}{2}\sqrt{(\beta_1^2 + 4\beta_2)}$$

and

$$r_2 = \frac{1}{2}\beta_1 - \frac{1}{2}\sqrt{(\beta_1^2 + 4\beta_2)} \ , \tag{5.3.21}$$

which may be complex.

If these roots are distinct, then a solution of Eq. (5.3.19) may be represented in the form:

$$\gamma_v = c_1 r_1^v + c_2 r_2^v , \tag{5.3.22}$$

where the constants c_1 and c_2 are the solution of the equations,

$$1 = c_1 + c_2$$

$$\beta_1 = c_1 r_1 + c_2 r_2 . \tag{5.3.23}$$

Therefore, if the roots r_1 and r_1 lie in the unit circle, i.e. $|r_1| < 1$ and $|r_2| < 1$, the infinite series in Eq. (5.3.17) will converge. If $r_1 = r_2 = r$, then it can be shown that this series will also be convergent if $|r| < 1$. When numerically specifying a model for computer experiments, it may be of interest to specify the roots r_1 and r_2 such that they lie in the unit circle. Then,

$$(x - r_1)(x - r_2) = x^2 - (r_1 + r_2)x + r_1 r_2 , \tag{5.3.24}$$

which yields the values $\beta_1 = r_1 + r_2$ and $\beta_2 = -r_1 r_2$ for the β-parameters.

When the roots of Eq. (5.3.20) lie in the unit circle, the autocovariance function of the process is given by the convergent series:

$$\Gamma(h) = \sum_{v=0}^{\infty} \gamma_v \gamma_{v+h} \sigma_\epsilon^2 \tag{5.3.25}$$

for $h \geq 0$, which may not be a desirable form for computing values. By observing that

$$\Gamma(h) = E\left[Y(t-h)Y(t)\right] \tag{5.3.26}$$

for all $h \geq 0$ and t, it can be shown that this function also satisfies a second order difference equation such that:

$$\Gamma(0) = \beta_1 \Gamma(1) + \beta_2 \Gamma(2) + \sigma_\epsilon^2$$

$$\Gamma(1) = \beta_1 \Gamma(0) + \beta_2 \Gamma(1)$$

$$\Gamma(h) = \beta_1\Gamma(h-1) + \beta_2\Gamma(h-1) \tag{5.3.27}$$

for $h \geq 2$.

For $h = 2$, this is a system in three unknowns, and a call to MAPLE yields the symbolic solution,

$$\Gamma(0) = (-1+\beta_2)\frac{\sigma_\epsilon^2}{(1+\beta_2)(\beta_1-1+\beta_2)(\beta_1+1-\beta_2)},$$

$$\Gamma(1) = -\beta_1\frac{\sigma_\epsilon^2}{(1+\beta_2)(\beta_1-1+\beta_2)(\beta_1+1-\beta_2)},$$

$$\Gamma(2) = -\sigma_\epsilon^2\frac{\beta_1^2+\beta_2-\beta_2^2}{(1+\beta_2)(\beta_1-1+\beta_2)(\beta_1+1-\beta_2)}. \tag{5.3.28}$$

From inspection of this symbolic system, it can be seen that the case $\beta_2 = -1$ must be excluded to ensure all the above formulas yield finite numbers. Similarly, to ensure that the process has a non-zero variance, i.e., $\Gamma(0) \neq 0$, the case $\beta_2 = 1$ must be excluded. Given numerical values of $\Gamma(0)$ and $\Gamma(1)$, values of $\Gamma(h)$ for $h \geq 0$ may be computed recursively.

These examples, based on first-order and second-order auto-regressive models, may be generalized in countless ways and belong to a vast literature on time series. For example, a model of the form,

$$Y(t) = \beta Y(t-1) + \epsilon(t) + \alpha\epsilon(t-1) \tag{5.3.29}$$

is known as first order auto-regressive moving average process, where α and β are constant parameters and the ϵ's are Gaussian noise. Books on the subject include those of Brillinger,[8] Brockwell and Davis,[9] and Fuller.[14] Stochastic difference equations had been treated in the literature on stochastic processes for several decades, but it was not until the book by Box and Jenkins[7] was published that variations of auto-regressive models were widely used not only in analyzing data on time series, but also in attempts to deduce a model that may have generated the data.

5.4 Stationary Log-Gaussian Processes

Transformations of Gaussian processes, in either continuous or discrete time, may be used to yield other stationary processes of potential interest as models of some phenomenon. Let $Z(t)$ be a stationary Gaussian process defined for $t \in \mathbb{R}$ with mean μ and auto-covariance function $\Gamma(h)$ for $h \in \mathbb{R}$. To simplify the notation, let $\sigma^2 = \Gamma(0) > 0$ be the variance of the process. A process,

$$\{X(t) \mid t \in \mathbb{R}\} \tag{5.4.1}$$

defined by

$$X(t) = e^{Z(t)} \tag{5.4.2}$$

with range $\mathbb{R}^+ = (0, \infty)$ is called a log-Gaussian or log-normal process. Observe that for every t, $\log X(t) = Z(t)$ has a normal distribution with mean μ and variance σ^2. For $n \geq 2$ and points $t_1 < t_2 < \cdots < t_n$, the $1 \times n$ vector random variable,

$$\mathbf{Z}_n' = (\log X(t_1), \cdots, \log X(t_n)) \tag{5.4.3}$$

has a multivariate normal distribution with mean vector $\boldsymbol{\mu}_n' = (\mu, \cdots, \mu)$ and covariance matrix,

$$\boldsymbol{\Gamma}_n = (\Gamma(t_j - t_i) \mid i, j = 1, 2, \cdots, n) \ . \tag{5.4.4}$$

In symbols, $X(t) \sim N(\mu, \sigma^2)$ and

$$\mathbf{Z}_n \sim \mathbf{N}_n(\boldsymbol{\mu}_n, \boldsymbol{\Gamma}_n) \ . \tag{5.4.5}$$

The moment generating functions of the normal and multivariate normal distributions play a basic role in deducing formulas for the mean and auto-covariance functions of a log-Gaussian process. If $Z \sim N(\mu, \sigma^2)$, then the moment generating function of the random variable. Z is:

$$M_Z(s) = E\left[e^{sZ}\right]$$

$$= \frac{1}{\sqrt{2\pi}\sigma} \int_{-\infty}^{\infty} e^{sz} \exp\left[-\frac{(z-\mu)^2}{2\sigma^2}\right] dz$$

$$= \exp\left[s\mu + \frac{s^2\sigma^2}{2}\right] \tag{5.4.6}$$

for all $s \in \mathbb{R}$. Let $\mathbf{s}_n$ be a $n \times 1$ vector in $\mathbb{R}^n$, n-dimensional real Euclidean space, $n \geq 2$. Then, if $\mathbf{Z}_n \sim \mathbf{N}_n\left(\boldsymbol{\mu}_n, \boldsymbol{\Gamma}_n\right)$, the moment generating function of the random vector $\mathbf{Z}_n$ is:

$$M_n(\mathbf{s}_n) = E\left[\exp(\mathbf{s}_n'\mathbf{Z}_n)\right]$$

$$= \exp\left[\mathbf{s}_n'\boldsymbol{\mu}_n + \frac{1}{2}\mathbf{s}_n'\boldsymbol{\Gamma}_n\mathbf{s}_n\right] \tag{5.4.7}$$

for all $\mathbf{s}_n \in \mathbb{R}^n$.

From these formulas, it can be seen that the mean of the X-process is:

$$E\left[X(t)\right] = E\left[\exp(Z(t))\right]$$

$$= M_Z(1) = \exp\left[\mu + \frac{\sigma^2}{2}\right] \tag{5.4.8}$$

and the second moment is:

$$E\left[X^2(t)\right] = M_Z(2)$$

$$= \exp\left[2\mu + 2\sigma^2\right] \tag{5.4.9}$$

for all $t \in \mathbb{R}$. Hence, the variance function is constant and has the form,

$$var\left[X(t)\right] = \Gamma_X(0)$$

$$= E\left[X^2(t)\right] - \left(E\left[X(t)\right]\right)^2$$

$$= e^{2\mu+\sigma^2}\left(e^{\sigma^2} - 1\right) . \tag{5.4.10}$$

To deduce a formula for $\Gamma_X(h)$, the auto-covariance function of the process, observe that for $h \geq 0$,

$$E\left[X(t)X(t+h)\right]$$

$$= E\left[\exp\left(Z(t) + Z(t+h)\right)\right] = M_2(\mathbf{1}_2)$$

$$= \exp\left[2\mu + \sigma^2 + \Gamma(h)\right] , \tag{5.4.11}$$

where $\mathbf{1}_2 = (1, 1)$. It then follows that the auto-covariance function of the X-process has the form,

$$\begin{aligned}\Gamma_X(h) &= E[X(t)X(t+h)] - (E[X(t)])^2 \\ &= \exp\left[2\mu + \sigma^2\right](\exp[\Gamma(h)] - 1) . \end{aligned} \tag{5.4.12}$$

As it should, this formula reduces to that of the variance when $h = 0$. From these formulas, it follows that the auto-correlation function of the X-process is:

$$\begin{aligned}\rho_X(h) &= \frac{\Gamma_X(h)}{\Gamma_X(0)} \\ &= \frac{e^{\Gamma(h)} - 1}{e^{\sigma^2} - 1}\end{aligned} \tag{5.4.13}$$

for $h \in \mathbb{R}$. The sign of this function depends on the sign of $\Gamma(h)$; if $\Gamma(h) < 0$, then $\rho_X(h) < 0$, but if $\Gamma(h) > 0$, then $\rho_X(h) > 0$.

The log-Gaussian process has many potential applications, and among them is that of a model for describing variability in $CD4^+$ counts over time in healthy patients. This will be considered in the next section. Another potential use of this stationary process is given by the following example. Suppose one wants to consider $n \geq 2$ random variables $X_1, X_2, \cdots, X_n$, representing positive waiting times among events that are identically distributed but not independent. A useful candidate and tractable model for these random variables would be a log-Gaussian process.

But, a transformation of a stationary Gaussian process taking values in $\mathbb{R}^+$ is not the only range of interest for many random variables. Among these ranges is the interval $(0, 1)$, which arises in the consideration of probabilities conditioned on some process. One possible choice of a transformation from $\mathbb{R}$ to $(0, 1)$ is the logistic distribution function. Thus, a stationary logistic-Gaussian process defined by the collection of random variables,

$$\left\{ Y(t) = \frac{e^{Z(t)}}{1 + e^{Z(t)}} \mid t \in \mathbb{R} \right\} . \tag{5.4.14}$$

could be considered. It does not appear easy to deduce simple formulas for the mean and auto-covariance function of this process, but in this computer age the properties of this process may be investigated by numerical methods, including numerical integration and Monte Carlo simulation.

As will be illustrated in subsequent chapters, stochastic models are very sensitive numerically to changes in probabilities. Suppose, for example, it is known that the range of a probability should lie in a sub-interval $(\theta_1, \theta_2) \subset (0, 1)$. Then, a possible candidate for a model of this random probability is the linear transformation,

$$\{W(t) = \theta_1 + (\theta_2 - \theta_1)Y(t) \mid t \in \mathbb{R}\} \tag{5.4.15}$$

of a logistic normal process.

5.5 HIV Latency Based on a Stationary Log-Gaussian Process

Berman[5] introduced a model of the HIV latency period based on a modification of a stationary log-Gaussian process. Suppose that among healthy patients the $CD4^+$ cell count per milliliter ($CD4^+$ cells/ml) may be described by $X(t) = \exp[Z(t)]$, where $Z(t)$ is a stationary Gaussian process with mean parameter μ and auto-covariance function $\Gamma(h)$ with $\Gamma(0) = \sigma^2$. Let the random function $W(t)$ represent the count of $CD4^+$ cells/ml at time $t \in \mathbb{R}^+ = (0, \infty)$ among patients who were infected with HIV at time $t = 0$. Then, according to the model introduced by Berman, the random function $W(t)$ is given by:

$$W(t) = e^{-\delta t} X(t) , \tag{5.5.1}$$

where the parameter $\delta > 0$ represents the rate of decline in $CD4^+$ cells/ml per unit time. An advantage of this formulation is that it is no longer necessary to group $CD4^+$ counts into intervals as was the case for the Walter-Reed system.

Among patients infected with HIV at time $t = 0$, the mean $CD4^+$ count at time $t > 0$ is given by:

$$\begin{aligned} E[W(t)] &= e^{-\delta t} E[X(t)] \\ &= \exp\left[-\delta t + \mu + \frac{\sigma^2}{2}\right] , \end{aligned} \tag{5.5.2}$$

and for $h \geq 0$, the covariance function of the W-process has the form,

$$\begin{aligned} &cov\left[W(t), W(t+h)\right] \\ &= e^{-2\delta t-\delta h} cov\left[X(t), X(t+h)\right] \\ &= \exp\left[-2\delta t - \delta h + 2\mu + \sigma^2\right]\left(\exp\left[\Gamma(h)\right] - 1\right) . \end{aligned} \tag{5.5.3}$$

Because the function $\exp\left[-\delta t\right]$ is non-random or constant for every $t > 0$, the auto-correlation function of the W-process is the same as that of the X-process; namely

$$\rho_W(h) = \frac{e^{\Gamma(h)} - 1}{e^{\sigma^2} - 1} . \tag{5.5.4}$$

Apart from health care workers, who know the time they were infected with HIV through needle pricks or cuts while working with infected people, or patients who have been infected with HIV by transfusions with contaminated blood or by the use blood products, the times of infection are unknown for the vast majority of people infected with the virus. Most people become aware that they are infected with HIV when a blood test reveals they are seropositive. Accordingly, let the random variable T represent the time from infection to the time the infection is discovered and assume it is independent of the W-process. Instead of working directly with the $CD4^+$ count $W(t)$, it will be convenient to consider the log of the $CD4^+$ count described by the random function,

$$R(t) = \log W(t) = Z(t) - \mu - \delta t . \tag{5.5.5}$$

The R-process is also Gaussian with mean function $E\left[R(t)\right] = \mu - \delta t$, but has the same covariance function $\Gamma(h)$ as the Z-process. Because it was assumed T is independent of the W-process, it is also independent of the R-process.

When applying the model to data, one must not only estimate the parameters μ, σ^2 and δ, but usually also make some assumptions about the auto-covariance function $\Gamma(h)$ and $f(t)$, the probability density function of the random variable T. The parameters μ and σ^2 may be estimated from data on healthy patients, and given such estimates, attention may be focused on the parameter $\delta > 0$. By definition of the random variable T, the random variable $R(T)$ represents the log CD4$^+$ count when the infection is discovered at some clinic and $R(0)$ is the value of this random variable at the time of infection. Now suppose a second visit to a clinic occurs at time $T+h$. Then, the random variable,

$$U(h) = \frac{R(T) - R(T+h)}{h} \tag{5.5.6}$$

is the change in log CD4$^+$ count per unit time.

Given that $T = t$, the conditional distribution of the random variables $R(t)$ and $R(t+h)$ is that of a bivariate normal with mean vector,

$$\boldsymbol{\mu}_R' = (\mu - \delta t,\ \mu - \delta(t+h)) \tag{5.5.7}$$

and covariance matrix

$$\boldsymbol{\Gamma}_R = \begin{bmatrix} \sigma^2 & \Gamma(h) \\ \Gamma(h) & \sigma^2 \end{bmatrix}. \tag{5.5.8}$$

It follows that, given $T = t$, the random variable $U(h)$ in Eq. (5.5.6) has a conditional normal distribution with expectation,

$$E\left[U(h) \mid T = t\right] = \delta \tag{5.5.9}$$

and variance,

$$var\left[U(h) \mid T = t\right] = \frac{2\left(\sigma^2 - \Gamma(h)\right)}{h^2}. \tag{5.5.10}$$

Since the normal distribution is completely determined by its mean and variance, and the above conditional expectation and variance do not depend on t, the conditional and unconditional distributions of $U(h)$ are the same.

By a similar argument, the random variable $R(T) = Z(T) - \delta T$ has the same distribution as the random variable $Z(0) - \delta T$, where, by assumption, $Z(0)$ and T are independent. From this observation and the additional assumption that T has a finite variance, a formula for the correlation coefficient of $R(T)$ and T may be derived. The expectation and variance of $R(T)$ are given by:

$$E\left[R(T)\right] = E\left[Z(0) - \delta T\right] = \mu - \delta E\left[T\right] \tag{5.5.11}$$

and

$$var\,[R(T)] = var\,[Z(0) - \delta T] = \sigma^2 + \delta^2 var\,[T]\ . \tag{5.5.12}$$

Similarly,

$$cov\,[R(T), T] = cov\,[Z(0) - \delta T,\ T] = -\delta var\,[T]\ . \tag{5.5.13}$$

From these formulas, it can be shown that the desired correlation coefficient may be expressed in the form:

$$\rho_{R,T} = \frac{cov\,[R(T),\ T]}{\sqrt{var[R(T)]\ var\,[T]}}$$

$$= -\left(\frac{var\left[\dfrac{\delta T}{\sigma}\right]}{1 + var\left[\dfrac{\delta T}{\sigma}\right]}\right)^{\frac{1}{2}} . \tag{5.5.14}$$

Curiously, this correlation, which is always negative, depends on the Z-process only through the parameter σ. For every fixed value of the ratio δ/σ, the larger the value of $var\,[T]$, the closer the correlation is to -1.

Because the parameters μ, σ and δ may be estimated easily from data, it will be assumed that they are known in the derivation of the joint density of the random variables $R(T)$ and T. In this derivation, it will be convenient to work with the random variables,

$$X = \frac{R(T) - \mu}{\sigma} = \frac{Z(T) - \mu}{\sigma} - \frac{\delta}{\sigma}T = V_1 - V_2\ . \tag{5.5.15}$$

Given $V_2 = (\delta/\sigma)T = v$, the conditional *p.d.f.* of the random variable X is normal with mean $-v$ and variance 1. Let $g(v)$ be the *p.d.f.* of the random variable V_2. Then, the joint *p.d.f.* of the random variables X and V_2 is:

$$h(x, v) = \frac{1}{\sqrt{2\pi}} \exp\left[-\frac{(x+v)^2}{2}\right] g(v) \tag{5.5.16}$$

for $x \in \mathbb{R}$ and $v \in \mathbb{R}^+$, so that the unconditional density of X is the marginal density,

$$h_1(x) = \frac{1}{\sqrt{2\pi}} \int_0^\infty \exp\left[-\frac{(x+v)^2}{2}\right] g(v)dv \tag{5.5.17}$$

for $x \in \mathbb{R}$. Given $X = x$, the posterior density of V_2 is:

$$h(v \mid x) = \frac{h(x,v)}{h_1(x)}, \tag{5.5.18}$$

provided that $h_1(x) \neq 0$.

The density $h_1(x)$ in Eq. (5.5.17) is uniquely determined by the density $g(v)$, and conversely, given the density $h_1(x)$, the density $g(v)$ is determined. The proof of this statement will be omitted, but the technical details entail passing to Fourier transforms in Eq. (5.5.17). From a sample $X_1, X_2, \cdots, X_n$ of independent observations on the random variable $X = (R(T) - \mu)/\sigma$, the statistical problem is that of drawing inferences about the distribution of the random variable $V_2 = (\delta/\sigma)T$. As one might expect, the moments of the density $h_1(x)$ in Eq. (5.5.17) are closely related to those of the density $g(v)$, as one can see by appealing to Hermite polynomials.

To simplify the writing let

$$\phi(x) = \frac{1}{\sqrt{2\pi}} e^{-\frac{x^2}{2}}, \tag{5.5.19}$$

for $x \in \mathbb{R}$, be the standard normal density. Then, the Hermite polynomials are a sequence of functions $\{H_m(x)\}$ defined as $H_0(x) = 1$ and, for $m \geq 1$, $H_m(x)$ is a polynomial of degree m defined by the relation,

$$\left(\frac{d}{dx}\right)^m \phi(x) = (-1)^m H_m(x)\phi(x), \tag{5.5.20}$$

for $x \in \mathbb{R}$ (see Cramér[10] page 133 for details). These polynomials have the property,

$$\int_{-\infty}^{\infty} H_m(x)\phi(x-t)dx = t^m, \tag{5.5.21}$$

for $m = 0, 1, 2, \cdots$. From this relationship, it follows that:

$$E\left[H_m(X) \mid V_2\right] = \int_{-\infty}^{\infty} H_m(x)\phi(x + V_2)dx = (-1)^m V_2^m \quad (5.5.22)$$

for $m = 0, 1, 2, \cdots$. Therefore, by taking expectations in this expression, it can be seen that for $m = 0, 1, 2, \cdots$

$$E\left[H_m(X)\right] = E\left[E\left[H_m(X) \mid V_2\right]\right]$$

$$= (-1)^m E\left[V_2^m\right] = (-1)^m E\left[\left(\frac{\delta T}{\sigma}\right)^m\right] . \quad (5.5.23)$$

To summarize the procedures for estimating the parameters μ and σ^2, let $Z_1, Z_2, \cdots, Z_{n_1}$ be a random sample of $\log \mathrm{CD4}^+$ counts in n_1 healthy patients, who have not been infected with HIV. Then, according to the model under consideration, these random variables are a sample from a normal population $N(\mu, \sigma^2)$. It is well-known that the statistics,

$$\widehat{\mu} = \overline{Z}_{n_1} = \frac{1}{n_1}\sum_{i=1}^{n_1} Z_i$$

$$\widehat{\sigma^2} = \frac{1}{n_1}\sum_{i=1}^{n_1}\left(Z_i - \overline{Z}_n\right)^2 \quad (5.5.24)$$

are the maximum likelihood as well as the moment estimators of the unknown parameters μ and σ^2. If the sample size n_1 is sufficiently large, an investigator may wish to test the hypothesis that this is indeed a sample from the normal distribution, and thus provide a partial validation of the model.

To estimate δ, let the random variables $U_1(h_1), \cdots, U_{n_2}(h_{n_2})$, be a random sample of changes per unit time of $\log \mathrm{CD4}^+$ counts of n_2 patients who visited a clinic twice (see Eq. (5.5.6)). Then, by the method of moments and Eq. (5.5.9), the sample mean,

$$\overline{U}_{n_2} = \widehat{\delta} = \frac{1}{n_2}\sum_{i=1}^{n_2} U_i(h_i) \quad (5.5.25)$$

is an unbiased estimator of the parameter δ.

By way of estimating the first four moments of the random variable T, observe that the first four Hermite polynomials are:

$$H_1(x) = -x \ , \ H_2(x) = x^2 - 1 \ ,$$

$$H_3(x) = -\left(x^3 - 3x\right) \ , \ H_4(x) = x^4 - 6x + 3 \ . \tag{5.5.26}$$

Now suppose one has a random sample of n_3 independent observations, say $X_1, X_2, \cdots, X_{n_3}$, on the random variable,

$$X = \frac{R(T) - \widehat{\mu}}{\widehat{\sigma}} \tag{5.5.27}$$

of standardized $\log \mathrm{CD4}^+$ counts. Then, by the method of moments and Eq. (5.5.23), the sample means,

$$\overline{H}_\nu = \frac{1}{n_3} \sum_{i=1}^{n_3} H_\nu(X) \tag{5.5.28}$$

are estimators of the expectations,

$$(-1)^\nu \left(\frac{\widehat{\delta}}{\widehat{\sigma}}\right)^\nu E\left[T^\nu\right] \ , \tag{5.5.29}$$

for $\nu = 1, 2, 3, 4$. More precisely, a moment estimator of the νth moment of T is:

$$\widehat{E\left[T^\nu\right]} = (-1)^\nu \left(\frac{\widehat{\sigma}}{\widehat{\delta}}\right)^\nu \overline{H}_\nu \ . \tag{5.5.30}$$

As will be illustrated in the next section, by having a knowledge of the first four moments of the random variable T, it will be possible to draw some inferences about its unknown distribution.

Other papers dealing with HIV latency are those of Berman.[6,4] Related papers dealing with drug therapies for HIV are Berman.[3,2] And finally, a Markov process with continuous diffusion and discrete components is discussed in Berman.[1]

5.6 HIV Latency Based on the Exponential Distribution

If one assumes some parametric form of the $p.d.f.$ of the random variable T, the waiting time from infection with HIV to the time of its discovery at a clinic by a seropositive test for the virus, then some explicit formulas may derived for the marginal density $h_1(x)$ in Eq. (5.5.17) and the conditional density in Eq. (5.5.18). In applying the model to data, Berman[5] assumed the random variable T followed an exponential distribution with a $p.d.f.$ of the form,

$$f(t) = \frac{1}{\theta} \exp\left[-\frac{t}{\theta}\right] \tag{5.6.1}$$

for $t \in \mathbb{R}^+$, where $\theta > 0$. It should be mentioned that $\delta T/\sigma$ is actually the random variable under consideration, but to lighten the notation, the ratio δ/σ will be dropped in what follows.

Under this assumption, the joint density of the random variable T and

$$X = \frac{Z(T) - \mu - \delta T}{\sigma} \tag{5.6.2}$$

is:

$$h(x,t) = \frac{1}{\sqrt{2\pi}} \exp\left[-\frac{(x+t)^2}{2}\right] \theta^{-1} \exp\left[-\theta^{-1}t\right] . \tag{5.6.3}$$

And, after some algebraic simplification, this density may be expressed in the form,

$$h(x,t) = \frac{1}{\sqrt{2\pi}} \exp\left[-\frac{x^2+t^2}{2}\right] \theta^{-1} \exp\left[-(\theta^{-1}+x)t\right] , \tag{5.6.4}$$

which is equivalent to

$$h(x,t) = \sqrt{2\pi}\phi(x)\phi(t)\theta^{-1} \exp\left[-(\theta^{-1}+x)t\right] , \tag{5.6.5}$$

where $\phi(\cdot)$ is the standard normal density

$$\phi(z) = \frac{1}{\sqrt{2\pi}} \exp\left[-\frac{z^2}{2}\right] . \tag{5.6.6}$$

Therefore, the marginal density of the random variable X is:

$$h_1(x) = \sqrt{2\pi}\phi(x) \int_0^\infty \phi(t)\theta^{-1} \exp\left[-(\theta^{-1}+x)t\right] dt . \tag{5.6.7}$$

To evaluate this integral and simplify the notation, let $r = \theta^{-1} + x$. Then, by completing the square in the exponent, it can be seen that:

$$\begin{aligned}\theta^{-1} &\int_0^\infty \phi(t) \exp\left[-rt\right] dt \\ &= \theta^{-1} \exp\left[\frac{r^2}{2}\right] \int_0^\infty \phi(t+r)dt \\ &= \theta^{-1} \exp\left[\frac{r^2}{2}\right] \int_r^\infty \phi(s)ds \, . \end{aligned} \tag{5.6.8}$$

This integral may be expressed in terms of the distribution function of the standard normal distribution

$$\Phi(z) = \int_{-\infty}^{z} \phi(s)ds \, , \tag{5.6.9}$$

defined for $z \in \mathbb{R}$. Thus, by letting $\Psi(z) = 1 - \Phi(z)$, it follows that the marginal density takes the form,

$$h_1(x) = \sqrt{2\pi}\theta^{-1}\phi(x) \exp\left[\frac{(\theta^{-1}+x)^2}{2}\right] \Psi(\theta^{-1}+x) \tag{5.6.10}$$

for $x \in \mathbb{R}$. Because many software packages contain routines for computing the standard normal distribution function, this density may be evaluated numerically with relative ease.

Having derived an explicit form of the marginal density of the random variable X, it follows that the conditional density of T, given that $X = x$, is:

$$\begin{aligned} h\left(t \mid x\right) = \frac{h(x,t)}{h_1(x)} &= \frac{\phi(t) \exp\left[-\frac{(\theta^{-1}+x)^2}{2} - (\theta^{-1}+x)t\right]}{\Psi(\theta^{-1}+x)} \\ &= \frac{\phi(t+\theta^{-1}+x)}{\Psi(\theta^{-1}+x)} \end{aligned} \tag{5.6.11}$$

for $t \in \mathbb{R}^+$. This conditional density is sometimes referred to as a censored normal distribution, and can be dealt with in terms of well-known functions. It can be shown that the conditional expectation of

T, given $X = x$, is:

$$M(x) = E\left[T \mid X = x\right] = \frac{\phi(\theta^{-1} + x)}{\Psi(\theta^{-1} + x)} - (\theta^{-1} + x) \tag{5.6.12}$$

and the conditional variance is:

$$V(x) = var\left[T \mid X = x\right]$$

$$= 1 + \frac{(\theta^{-1} + x)^2}{4} - \left\{\frac{\theta^{-1} + x}{2} - \frac{\phi(\theta^{-1} + x)}{\Psi(\theta^{-1} + x)}\right\}^2 . \tag{5.6.13}$$

Moreover, it can be shown that:

$$\frac{dM(x)}{dx} = -V(x) \leq 0 \tag{5.6.14}$$

so that $M(x)$ is a non-increasing function of x.

5.7 Applying the Model to Data in a Monte Carlo Experiment

Applications of the model discussed in the preceding two sections have been reported by Berman[5] and Dubin et al.[12] The sample analyzed by Berman consisted of cohorts of IVDU's in detoxification and methadone maintenance programs in New York City (NYC). Among those studied, 191 were HIV-free subjects and were used to estimate the parameters μ and σ. Estimates of the parameter δ and the moments of the random variable T were based on 59 HIV-infected individuals who had tested positive on the first visit and had returned to the clinic at least once.

A second sample consisted of 1072 homosexual/bisexual men in Sydney, Australia, who had enrolled in the Sydney AIDS Prospective Study (SAPS) between February 1984 and January 1985 (see Dubin et al.[12] for more details on both samples). Data were collected up to March 1991 and 892 subjects had returned for at least one follow-up visit, with a median time of 6.7 months between the first and second visits. Among those enrolled, there were 564 subjects who tested negative for HIV-1 antibodies at enrollment and remained HIV-1 antibody-free at subsequent follow-ups that were used to estimate the parameters μ

and σ. Data on 355 subjects who were consistently positive for HIV-1 and had returned for at least one follow-up visit were used to estimate the parameters δ and the first four moments of the random variable T.

Presented in Table 5.7.1 are estimates of the parameters μ, σ and δ, as well as the correlation coefficient ρ_{RT} for the sample of NYC intravenous drug users (IVDU's) and the sample of homosexual/bisexual men in the SAPS. It is interesting to observe that the estimates of the parameters μ and σ were fairly close for the two samples. But the estimate of δ for the NYC IVDU's was $0.0335/0.0158 = 2.1203$ times greater than that for the Australian homosexual/bisexual men, suggesting that $\log \mathrm{CD4}^+$ count declined more rapidly among IVDU's than among non-IVDU's for SAPS cohorts. It was also observed by Dubin et al.[12] that among those subjects who seroconverted while under study, the $\mathrm{CD4}^+$ count approximately six months after seroconversion exceeded that of the hypothesized log-linear decline, a result that suggests the model may have to modified. Another observation of interest is that the magnitude of the correlation of the random variables R and T was $0.9022/0.6600 = 1.3670$ times greater for IVDU's than for SAPS cohorts.

Table 5.7.1. Estimates of the Parameters μ, σ, δ, and the Correlation Coefficient ρ_{RT} Based on NYC IVDU's and Australian Homosexual/Bisexual Men

	μ	σ	δ	ρ_{RT}
NYC IVDU's	6.966	0.354	0.0335	−0.9022
SAPS	6.550	0.419	0.0158	−0.6600

A question that naturally arises is whether evidence based on the data is consistent with the assumption that the random variable T follows an exponential distribution. One approach to answering this question is to compare the theoretical moments of the exponential distribution with those estimated from the Hermite polynomials. The nth moment of the exponential distribution is:

$$\alpha_n = E\left[T^n\right] = \frac{1}{\theta}\int_0^\infty t^n e^{-\frac{t}{\theta}} dt = \theta^n \Gamma(n+1) = \theta^n n! \,. \tag{5.7.1}$$

As reported by Berman,[5] the estimates of the first four moments of the distribution of the random variable $\delta T/\sigma$ based on the first four Hermite polynomials for the NYC IVDU's are:

$$-\overline{H}_1 = 2.3744,\ \overline{H}_2 = 10.0125,\ -\overline{H}_3 = 75.8390,\ \overline{H}_4 = 857.9250\,. \tag{5.7.2}$$

From Eq. (5.7.1), it may be seen that $\widehat{\theta} = 2.3744$ is the moment estimate of the parameter θ. Given this estimate, and by applying Eq. (5.7.1), it can be seen that the estimates of the first four moments of the exponential distribution are:

$$\widehat{\alpha}_1 = 2.3744,\ \widehat{\alpha}_2 = 11.2760,\ \widehat{\alpha}_3 = 80.3180,\ \widehat{\alpha}_4 = 762.8300\,. \tag{5.7.3}$$

Because the estimates in Eqs. (5.7.2) and (5.7.3) are quite close and are probably within sampling error, the data suggest that the exponential is a plausible candidate for the distribution of the random variable $\delta T/\sigma$. Similar conclusions were reached by Dubin et al.,[12] using data on Australian cohorts of homosexual/bisexual men. Further evidence that the exponential is a plausible candidate for the distribution of $\delta T/\sigma$ may be obtained by comparing a histogram of the sample of the random variable $(R-\mu)/\sigma$ with the theoretical marginal density $h_1(x)$ (see Eq.(5.6.10)). Dubin et al.[12] also displays graphs which suggest that the plot of this density compares favorably with the histograms for both sets of data.

Another quantity of interest is the unconditional expectation of the random variable T, the waiting time from infection with HIV to discovery of the infection at a clinic. Let $V = \delta T/\sigma$, then the unconditional expectation of T is:

$$E[T] = \frac{\sigma}{\delta} E[V]\,, \tag{5.7.4}$$

where the time unit is a month. By applying this formula to the NYC IVDU's (see Tables 5.7.1 and 5.7.2), it can be seen that an estimate of this expectation is $(0.3540/.0335)2.3744 = 25.0910$ months. A similar calculation based the Australian data, for which the estimate of $E[V]$ was 1.0, yielded an estimate of 26.5190 months, indicating that the two estimates of $E[T]$ are close in the two samples.

A basic ingredient of any stochastic model for projecting the spread of HIV infection in a population is the distribution of the waiting time from infection to the diagnosis of an AIDS defining disease. Because the formulation under consideration deals only with the evolution of the $CD4^+$ count of an infected individual, and this count is only one of the indicators of AIDS, the distribution in question cannot be deduced directly from the model.

Nevertheless, it is of interest to study the distribution of the waiting time from infection to the time the $CD4^+$ count falls below 200, one of the indicators of AIDS. A useful approach to deducing some information about this distribution based on parameter estimates in the two samples is to do some Monte Carlo experiments in which realizations of a log-Gaussian process are simulated. To conduct such experiments, it is necessary to make some further assumptions about the stationary Z process so that its auto-covariance function is specified. As in Section 5.3, suppose the Z process has the form,

$$Z(t) = \mu + Y(t) , \tag{5.7.5}$$

where the Y process is stationary and Gaussian with expectation 0. One of the simplest choices for a model of the Y process is a discrete time first-order auto-regressive model of the form,

$$Y(t) = \beta Y(t-1) + \epsilon(t) , \tag{5.7.6}$$

where $|\beta| < 1$ and the ϵ's are independently and normally distributed random variables with common expectation of 0 and variance σ_ϵ^2.

According to Section 5.3, in this case, the variance of the Z process is

$$\sigma^2 = \Gamma(0) = \frac{\sigma_\epsilon^2}{1-\beta^2} . \tag{5.7.7}$$

Therefore, given an estimate of σ and a specified value of β, a value of σ_ϵ may be computed, and Eqs. (5.7.5) and (5.7.6) may be used to compute Monte Carlo realizations of the Z process on a monthly time scale. The formula,

$$W(t) = \exp\left[Z(t) - \delta t\right] \tag{5.7.8}$$

may then be used to compute realizations of the $CD4^+$ count following an infection at time $t = 0$. The smallest value of t such that $W(t) < 200$ is the waiting time for the $CD4^+$ count to fall below 200. Presented in Table 5.7.2 are the results of several Monte Carlo experiments based on selected values of β and estimates of the parameters μ, σ, and δ in the two samples.

Table 5.7.2. Monte Carlo Estimates of the Waiting Times in Months for the $CD4^+$ Counts to Fall Below 200

NYC IVDU's

Beta	*Min*	*Mean*	*Max*
0.25	46	50.15	54
0.50	46	50.26	54
0.90	45	50.38	55

Australian Homosexual/Bisexual Men

Beta	*Min*	*Mean*	*Max*
0.25	71	79.10	87
0.50	72	79.73	88
0.90	69	79.32	92

For each value of β in Table 5.7.2, 100 Monte Carlo realizations of the W-process were computed and the lengths of all realizations were chosen to assure that all sample functions fell below 200. The minimum, mean, and maximum of the 100 simulated times for the $CD4^+$ count to fall below 200 were computed for each value of β and are presented in the table. The most striking feature of the table is the difference in the mean time since infection for the $CD4^+$ count to fall below 200. For the NYC IVDU's, the mean was about 50 months with little variation about this value as indicated by the minimum and maximum values, but for the Australian homosexual/bisexual men, the mean was a little less than 80 months with somewhat greater variation about the mean. The results presented in Table 5.7.2 did not change significantly when the corresponding negative values of β were used in similar experiments. These simulation experiments also suggest that the model may be insensitive to assumptions about the form of the auto-covariance function of the process, because in both samples the estimates of σ were rather small.

Whether the proposed log-linear decline in $\log \text{CD4}^+$ count is a valid model for the data remains an open question. However, the possibility that the latency period of HIV may differ among IVDU's and non-IVDU's raises questions worthy of further investigation and of potential importance when considering models to project an HIV/AIDS epidemic within these sub-populations. In summary, the model considered in this and the preceding section may be modified in many ways. Among them is the assumption that the mean function for the $\log \text{CD4}^+$ count is a linear function of t. For example, a mean function of the form,

$$\mu(t) = \mu \exp\left[-\left(\frac{t}{\theta}\right)^{\alpha}\right] \tag{5.7.9}$$

would produce a non-linear decline, where α and θ are positive parameters and μ is the mean in a non-infected population or perhaps some baseline population of persons at high risk for being infected with HIV. Whatever the value of μ, the convergence of this function to 0 as $t \to \infty$ may be slow, particularly for values of α such that $0 < \alpha < 1$. Survival functions other than the Weibull could also be considered in the search for models that permit non-linear declines in the mean function. Because the data in the two samples described in this section suggest the variance of the process is rather small, it may be plausible to assume that the variance-covariance structure of the process remains stationary in time.

To estimate the parameters in this case, it would be necessary to specify a form for the auto-correlation function of the process as outlined in the previous sections of this chapter. Furthermore, if it is suspected that the decline in $\log \text{CD4}^+$ count may be nonlinear, it would advisable to have data on patients who visit a clinic at least three times. Then, it may be possible to estimate the unknown parameters by the method of maximum likelihood under Gaussian assumptions.

For example, suppose that a patient visits a clinic at times $t_1 < t_2 < \cdots < t_n$, where $n \geq 3$. Then, let $\mathbf{r} = (r(t_i) \mid i = 1, 2, \cdots, n)$ be a $n \times 1$ vector of $\log \text{CD4}^+$ counts at these times, and finally, let the $n \times 1$ vector $\boldsymbol{\mu} = (\mu(t_i) \mid i = 1, 2, \cdots, n)$ be the means expressed as functions of the unknown parameters. The covariance matrix associated with these observations would have the form,

$$\mathbf{\Gamma}_n = \left(\sigma^2 \rho(t_j - t_i \mid i, j = 1, 2, \cdots, n)\right) , \tag{5.7.10}$$

where $\rho(\cdot)$ is some specified form of an auto-correlation function that may depend on one or more unknown parameters. If the matrix in Eq. (5.7.10) is non-singular, then the likelihood function associated with this patient would have the form of the familiar multivariate normal density,

$$L_n = \frac{1}{(2\pi)^{\frac{n}{2}} \left|\mathbf{\Gamma}_n\right|^{\frac{1}{2}}} \exp\left[-\frac{(\mathbf{r}-\boldsymbol{\mu})' \mathbf{\Gamma}_n^{-1} (\mathbf{r}-\boldsymbol{\mu})}{2}\right] , \tag{5.7.11}$$

where $|\mathbf{\Gamma}_n|$ stands for the determinant of the matrix $\mathbf{\Gamma}_n$. If data of this form are available for $N \geq 2$ patients, then, under the assumption that data on the patients are independent, the likelihood function of the sample would be a N-fold product of functions of form Eq. (5.7.11). In principle, unknown parameters could be estimated by the method of maximum likelihood, using computer intensive techniques.

One could also use Bayesian notions and let the random variable T be the waiting time from infection to the time of discovery of the infection at some clinic. Then, the times a patient visits a clinic would be random variables of the form $t_1 = T$, $t_2 = T + h_2, \cdots, t_n = T + h_n$, where the h's are known values. With the help of numerical and computer intensive methods, it may be possible to find Bayesian estimates of all the parameters under consideration as well as the posterior distribution of the random variable T, given the data and perhaps some other prior distribution of the unknown parameters. However, such a program of research will be left to other investigators and will not be pursued here. An informative exposition of Bayesian principles, models, and applications has been given by Press.[18]

The idea of using Bayesian methods to deduce some information about the conditional distribution of the random variable T, given some observable quantity such as the log CD4$^+$ count, is very intriguing. But, the range of applicability of statistical inferences based on this approach to the population as a whole should be interpreted with some caution for several reasons. One such reason is that for the vast majority of persons infected with HIV, the time of infection is not known, making it difficult to empirically validate some candidate for the prior distribution of T. Another is that patients participating in some program may be self-selected and not representative of that segment of the population that is at highest risk for becoming infected with HIV.

For example, those who present themselves a clinic may have higher rates of decline in $CD4^+$ counts that result in shorter latency periods than those who may have some natural resistance to the virus and thus do not perceive a need to seek medical advice and treatment. Therefore, samples of the type discussed in this section may be biased toward short latency periods. Nevertheless, the methods discussed in this chapter are interesting and worthy of further development.

5.8 References

1. S. M. Berman, A Bivariate Markov Process with Diffusion and Discrete Components, *Communications in Statistics - Stochastic Models* **10:** 271-308, 1994.
2. S. M. Berman, Conditioning a Diffusion at First-Passage and Last-Exit Times, and a Mirage Arising in Drug Therapy for HIV, *Mathematical Biosciences* **116:** 45-87, 1993.
3. S. M. Berman, Is Earlier Better for AZT Therapy in HIV Infection? - A Mathematical Model, N. P. Jewell, K. Dietz and V. Farewell (eds.), *AIDS Epidemiology: Methodological Issues,* Birkhauser, Boston, 1992, pp. 366-383.
4. S. M. Berman, Perturbation of Normal Random Vectors by Non-Normal Translation, and an Application to HIV Latency Time Distributions, *The Annals of Applied Probability* **4:** 968-980, 1994.
5. S. M. Berman, A Stochastic Model for the Distribution of HIV Latency Time Based on T4 Counts, *Biometrika* **77:** 733-741, 1990.
6. S. M. Berman, The Tail of the Convolution of Densities and Its Application to a Model of HIV-Latency Time, *The Annals of Applied Probability* **2:** 481-502, 1992.
7. G. E. P. Box and G. M. Jenkins, *Time Series Analysis - Forecasting and Control,* Holden-Day, Oakland, California, 1976.
8. D. R. Brillinger, *Time Series - Data Analysis and Theory,* Holden-Day,

Inc. San Francisco, London, 1981.

9. P. J. Brockwell and R. A. Davis, *Time Series - Theory and Methods,* 2nd ed., Springer-Verlag, New York, Berlin, Heidelberg, 1991.
10. H. Cramér, *Mathematical Methods of Statistics,* Princeton University Press, Princeton, New Jersey, 1946.
11. J. L. Doob, *Stochastic Processes,* John Wiley and Sons, Inc. New York, London, 1953.
12. N. Dubin and S. M. Berman et al., Estimation of Time Since Infection Using Longitudinal Disease-Marker Data, *Statistics in Medicine* **13:** 231-244, 1994.
13. W. Feller, *An Introduction to Probability Theory and Its Applications, II,* John Wiley and Sons, Inc., New York, London, Sydney, 1966.
14. W. A. Fuller, *Introduction to Statistical Time Series,* John Wiley and Sons, New York, London, 1976.
15. W. J. Kennedy, Jr. and J. E. Gentle, *Statistical Computing,* Marcel Dekker, Inc., New York and Basel, 1980.
16. M. Loève, *Probability Theory,* 2nd ed., Van Nostrand Company, Inc., Princeton, New Jersey, New York, London, 1960.
17. N. U. Prabhu, *Stochastic Processes - Basic Theory and Applications,* The Macmillan Company, New York and London, 1965.
18. S. J. Press, *Bayesian Statistics - Principles, Models, and Applications,* John Wiley and Sons, Inc. New York, London, 1989.

Chapter 6
THE THRESHOLD PARAMETER OF ONE-TYPE BRANCHING PROCESSES

6.1 Introduction

A quantity of importance in studying epidemics of infectious diseases is the basic reproduction number R_0, which is defined roughly as the expected number of secondary cases produced by one infected individual in a large population of susceptibles throughout his or her infectious period. Key threshold results of epidemic theories, in both deterministic and stochastic formulations, associate the outbreaks of epidemics and the persistence of endemic levels with values of R_0 greater than one. When $R_0 \leq 1$, then the epidemic dies out or becomes extinct. Anderson and May[1] may be consulted for extensive discussion of this threshold parameter, which they define in various ways. Among the reported uses of R_0 is the estimation of the amount of effort necessary to either prevent an epidemic or to eliminate an infection from a population. There is a rather large literature related to this basic quantity, dating back at least a century, which has been reviewed by Dietz.[12] Other recent works on this quantity include Diekmann et al.[11,10]

Among the classes of stochastic processes used to approximate real epidemics, particularly in their early stages, are various kinds of one-type and multi-type branching processes. Examples of applications of a multi-type Bienaymé-Galton-Watson process (BGW-process) to epidemic theory may be found in the paper of Becker and Marschner[7]. These authors also cite some earlier work of Whittle[20] on the application of branching processes to epidemic theories. Bartoszynski[6] was also among the earlier workers who applied ideas from branching processes to stochastic models of epidemics. An interesting historical account of I. J. Bienaymé's early work in branching processes, justifying the term BGW-processes, may be found in Heyde[14]. A limitation of any BGW-process is that only successive generations of "offspring" are accommodated in a discrete time formulation. For example, in the context of epidemics of infectious diseases, an "offspring" of an infectious individual is a person infected by this individual and the generation of "offspring" produced by this individual is the total number of people he or she infects during the infectious period.

For many diseases, such as HIV/AIDS, infectious periods are of random duration and throughout these periods an infectious individual may infect others at random points in time. To accommodate such real life phenomena, BGW-processes were extended independently by Crump and Mode[8,9] and Jagers[17] to accommodate the case of individuals producing "offspring" at random points throughout their lifetimes. Subsequently, these generalized age-dependent branching processes have become known as CMJ-processes.

Rather than referring to these classes of processes as generalized age-dependent branching processes, which in retrospect are not very general, the shortened acronym, CMJ-processes, will be used throughout this book. For extensive accounts of these classes of processes, the book Jagers[16] may be consulted for the one-type case; the multi-type case is discussed in the book Mode[18]. For a one-type CMJ-process, the threshold parameter R_0 in an epidemic setting, as we shall see, is indeed the expected number of individuals infected by an infectious person throughout the infectious period and in a demographic setting R_0 is called the net fertility rate (see Mode[19]).

Thanks to recent and very interesting work by Ball and his colleagues, it is becoming clear that CMJ-processes may be viewed as approximations to an extensively studied class of stochastic models of epidemics in closed populations known as SIR-processes. Briefly, the acronym SIR refers to a closed population of fixed size in which there are susceptibles, infectives, and those who have been removed from the epidemic by either recovery with immunity or death. Under rather general conditions, it can be shown that as the initial number n of susceptibles becomes large, the sample functions of a SIR-process converge strongly, i.e., with probability one, to those of a CMJ-process. Some of the initial ideas leading to the branching process approximations, as well as historical references, may be found in Ball.[2] For more recent results, the papers Ball and O'Neill[5] and Ball and Donnelly[4] may be consulted.

The overall purpose of this chapter is to provide a means of studying threshold phenomena within the framework of a one-type CMJ-process. More specifically, the objective of this chapter is five-fold; namely, to supply an overview of the theoretical structure underlying one-type CMJ-processes; to outline some concrete and simple examples as to how CMJ-process may be applied to simple epidemics; to demonstrate the application of a simple case in the estimation of infectivity of HIV; to extend the model to accommodate several stages of the infectious period such as that of HIV disease; and to briefly review the work of Ball and his colleagues.

6.2 Overview of a One-Type CMJ-Process

Even though the evolution of an epidemic in continuous time may be accounted for in a one-type CMJ-process, all such processes have a discrete time BGW-process embedded in them. Consequently, it is appropriate to begin the discussion with a brief overview of a one-type BGW-process within the context of a stochastic model of an epidemic. To this end, consider one infective individual in a large population of susceptibles at the beginning of his or her infectious period. Then, let the random variable $\boldsymbol{\xi}$ with range:

$$\mathbb{N}^+ = \{n \mid n = 0, 1, 2, \cdots\} \ , \tag{6.2.1}$$

the set of non-negative integers, represent the total number of susceptibles in the population infected by the initial infective throughout his or her infectious period. Suppose the *p.d.f.* of $\boldsymbol{\xi}$ is:

$$\mathbb{P}[\boldsymbol{\xi} = n] = f(n) \tag{6.2.2}$$

for $n \in \mathbb{N}^+$ and let

$$h(s) = E\left[s^{\boldsymbol{\xi}}\right] = \sum_{n=0}^{\infty} f(n)s^n, \ s \in [0,1] \tag{6.2.3}$$

be its probability generating function (*p.g.f.*). The total number of susceptibles infected by the initial infective constitutes the first generation of a BGW-process.

A central focus of attention in a one-type BGW-process is the sequence of random variables $(\mathbf{X}_n \mid n \in \mathbb{N}^+)$, representing generation sizes with $\mathbf{X}_0 = 1$. For example, if the total number of infectives in generation n is $\mathbf{X}_n$, then the total number of susceptibles infected by these infectives is $\mathbf{X}_{n+1}$. It is assumed that all infectives in the population act independently in a probabilistic sense. To state this assumption formally, for every $n \in \mathbb{N}^+$and a given $\mathbf{X}_n$, let $\left(\boldsymbol{\xi}_{n,k} \mid k = 1, 2, \cdots, \mathbf{X}_n\right)$ be a collection of conditionally independent and identically distributed random variables whose common distribution is that of $\boldsymbol{\xi}$. Then, successive generation sizes are given by:

$$\mathbf{X}_{n+1} = \sum_{k=1}^{\mathbf{X}_n} \boldsymbol{\xi}_{n,k} \ , \tag{6.2.4}$$

a random sum of random variables such that $\mathbf{X}_{n+1} = 0$ if $\mathbf{X}_n = 0$.

In view of Eq. (6.2.4), it seems natural to formulate the finite dimensional distributions of the generation sizes as a Markov chain with infinite state space $\mathfrak{S} = \mathbb{N}^+$ and stationary transition probabilities:

$$\mathbb{P}\left[\mathbf{X}_{n+1} = j \mid \mathbf{X}_n = i\right] = p_{ij} \tag{6.2.5}$$

determined as follows for $n \geq 0$. Given that $\mathbf{X}_n = i$, it follows from Eq. (6.2.4) that $\mathbf{X}_{n+1}$ is a sum of i independently and identically distributed random variables whose common distribution is that of $\boldsymbol{\xi}$. Therefore, the conditional probability generating function of $\mathbf{X}_{n+1}$ is:

$$E\left[s^{\mathbf{X}_{n+1}} \mid X_n = i\right] = \sum_{j=0}^{\infty} p_{ij} s^j = h^i(s), \ s \in [0,1] \ . \tag{6.2.6}$$

From this expression, it follows that the transition probability p_{ij} is the coefficient of s^j in the power series expansion of $h^i(s)$. In particular, if $i = 0$, then the right hand side of Eq. (6.2.6) is 1 for all $s \in [0,1]$. Therefore, $p_{00} = 1$ and $p_{0j} = 0$ for all $j \geq 1$ so that 0 is an absorbing state. In models considered in this chapter, the *p.d.f.* of the random variable $\boldsymbol{\xi}$, $f(n)$, will be chosen such that all states in the set $\mathfrak{S}_2 = \{n \mid n = 1, 2, \cdots\}$ communicate. Furthermore, this density will always be chosen such that $f(0) > 0$ so that any infective may infect no susceptibles with positive probability. Unlike the Markov chains discussed in Chapter 3, a BGW-process $\{\mathbf{X}_n \mid n \in \mathbb{N}^+\}$ has an infinite state space $\mathfrak{S}$ partitioned into a set $\mathfrak{S}_1 = \{0\}$, consisting of one absorbing state and an infinite set $\mathfrak{S}_2$ of transient states.

When a BGW-process is viewed as a model of an epidemic in a large population of susceptibles, entrance of the process into the absorbing state 0 is of fundamental importance, for it signals the end of the epidemic in the sense that for some generation $n \geq 1$ the infectives of this generation infect no susceptibles. One is thus led to consider the conditional probability of extinction,

$$q = \mathbb{P}\left[\mathbf{X}_n = 0 \text{ for some } n > 0 \mid \mathbf{X}_0 = 1\right] . \tag{6.2.7}$$

As a first step towards developing methods for calculating this probability, it will be convenient to think of a probability space $(\boldsymbol{\Omega}, \mathfrak{A}, \mathbb{P})$ underlying the process and define ω-sets as $[\mathbf{X}_n = 0] = [\omega \in \boldsymbol{\Omega} \mid \mathbf{X}_n(\omega) = 0]$ for $n \geq 1$. Then, because $\mathbf{X}_n = 0$ implies $\mathbf{X}_{n+1} = 0$ for all $n \geq 1$, it follows that $[\mathbf{X}_n = 0] \subset [\mathbf{X}_{n+1} = 0]$ for all $n \geq 1$. Therefore,

$$\begin{aligned} q &= \lim_{n \uparrow \infty} \mathbb{P}\left[\bigcup_{k=1}^{n} [\mathbf{X}_k = 0] \mid \mathbf{X}_0 = 1\right] \\ &= \lim_{n \uparrow \infty} \mathbb{P}\left[\mathbf{X}_n = 0 \mid \mathbf{X}_0 = 1\right] . \end{aligned} \tag{6.2.8}$$

To determine this conditional probability, it will be useful to consider the probability generating function,

$$g_n(s) = E\left[s^{\mathbf{X}_n} \mid \mathbf{X}_0 = 1\right] \tag{6.2.9}$$

of the size of the nth generation. Because

$$E\left[s^{\mathbf{X}_n} \mid \mathbf{X}_{n-1},\ \mathbf{X}_0 = 1\right] = h^{\mathbf{X}_{n-1}}(s) , \tag{6.2.10}$$

it follows that,

$$g_n(s) = E\left[h^{\mathbf{X}_{n-1}}(s)\right] = g_{n-1}(h(s)) \tag{6.2.11}$$

for $n \geq 1$, where by definition $g_0(s) = s$. By construction $g_1(s) = h(s)$, and if we define a sequence of functional iterates of $h(s)$ by setting $h^{(1)}(s) = h(s)$ and define $h^{(n)}(s)$ recursively by $h^{(n)}(s) = h(h^{(n-1)}(s))$ for $n \geq 2$, then it can be seen from Eq. (6.2.11) that:

$$g_n(s) = h^{(n)}(s) = h(g_{n-1}(s)) \tag{6.2.12}$$

for $n \geq 1$.

As we shall see, Eq. (6.2.12) provides a basis for calculating the probability of extinction q by first observing that:

$$q_n = \mathbb{P}\left[\mathbf{X}_n = 0 \mid \mathbf{X}_0 = 1\right] = g_n(0) \tag{6.2.13}$$

for $n \geq 1$. Furthermore, from Eq. (6.2.12) it can be seen that the sequence (q_n) satisfies the equation,

$$q_n = h(q_{n-1}) \tag{6.2.14}$$

for $n \geq 2$. Finally, by letting $n \to \infty$ in Eq. (6.2.14) and using the continuity of $h(s)$ on $[0,1]$,it can be seen that $q = h(q)$ so that q is a root of the equation,

$$s = h(s) \tag{6.2.15}$$

belonging to the interval $[0,1]$.

If $q = 1$, then the epidemic dies out with certainty, which would be a desirable result from the point of view of public health. On the other hand, if $0 < q < 1$, then the extinction of the epidemic is not certain and it is well known from extensive theoretical investigations of BGW-processes that with probability $1 - q$, the epidemic amongst the susceptibles of the population would grow without bound. Finding conditions under which either $q = 1$ or $q < 1$ leads to what are generally referred to as threshold theorems when considering stochastic models of epidemics. As can be seen from the following theorem, for BGW-processes a threshold condition may easily be stated in terms of the

$$m = E\left[\boldsymbol{\xi}\right] = \sum_{n=0}^{\infty} nf(n) = h^{'}(1) < \infty \ , \tag{6.2.16}$$

the finite expectation of the total number of susceptibles infected by any infective throughout his infectious period, where $h^{'}(1)$ is the derivative of $h(s)$ at $s = 1$.

Theorem 6.2.1. Suppose $f(0) > 0$. (*i*) If $m \le 1$, then $q = 1$. (*ii*) But, if $m > 1$, then $0 < q < 1$ and is the smallest root of the equation $s = h(s)$ in $(0, 1)$.

Proof: A detailed proof of the theorem may be found in, among other places, in the book Jagers.[16] Because knowing q is the smallest root of the equation $s = h(s)$ in $(0, 1)$ is important in finding numerical values of the extinction probability when $m > 1$, a proof of this statement will be included here. Let s be any root of $s = h(s)$ in the open interval $(0, 1)$. Then, because $h(s)$ is strictly increasing on $(0, 1)$, $q_1 = h(0) < h(s) = s$ for $s > 0$. Hence, by the same reasoning $q_2 = h(q_1) < h(s) = s$ and by induction $q_n < s$ for all $n \ge 1$. By letting $n \to \infty$, it follows that $q \le s$.

As mentioned in the introduction to this chapter, continuous time CMJ-processes may be viewed as extensions of BGW-processes in the sense that the length of the infectious period is a random variable T and infectious contacts of infecteds with susceptibles occur at random points of time according to some point process K defined on $[0, \infty)$, which stops at some random time T, the end of infectious period. Thus, when a stochastic model of an epidemic is formulated within the framework of a CMJ-process, a life history $\mathcal{H} = (T, K)$ is associated with each infectious individual in the population and it is assumed that the life histories of all infectious individuals in the population are independent and identically distributed copies of $\mathcal{H}$. Models of life histories may be constructed in various ways as will be illustrated in subsequent sections of this chapter, and, depending of the methods used to construct $\mathcal{H}$, the random variable T and the point process K may, or may not, be independent. A discussion of a method for constructing a probability space $(\mathbf{\Omega}, \mathfrak{A}, \mathbb{P})$ underlying a multi-type CMJ-process, which may be specialized to the one-type case, can be found in the book Mode.[18]

Methods for constructing models of life histories will be discussed subsequently, but in the remainder of this section attention will be focused on the connections between a continuous time CMJ-process, an embedded discrete time BGW-process, and its connection with a fundamental threshold theorem regarding the extinction of the epidemic. Suppose at time $t = 0$, the process starts with one infectious individual at the beginning of his or her infectious period and suppose his or her life history, which evolves in continuous time, is governed by some $\mathcal{H}$-process. Let the random function $\mathbf{Z}(t)$ be the number of infecteds in the population at time $t \in [0, \infty)$ with $\mathbf{Z}(0) = 1$. It can be shown that if the collection of random variables $\{\mathbf{X}_n \mid n \in \mathbb{N}^+\}$, representing the total number of susceptibles infected in successive generations with $\mathbf{X}_0 = 1$, is an embedded BGW-process governed by some discrete distribution $\{f(n) \mid n \in \mathbb{N}^+\}$ with probability generating function $h(s)$ determined by a model $\mathcal{H}$ of life histories.

That the threshold behavior of a continuous time CMJ-process is governed by the embedded discrete time BGW-process follows from well-known theoretical results. Let the ω-set,

$$A = [\mathbf{Z}(t) = 0 \text{ for some } t > 0] \tag{6.2.17}$$

represent extinction of the continuous time process and let the ω-set,

$$B = [\mathbf{X}_n = 0 \text{ for some } n > 0] \tag{6.2.18}$$

represent extinction of the embedded BGW-process. Then, it can be shown (see Jagers[16]) that:

$$\mathbb{P}\left[A \mid \mathbf{Z}(0) = 1\right] = \mathbb{P}\left[B \mid \mathbf{X}_0 = 1\right]. \tag{6.2.19}$$

Consequently, when the probability generating function $h(s)$ is properly defined in terms of a $\mathcal{H}$-process, **Theorem 6.2.1** becomes a threshold result for a continuous time CMJ-process.

6.3 Life Cycle Models and Mean Functions

One approach to constructing a life cycle model $\mathcal{H} = (T, K)$ is to suppose the random variable T and the K-process are independent. Let the distribution function of the random variable T be

$$G(t) = \mathbb{P}\left[T \le t\right] \text{ for } t \in [0, \infty), \tag{6.3.1}$$

and let $g(t) = G'(t)$ be the *p.d.f.* of T. It will assumed that $G(0) = 0$, $G(t) \to 1$ as $t \to \infty$, and for all models considered in the chapter $g(t)$ will be continuous on $(0, \infty)$. Another function that will be of use is:

$$f(s,t) = E\left[s^{K(t)}\right] , \tag{6.3.2}$$

the *p.g.f.* of the K-process, defined for $s \in [0,1]$ and $t \in [0, \infty)$. The K-process continues until it is stopped at the end of the infectious period, and to take this stoppage into account, let the random function $N(t)$ be defined as follows for all $t \in [0, \infty)$. Fix a $t \in (0, \infty)$. If $T > t$, then

$$N(t) = K(t) . \tag{6.3.3}$$

But, if $T \leq t$, then

$$N(t) = K(T) . \tag{6.3.4}$$

For $s \in [0,1]$ and $t \in [0, \infty)$, let

$$h(s,t) = E\left[s^{N(t)}\right] \tag{6.3.5}$$

be the *p.g.f.* of $N(t)$.

An equation connecting the *p.g.f.*'s in Eqs. (6.3.2) and (6.3.5) may derived by an intuitive conditioning argument. The probability of the event $[T > t]$ is $1 - G(t)$, and given this event, the *p.g.f.* of $N(t)$ is $f(s,t)$ (see Eq. (6.3.3)). Given the event $[T \leq t]$, the probability T falls in a small interval containing $x \in [0, t]$ is approximately $g(x)dx$ and the *p.g.f.* of $N(x)$ is, by Eq. (6.3.4), $f(s,x)$. Integrating on x and summing over these two disjoint events leads to the equation,

$$h(s,t) = (1 - G(t))f(s,t) + \int_0^t f(s,x)g(x)dx . \tag{6.3.6}$$

For $t \in [0, \infty)$, let

$$\nu(t) = E\left[K(t)\right] \tag{6.3.7}$$

be the mean function of the K-process, and let

$$m(t) = E\left[N(t)\right] \tag{6.3.8}$$

be the mean function of the N-process. In all models to be considered in this chapter, these non-decreasing mean functions are finite, continuous, and differentiable for all $t \in (0, \infty)$. By a conditioning argument similar to that used in the derivation of Eq. (6.3.6), it can be shown that for any $t \in (0, \infty)$,

$$m(t) = (1 - G(t))\nu(t) + \int_0^t \nu(x)g(x)dx \ . \tag{6.3.9}$$

A continuous function defined for $t \in (0, \infty)$ that plays an important role in threshold theorems is

$$b(t) = \frac{d\nu(t)}{dt} \ , \tag{6.3.10}$$

the density for the mean function of the K-process. In the context of a stochastic model of an epidemic, it may be referred to as the rate infecteds whose duration of infection is t infect susceptibles. An integration by parts in Eq. (6.3.9) leads to the equivalent representation,

$$m(t) = \int_0^t b(x)(1 - G(x))dx \tag{6.3.11}$$

of the mean function of the N-process defined for $t \in (0, \infty)$.

The total number of susceptibles infected by any infectious individual throughout his or her infectious period is given by the random variable,

$$N = \lim_{t \uparrow \infty} N(t) \ . \tag{6.3.12}$$

Because convergence in Eq. (6.3.12) in monotone increasing, by applying the monotone convergence theorem in Eq. (6.3.6), it can be shown that the $p.g.f.$ of N is:

$$h(s) = E\left[s^N\right] = \lim_{t \uparrow \infty} h(s, t)$$

$$= \int_0^\infty f(s, x)g(x)dx \ . \tag{6.3.13}$$

Another application of the monotone convergence theorem together with Eq. (6.3.11) leads to the conclusion that the expectation of N is:

$$m = E[N] = \int_0^\infty b(x)(1 - G(x))dx \ . \tag{6.3.14}$$

Let $\{\mathbf{X}_n \mid n \in \mathbb{N}^+\}$ be the discrete time BGW-process embedded in the continuous time CMJ-process $\{\mathbf{Z}(t) \mid t \in [0, \infty)\}$ under consideration. Then, for this embedded process, the random variable N plays the role of the random variable $\boldsymbol{\xi}$ that was used in the construction of the BGW-process as described in Section 6.2. Therefore, according to **Theorem 6.2.1** and the subsequent discussion in that section, the threshold parameter for the continuous time CMJ-process is the expectation in Eq. (6.3.14). Because it has become customary in discussing mathematical models of epidemics to call this expectation R_0, henceforth in this section this symbol will be used for the expectation so that by definition:

$$R_0 = E[N] = \int_0^\infty b(x)(1 - G(x))dx \ . \tag{6.3.15}$$

In terms of the notation of this section, the threshold theorem for a one-type CMJ-process may be stated as follows:

Theorem 6.3.1. Let $h(s)$ be the *p.g.f.* in Eq. (6.3.14), suppose that $\mathbb{P}[N = 0] = h(0) > 0$, and let q be the probability the continuous time CMJ-process becomes extinct, given that $\mathbf{Z}(0) = 1$. (*i*) If $R_0 \leq 1$, then $q = 1$. (*ii*) But, if $R_0 > 1$, then q is the smallest root of the equation $s = h(s)$ in $(0, 1)$.

When considering stochastic models of epidemics, two other random functions of interest may be defined in connection with any one-type CMJ-process. Suppose $\mathbf{Z}(0) = 1$ and for $t > 0$ let the random function $\mathbf{Z}_I(t)$ be the total number of susceptibles infected during the time interval $(0, t]$ and let the random function $\mathbf{Z}_R(t)$ be the total number of infectives that have been removed by either recovery or death during this time interval. Then, the total number of infectives in the population at time $t > 0$ is $\mathbf{Z}(t) = \mathbf{Z}_I(t) - \mathbf{Z}_R(t)$. It can be shown, under rather general conditions, that all these random functions have continuous finite expectations of all $t > 0$ and satisfy renewal type integral equations. That these expectations satisfy renewal type integral equations can be seen by the following intuitive argument.

For $t > 0$, let

$$M(t) = E[\mathbf{Z}(t)] \tag{6.3.16}$$

be the mean of the random function $\mathbf{Z}(t)$ and define the expectation functions $M_I(t)$ and $M_R(t)$ similarly for the random functions $\mathbf{Z}_I(t)$ and $\mathbf{Z}_R(t)$. To simplify the notation, let $S(t) = 1 - G(t)$ be the survival function for the duration of the infectious period and consider $M(t)$, the expected number of infectives in the population at time $t > 0$ that have evolved from an initial infective at time $t = 0$.

At time $t > 0$ the initial infective is still infectious with probability $S(t)$. Moreover, during the time interval $(0, t]$ the initial infective may make infectious contacts with susceptibles. If such a contact is made at $x \in (0, t]$, then the expected number of infectious individuals at time t evolving from this contact is $M(t - x)$ and the mean number of such contacts in a small interval containing x is $b(x)S(x)dx$ (see Eq. (6.3.15)). Integrating on x for $t > 0$ and adding these two possibilities results in the renewal type integral equation,

$$M(t) = S(t) + \int_0^t b(x)S(x)M(t - x)dx \ . \tag{6.3.17}$$

Similar renewal type arguments may be used to show that the expectation functions $M_I(t)$ and $M_R(t)$ satisfy the equations

$$M_I(t) = 1 + \int_0^t b(x)S(x)M_I(t - x)dx \tag{6.3.18}$$

and

$$M_R(t) = G(t) + \int_0^t b(x)S(x)M_R(t - x)dx \tag{6.3.19}$$

for $t > 0$. From these equations, $M(t) = M_I(t) - M_R(t)$.

When $R_0 > 1$ it would be of interest to have some information on the rate at which an epidemic may spread amongst a large population of susceptibles, given that the epidemic does not become extinct.

As is well known, some key limit theorems from renewal theory may be applied to obtain the desired information. For the case of continuous time, these limit theorems have been discussed in detail by Jagers.[16] Related discussions for the case of discrete time, which is sometimes called the lattice case, may be found in Mode[19] (see Chapter 7). Let r be a positive number such that:

$$\int_0^\infty e^{-rx} b(x) S(x) dx = 1 , \tag{6.3.20}$$

and suppose the integral,

$$\int_0^\infty x e^{-rx} b(x) S(x) dx \tag{6.3.21}$$

is finite. Then, it can be shown that the solution of Eq. (6.3.17) has the property

$$\lim_{t \uparrow \infty} e^{-rt} M(t) = \frac{\int_0^\infty e^{-rt} S(t) dt}{\int_0^\infty t e^{-rt} b(x) S(x) dx} = c \neq 0 . \tag{6.3.22}$$

Hence, for large t,

$$M(t) \approx c e^{rt} \tag{6.3.23}$$

so that the mean function of the epidemic grows exponentially at rate r per unit time. In view of Eq. (6.3.23), the parameter r will be called the intrinsic growth rate of the epidemic. It can also be shown, by another application of renewal limit theorems, that the mean functions $M_I(t)$ and $M_R(t)$ grow exponentially at rate $r > 0$ when t is large.

The structure set forth in this and the preceding section is quite general, but in subsequent sections of this chapter specific parametric examples belonging to this structure will be developed.

6.4 On Modeling Point Processes

As will be illustrated in subsequent sections of this chapter, several approaches may be used to develop models of the K-process discussed in the previous section. Among these approaches is that of applying renewal theory. To this end, let $\{X_n \mid n = 1, 2, \cdots\}$ be a sequence of *i.i.d.* random variables, with common range $[0, \infty)$, representing waiting times among contacts. Suppose the common distribution of these random variables is that of a random variable X with a continuous *p.d.f.* $f(x)$ on $(0, \infty)$ and distribution function $F(x)$.

If an infection occurs at $t = 0$, then the waiting time to the first contact is $T_1 = X_1$, the waiting time to the second contact is $T_2 = X_1 + X_2$, and, in general for $n \geq 1$, the waiting time to the nth contact is given by the sum,

$$T_n = X_1 + X_2 + \cdots + X_n \tag{6.4.1}$$

of *i.i.d.* random variables. Let $f_n(t)$ be the *p.d.f.* of the random variable T_n. Then, for $t > 0$ the distribution function of this random variable is:

$$F_n(t) = \mathbb{P}\left[T_n \leq t\right] = \int_0^t f_n(x)dx \ . \tag{6.4.2}$$

Because T_n is a sum of *i.i.d.* random variables, $f_n(t)$ is the n-fold convolution of $f(x)$ with itself. For if we let $f_1(x) = f(x)$, then for $n > 1$ a sequence of convolutions $\{f_n(t) \mid n = 1, 2, \cdots\}$ may be determined recursively for $t > 0$ according to the formula,

$$f_n(t) = \int_0^t f_{n-1}(t - x)f(x)dx \ . \tag{6.4.3}$$

A random function of basic importance in defining the K-process discussed in the previous section is defined as follows. For an individual infected at $t = 0$, let the random function $C(t)$ represent the number of contacts with susceptibles during the time interval $(0, t]$ for $t > 0$. Then, $C(t) \geq n$, if, and only if, $T_n \leq t$. Therefore, for $n \geq 1$,

$$\mathbb{P}\left[C(t) \geq n\right] = \mathbb{P}\left[T_n \leq t\right] = F_n(t) \ . \tag{6.4.4}$$

But,

$$\mathbb{P}\left[C(t) \geq n\right] = \mathbb{P}\left[C(t) = n\right] + \mathbb{P}\left[C(t) \geq n + 1\right] \ , \tag{6.4.5}$$

which implies

$$\mathbb{P}\left[C(t) = n\right] = F_n(t) - F_{n+1}(t) \tag{6.4.6}$$

is valid for $n \geq 1$. To extend this formula to the case $n = 0$, observe that $C(t) = 0$ if, and only if, $T_1 = X_1 > t$ so that:

$$\mathbb{P}[C(t) = 0] = \mathbb{P}[T_1 > t] = 1 - F_1(t) . \tag{6.4.7}$$

Therefore, if a function $F_0(t)$ is defined as

$$F_0(t) = 1 \tag{6.4.8}$$

for all $t > 0$, then Eq. (6.4.6) holds for all $n = 0, 1, 2, \cdots$, and $t > 0$.

All contacts between infecteds and susceptibles may not lead to infection. Accordingly, for contacts between infecteds and susceptibles, let $p \in (0, 1)$ be the probability per contact that infection results, let $\{\eta_i \mid i = 1, 2, \cdots\}$ be a sequence of *i.i.d.* Bernoulli indicators such that $\eta_i = 1$ if the ith contact results in infection with $\eta_i = 0$ otherwise, and suppose the C-process and the sequence of Bernoulli indicators are independent. Then, the K-process discussed in the previous section may be defined as the random sum,

$$K(t) = \sum_{i=1}^{C(t)} \eta_i , \tag{6.4.9}$$

where $K(t) = 0$ if $C(t) = 0$. From the observation $E[\eta_i] = p$ for all $i \geq 1$, it can be seen that:

$$E[K(t) \mid C(t)] = C(t)p . \tag{6.4.10}$$

Furthermore,

$$\begin{aligned} E[C(t)] &= \sum_{n=1}^{\infty} \mathbb{P}[C(t) \geq n] \\ &= \sum_{n=1}^{\infty} F_n(t) , \end{aligned} \tag{6.4.11}$$

and it can be shown that the series on the right converges for all $t \in (0, \infty)$. Therefore, by taking the expectation in Eq. (6.4.10), the formula,

$$\nu(t) = \left(\sum_{n=1}^{\infty} F_n(t) \right) p \tag{6.4.12}$$

arises so that the density of this expectation function has the form,

$$b(t) = \frac{d\nu(t)}{dt} = \left(\sum_{n=1}^{\infty} f_n(t) \right) p \text{ for } t \in (0, \infty). \tag{6.4.13}$$

For the case of discrete time, say $t = 0, 1, 2, \cdots$, the infinite series on the right in Eq. (6.4.13) contains only finitely many non-zero terms when the $p.d.f.$ satisfies the condition $f(0) = 0$. Consequently, it is feasible in this case to use the algorithms described in Chapter 4 to compute the density in Eq. (6.4.13) on finitely many points. However, in the case of continuous time, this density has a very simple constant form, when $f(x)$, the $p.d.f.$ of the waiting times among contacts, has an exponential distribution. As a first step in deriving this simple form, for $u \in [0, 1]$ and $t \in [0, \infty)$ let

$$f_C(u, t) = E\left[u^{C(t)}\right] \tag{6.4.14}$$

be the $p.g.f.$ of the C-process. Let $q = 1 - p$. Then, because

$$E\left[s^{\eta_i}\right] = pu + q \tag{6.4.15}$$

for all $i = 1, 2, \cdots$, it can be seen from Eq. (6.4.9) that:

$$E\left[s^{K(t)} \mid C(t)\right] = (pu + q)^{C(t)}, \tag{6.4.16}$$

and, by taking expectations, it follows that the $p.g.f.$ of the K-process is:

$$f(u, t) = E\left[(pu + q)^{C(t)}\right] = f_C(pu + q, t) \tag{6.4.17}$$

Now suppose

$$f(x) = \lambda e^{-\lambda x} \tag{6.4.18}$$

for $x \in [0, \infty)$ and $\lambda > 0$, and observe that the Laplace transform of this $p.d.f.$ is:

$$\widehat{f}(s) = \int_0^{\infty} e^{-sx} f(x) dx = \frac{\lambda}{\lambda + s} \tag{6.4.19}$$

for $s \geq 0$. Recall that a random variable X has a gamma distribution if its $p.d.f.$ with index parameter $\alpha > 0$ and scale parameter $\gamma > 0$ has the form

$$g(x) = \frac{\gamma^{\alpha}}{\Gamma(\alpha)} x^{\alpha - 1} e^{-\gamma x} \text{ for } x \in (0, \infty). \tag{6.4.20}$$

From this formula, it can be seen that the Laplace transform of this density is

$$\widehat{g}(s) = \int_0^\infty e^{-sx} g(x)dx = \left(\frac{\gamma}{\gamma + s}\right)^\alpha, \tag{6.4.21}$$

which is defined for $s \geq 0$.

By definition, for $s \geq 0$ the Laplace transform of the sum T_n of *i.i.d.* random variables is:

$$\begin{aligned}
\widehat{f}_n(s) &= \int_0^\infty e^{-st} f_n(t)dt = E\left[e^{-rT_n}\right] \\
&= E\left[\exp\left(-s\left(X_1 + X_2 + \cdots + X_n\right)\right)\right] \\
&= E\left[\prod_{i=1}^n e^{-sX_i}\right] = \prod_{i=1}^n E\left[e^{-sX_i}\right] \\
&= \prod_{i=1}^n \frac{\lambda}{\lambda + s} = \left(\frac{\lambda}{\lambda + s}\right)^n.
\end{aligned} \tag{6.4.22}$$

It follows, therefore, that the *p.d.f.* of the random variable T_n is that of a gamma distribution with index parameter $\alpha = n$, scale parameter $\gamma = \lambda$, and *p.d.f.*

$$f_n(t) = \frac{\lambda^n}{\Gamma(n)} t^{n-1} e^{-\lambda t} \tag{6.4.23}$$

where $t \in [0, \infty)$ and $n = 1, 2, \cdots$.

The distribution function corresponding to this density for $t > 0$ is, by definition,

$$\mathbb{P}\left[T_n \leq t\right] = F_n(t) = \frac{\lambda^n}{\Gamma(n)} \int_0^t x^{n-1} e^{-\lambda x} dx\ . \tag{6.4.24}$$

When $n = 1$, this integral reduces to

$$F_1(t) = 1 - e^{-\lambda t}. \tag{6.4.25}$$

By using this observation, induction, and integration by parts, it can be shown that for all $n \geq 1$ the formula,

$$F_n(t) = 1 - e^{-\lambda t} \sum_{\nu=0}^{n-1} \frac{(\lambda t)^\nu}{\nu!}, \tag{6.4.26}$$

is valid for all $t \geq 0$.

From this result, it can be seen that the formula in Eq. (6.4.6) takes the simple form,

$$\mathbb{P}\left[C(t) = n\right] = e^{-\lambda t} \frac{(\lambda t)^n}{n!} \tag{6.4.27}$$

for $n = 0, 1, 2, \cdots$. Hence, the *p.g.f.* of th C-process is:

$$f_C(u,t) = \sum_{n=0}^{\infty} e^{-\lambda t} \frac{(\lambda t)^n s^n}{n!} = e^{\lambda t(u-1)} . \tag{6.4.28}$$

One thus reaches the conclusion that, under the assumption that the waiting times among contacts are *i.i.d.* exponential random variables, the C-process is Poisson with intensity parameter $\lambda > 0$. That the K-process is also Poisson may be seen by the following observation. According to Eq. (6.4.17), the *p.g.f.* of the K-process is:

$$f(u,t) = e^{\lambda t(pu+q-1)} = e^{\lambda pt(u-1)} \tag{6.4.29}$$

for all $u \in [0,1]$ and $t \in [0,\infty)$. Hence, the K-process is also Poisson. Given this result, it is easy to see that the mean function of the K-process is

$$\nu(t) = \lambda pt \tag{6.4.30}$$

with the constant density

$$b(t) = \frac{d\nu(t)}{dt} = \lambda p . \tag{6.4.31}$$

As will be seen in the next section, the case this density is constant coincides with widely used definitions of R_0. The procedure just outlined is just one of many possible ways of constructing a point process. Further references on point processes may be found in Jagers.[16]

6.5 Examples with a Constant Rate of Infection

Let $\mathcal{H} = (T, K)$ be a life cycle model underlying a one-type CMJ-process, and let $G(t)$ be the distribution function, with *p.d.f.* $g(t)$, of the random variable T, representing the length of the infectious period.

In Section 6.4, it was shown that when the K-process is Poisson, the infection rate density $b(t)$ was the constant λp, where λ is the expected number of contacts per unit time between an infected individual and susceptibles and p is the probability per contact an infectious individual infects a susceptible. When $b(t) = \lambda p$ for all $t \geq 0$, then the threshold parameter R_0 takes the form,

$$R_0 = \lambda p \int_0^\infty (1 - G(t))\, dt \ , \tag{6.5.1}$$

(see Eq. (6.3.15)). But, as is well known, if the expectation,

$$\mu = E\,[T] = \int_0^\infty tg(t)dt \tag{6.5.2}$$

is finite, then, by using integration by parts, it can be shown that

$$\mu = \int_0^\infty (1 - G(t))\, dt \ . \tag{6.5.3}$$

Therefore, when the infection rate density is constant, R_0 has the simple form,

$$R_0 = \lambda p \mu \ , \tag{6.5.4}$$

a form that has been used widely in the literature on mathematical models of epidemics (see Anderson and May[1]).

A number of other interesting and useful formulas may be derived when the distribution function $G(t)$ has certain parametric forms. For example, if the random variable T has an exponential distribution with scale parameter $\gamma > 0$, then

$$\mathbb{P}\,[T \leq t] = G(t) = 1 - e^{-\gamma t} \text{ for } t \in [0, \infty) \ , \tag{6.5.5}$$

and R_0 takes the form,

$$R_0 = \lambda p \int_0^\infty e^{-\gamma t} dt = \frac{\lambda p}{\gamma} \ . \tag{6.5.6}$$

In this case, the $p.g.f.$ of the random variable N, representing the total number of susceptibles infected by a typical infective throughout his or her infectious period, has a simple form. For, if the *p.g.f.* of the K-process is:

$$f(s,t) = e^{\lambda pt(s-1)} , \tag{6.5.7}$$

then, by Eq. (6.3.14), the *p.g.f.* of N takes the form,

$$\begin{aligned} h(s) &= \gamma \int_0^\infty e^{\lambda pt(s-1)} e^{-\gamma t} dt \\ &= \gamma \int_0^\infty \exp\left[-\left(\gamma + \lambda p\left(1-s\right)\right)t\right] dt \\ &= \frac{\gamma}{\gamma + \lambda p\left(1-s\right)} . \end{aligned} \tag{6.5.8}$$

But, in view of Eq. (6.5.6), it can be seen that this *p.g.f.* may also be expressed in the form,

$$h(s) = \frac{1}{1 + R_0\left(1-s\right)} . \tag{6.5.9}$$

By inspection, when $h(s)$ has this form, it can be seen that the equation $h(s) = s$ has two roots; namely 1 and $1/R_0$. Let q be the probability of extinction for the continuous time CMJ-process. According to **Theorem 6.3.1**, if $R_0 \leq 1$, then $q = 1$, but, if $R_0 > 1$, then q has the simple form,

$$q = \frac{1}{R_0} . \tag{6.5.10}$$

When the length of the infectious period has an exponential distribution, a simple formula may also be derived for r, the intrinsic growth rate of the epidemic. For, when

$$1 - G(t) = e^{-\gamma t} , \tag{6.5.11}$$

Eq. (6.3.20) take the form,

$$\lambda p \int_0^\infty e^{-(r+\gamma)t} dt = \frac{\lambda p}{r+\gamma} = 1 , \tag{6.5.12}$$

so that r becomes

$$r = \lambda p - \gamma = \frac{\lambda p\mu - 1}{\mu} = \frac{R_0 - 1}{\mu} . \tag{6.5.13}$$

Eq. (6.5.13) connecting r, R_0 and μ, the expected length of the infectious period, has been used quite extensively in the literature (see, for example, Anderson and May[1] page 19 for an intuitive interpretation of this formula). But, as will be illustrated by example, it appears to be valid only in this special case under consideration.

For the case under consideration, the integral equations that appear in Eqs. (6.3.17), (6.3.18), and (6.3.19) for the mean functions of a CMJ-process take simple forms, which yield explicit solutions, for an epidemic which evolves from one infectious individual at $t = 0$. The equation for $M(t)$, the expected number of infectious individuals in the population at time $t > 0$, is:

$$M(t) = e^{-\gamma t} + \lambda p \int_0^t e^{-\gamma x} M(t-x)dx \,. \tag{6.5.14}$$

Similarly, $M_I(t)$, the expected total number of susceptibles that have been infected during the time interval $(0, t]$, satisfies the equation,

$$M_I(t) = 1 + \lambda p \int_0^t e^{-\gamma x} M_I(t-x)dx \,. \tag{6.5.15}$$

And lastly, $M_R(t)$, the expected total number of infecteds that have been removed during the time interval $(0, t]$, satisfies the equation,

$$M_R(t) = 1 - e^{-\gamma t} + \lambda p \int_0^t e^{-\gamma x} M_R(t-x)dx \,. \tag{6.5.16}$$

For $s > r = \lambda p - \gamma > 0$, it can be shown that the Laplace transform,

$$\widehat{M}(s) = \int_0^\infty e^{-st} M(t)dt \tag{6.5.17}$$

converges. The same can be said for the Laplace transforms $\widehat{M_I}(s)$ and $\widehat{M_R}(s)$ of the mean functions $M_I(t)$ and $M_R(t)$. By passing to Laplace transforms in Eq. (6.5.14), it can be shown that $\widehat{M}(s)$ satisfies the linear equation,

$$\widehat{M}(s) = \frac{1}{\gamma + s} + \frac{\lambda p}{\gamma + s}\widehat{M}(s) \,, \tag{6.5.18}$$

which has the solution,

$$\widehat{M}(s) = \frac{1}{s-r} \,. \tag{6.5.19}$$

Similar operations on Eqs. (6.5.15) and (6.5.16) yield the formulas,

$$\widehat{M_I}(s) = \frac{\gamma}{s\,(s-r))} + \frac{1}{s-r} \tag{6.5.20}$$

and

$$\widehat{M_R}(s) = \frac{\gamma}{s\,(s-r)} \tag{6.5.21}$$

for Laplace transforms of the mean functions $M_I(t)$ and $M_R(t)$.

Given these formulas, it may easily be verified that the mean functions,

$$M(t) = e^{rt} \,, \tag{6.5.22}$$

$$M_I(t) = e^{rt} + \frac{\gamma}{r}\left(e^{rt} - 1\right) \,, \tag{6.5.23}$$

and

$$M_R(t) = \frac{\gamma}{r}\left(e^{rt} - 1\right) \tag{6.5.24}$$

have, respectively, the Laplace transforms in Eqs. (6.5.19), (6.5.20) and (6.5.21), when $r > 0$. They are, therefore, the unique solutions of the integral equations in Eqs. (6.5.14), (6.5.15) and (6.5.16) for $t \in [0, \infty)$ in this case. Observe when $r > 0$, all these functions increase without bound as $t \uparrow \infty$. The cases $r = 0$ and $r < 0$ will be left as exercises for the reader.

All these formulas change significantly when the distribution of the length of the infectious period has a different parametric form. For example, if the random variable T has a gamma density,

$$g(t) = \frac{\gamma^{\alpha}}{\Gamma(\alpha)} t^{\alpha-1} e^{-\gamma t} \text{ for } t \in (0, \infty) \,, \tag{6.5.25}$$

where $\alpha > 0$ and $\gamma > 0$, then R_0 has the explicit form,

$$R_0 = \frac{\lambda p \alpha}{\gamma} \,. \tag{6.5.26}$$

Moreover, $h(s)$, the *p.g.f.* of the random variable N, representing the total number of susceptibles infected by an infective throughout his or her infectious period, has the form,

$$h(s) = \int_0^\infty e^{\lambda pt(s-1)} g(t)dt = \left(\frac{\gamma}{\gamma + \lambda p(1-s)}\right)^\alpha \tag{6.5.27}$$

for $s \in [0,1]$.

Just as in the simpler case, if $R_0 \leq 1$, then the continuous time CMJ-process becomes extinct with probability $q = 1$. But, if $R_0 > 1$, then q does not have a simple formula but may be estimated by a recursive procedure. Let $q_1 = h(0)$, and for $n \geq 2$ define the sequence (q_n) recursively by $q_n = h(q_{n-1})$. Then, $q_n \uparrow q$ as $n \uparrow \infty$ and in many cases the convergence is rapid. Furthermore, it can be shown that q so calculated is the smallest solution of $s = h(s)$ in $(0,1)$.

Unlike the case where the random variable T has a simple exponential distribution, finding the intrinsic growth rate of the epidemic in this case leads to a more complicated equation for computing r. To derive this equation, one needs to consider the Laplace transform,

$$\int_0^\infty e^{-st}(1 - G(t))\,dt \tag{6.5.28}$$

for $s > 0$, where $G(t)$ is an arbitrary continuous distribution function on $(0,\infty)$ with the continuous density $g(t)$. For $s > 0$, let $\widehat{g}(s)$ be the Laplace transform of $g(t)$. Integration by parts may be used to show that:

$$\int_0^\infty e^{-st} G(t)dt = \frac{\widehat{g}(s)}{s} \tag{6.5.29}$$

for $s > 0$. Then, for $s > 0$ it can easily be seen that the integral in Eq. (6.5.28) reduces to:

$$\int_0^\infty e^{-st}(1 - G(t))\,dt = \frac{1 - \widehat{g}(s)}{s}\,. \tag{6.5.30}$$

For a distribution function determined by the gamma density in Eq. (6.5.25),it can be seen, by consulting Eq. (6.4.21) for the Laplace gamma density, that equation defining r becomes:

$$\lambda p \int_0^\infty e^{-rt}(1 - G(t))\,dt$$

$$= \frac{\lambda p}{r}\left(1 - \left(\frac{\gamma}{\gamma + r}\right)^{\alpha}\right) = 1 \ . \tag{6.5.31}$$

If $R_0 > 1$, then there is a $r > 0$ satisfying this equation. Even though this equation yields no simple formula connecting r, R_0 and μ as in Eq. (6.5.13), numerical procedures may be used to calculate r.

Both forms of the $p.g.f.$ of the random variable N encountered in this section belong to a canonical family. Let $\alpha > 0$ be a positive parameter, let $p_1 \in (0,1)$, and put $q_1 = 1 - p_1$. For $n = 0, 1, 2, \cdots$, define the function $\alpha^{(n)}$ by:

$$\alpha^{(n)} = \frac{\Gamma(\alpha + n)}{\Gamma(n)} \ . \tag{6.5.32}$$

A random variable N with range $\mathbb{N}^+$ is said to have a negative binomial distribution if its $p.g.f.$ has the form,

$$h(s) = E\left[s^N\right] = \left(\frac{p_1}{1 - q_1 s}\right)^{\alpha} = \sum_{n=0}^{\infty} \mathbb{P}\left[N = n\right] s^n \tag{6.5.33}$$

for $s \in [0, 1]$. By expanding this function in Taylor series about $s = 0$, it can be shown that N had the $p.d.f.$,

$$\mathbb{P}\left[N = n\right] = \frac{\alpha^{(n)}}{n!} p_1^{\alpha} q_1^n \tag{6.5.34}$$

for $n = 0, 1, 2, \cdots$. For $\alpha = 1$, this density reduces to that of a geometric distribution; namely

$$\mathbb{P}\left[N = n\right] = p_1 q_1^n \tag{6.5.35}$$

for $n = 0, 1, 2, \cdots$. By letting

$$p_1 = \frac{\gamma}{\gamma + \lambda p} \tag{6.5.36}$$

in Eq. (6.5.27), it can be seen that this generating function may be put in the canonical form (6.5.33) of a negative binomial distribution. Similarly, with p_1 defined as in Eq. (6.5.36), then generating function in Eq. (6.5.8) may be put in the canonical form of a geometric distribution with $p.d.f.$ in Eq. (6.5.35). These canonical forms will be useful in studying the distribution of the total size of an epidemic as we shall see in the next section.

6.6 On the Distribution of the Total Size of an Epidemic

Let $\{\mathbf{X}_n \mid n \in \mathbb{N}^+\}$ be a BGW-process embedded in the continuous time $\{\mathbf{Z}(t) \mid t \in [0, \infty)\}$ CMJ-process. Then, the random variable,

$$Y = \sum_{n=0}^{\infty} \mathbf{X}_n \tag{6.6.1}$$

is defined as the total size of the epidemic and is either integer-valued or infinite. For every integer $k = 1, 2, \cdots$, let

$$\mathbb{P}\left[Y = k\right] = \rho(k) \; . \tag{6.6.2}$$

Then, because

$$\mathbb{P}\left[Y < \infty\right] = q \tag{6.6.3}$$

the probability the continuous time CMJ-process becomes extinct, it follows that

$$\sum_{k=1}^{\infty} \rho(k) = q \; . \tag{6.6.4}$$

Clearly, the probability that Y is infinite is $1 - q$. For $s \in [0, 1]$ let

$$r(s) = E\left[s^Y\right] = \sum_{k=1}^{\infty} \rho(k) s^k \tag{6.6.5}$$

be the *p.g.f.* of Y.

One approach to determining the probabilities in Eq. (6.6.2) is to attempt a derivation of a formula for the *p.g.f.* $r(s)$. Toward this end, for $n = 1, 2, \cdots$, consider the sequence of partial sums,

$$Y_n = \sum_{k=0}^{n} \mathbf{X}_n \uparrow Y \; , \tag{6.6.6}$$

and, for $s \in [0, 1]$, let

$$r_n(s) = E\left[s^{Y_n}\right] \tag{6.6.7}$$

be the *p.g.f.* of the random variable Y_n. As in previous sections, let the random variable N with range $\mathbb{N}^+$ be the total number of susceptibles infected by any infectious individual throughout his or her infectious period, and let $h(s)$ be its *p.g.f.*

Because $Y_1 = 1 + \mathbf{X}_1$, it can be seen that:

$$r_1(s) = E\left[s^{1+\mathbf{X}_1}\right] = sE\left[s^{\mathbf{X}_1}\right] = sh(s)\,. \tag{6.6.8}$$

In general, with the "birth" of each individual a new branching process begins and these processes are, by assumption, independent. Thus, let $\{Y_{nk} \mid k = 1, 2, \cdots, \mathbf{X}_1\}$ be a collection of *i.i.d.* copies of Y_n. If $\mathbf{X}_1 = 0$, then this collection is empty. It follows, therefore, that for every $n \geq 1$,

$$Y_{n+1} = 1 + \sum_{k=1}^{\mathbf{X}_1} Y_{nk}\,. \tag{6.6.9}$$

Hence,

$$E\left[s^{Y_{n+1}} \mid \mathbf{X}_1\right] = s\left(r_n(s)\right)^{\mathbf{X}_1}\,. \tag{6.6.10}$$

And, by taking expectations in this equation, it follows that:

$$r_{n+1}(s) = sh\left(r_n(s)\right) \tag{6.6.11}$$

for $n \geq 1$. By applying the dominated convergence theorem, it can be seen that:

$$\lim_{n\uparrow\infty} r(s) = r(s) = E\left[s^Y\right] \tag{6.6.12}$$

for all $s \in [0, 1]$, and a passage to the limit in Eq. (6.6.8) leads to the conclusion that the *p.g.f.* of the random variable Y satisfies the functional equation,

$$r(s) = sh\left(r(s)\right) \tag{6.6.13}$$

for $s \in [0, 1]$. It is known that there is a unique function with domain $[0, 1]$ and range $[0, 1]$ satisfying this equation (see Jagers[16] for details). Feller[13] has shown that $r(s)$ is the unique positive solution of Eq. (6.6.13) satisfying the condition $r(s) \leq q$ for all $s \in [0, 1]$. From Eq. (6.6.5), it can also be seen that $r(0) = 0$.

In general, it will be very difficult to find the required solution $r(s)$ of Eq. (6.6.13), but for some choices of $h(s)$ an explicit form of $r(s)$ may be found. One such choice is the function,

$$h(s) = \frac{1}{1 + R_0\left(1 - s\right)}\,, \tag{6.6.14}$$

(see Eq. (6.5.9)), which arose when the infection rate was the constant λp and the length of the infectious period followed an exponential distribution with parameter $\gamma > 0$ so that $R_0 = \lambda p/\gamma$. In this case, $r(s)$ is a solution of the quadratic equation,

$$x = \frac{s}{1 + R_0(1-x)} . \tag{6.6.15}$$

An application of the quadratic formula leads to the formula,

$$r(s) = \frac{1 + R_0 - \sqrt{(1+R_0)^2 - 4R_0 s}}{2R_0} . \tag{6.6.16}$$

As it should, this function satisfies the conditions $r(0) = 0$, $r(1) = 1$ if $R_0 \le 1$, but if $R_0 > 1$, then $r(1) = q = 1/R_0$, the probability of extinction.

For $k \ge 1$, let $r^{(k)}(s)$ be the kth derivative of $r(s)$, and let the sequence (c_k) of constants is determined recursively by:

$$c_{k+1} = 2(2k-1)c_k , \tag{6.6.17}$$

where $c_1 = 1$. Then, by using mathematical induction, it can be shown that

$$r^{(k)}(s) = c_k R_0^{k-1} \left((1+R_0)^2 - 4R_0 s\right)^{-\left(\frac{2k-1}{2}\right)} \tag{6.6.18}$$

is valid for all $k \ge 1$ and $s \in [0,1]$. A Taylor series expansion of the *p.g.f.* $r(s)$ about 0 results in the formula,

$$\mathbb{P}[Y = k] = \rho(k) = \frac{c_k R_0^{k-1}}{k!\,(1+R_0)^{2k-1}} , \tag{6.6.19}$$

$k = 1, 2, 3, \cdots$ for the *p.d.f.* of the random variable Y.

If $\mathbf{X}_0 = 1$, then the expected size of the nth generation of a BGW-process is

$$E[\mathbf{X}_n] = R_0^n . \tag{6.6.20}$$

By using this formula, it can be seen from Eq. (6.6.1) that if $R_0 < 1$, then the expected total size of the epidemic is:

$$E[Y] = \frac{1}{1 - R_0} . \tag{6.6.21}$$

By making the observation,

$$r^{(2)}(1) = E\left[Y\left(Y-1\right)\right] = \frac{2R_0}{\left(1-R_0\right)^3}\,, \tag{6.6.22}$$

it can be shown that the variance of Y is:

$$var\left[Y\right] = \frac{R_0\left(R_0+1\right)}{\left(1-R_0\right)^3}\,. \tag{6.6.23}$$

When R_0 is close to 1, this expectation and variance can be very large, and when $R_0 = 1$, the expected total size of the epidemic is infinite so that in this case the *p.d.f.* in Eq. (6.6.19) would have no finite expectation and variance.

One may, however, in principle compute values of this *p.d.f.* to provide some insights into the distribution of the random variable Y. A useful approach to doing such computations is to observe that the *p.d.f.* in Eq. (6.6.19) satisfies the recursive relationship,

$$\rho(k+1) = \left(\frac{2\left(2k-1\right)}{k+1}\right)\left(\frac{R_0}{\left(1+R_0\right)^2}\right)\rho(k) \tag{6.6.24}$$

for $k \geq 1$, where

$$\rho(1) = \frac{1}{1+R_0}\,. \tag{6.6.25}$$

Before presenting some sample calculations, it is of interest to observe that when $R_0 \leq 1$, $\rho(1)$ is the probability the epidemic stops with the initial infected individual so that

$$1-\rho(1) = \frac{R_0}{1+R_0} \tag{6.6.26}$$

is the probability the initial infective infects at least one susceptible. On the other hand, if $R_0 > 1$, then $q = 1/R_0$ is the probability that the epidemic becomes extinct, and for $k = 1, 2, \cdots$,

$$\rho_1(k) = \frac{\rho(k)}{q} = R_0\rho(k) \tag{6.6.27}$$

is the conditional *p.d.f.* of the size of the epidemic, given that extinction occurs.

Given extinction,

$$\rho_1(1) = \frac{R_0}{1 + R_0} \tag{6.6.28}$$

is the conditional probability the epidemic stops with the initial infective, and

$$1 - \rho_1(1) = \frac{1}{1 + R_0} \tag{6.6.29}$$

is the conditional probability the initial infective infects at least one susceptible. One can also show, using the formula in Eq. (6.6.18), that if $R_0 > 1$, then, conditional on extinction, the expectation and variance of the size Y of the epidemic when $\mathbf{X}_0 = 1$ are:

$$E\left[Y\right] = \frac{R_0}{R_0 - 1} \tag{6.6.30}$$

and

$$var\left[Y\right] = \frac{R_0\left(R_0 + 1\right)}{\left(R_0 - 1\right)^3} \ . \tag{6.6.31}$$

A certain duality exists between the cases $R_0 < 1$ and $R_0 > 1$. Let R_0^* be a number such that:

$$R_0^* R_0 = 1 \ , \tag{6.6.32}$$

and to emphasize that the *p.d.f.* in Eq. (6.6.19) depends on the threshold parameter R_0, let $\rho(k) = \rho(k; R_0)$. Then, it can be seen from Eq. (6.6.27) that:

$$\rho(k; R_0) = \rho\left(k; \frac{1}{R_0^*}\right) = \rho_1(k; R_0^*) \ . \tag{6.6.33}$$

Therefore, whenever $R_0 < 1$ and $\rho(k; R_0)$ is calculated for $k = 1, 2, \cdots$, it may also be interpreted as the case $R_0^* = 1/R_0 > 1$ so that $\rho_1(k; R_0^*)$ is the conditional density of the total size of the epidemic, given that extinction occurs with probability $q = 1/R_0^* = R_0$.

Table 6.6.1. Values of the Distribution Function of the Total Size an Epidemic for Selected Values of R_0.

$P[Y \leq y]$	$R_0 = 1$	$R_0 = 0.95$	$R_0 = 0.75$	$R_0 = 0.5$
1	0.500	0.513	0.571	0.667
2	0.625	0.641	0.711	0.815
3	0.688	0.705	0.780	0.881
4	0.727	0.745	0.822	0.917
5	0.754	0.773	0.851	0.940
6	0.774	0.794	0.872	0.955
7	0.791	0.810	0.888	0.966
8	0.804	0.824	0.901	0.973
9	0.815	0.835	0.912	0.979
10	0.823	0.844	0.920	0.983

Presented in Table 6.6.1 are illustrative values of the distribution function $P[Y \leq y]$ of the total size Y of an epidemic for chosen values of y and R_0. As can be seen from Table 6.6.1, when $R_0 = 1$ so that the distribution does not have a finite expectation or variance, the right hand tail is heavy and the probability that the size of the epidemic exceeds 10 is about $P[Y > 10] = 1 - 0.823 = 0.177$, even though extinction occurs with probability one. For the other values of R_0, the distribution of Y would have a finite expectation and variance, and the probabilities that the size of the epidemic exceeds 10 for the cases $R_0 = 0.95, 0.75$, and 0.5 are about $1 - 0.844 = 0.156$, $1 - 0.920 = 0.08$, and $1 - 0.983 = 0.017$, respectively. This suggests that the probability of the size of the epidemic exceeding 10 becomes negligible only for values of $R_0 < 0.5$. For $R_0^* = 1/0.95 = 1.0526$, $1/0.75 = 1.3333$, and $1/0.5 = 2.0$, the values in the table have a dual interpretation as the conditional probabilities of the events $[Y \leq y]$, given that extinction occurs with probabilities 0.95, 0.75, and 0.5. Thus, given extinction with probability 0.95, there is a significant probability of 0.156 that the total size of the epidemic exceeds 10.

All of the above formulas were derived under the assumption that the random variable N, the total number of susceptibles infected by an infective follows a geometric distribution with *p.g.f.* in Eq. (6.6.14).

Thanks to a result of Dwass, there is a relatively simple general formula for the distribution of the total size of the epidemic, which may be written down without solving Eq. (6.6.13) explicitly for $r(s)$. Let (p_{ij}) be the transition matrix for the BGW-process embedded in the continuous time CMJ-process. Then, for $k \geq j$,

$$\mathbb{P}[Y = k \mid \mathbf{X}_0 = j] = \frac{j}{k} p_{k,k-j} \,. \tag{6.6.34}$$

Jagers[16] (page 40) may be consulted for a proof of this result. Another way of viewing this formula is to let (N_ν) be *i.i.d.* copies of the random variable N. Then,

$$\mathbb{P}[Y = k \mid \mathbf{X}_0 = j] = \frac{j}{k} \mathbb{P}[N_1 + N_2 + \cdots + N_k = k - j] \,. \tag{6.6.35}$$

For the case the distribution of N follows a negative binomial distribution with *p.g.f.* of the form

$$h(s) = \left(\frac{p_1}{1 - q_1 s} \right)^\alpha , \tag{6.6.36}$$

an explicit formula may be written down for the probability in (6.6.35). Such a form arose in section 6.5 under the assumption the length of the infectious period followed a gamma distribution with positive parameters α and γ. In this case,

$$p_1 = \frac{\gamma}{\gamma + \lambda p} \tag{6.6.37}$$

(see Eq. (6.5.36)). When N has the *p.g.f.* in Eq. (6.6.36), the generating function of the sum in Eq. (6.6.35) is:

$$\begin{aligned} E\left[s^{N_1+N_2+\cdots+N_k}\right] &= \prod_{\nu=1}^{k} E\left[s^{N_\nu}\right] \\ &= \prod_{\nu=1}^{k} h(s) \\ &= \left(\frac{p_1}{1 - q_1 s} \right)^{\alpha k} . \end{aligned} \tag{6.6.38}$$

Because this is a *p.g.f.* of a negative binomial distribution with parameters αk and p_1 , it follows from Eq. (6.6.35) that:

$$\mathbb{P}\left[Y = k \mid \mathbf{X}_0 = j\right] = \frac{(\alpha k)^{(k-j)}}{(k-j)!} p_1^{\alpha k} q_1^{k-j} . \tag{6.6.39}$$

This formula may easily be evaluated numerically for moderate values of k and j such that $k \geq j \geq 1$.

6.7 Estimating HIV Infectivity in the Primary Stage of Infection

As was described in Chapter 2, during stage 1 of HIV disease infected individuals are not seropositive, and thus may not be aware that they are infected with HIV. Because during stage 1 the immune system has not yet generated sufficient antibodies to combat the virus, the concentration of virus particles in the blood and other body fluids, such as semen, is believed to be high. Consequently, due to this high concentration of virus particles, the probability per sexual contact that an infective infects a susceptible may be higher than in later stages of the disease when the action of the immune system has reduced the concentration of virus particles in body fluids. Among homosexual men, genital-anal sexual contacts have been reported to be prevalent, and it is believed that in such cases the probability of infection per contact is high, because the semen of the infective may come into direct contact with the blood of the susceptible due to damaged mucous membranes.

Jacquez et al.[15] have reviewed the data on infectivity per sexual contact for the transmission of HIV among US cohorts of homosexual men that had been reported since the late seventies and early eighties up to 1993 in the San Francisco hepatitis B vaccine trial and from cohorts in Chicago, Baltimore, Los Angeles, and Pittsburgh. When expressed as a percentage of the sample size of the cohort, the number that were seropositive for HIV rapidly increased initially then leveled off in approximately the mid-eighties. This initial steep rise in the percentage of seropositives suggested a pattern of high contagiousness during the primary stage of infection followed by a decrease in infectiousness in the early years of the HIV/AIDS epidemic among US cohorts of homosexual men. To test for evidence of this pattern of high contagiousness, it was necessary to obtain estimates of the probability p of infection per contact during the early stages of HIV infection.

The method used to obtain estimates of p was essentially an application of the theory outlined in Section 6.5. From the relationship,

$$r = \frac{R_0 - 1}{\mu}, \tag{6.7.1}$$

(see Eq. (6.5.13)), connecting the intrinsic growth rate r of the epidemic with R_0 and μ, the expected length of the infectious period, it can be seen that:

$$R_0 = r\mu + 1 . \tag{6.7.2}$$

Thus, if estimates of r and μ are available, then R_0 may be estimated. But, as shown in Section 6.5, if λ is the rate of sexual contacts per unit time for a Poissonian K-process, then $R_0 = \lambda p\mu$. So if estimates of R_0, λ, and μ are available, then p may also be estimated. At this point it should be recalled that the validity of these relationships depends on the assumptions that the K-process is Poissonian and the length of the infectious period has an exponential distribution with expectation μ.

To illustrate the ideas used by Jacquez et al. to obtain estimates of p, the incidence data, representing the number of seroconversions per month in the San Francisco hepatitis B study, were plotted on a log-scale and the first four points were observed to lie on an approximately straight line, which yielded a least-squares estimate of $\widehat{r} = 0.156$ per month. Given this estimate of r and an estimate of $\widehat{\mu} = 2$ months for the length of stage 1 of the infectious period, the estimated value of R_0 was:

$$\widehat{R_0} = (0.156)2 + 1 = 1.312 . \tag{6.7.3}$$

But, if one assumes that the length of stage 1 is shorter, say $\widehat{\mu} = 1.5$ months, then

$$\widehat{R_0} = (0.156)1.5 + 1 = 1.234 . \tag{6.7.4}$$

Let $\widehat{\lambda}$ be an estimate of the contact rate per unit time. Then, given this estimate, the equation,

$$\widehat{p} = \frac{\widehat{R_0}}{\widehat{\lambda}\widehat{\mu}} \tag{6.7.5}$$

may be used to estimate p, the probability of infection per sexual contact in stage 1 of HIV disease. Estimates of λ in the range 5 to 10 per month were reported in the literature reviewed by Jacquez et al. For $\widehat{\mu}$ = 2, this range of estimates for λ yielded estimates of p in the interval,

$$\widehat{p} \in \left[\frac{1.312}{(10)2} = 0.0656, \frac{1.312}{(5)2} = 0.1312\right] . \tag{6.7.6}$$

But, for $\widehat{\mu} = 1.5$, this range of estimates for λ yielded estimates of p in the range,

$$\widehat{p} \in \left[\frac{1.234}{(10)1.5} = 0.082267, \frac{1.234}{(5)1.5} = 0.16453\right] . \tag{6.7.7}$$

These estimates of p appear to high in relation to those reported for this value in other stages of HIV disease. In a subsequent chapter, the implications of these estimates, as well as other estimates that have been reported in the literature, will be explored more thoroughly.

6.8 Threshold Parameters for Staged Infectious Diseases

As described in Chapter 2, HIV disease, as well as some other infectious diseases, progress in stages. Accordingly, a need arises to extend the ideas developed in the previous sections of this chapter to the case where a disease progresses through $k \geq 2$ stages. Let E_j represent the jth stage of a disease, and suppose progression through the stages is linear as symbolized by:

$$E_1 \rightarrow E_2 \rightarrow \cdots \rightarrow E_k . \tag{6.8.1}$$

Entrance into stage E_1 signals the event that a susceptible is infected by contacts with an infective individual, and following this infection, the times spent in the successive stages of the disease are random variables. An exit from stage E_k indicates that an infective individual is removed from the population by immunity or death. Table 2.9.1 may be consulted for a classification of the stages of HIV disease based on $CD4^+$ cell count.

Let the random variable X_j represent the time spent in stage j of the disease, and let $G_j(t)$ be the distribution function of X_j with *p.d.f.* $g_j(t)$, where $j = 1, 2, \cdots, k$, and $t \in (0, \infty)$. In all the examples considered in this section, these and similar functions will be continuous on $(0, \infty)$. It will also be assumed that the random variables $X_1, \cdots, X_k$ are independent. After a random length of time X_1 in stage 1, stage 2 is entered at time $T_2 = X_1$, and in general, the time stage i is entered is given by the random variable,

$$T_i = X_1 + X_2 + \cdots + X_{i-1} \tag{6.8.2}$$

for $i = 2, 3, \cdots, k+1$, with the proviso that T_{k+1} is the time an infective exits the population. To extend the structure of CMJ-processes developed in Section 6.3 to the case a disease may have several stages, the densities $c_i(t)$ of the random variable in Eq. (6.8.2) will be required. By definition $c_2(t) = g_1(t)$ and, in general, the required densities may be computed recursively by the formula,

$$c_i(t) = \int_0^t c_{i-1}(x) g_{i-1}(t-x) dx \tag{6.8.3}$$

for $i = 3, \cdots, k+1$, and $t \in (0, \infty)$.

Conditional on stage $j \geq 2$ being entered at time $t = 0$, let the random function $K_j(t)$ be the number of susceptibles infected by an infective individual during the time interval $(0, t]$ for $t > 0$. By definition, the mean function of this process is:

$$\nu_j(t) = E\left[K_j(t)\right] , \tag{6.8.4}$$

with infection rate density,

$$b_j(t) = \frac{d\nu_j(t)}{dt} . \tag{6.8.5}$$

In all the examples considered in this section, these, and similar functions, will be finite and continuous on $t \in (0, \infty)$. Again, conditional on stage $j = 2, \cdots, k$, being entered at $t = 0$, let the random function $K_j^*(t)$ the random function $K_j(t)$ stopped at the random time X_j, and let

$$\mu_j(t) = E\left[K_j^*(t)\right] \tag{6.8.6}$$

for $t \in (0, \infty)$. Then, just as in Section 6.3, it can be shown that for $t \in (0, \infty)$ and $j = 2, \cdots, k$,

$$\mu_j(t) = \int_0^t b_j(x)(1 - G_j(x))dx \, . \tag{6.8.7}$$

Observe that when $j = 1$, there is no need to introduce the random function $K_1^*(t)$, because by definition entrance into stage 1 occurs at $t = 0$ so that conditioning on the random time of entrance is not required. Consequently, Eq. (6.8.7) also holds for $j = 1$. Given that an infective individual is infected at $t = 0$, let the random function $N_j(t)$ be the number of susceptibles infected by this infective during the time interval $(0, t]$, $t > 0$, and let

$$m_j(t) = E\left[N_j(t)\right] \tag{6.8.8}$$

be its mean function defined for $j = 1, 2, \cdots, k$. Then, $m_1(t) = \mu_1(t)$, which is given by Eq. (6.8.7), but for $j \geq 2$, the random time T_i of entrance into stage i must be taken into account. By a renewal argument, it can be seen that for $j = 2, \cdots, k$ and $t \in (0, \infty)$,

$$m_j(t) = \int_0^t c_j(x)\mu_j(t - x)dx \, . \tag{6.8.9}$$

Given that an infective is infected at $t = 0$, the random function

$$N(t) = \sum_{j=1}^{k} N_j(t) \tag{6.8.10}$$

is the number of susceptible infected by this infective during the time interval $(0, t]$, $t > 0$, and the corresponding mean function is

$$m(t) = \sum_{j=1}^{k} m_j(t) \, . \tag{6.8.11}$$

In this formulation, the threshold parameter R_0 will be defined in terms of the random variable,

$$N = \lim_{t \uparrow \infty} N(t) \, , \tag{6.8.12}$$

which is the total number of susceptibles infected by an infective that was infected at $t = 0$. By definition,

$$R_0 = E[N] = \lim_{t \uparrow \infty} m(t) < \infty. \tag{6.8.13}$$

To express R_0 in terms of the basic components of the model and derive a formula for computing r, the intrinsic growth rate of the epidemic, it will be convenient to the consider the Laplace–Stieltjes transform,

$$H(s) = \int_0^\infty e^{-st} m(dt) \tag{6.8.14}$$

for $s \geq 0$. Observe that $R_0 = H(0)$ and r is a solution of the equation $H(s) = 1$, where if s is a solution such that $s \neq r$, then $| s | < r$.

As a first step in deriving a formula for this transform, for $s \geq 0$ and $j = 1, 2, \cdots, k$, let

$$\widehat{\mu}_j(s) = \int_0^\infty e^{-st} \mu_j(dt)$$

$$= \int_0^\infty e^{-st} b_j(t)(1 - G_j(t))dt \tag{6.8.15}$$

and

$$\widehat{c}_j(s) = \int_0^\infty e^{-st} c_j(t)dt\ . \tag{6.8.16}$$

Then, from Eq. (6.8.9) it follows that:

$$H_j(s) = \int_0^\infty e^{-st} m_j(dt) = \widehat{c}_j(s)\widehat{\mu}_j(s)\ , \tag{6.8.17}$$

an equation that holds for all $j = 1, 2, \cdots, k$, provided $\widehat{c}_1(s) = 1$ for all $s \geq 0$. From this result, it can be seen that the desired formula for $H(s)$ is:

$$H(s) = \sum_{j=1}^{k} H_j(s) = \sum_{j=1}^{k} \widehat{c}_j(s)\widehat{\mu}_j(s)\ . \tag{6.8.18}$$

Therefore, because $\widehat{c}_j(0) = 1$ for all $j = 1, 2, \cdots, k$, the formula for R_0, by Eq. (6.8.15) takes the form,

$$R_0 = \sum_{j=1}^{k} \widehat{\mu}_j(0)$$

$$= \sum_{j=1}^{k} \int_0^\infty b_j(t)(1 - G_j(t))dt \,. \tag{6.8.19}$$

Hence, if R_{0j} for the jth stage is defined by:

$$R_{0j} = \int_0^\infty b_j(t)(1 - G_j(t))dt \,, \tag{6.8.20}$$

then Eq. (6.8.19) justifies the statement,

$$R_0 = \sum_{j=1}^{k} R_{0j} \,, \tag{6.8.21}$$

that threshold parameters are additive over stages. Among other authors, Jacquez et al.[15] have used a special case of this formula.

To develop formulas for finding q, the probability of extinction, it will be necessary to derive a formula of the $p.g.f.$ of the random variable N. In this connection, it will be useful to write N in the form,

$$N = \sum_{j=1}^{k} K_j(X_j) \,. \tag{6.8.22}$$

Given the collection of random variables $\mathbb{C} = \{X_j,\ j = 1, 2, \cdots, k\}$ assume that the random variables $K_j(X_j),\ j = 1, 2, \cdots, k$, are conditionally independent, and let

$$f_j(s,t) = E\left[s^{K_j(t)}\right] \,. \tag{6.8.23}$$

Then,

$$E\left[s^N \mid \mathbb{C}\right] = \prod_{j=1}^{k} f_j(s, X_j) \,. \tag{6.8.24}$$

Therefore, since $\mathbb{C}$ is a collection of independent random variables, one may conclude that:

$$h(s) = E\left[E\left[s^N \mid \mathbb{C}\right]\right] = \prod_{j=1}^{k} E\left[f_j(s, X_j)\right] \,. \tag{6.8.25}$$

But, if $g_j(t)$ is the *p.d.f.* of X_j, then

$$h_j(s) = E\left[f_j(s, X_j)\right] = \int_0^\infty f_j(s,t)g_j(t)dt \qquad (6.8.26)$$

Consequently, under the assumptions just stated, the *p.g.f.* of N has the form,

$$h(s) = \prod_{j=1}^{k} h_j(s) \qquad (6.8.27)$$

for $s \in [0, 1]$.

All the above formulas take simple forms under the following assumptions. Suppose for $j = 1, 2, \cdots, k$ the K_j-process is Poissonian with parameter $\lambda_j p_j$, where λ_j is the contact rate per unit time and p_j is the probability of infection per contact between a susceptible and infective. Also suppose that the duration of stay X_j in stage j has an exponential distribution with distribution function

$$G_j(t) = 1 - e^{-\gamma_j t}\ , \qquad (6.8.28)$$

where $\gamma_j > 0$, $j = 1, 2, \cdots, k$, and $t \in [0, \infty)$. Then, the threshold parameter R_0 has the form

$$R_0 = \sum_{j=1}^{k} \frac{\lambda_j p_j}{\gamma_j}\ , \qquad (6.8.29)$$

and, by definition, $R_{0j} = \lambda_j p_j/\gamma_j$.

Under these assumptions, the equation defining r also takes a relatively simple form. For $j = 1, 2, \cdots, k$, and $s \in [0, \infty)$, the Laplace transform of X_j is:

$$\widehat{g}_j(s) = E\left[e^{-sX_j}\right] = \frac{\gamma_j}{\gamma_j + s}\ . \qquad (6.8.30)$$

Hence, $\widehat{c}_1(s) = \widehat{g}_1(s)$ and for $i = 2, 3, \cdots, k$,

$$\widehat{c}_i(s) = \prod_{j=1}^{i-1} \frac{\gamma_j}{\gamma_j + s}\ . \qquad (6.8.31)$$

Moreover, for $j = 1, 2, \cdots, k$

$$\widehat{\mu}_j(s) = \frac{\lambda_j p_j}{\gamma_j + s} = R_{0j}\widehat{g}_j(s) \ . \tag{6.8.32}$$

With these definitions for $s \in [0, \infty)$, the Laplace-Stieltjes transform in Eq. (6.6.18) has the form,

$$H(s) = \sum_{j=1}^{k} R_{0j} \prod_{i=1}^{j} \left(\frac{\gamma_i}{\gamma_i + s} \right) \ . \tag{6.8.33}$$

In principle, this formula may be used to find numerical values of r, and when $R_0 > 1$, then $r > 0$.

To derive a formula for the $p.g.f.$ of N, observe that when the K_j-process is Poissonian, then its $p.g.f.$ is:

$$f_j(s, t) = e^{\lambda_j p_j t(s-1)} \ , \tag{6.8.34}$$

and Eq. (6.8.26) has the form,

$$h_j(s) = \frac{\gamma_j}{\gamma_j + \lambda_j p_j (1 - s)}$$

$$= \frac{1}{1 + R_{0j}(1 - s)} \tag{6.8.35}$$

for $j = 1, 2, \cdots, k$. Therefore, given these assumptions, for $s \in [0, 1]$ the $p.g.f.$ of N is:

$$h(s) = \prod_{j=1}^{k} \left(\frac{1}{1 + R_{0j}(1 - s)} \right) \ . \tag{6.8.36}$$

If $R_0 \leq 1$, then $q = 1$, but if it is the case that $R_0 > 1$, then q is the smallest root of $s = h(s)$ in $(0, 1]$. The possibility of deriving a formula for q seems remote, but by using numerical methods, it would be feasible to calculate values of q, given values of the parameters.

6.9 Branching Processes Approximations

In all the preceding sections of this chapter, it has been assumed that a CMJ-process was, in some sense, an approximation to an epidemic evolving within a large population of susceptibles, but the sense in which the branching process approximated the epidemic was not made clear. Accordingly, the purpose of this section is to outline a structure, inspired by the work of Ball[3] and the references contained therein, in which a branching process approximation to an epidemic is made more precise. The papers of Ball and O'Neill[5] and Ball and Donnelly[4] may also be consulted. The mathematics presented in this section is more advanced than that of the previous sections, and may be skipped by readers primarily interested in applications of the theory rather than in the mathematics underlying it.

Consider a population of some fixed size, say m, and let the random functions $X(t), Y(t)$, and $Z(t)$ denote, respectively, the number of susceptibles, infectious, and removed individuals at time $t \in [0, \infty)$. Suppose the initial values are $(X(0),\ Y(0),\ Z(0)) = (n, a, 0)$, where $n + a = m$. It will be assumed that infectious individuals have *i.i.d.* life histories $\mathcal{H} = (T, K)$, which may be used to construct a CMJ-process in continuous time. As before, the random variable T is the time elapsing between an individual's infection and the individual's removal or death, and K is a point process of times at which infectious contacts with susceptibles occur. In all the models $\mathcal{H}$ of life histories considered so far in this chapter T and K have been assumed to be independent, but as will be illustrated in subsequent chapters, models of $\mathcal{H}$ may be constructed such that the independence assumption does not hold.

Within this finite population of n susceptibles and a infectives, let $\mathbb{E}_{n,a}$ denote an epidemic model that evolves as follows. Each contact between infectives and susceptibles is chosen independently and uniformly from the n initial infectives, and after death or removal an individual is immune to further infection. When an infective contacts a susceptible, an infection occurs according to the K-process, but otherwise nothing happens. When there are no more infectives in the population, the epidemic ceases. In principle, the K-process may be modified so that the possibility of contacts with oneself and the lack of contacts with the a initial infectives involves no loss of generality.

In order to examine the asymptotic behavior of the model, it will be useful to introduce a sequence of models,

$$\{\mathbb{E}_{n,a} \mid n = 1, 2, \cdots\} \tag{6.9.1}$$

defined on some probability space $(\Omega, \mathfrak{A}, \mathbb{P})$ with the following random entities defined on it.

Label the initial a infectives as $i = -(a-1), -(a-2), \cdots, -1, 0$, and the initial susceptibles as $i = 1, 2, \cdots, n$. Then, let the collection of life histories,

$$\{\mathcal{H}_i \mid i = -(a-1), -(a-2), \cdots, 0, 1, 2, \cdots, n\} \tag{6.9.2}$$

be *i.i.d.* copies of $\mathcal{H} = (T, K)$. Moreover, let $U_1, U_2, \cdots$, be a sequence of *i.i.d.* uniform random variables on $(0, 1)$.

For $i = -(a-1), -(a-2), \cdots, 0$, the ith initial infective makes contacts during $(0, T_i)$ according to the time points of the K_i-process. The individual contacted at the jth contact is the random variable,

$$\chi_j^{(n)} = [nU_j] + 1 \ , \tag{6.9.3}$$

where $[\cdot]$ is the greatest integer function. If this individual is susceptible, then he or she becomes infected according to the K_i-process and follows life history $\mathcal{H}_k$, where, for $k \geq 1$, $k-1$ is the number of susceptibles that have been previously infected. Hence, the life histories $\mathcal{H}_i$, $i = 1, 2, \cdots, n$, are assigned sequentially to the susceptibles in the order in which they are infected. When contacts among infectives occur, nothing happens. To emphasize that the process depends on n, let the random functions $X_n(t), Y_n(t)$ and $Z_n(t)$ denote, respectively, the number of susceptible, infectious, and removed individuals in the $\mathbb{E}_{n,a}$-process at time $t \in [0, \infty)$. For $t > 0$, let $W_n(t)$ be the total number of susceptibles that have been infected during $(0, t]$.

The collection of life histories,

$$\{\mathcal{H}_i \mid i = -(a-1), -(a-2), \cdots, 0, 1, \cdots\} \tag{6.9.4}$$

could also be used to define a CMJ-process $\mathfrak{B}_{CJM}$ on the same probability space $(\Omega, \mathfrak{A}, \mathbb{P})$, in which a typical individual lives to age T and reproduces according to a K-process.

It will be assumed all a initial individuals are born at $t = 0$ and follow the life histories $\mathcal{H}_j,\ j = -(a-1), -(a-2), \cdots, 0$. For $i = 1, 2, \cdots, \mathcal{H}_i$ is the life history of the ith individual born in the branching process $\mathfrak{B}_{CJM}$. The assumption that all initial individuals are born at $t = 0$, may be strong or weak, depending on the model chosen for a typical life history $\mathcal{H}$. In a demographic context, the initial age distribution is of fundamental importance in projecting the subsequent course of a population projection (see Mode[19] for details). However, with regard to the results that follow, it seems plausible that the assumption that all initial individuals in the branching process are born at $t = 0$ can and will be removed sometime in the future. For $t > 0$, let the random function $Z(t)$ be the number of live individuals in the branching process $\mathfrak{B}_{CJM}$ at time t, and let $Z_I(t)$ and $Z_R(t)$, respectively, denote the total numbers of individuals that have born (infected) and removed in the $\mathfrak{B}_{CJM}$-process during $(0, t]$.

To make clear the sense in which the $\mathfrak{B}_{CJM}$-process is an approximation to the $\mathbb{E}_{n,a}$-process as $n \to \infty$, it will be useful to consider the following ω-sets in the σ-algebra $\mathfrak{A}$. Let

$$A = \left[\omega \in \Omega \mid \lim_{t\uparrow\infty} Z(t,\omega) = 0\right] \tag{6.9.5}$$

be the set on which the $\mathfrak{B}_{CMJ}$-process becomes extinct; let

$$B = [\omega \in \Omega \mid U_i(\omega) \neq U_j(\omega), \text{ for all } i \neq j] \ ; \tag{6.9.6}$$

and let

$$C = [\omega \in \Omega \mid Z_I(t,\omega) < \infty, \text{ for all } t \in (0,\infty)] \tag{6.9.7}$$

be the set on which the branching process is non-explosive. For all branching processes considered in this chapter, it can be shown that $\mathbb{P}[C] = 1$. By way of preparation for the main results, a proof of the following lemma will be needed.

Lemma 6.9.1. *(i)* $\mathbb{P}[B] = 1$. *(ii)* If D is any set in $\mathfrak{A}$, then it is the case that $\mathbb{P}[D \cap B] = \mathbb{P}[D]$.

Proof: To prove assertion (i), for $n = 1, 2, \cdots$, let

$$B_n = [\omega \in \Omega \mid U_i(\omega) \neq U_j(\omega) \text{ for all } 1 \leq i < j \leq n] \; . \tag{6.9.8}$$

Then

$$B = \bigcap_{n=1}^{\infty} B_n \; . \tag{6.9.9}$$

Let B^c be the complement of B. Because finitely many *i.i.d.* uniform random variable on $(0, 1)$ are equal with probability zero, $\mathbb{P}[B_n^c] = 0$ for all $n = 1, 2, \cdots$. Therefore,

$$\begin{aligned} 0 \leq \mathbb{P}[B^c] &= \mathbb{P}\left[\bigcup_{n=1}^{\infty} B_n^c\right] \\ &\leq \sum_{n=1}^{\infty} \mathbb{P}[B_n^c] = 0 \; . \end{aligned} \tag{6.9.10}$$

Hence, $\mathbb{P}[B] = 1$. To prove the second assertion, observe that:

$$(D \cap B)^c = D^c \cup B^c = D^c \cup (B^c \cap D) \; . \tag{6.9.11}$$

But, $\mathbb{P}[B^c \cap D] \leq \mathbb{P}[B^c] = 0$, and it follows that

$$\mathbb{P}[(D \cap B)^c] = \mathbb{P}[D^c] \; . \tag{6.9.12}$$

From this result, it can be seen that $\mathbb{P}[D \cap B] = \mathbb{P}[D]$, which completes the proof of the lemma.

The first theorem makes precise the sense in which the number of infectives in the epidemic process $\mathbb{E}_{n,a}$ is approximated by the number alive in the branching process $\mathfrak{B}_{CJM}$.

Theorem 6.9.1. At time $t > 0$, let $Y_n(t)$ be the number of infectives is the $\mathbb{E}_{n,a}$-process and let $Z(t)$ be the number alive in the $\mathfrak{B}_{CJM}$-process. Then,

$$(i) \; \lim_{n \uparrow \infty} \sup_{0 \leq t < \infty} \mid Y_n(t, \omega) - Z(t, \omega) \mid = 0 \tag{6.9.13}$$

for $\mathbb{P}$-almost all $\omega \in A$, and

$$(ii) \lim_{n\uparrow\infty} \sup_{0\le t<t_0} | Y_n(t,\omega) - Z(t,\omega) | = 0 \tag{6.9.14}$$

for $\mathbb{P}$-almost all $\omega \in A^c$, where $t_0 > 0$.

Proof: Let $\tau_n(\omega)$ be the first time a previously infected individual in the $\mathbb{E}_{n,a}$-process is contacted. Then, $Y_n(t,\omega) = Z(t,\omega)$ for all $0 \le t < \tau_n(\omega)$. Now fix $\omega \in A \cap B$. Then, for this ω, the total number of births in the $\mathfrak{B}_{CJM}$-process,

$$\lim_{t\uparrow\infty} Z_I(t,\omega) = Z_I(\omega) , \tag{6.9.15}$$

is finite. Because $\omega \in B$,

$$\varepsilon(\omega) = \min\{| U_i(\omega) - U_j(\omega) | \mid i \neq j = 1, 2, \cdots, Z_I(\omega)\} > 0 . \tag{6.9.16}$$

Next consider the partition,

$$\left\{[0, \frac{1}{n}), [\frac{1}{n}, \frac{2}{n}), \cdots, [\frac{n-1}{n}, 1)\right\} \tag{6.9.17}$$

of the interval $[0,1)$, and note that the length of each sub-interval is n^{-1}. If for some j, there is a $k \ge 1$ such that:

$$\frac{k-1}{n} \le U_j(\omega) < \frac{k}{n} , \tag{6.9.18}$$

then $k - 1 \le nU_j(\omega) < k$, so that $[nU_j(\omega)] = k - 1$ and

$$\chi_j^{(n)}(\omega) = [nU_j(\omega)] + 1 = k . \tag{6.9.19}$$

Therefore, if n is chosen such the $n^{-1} < \varepsilon(\omega)$, or equivalently $n > \varepsilon^{-1}(\omega)$, then the subset,

$$\left\{\chi_1^{(n)}(\omega), \cdots, \chi_{Z_I(\omega)}^{(n)}(\omega)\right\} \tag{6.9.20}$$

of integers will be distinct. Consequently, all births in the $\mathfrak{B}_{CMJ}$-process will correspond to infections in the $\mathbb{E}_{n,a}$-process. By noting **Lemma 6.9.1** implies $\mathbb{P}[A \cap B] = \mathbb{P}[A]$, assertion (i) follows.

To prove assertion (ii), fix $\omega \in A^c \cap B \cap C \subset C$. Since $\omega \in C$, there is a t_0 such that $Z_I(t_0, \omega) < \infty$. The argument used in proving (i) may now be repeated with $Z_I(\omega)$ replaced by $Z_I(t_0, \omega)$. The proof of (ii) is completed by observing **Lemma 6.9.1** implies $\mathbb{P}[A^c \cap B \cap C] = \mathbb{P}[A^c]$.

For $n = 1, 2, \cdots$, the total number of susceptibles infected in the $\mathbb{E}_{n,a}$-process is given by the random variable,

$$\lim_{t \uparrow \infty} W_n(t) = W_n, \tag{6.9.21}$$

and according to Eq. (6.9.12), Z_I is the number of births (susceptibles infected) in the $\mathfrak{B}_{CMJ}$-process. As shown in the next theorem, when n is large, Z_I is an approximation to the random variable W_n.

Theorem 6.9.2. Let

$$D = \left[\omega \in \Omega \mid \lim_{n \uparrow \infty} W_n(\omega) = Z_I(\omega) \right] . \tag{6.9.22}$$

Then, $\mathbb{P}[D] = 1$.

Proof: If $\omega \in A \cap B$, then by **Theorem 6.9.1** (i), $Z_I(\omega) < \infty$ and for n sufficiently large $Y_n(\cdot, \omega)$ and $Z(\cdot, \omega)$ coincide so that:

$$\lim_{n \uparrow \infty} W_n(\omega) = Z_I(\omega) . \tag{6.9.23}$$

If $\omega \in A^c \cap B \cap C$, then $Z_I(\omega) = \infty$, and for $k = 1, 2, \cdots$ let

$$\tau_k^*(\omega) = \inf \{ t \mid Z_I(t, \omega) \geq k \} . \tag{6.9.24}$$

Then, $\tau_k^*(\omega) < \infty$ and, as in the proof of (ii) in **Theorem 6.9.1**, $Y_n(t, \omega) = Z(t, \omega)$ for all n sufficiently large and t such that it is the case that $0 \leq t \leq \tau_k^*(\omega)$. Therefore, $\lim_{n \uparrow \infty} W_n(\omega) \geq k$ for $k = 1, 2, \cdots$. Hence, $\lim_{n \uparrow \infty} W_n(\omega) = \infty$. Now observe that:

$$D = (A \cap B) \cup (A^c \cap B \cap C) . \tag{6.9.25}$$

To complete the proof of the theorem, observe that by **Lemma 6.9.1**, it follows that:

$$\mathbb{P}[D] = \mathbb{P}[A] + \mathbb{P}[A^c] = 1 . \tag{6.9.26}$$

The final theorem of this section makes precise the sense in which all branching processes discussed in the foregoing sections are approximations to $\mathbb{E}_{n,a}$-processes of the type under consideration. An epidemic will be called minor or major, respectively, according to whether extinction occurs or does not occur. It should be emphasized that this is an operational definition and it is advised that for any designation of a model $\mathcal{H} = (T, K)$ of the life histories, a more detailed meaning of the terms minor and major should be sought by either mathematical analysis or computer simulations (see Section 6.6 for an illustrative example).

Theorem 6.9.3. Let the random variable N be the total number of susceptibles infected by a typical infective throughout his infectious period in the $\mathbb{E}_{n,a}$-process, define R_0 as $R_0 = E[N]$, and let $h(s) = E\left[s^N\right]$ be the *p.g.f.* of N. Then, as $n \uparrow \infty$,

(*i*) a minor or major epidemic occurs according to whether $R_0 \leq 1$ or $R_0 > 1$, and

(*ii*) the probabilities of a minor or major epidemic are q^a and $1 - q^a$, respectively, where q is the smallest solution of $s = h(s)$ in $[0, 1]$.

(*iii*) Let $r_a(s) = E\left[s^W\right]$ be the *p.g.f.* of W, the total number of susceptibles infected in the epidemic. Then, $r_a(s) = (r(s))^a$, where $r(s)$ is a solution of the functional equation,

$$r(s) = h(sr(s)) \tag{6.9.27}$$

and for $k = 0, 1, 2, \cdots$

$$\mathbb{P}[W = k]$$

$$= \frac{a}{a+k}\mathbb{P}[N_1 + N_2 + \cdots + N_{a+k} = k] , \tag{6.9.28}$$

where $N_1, N_2, \cdots$ are *i.i.d.* copies of N.

Proof: By **Theorem 6.9.2**, $W_n \to W = Z_I$ as $n \to \infty$ with probability one, where Z_I is the total number of births (susceptibles infected) in the $\mathfrak{B}_{CJM}$-process. The random variable Z_I is also the total number of births in the BGW-process embedded in $\mathfrak{B}_{CJM}$.

Therefore, assertions (i) and (ii) follow from well-known results regarding BGW-processes. The proof of Eq. (6.9.27) is a slight variant of the proof of Eq. (6.6.26). Suppose X_1 is the number of susceptibles infected in the first generation of the embedded BGW-process, and let $Z_{I,\nu}$, $v = 1, 2, \cdots, X_1$ be *i.i.d.* copies of the random variable Z_I. Then,

$$Z_I = X_1 + \sum_{\nu=1}^{X_1} Z_{I,\nu} \tag{6.9.29}$$

so that

$$E\left[s^{Z_I} \mid X_1\right] = s^{X_1} \left(r(s)\right)^{X_1} \ . \tag{6.9.30}$$

Eq. (6.9.27) now follows by taking expectations. To complete the proof of assertion (iii) let $j = a$ and substitute $a + k$ for k in Eq. (6.6.33).

In projecting an epidemic based on a $\mathbb{E}_{n,a}$-process, one is often interested in the random functions $X_n(t), Y_n(t)$, and $Z_n(t)$ denoting, respectively, the number of susceptible, infective, and removed individuals at time $t \geq 0$. For n sufficiently large, these random functions may be approximated by a $\mathfrak{B}_{CJM}$-process as $X_n(t) \simeq n - Z_I(t)$, $Y_n(t) \simeq Z(t)$, and $Z_n(t) \simeq Z_R(t)$.

6.10 References

1. R. M. Anderson and R. M. May, *Infectious Diseases of Humans - Dynamics and Control,* Oxford University Press, Oxford, New York, Tokyo, 1992.
2. F. Ball, The Threshold Behavior of Epidemic Models, *Journal of Applied Probability* **20:** 227-241, 1983.
3. F. Ball, The Threshold Behaviour of Stochastic Epidemics, *Series in Mathematical Biology and Medicine* **6:** 407-424, O. Arino, D. Axelrod and M. Kimmel (eds.), *Advances in Mathematical Population Dynamics - Molecules, Cells, and Man,* World Scientific Publishing Company, Singapore, New Jersey, London, Hong Kong, 1997.
4. F. Ball and P. Donnelly, Strong Approximations for Epidemic Models, *Stochastic Processes and Their Applications* **55:** 1-21, 1995.

5. F. Ball and P. O'Neill, Strong Convergence of Stochastic Epidemics, *Advances in Applied Probability* **26:** 629-655, 1994.

6. R. Bartoszynski, On a Certain Model of an Epidemic, *Applications Mathematicae* **XIII (2)**: 139-151, 1975.

7. N. Becker and I. Marschner, The Effect of Heterogeneity on the Spread of Disease, *Lecture Notes in Biomathematics* **86:** 90-103, J.-P. Gabriel, C. Lefèvre and P. Picard (eds.), *Stochastic Processes in Epidemic Theory,* Springer-Verlag, Berlin, Heidelberg, New York, 1990.

8. K. S. Crump and C. J. Mode, A General Age-Dependent Branching Process I, *Journal of Mathematical Analysis and Applications* **24**: 494-508, 1968.

9. K. S. Crump and C. J. Mode, A General Age-Dependent Branching Process II, *Journal of Mathematical Analysis and Applications* **25**: 8-17, 1969.

10. O. Diekmann, K. Dietz, and J.A.P. Heesterbeek, The Basic Reproduction Ratio for Sexually Transmitted Diseases I, Theoretical Considerations, *Mathematical Biosciences* **107:** 325-339, 1991.

11. O. Diekmann, J.A.P. Heesterbeek, and J.A.J. Metz, On the Definition and the Calculation of the Basic Reproduction Ratio R_0 in Models for Infectious Diseases in Heterogeneous Populations, *Journal of Mathematical Biology* **28:** 365-382, 1990.

12. K. Dietz, The Estimation of the Basic Reproduction Number for Infectious Diseases, *Statistical Methods in Medical Research* **2:** 23-41, 1993.

13. W. Feller, *An Introduction to Probability Theory and Its Applications, I,* 3rd ed., John Wiley and Sons, Inc., New York, London, 1968.

14. C. C. Heyde and E. Seneta, *I. J. Bienaymé Statistical Theory Anticipated,* Springer-Verlag, New York, Heidelberg, Berlin, 1977.

15. J. A. Jacquez, J. S. Koopman, C. P. Simon and I. M. Longini, Jr., Role of the Primary Infection in Epidemics of HIV Infection in Gay Cohorts, *Journal of Acquired Immune Deficiency Syndromes* **7:** 1169-1184, 1994.

16. P. Jagers, *Branching Processes with Biological Applications,* John Wiley and Sons, London and New York, 1975.

17. P. Jagers, A General Stochastic Model for Population Development, *Skandinavisk Aktuarietidskift* 84-103, 1969.

18. C. J. Mode, *Multitype Branching Processes - Theory and Applications,* American Elsevier, New York, 1971.

19. C. J. Mode, *Stochastic Processes in Demography and Their Computer*

Implementation, Springer-Verlag, Berlin, 1985.

20. P. Whittle, The Outcome of a Stochastic Epidemic - A Note on Bailey's Paper, *Biometrika* **42:** 116-122, 1955.

Chapter 7
A STRUCTURAL APPROACH TO SIS AND SIR MODELS

7.1 Introduction

Although the focus of attention in Chapter 6 was epidemics in a large population of susceptibles, it is of interest to explore stochastic models of epidemics in small populations. Examples of such populations include a community consisting of a few households, a set of people who meet regularly at some designated time and place, such as a class meeting in some school or university or some cohort of individuals under observation in a clinical study. There is a large literature on such models, consisting of deterministic and stochastic formulations, which dates in part from the 19th century. An excellent comprehensive review of the literature up to about 1975 may be found in the book Bailey.[1] Among the pioneering works mentioned is the paper of Kermack and McKendrick,[9] as well as other works such as Ross.[18] Briefly, the models receiving attention is this chapter are those belonging to the classes designated as simple and general epidemics by Bailey and discussed in his Chapters 5 and 6.

More than two decades have elapsed since the publication of Bailey's book, but the literature on stochastic models of epidemics has continued to grow. A more recent account of this literature from the perspective of the analysis of infectious disease data has been given by Becker.[2] Lefèvre,[12] in a lead-off paper of a conference volume devoted to stochastic models in epidemic theory, provides a survey of more recent literature. Classes of stochastic models designated as simple and general in the older literature have, with the passage of time, been reclassified in terms of the acronyms SI, SIS and SIR, models which are now widely used. Briefly, in a SI model, sometimes referred to as the simple epidemic, only transitions from the susceptible to infectious state are considered so that once infected an individual remains infectious throughout his or her life span. In SIS models, one considers the situation in which a population consists of susceptible and infectious individuals, but an infectious person may return to the susceptible state and can again be infected through contacts with infectious individuals. Evidently, the common cold and some types of influenza are examples of such infectious diseases. SIR models, on the other hand, are designed for those situations in which susceptibles become infected and infectives are removed from the population by either immunity or death. Even though the branching process approximation to the class of models discussed in Section 9 of Chapter 6 applied to a large population of susceptibles, the stochastic models described there, and in most of the other sections of Chapter 6, belong to the SIR class.

For the most part, the literature on SIS and SIR models of epidemics consists of detailed and often clever mathematical analyses of models, which, when viewed from the perspective of general classes of stochastic processes, appear rather specialized. Because, as mentioned above, reviews of the literature on these classes of processes have recently been published, no attempt will be made to review this literature here. Rather, attention in this chapter will be focused on the simple semi-Markovian structure underlying these classes of stochastic models and how this structure may be exploited to obtain useful numerical results in this computer age. Attention will also be given to discrete time approximations to models with a continuous time parameter and techniques for embedding deterministic models in stochastic processes. Historically, most mathematical analyses of SIS and SIR processes have been based on various versions of the forward Kolmogorov differential equations. But, in this chapter attention will be focused on the structure of SIS and SIR processes from a semi-Markov perspective.

7.2 Structure of SIS Stochastic Models

Consider a population classified by two types of individuals, susceptible and infectious. Let the random functions $X(t)$ and $Y(t)$, respectively, denote the number of susceptibles and infectives at time $t \in [0, \infty)$. Furthermore, suppose the total population size $m \geq 2$ is constant so that

$$X(t) + Y(t) = m \tag{7.2.1}$$

for all $t \in [0, \infty)$, and the initial conditions are $X(0) = n \geq 1$ and $Y(0) = a \geq 1$ such that $n + a = m$. As long as there are infectives in the population, susceptibles may be infected through contacts, but the epidemic stops when there are no infectives, i.e., when there is a $t > 0$ such that $Y(t) = 0$.

In view of Eq. (7.2.1), one may describe the evolution of the epidemic in terms of either of the random functions $X(t)$ or $Y(t)$; however, many authors have chosen to describe the epidemic in terms of the random function $Y(t)$. Then, the one-dimensional state space of the model is the set,

$$\mathfrak{S} = \{y \mid y = 0, 1, 2, \cdots, m\} \tag{7.2.2}$$

of non-negative integers, representing the number of infectives in the population at any time. Because the epidemic stops when $y = 0$, the set $\mathfrak{S}_1$ of absorbing states consists of the singleton $\{0\}$, and the set $\mathfrak{S}_2$ of transient states is:

$$\mathfrak{S}_2 = \{y \mid y = 1, 2, \cdots, m\} \ . \tag{7.2.3}$$

A customary approach to formulating a SIS stochastic model of an epidemic is to suppose it evolves according to a continuous time parameter Markov jump process such that for every $y \in \mathfrak{S}_2$ there are positive rate constants γ_y and β_y with the following properties. Given $Y(t) = y$, during a small time interval $(t, t + h]$, for $t, h > 0$, the conditional probability the number of infectives increases by one is:

$$\mathbb{P}\left[Y(t + h) = y + 1 \mid Y(t) = y\right] = \beta_y h + o(h) \ , \tag{7.2.4}$$

and the conditional probability an infective recovers and returns to the susceptible state is:

$$\mathbb{P}\left[Y(t + h) = y - 1 \mid Y(t) = y\right] = \gamma_y h + o(h) \ . \tag{7.2.5}$$

Furthermore, during any small time interval of length h the conditional probability of any other transition has the property,

$$\mathbb{P}\left[Y(t+h) = k \mid Y(t) = y\right] = o(h) \tag{7.2.6}$$

for $k \neq y-1$ or $k \neq y+1$. Given these explicit assumptions, it is a straightforward exercise to write down either the forward or backward Kolmogorov differential equations. Rather than proceeding in this customary manner, the model will be formulated within a semi-Markovian structure.

In this structure, the rate constants β_y and γ_y will be viewed as elements in the $(m+1) \times (m+1)$ matrix $\mathbf{\Theta} = (\theta_{ij})$ of latent risks, which has the partitioned form,

$$\mathbf{\Theta} = \begin{bmatrix} \mathbf{\Theta}_{11} & \mathbf{\Theta}_{12} \\ \mathbf{\Theta}_{21} & \mathbf{\Theta}_{22} \end{bmatrix}, \tag{7.2.7}$$

corresponding to the sets of absorbing and transient states $\mathfrak{S}_1$ and $\mathfrak{S}_2$ (see Section 3.7). For the SIS-model under consideration, $\mathbf{\Theta}_{11} = (0)$ and $\mathbf{\Theta}_{12}$ is a $1 \times m$ matrix of zeroes. The $m \times 1$ matrix $\mathbf{\Theta}_{21}$ has the form,

$$\mathbf{\Theta}_{21} = \begin{bmatrix} \gamma_1 \\ 0 \\ \vdots \\ 0 \end{bmatrix}, \tag{7.2.8}$$

and governs transitions from the set $\mathfrak{S}_2$ of transient states to the absorbing state 0. Finally, the $m \times m$ matrix $\mathbf{\Theta}_{22}$, governing transitions among the transient states, has the form,

$$\mathbf{\Theta}_{22} = \begin{bmatrix} 0 & \beta_1 & 0 & 0 & 0 & \cdots & 0 \\ \gamma_2 & 0 & \beta_2 & 0 & 0 & \cdots & 0 \\ \vdots & \vdots & \vdots & \vdots & \vdots & \vdots & \vdots \\ 0 & 0 & 0 & \cdots & \gamma_{m-1} & 0 & \beta_{m-1} \\ 0 & 0 & 0 & \cdots & 0 & \gamma_m & 0 \end{bmatrix}. \tag{7.2.9}$$

According to Section 3.7, the $(m+1) \times (m+1)$ transition matrix $\mathbf{P} = (p_{ij})$ for the Markov chain embedded in the continuous time semi-Markov process can be very useful in the analysis of the model. For

$i = 1, 2, \cdots, m$, the ijth element of this matrix has the form,

$$p_{ij} = \frac{\theta_{ij}}{\theta_i}, \tag{7.2.10}$$

where $\theta_i = \sum_j \theta_{ij} > 0$. By applying this formula to the matrix $\mathbf{\Theta}$, it can be seen that the transition matrix $\mathbf{P}$ has the form,

$$\mathbf{P} = \begin{bmatrix} 1 & 0 & 0 & 0 & 0 & \cdots & 0 \\ p_{10} & 0 & p_{12} & 0 & 0 & \cdots & 0 \\ 0 & p_{21} & 0 & p_{23} & 0 & \cdots & 0 \\ \vdots & \vdots & \vdots & \vdots & \vdots & \vdots & \vdots \\ 0 & 0 & \cdots & 0 & p_{m-1,m-2} & 0 & p_{m-1,m} \\ 0 & 0 & \cdots & 0 & 0 & 1 & 0 \end{bmatrix}, \tag{7.2.11}$$

where for $i \geq 1$, $p_{i,i-1} = \gamma_i/(\gamma_i + \beta_i)$ and $p_{i,i+1} = \beta_i/(\gamma_i + \beta_i)$. By definition, $\beta_m = 0$. From this form, it can be seen that $\mathbf{P}$ is the transition matrix of a random walk on the integers $0, 1, 2, \cdots, m$, with 0 as an absorbing barrier and m a reflecting barrier.

The formulation just described depends on $2m$ parameters and it is natural to ask whether some simplifying, but acceptable, assumptions can be made so as to reduce the dimension of the parameter space. As was seen in Chapter 6, a basic assumption underlying any branching process is that life cycles among individuals in a population are independent in a probabilistic sense. When one inspects the conditions in Eqs. (7.2.4), (7.2.5), and (7.2.6), it is not clear whether such an independence condition would hold, but, as we shall see, if some widely used forms of the γ's and β's are chosen, then the assumption that the life cycles among individuals in the population are independent is consistent with these choices. As a first step to demonstrating this consistency, the following well-known property of the exponential distribution will be needed repeatedly.

Suppose $X_1, X_2, \cdots, X_n$ are independent exponential random variables with scale parameters $\delta_1, \delta_2, \cdots, \delta_n$. Then, the random variable,

$$Y = \min_{1 \leq i \leq n} \{X_1, X_2, \cdots, X_n\} \tag{7.2.12}$$

has an exponential distribution with parameter $\delta = \delta_1 + \delta_2 + \cdots + \delta_n$. To prove this assertion observe that $Y > y > 0$ if, and only if, $X_i > y$ for all $i = 1, 2, \cdots, n$. Therefore, by independence, it follows that:

$$\begin{aligned} \mathbb{P}[Y > y] &= \mathbb{P}[X_1 > y, X_2 > y, \cdots, X_n > y] \\ &= \prod_{i=1}^{n} \mathbb{P}[X_i > y] = \prod_{i=1}^{n} e^{-\delta_i y} = e^{-\delta y} \,. \end{aligned} \tag{7.2.13}$$

Now suppose for some time $t > 0$ the number of infectives in the population is $Y(t) = y \geq 1$ and any susceptible makes contacts with the y infectives according to a Poisson process with parameter $\lambda > 0$. At each contact, any infective is chosen with probability y/m and the probability this susceptible is infected per contact is p. Thus, py/m is the probability per contact that a susceptible becomes infected by contacting some infective. By reasoning as in Section 6.4 and assuming the contacts are independent, it follows that the number of infectious contacts made by a susceptible during the time interval $(t, t + t_1]$ is a Poisson process, which implies $\lambda p y t_1/m$ is the expected number of infectious contacts made during this time interval.

But, any susceptible becomes infected at the first infectious contact with an infective. Hence, the latent distribution of the waiting time per susceptible to become infected is exponential with parameter $\lambda py/m$. But, at time t there are $m-y$ susceptibles in the population and under the assumption these individuals make contacts independently, the latent distribution of the transition $y \to y + 1$ in the population is that of the minimum of $m - y$ exponential random variables with a common parameter $\lambda py/m$. Therefore, according to Eq. (7.2.13), the latent risk for the transition $y \to y + 1$ in the population is:

$$\beta_y = (m - y)\left(\frac{\lambda p y}{m}\right) = \lambda p y \left(1 - \frac{y}{m}\right) \tag{7.2.14}$$

For $y \geq 1$, the transition $y \to y - 1$ in the population may be modelled in a similar way. Suppose the length of the infectious period for each infective follows an exponential distribution with parameter $\gamma > 0$, and assume the lengths of infectious periods among individuals are independent. Then, if at time $t > 0$ the number of infectives in the population is $Y(t) = y$, the latent distribution for the transition $y \to y-1$ in the population is that of y independent exponential random variables with common parameter γ. Therefore, under these assumptions and according to Eq. (7.2.13), the latent risk for the transition $y \to y-1$ in the population takes the form,

$$\gamma_y = y\gamma \,. \tag{7.2.15}$$

Many authors have used the risk functions in Eqs. (7.2.14) and (7.2.15) in investigations of SIS-models, which are sometimes referred to as logistic birth and death processes. Among these authors are Jacquez and Simon[8] and Kryscio and Lefèvre.[10] The references cited in these papers may also be consulted. Related models, which are quite often referred to as simple epidemics, have been studied by Bailey.[1] In the stochastic model for a simple epidemic, however, the latent risk function in Eq. (7.2.14) is chosen as:

$$\beta_y = \lambda p y(m-y) \,. \tag{7.2.16}$$

This form of the latent risk β_y could also be derived under an assumption of independence among life cycles of individuals in the population.

When using any of these parameterized forms of latent risk functions, one should be mindful that they depend significantly on the property in Eq. (7.2.13) of independent exponential random variables and the assumption that life cycles among individuals in the population are independent, an assumption that also underlies models based on branching processes. If the parameters γ, λ and p were used as in Section 6.5 to the construct a K-process underlying a CMJ-process, then the threshold parameters for the branching process would be:

$$R_0 = \frac{\lambda p}{\gamma} \,. \tag{7.2.17}$$

As will be demonstrated in a subsequent section, whether $R_0 \leq 1$ or $R_0 > 1$ will significantly affect the behavior of the logistic SIS-process under consideration.

7.3 Waiting Time Distributions for the Extinction of an Epidemic

When an epidemic of some infectious disease in a closed finite population evolves according to the class SIS-processes discussed in Section 7.2, it terminates or becomes extinct when there are no infectives in the population. Furthermore, when the model is formulated as a semi-Markov process with a finite state space $\mathfrak{S}$, consisting of $r \geq 2$ states with a set $\mathfrak{S}_1$ of $r_1 \geq 1$ absorbing states and a set $\mathfrak{S}_2$ of $r_2 \geq 2$ transient communicating states, such that $r_1 + r_2 = r$, then, as shown in Section 3.8, under rather general conditions the process will terminate with probability one in some absorbing state, given that it starts in some transient state. It is, therefore, natural to investigate the distribution of the waiting time to the extinction of an epidemic. From a practical point of view, if the waiting time to extinction may be shortened by the intervention of public health measures designed to impact some basic parameters of a model, a knowledge of the expected waiting time to the extinction of an epidemic could be of significant practical value.

Norden,[17] among other authors, has studied the distribution of the waiting time to the extinction of an epidemic, using the logistic parameterization of a SIS-process as discussed in Section 7.2. Let the random variable T denote the waiting time to extinction and define a parameter ρ by:

$$\rho = \frac{1}{R_0} = \frac{\gamma}{\lambda p} . \tag{7.3.1}$$

Then, the following formula for the conditional expectation of the waiting time to extinction:

$$E\left[T \mid Y(0) = y\right] = \frac{1}{\gamma} \sum_{k=1}^{m} \sum_{j=1}^{\min(k,y)} \eta_k \frac{(m-j)!}{(m\rho)^{m-j+1}} , \tag{7.3.2}$$

where $y \geq 1$ and

$$\eta_k = \frac{(m\rho)^{m-k+1}}{k\,(m-k)!} , \tag{7.3.3}$$

was derived by Norden.

More recently, Nasell[15] has also studied the distribution of the waiting time to the extinction of a SIS epidemic in connection with the concept of a quasi-stationary distribution. Such distributions arise when one conditions on the event of non-extinction of an epidemic by time t. Then, for the case of a SIS-process, by letting $t \uparrow \infty$, it can be shown by modifying the forward Kolmogorov differentials equations, that the conditional distribution of the state of the process converges to a $m \times 1$ probability vector $\mathbf{q}$ on the set $\mathfrak{S}_2$ of transient states. Moreover, $\mathbf{q}$ is a left eigenvector of a matrix corresponding to an eigenvalue, which is a simple explicit function of the parameters of the model. One may then proceed to show that if the quasi-stationary distribution $\mathbf{q}$ is the initial distribution for the unconditional process, then the waiting time to the extinction of the epidemic follows a simple exponential distribution, whose parameter may be determined. Thus, for those cases in which it is reasonable to assume that a SIS-epidemic has been evolving in a population for a long time and the epidemic has not become extinct so that it is reasonable to assume $\mathbf{q}$ is an appropriate initial distribution, then the waiting time to the extinction of an epidemic has a simple exponential form. However, the unconditional distribution of the waiting time to the extinction of a SIS-epidemic can be quite complex, and the interested reader should consult Nasell for details.

The results just described involve a great deal of ingenious mathematics and are very much worthwhile, because they provide an explicit formula for the expectation and variance of the waiting time to the extinction of an epidemic as a function of the basic parameters of the model. For in principle, given a numerical specification of the parameters γ, λ and p, one may evaluate the expectation numerically, provided that m is not too large. But, it is not immediately clear how these methods, which have been very successful in analyzing SIS-processes, may be extended to more complicated models of epidemics. Fortunately, in this day of powerful desktop computers that are increasingly user-friendly, an investigator can pay more attention to the structure of a model than in the past, and there is no longer a compelling need to confine investigations to mathematics that can be done only with paper and pencil. Consequently, in the remainder of this section, attention will be focused on a structural approach with a view towards writing software that would yield information on the expectation and variance of the waiting time to the extinction of an epidemic in a finite closed population.

Rather than confining attention to the SIS model, it will be more fruitful to return to a general semi-Markov process formulation with a set $\mathfrak{S}_1$ of $r_1 \geq 1$ absorbing states and a set $\mathfrak{S}_2$ of $r_2 \geq 1$ transient states. As in Section 3.8, let $f_{ij}(t)$ be the conditional density of the waiting time to absorption in state $j \in \mathfrak{S}_1$, and given that at $t = 0$, the process starts in state $i \in \mathfrak{S}_2$. Then,

$$f_i(t) = \sum_{j \in \mathfrak{S}_1} f_{ij}(t) \tag{7.3.4}$$

may be interpreted as the conditional probability density function of the waiting time to absorption in some absorbing state. It is interesting to note that a conditional density $f_{ij}(t)$ will not, in general, be a proper *p.d.f.*, i.e., its integral over the interval $(0, \infty)$ is not one. It can, however, be shown that the density $f_i(t)$ is a proper *p.d.f.* Let the random function $Z(t)$ denote the state of the process at time $t \geq 0$, and let the random variable T be the waiting time to absorption in some absorbing state. Then, the kth conditional moment of T is:

$$E\left[T^k \mid Z(0) = i\right] = \int_0^\infty t^k f_i(t)dt\,. \tag{7.3.5}$$

In principle, the conditional expectation in question may be obtained by letting $k = 1$ in Eq. (7.3.5), and for any $i \in \mathfrak{S}_2$ the general formula for the desired conditional variance is:

$$\begin{aligned} \tau_i &= var\left[T \mid Z(0) = i\right] \\ &= E\left[T^2 \mid Z(0) = i\right] - \left(E\left[T \mid X(0) = i\right]\right)^2\,. \end{aligned} \tag{7.3.6}$$

A useful method for deriving formulas for these conditional expectations and variances is to consider

$$\widehat{f_{ij}}(s) = \int_0^\infty e^{-st} f_{ij}(t)dt\,, \tag{7.3.7}$$

the Laplace transform, defined for $s \geq 0$, of the conditional density $f_{ij}(t)$. By formally taking the kth derivative of this transform with respect to s, it can be seen that:

$$\widehat{f_{ij}}^{(k)}(s) = (-1)^k \int_0^\infty t^k e^{-st} f_{ij}(t)dt \tag{7.3.8}$$

for $k \geq 1$. Therefore, if a formula for this collection of Laplace transforms can be derived, then the conditional expectation of the waiting time to absorption in some absorbing state is:

$$\nu_i = E\left[T \mid X(0) = i\right] = -\sum_{j \in \mathfrak{S}_1} \widehat{f}_{ij}^{(1)}(0) \tag{7.3.9}$$

for any $i \in \mathfrak{S}_2$. Similarly, the conditional second moment of T is:

$$\nu_i^{(2)} = E\left[T^2 \mid X(0) = i\right] = \sum_{j \in \mathfrak{S}_1} \widehat{f}_{ij}^{(2)}(0) \tag{7.3.10}$$

for any $i \in \mathfrak{S}_2$.

When the process is viewed from the semi-Markov perspective, it is easy to see that the $r_2 \times r_1$ matrices,

$$\widehat{\mathbf{f}}^{(k)}(s) = \left(\widehat{f}_{ij}^{(k)}(s)\right) \tag{7.3.11}$$

of derivatives of Laplace transforms, satisfy manageable systems of linear equations for $k = 1, 2$. For, let

$$\widehat{\mathbf{f}}(s) = \left(\widehat{f}_{ij}(s)\right) \tag{7.3.12}$$

be the $r_2 \times r_1$ matrix of Laplace transforms in Eq. (7.3.7). Then, as shown in Eq. (3.8.7), this matrix satisfies the linear matrix equation,

$$\widehat{\mathbf{f}}(s) = \widehat{\mathbf{r}}(s) + \widehat{\mathbf{q}}(s)\widehat{\mathbf{f}}(s)\,. \tag{7.3.13}$$

The discussion connected with Eqs. (3.8.2), (3.8.3), and (3.8.4) may be consulted for definitions and technical details. The formal solution of this equation is:

$$\widehat{\mathbf{f}}(s) = \left(\mathbf{I}_{r_2} - \widehat{\mathbf{q}}(s)\right)^{-1}\widehat{\mathbf{r}}(s)\,. \tag{7.3.14}$$

If Eq. (7.3.13) is formally differentiated with respect to s, then the matrix equation,

$$\widehat{\mathbf{f}}^{(1)}(s) = \widehat{\mathbf{r}}^{(1)}(s) + \widehat{\mathbf{q}}^{(1)}(s)\widehat{\mathbf{f}}(s) + \widehat{\mathbf{q}}(s)\widehat{\mathbf{f}}^{(1)}(s) \tag{7.3.15}$$

arises. Clearly, this equation is linear in the desired matrix of first derivatives, and by letting $s = 0$, it can be seen that:

$$\widehat{\mathbf{f}}^{(1)}(0) = (\mathbf{I}_{r_2} - \widehat{\mathbf{q}}(0))^{-1} \left(\widehat{\mathbf{r}}^{(1)}(0) + \widehat{\mathbf{q}}^{(1)}(0)\widehat{\mathbf{f}}(0) \right) \tag{7.3.16}$$

is, in principle, a formula for computing the conditional expectations in Eq. (7.3.9).

But, this formula may be simplified by considering sub-matrices of the transition matrix of the Markov chain embedded in the semi-Markov process (see Eq. (3.7.7)). For, according to Eq. (3.8.9)

$$\widehat{\mathbf{f}}(0) = \mathbf{MR} \,, \tag{7.3.17}$$

where

$$\mathbf{M} = (\mathbf{I}_{r_2} - \mathbf{Q})^{-1} = (\mathbf{I}_{r_2} - \widehat{\mathbf{q}}(0))^{-1} \,. \tag{7.3.18}$$

Therefore, Eq. (7.3.16) may be expressed in the form,

$$\widehat{\mathbf{f}}^{(1)}(0) = \mathbf{M} \left(\widehat{\mathbf{r}}^{(1)}(0) + \widehat{\mathbf{q}}^{(1)}(0)\mathbf{MR} \right) \,. \tag{7.3.19}$$

During the course of an analysis of a semi-Markov process, the matrix $\mathbf{M}$ may be computed. Hence, to compute that matrix in Eq. (7.3.19), it would be necessary to compute matrices of derivatives of Laplace transforms of the matrix-valued functions $\widehat{\mathbf{r}}(t)$ and $\widehat{\mathbf{q}}(t)$ at $s = 0$. In many formulations, these matrices of Laplace transforms have simple forms with elementary derivatives so that they may be easily computed.

By differentiating Eq. (7.3.15) with respect to s, the linear equation for the matrix of second derivatives of Laplace transforms takes the form,

$$\widehat{\mathbf{f}}^{(2)}(s) = \widehat{\mathbf{r}}^{(2)}(s) + \widehat{\mathbf{q}}^{(2)}(s)\widehat{\mathbf{f}}(s) + 2\widehat{\mathbf{q}}^{(1)}(s)\widehat{\mathbf{f}}^{(1)}(s) + \widehat{\mathbf{q}}(s)\widehat{\mathbf{f}}^{(2)}(s) \,. \tag{7.3.20}$$

Because the solution of this equation at $s = 0$ can be expressed in the form,

$$\widehat{\mathbf{f}}^{(2)}(0) = \mathbf{M} \left(\widehat{\mathbf{r}}^{(2)}(0) + \widehat{\mathbf{q}}^{(2)}(0)\mathbf{MR} + 2\widehat{\mathbf{q}}^{(1)}(0)\widehat{\mathbf{f}}^{(1)}(0) \right) \,, \tag{7.3.21}$$

the matrix in Eq. (7.3.19) may be used to compute the desired matrix of second order derivatives of the Laplace transforms. For many formulations, it will also be easy to compute matrices of second derivatives of

Laplace transforms evaluated at $s = 0$ so that the matrix in Eq. (7.3.21) may be computed with relative ease for state spaces of moderate size.

To summarize the above derivations in a succinct form that is convenient for computer programming, let $\boldsymbol{\nu}$ and $\boldsymbol{\nu}^{(2)}$ be a $r_2 \times 1$ vectors whose elements are, respectively, the conditional expectations ν_i and $\nu_i^{(2)}$ in Eqs. (7.3.9) and (7.3.10), and let $\mathbf{1}$ be a $r_2 \times 1$ vector of ones. Then, by Eqs. (7.3.9) and (7.3.10),

$$\boldsymbol{\nu} = -\widehat{\mathbf{f}}^{(1)}(0)\mathbf{1} \,, \tag{7.3.22}$$

and

$$\boldsymbol{\nu}^{(2)} = \widehat{\mathbf{f}}^{(2)}(0)\mathbf{1} \,. \tag{7.3.23}$$

Finally, let $\boldsymbol{\tau}$ be a $r_2 \times 1$ vector whose elements are the conditional variances τ_i in Eq. (7.3.6), and let $\boldsymbol{\nu}_{sq}$ be a $r_2 \times 1$ vector whose elements are ν_i^2. Then,

$$\boldsymbol{\tau} = \boldsymbol{\nu}^{(2)} - \boldsymbol{\nu}_{sq} \,. \tag{7.3.24}$$

Whenever the matrix $\mathbf{M}$ is computed in some application of the theory, it is often possible to glean other information of interest to an analysis of a model. Such is the case for a random variable V_j, denoting the total amount of time spent in transient state $j \in \mathfrak{S}_2$ prior to the termination of the process in some absorbing state. For any $j \in \mathfrak{S}_2$, let the indicator function $\delta_j(t) = 1$ if at time $t > 0$ the process is in state j and let $\delta_j(t) = 0$ otherwise. Then,

$$V_j = \int_0^\infty \delta_j(t)dt \,. \tag{7.3.25}$$

The integral makes sense, because for virtually all models of epidemics based on semi-Markov processes, $\delta_j(t)$ is a step function of $t \in (0, \infty)$ with probability one. Given that the process starts in some transient state $i \in \mathfrak{S}_2$ at time $t = 0$, the conditional expectation of $\delta_j(t)$ is

$$E\left[\delta_j(t) \mid Z(0) = j\right] = \mathbb{P}\left[Z(t) = j \mid Z(0) = i\right] = P_{ij}(t) \,, \tag{7.3.26}$$

(see Eqs. (3.8.18) through (3.8.20)). Further, according to Eq. (3.8.20), the $r_2 \times r_2$ matrix $\mathbf{P}(t) = (P_{ij}(t))$ satisfies a matrix-type renewal integral equation. For $i \in \mathfrak{S}_2$, the conditional expectation of V_j is:

$$\xi_{ij} = E\left[V_j \mid Z(0) = i\right] = E\left[\int_0^\infty \delta_j(t)dt \mid Z(0) = i\right]$$

$$= \int_0^\infty E\left[\delta_j(t) \mid Z(0) = i\right] dt = \int_0^\infty P_{ij}(t)dt \,. \tag{7.3.27}$$

Thus, to evaluate this conditional expectation, the integral must be computed.

To compute integrals of this type, it will again be useful to consider Laplace transforms. Let the matrix $\widehat{\mathbf{P}}(s) = \left(\widehat{P}_{ij}(s)\right)$ be the Laplace transform of the matrix $\mathbf{P}(t)$. Then, by passing to Laplace transforms in Eq. (3.8.20), it can be seen that this matrix satisfies the linear equation,

$$\widehat{\mathbf{P}}(s) = \widehat{\mathbf{D}}(s) + \widehat{\mathbf{q}}(s)\widehat{\mathbf{P}}(s) \,, \tag{7.3.28}$$

which has the formal solution

$$\widehat{\mathbf{P}}(s) = \left(\mathbf{I}_{r_2} - \widehat{\mathbf{q}}(s)\right)^{-1} \widehat{\mathbf{D}}(s) \,. \tag{7.3.29}$$

Next observe that

$$\lim_{s\downarrow 0} \widehat{P}_{ij}(s) = \lim_{s\downarrow 0} \int_0^\infty e^{-st} P_{ij}(t)dt = \int_0^\infty P_{ij}(t)dt \,. \tag{7.3.30}$$

Therefore, to derive a formula for the $r_2 \times r_2$ matrix $\mathbf{\Xi} = (\xi_{ij})$ of conditional expectations in Eq. (7.3.27), it suffices to let $s \downarrow 0$ in Eq. (7.3.29). But,

$$\lim_{s\downarrow 0} \left(\mathbf{I}_{r_2} - \widehat{\mathbf{q}}(s)\right)^{-1} = \left(\mathbf{I}_{r_2} - \mathbf{Q}\right)^{-1} = \mathbf{M} = (m_{ij}) \,, \tag{7.3.31}$$

and according to Eqs. (3.8.19) and (3.8.20), the diagonal matrix $\widehat{\mathbf{D}}(s)$ has the form,

$$\widehat{\mathbf{D}}(s) = \left(\delta_{ij}\left(\frac{1 - \widehat{A}_i(s)}{s}\right)\right) , \tag{7.3.32}$$

where δ_{ij} is the Kronecker delta and

$$\widehat{A}_i(s) = \int_0^\infty e^{-st} a_i(t)dt \,, \tag{7.3.33}$$

the Laplace transform of the density $a_i(t)$ of any sojourn time in transient state $i \in \mathfrak{S}_2$. Following any entrance into state i, the expected duration of the stay in this state is:

$$\mu_i = \int_0^\infty t a_i(t)dt = -\lim_{s\downarrow 0} \widehat{A}_i^{(1)}(s) \,. \tag{7.3.34}$$

As above, the first derivative of a Laplace transform has been denoted by the superscript "(1)". By an application of l'Hospital's rule, it can be seen that:

$$\lim_{s \downarrow 0} \widehat{\mathbf{D}}(s) = \left(\delta_{ij} \lim_{s \downarrow 0} \left(\frac{1 - \widehat{A}_i(s)}{s} \right) \right)$$

$$= \left(-\delta_{ij} \lim_{s \downarrow 0} \widehat{A}_i^{(1)}(s) \right) = (\delta_{ij}\mu_i) \ . \tag{7.3.35}$$

Therefore, from Eq. (7.3.29) it follows that the matrix of means Ξ takes the form,

$$\Xi = (\xi_{ij}) = \lim_{s \downarrow 0} \widehat{\mathbf{P}}(s) = \left(\sum_{k=1} m_{ik}\delta_{kj}\mu_k \right) = (m_{ij}\mu_j) \ . \tag{7.3.36}$$

This formula has a very simple and clear interpretation. Given that the process starts in transient state i at $t = 0$, m_{ij} is the expected number of visits to transient state j prior to the termination of the process in some absorbing state. For each visit to state j, the expected duration of stay is μ_j. Hence, given that the process starts in state i at time $t = 0$, $m_{ij}\mu_j$ is the expected duration of time spent in state j prior to termination of the process. For those applications in which the state of the process is the number of infectives in a population, a knowledge of the elements of the matrix Ξ may provide useful information on the average size of the epidemic prior to extinction.

7.4 Numerical Study of Extinction Time of Logistic SIS

Eqs. (7.3.22) and (7.3.24) for the vectors of expectations and variances of the waiting times to the extinction of a logistic SIS epidemic, conditioned on the initial number of infectives in the population, may be easily programmed in such array manipulating languages as APL. Such programs, which involve the computation of the inverse of a $m \times m$ matrix of the form $\mathbf{I} - \mathbf{Q}$, work very well when the population size m is not too large and lead to quick numerical insights on the behavior of the model at chosen points in the parameter space. In the illustrative examples presented in this section, the value of m was chosen as 100. For larger values of m, it may be advisable to compute the inverse of a matrix by solving triangular systems of linear equations that arise from the special algebraic structure of the model.

A major focus of attention in this section is that of studying the impact of $R_0 = \lambda p/\gamma$ on the expectations and standard deviations of the waiting times to extinction. Because in SIS models the epidemic always becomes extinct with probability one, R_0 is not a predictor of whether the epidemic becomes extinct as was the case in a branching process formulation. Nevertheless, as will be demonstrated in the following numerical examples, R_0 has value as a qualitative predictor of the magnitudes of the expectations and standard deviations of the waiting times to extinction of the epidemic, and it is also a useful indicator as to whether an epidemic will take off following the introduction of a few infective individuals.

As was shown in Section 7.3, to implement Eqs. (7.3.22) and (7.3.24) numerically, it is necessary to take Laplace transforms of transition densities of the form,

$$a_{ij}(t) = \theta_{ij} \exp\left[-\theta_i t\right] , \tag{7.4.1}$$

where $\theta_i = \sum_j \theta_{ij}$ and $t \in [0, \infty)$. For SIS models, when $i \geq 1$, $\theta_{ij} = 0$ unless $j = i - 1$ or $j = i + 1$. The Laplace transform of the function in Eq. (7.4.1), defined for $s \geq 0$, is:

$$\widehat{a}_{ij}(s) = \int_0^\infty e^{-st} a_{ij}(t)dt = \frac{\theta_{ij}}{\theta_i + s} . \tag{7.4.2}$$

Thus, $\widehat{a}_{ij}(0) = \theta_{ij}/\theta_i$ may be easily computed. The first derivative of this transform is evaluated at $s = 0$ is:

$$\frac{d\widehat{a}_{ij}(0)}{ds} = -\frac{\theta_{ij}}{\theta_i^2} , \tag{7.4.3}$$

and the second derivative evaluated at $s = 0$ is:

$$\frac{d^2\widehat{a}_{ij}(0)}{ds^2} = \frac{2\theta_{ij}}{\theta_i^3} . \tag{7.4.4}$$

When $\theta_{i,i-1} = i\gamma$ and $\theta_{i,i+1} = \lambda p i(1 - i/m)$, as in the logistic SIS model, it is a straightforward exercise to write APL programs that use the above formulas to compute expectations and standard deviations of waiting times to the extinction of an epidemic as functions of the parameters γ, λ, and p.

The behavior of the model is sensitive to the value of p, the probability of infection per contact. However, to simplify the presentation, the particular value of p was subsumed in the parameter λ throughout all computations. This does mean that the chosen value of p was $p = 1$. Values of the parameters γ and λ were chosen such that R_0 had the two values 2 and 1.25, and, for each value of R_0, two distinct values of γ and λ were chosen as shown in Table 7.4.1 to illustrate that the same values of R_0 will, in general, lead to quite different behaviors of the model, depending on the values of the parameters γ and λ.

For example, when $R_0 = 2$ in Case 1, the number of infectious contacts per unit time between infectious and susceptible individuals is $\lambda = 2$, and the expected length of the infectious period is $1/\gamma = 1$ time unit. Case 2 under $R_0 = 2$, denotes the situation in which the rate of contact per unit time among infectives and susceptibles is $\lambda = 0.5$ and the expected length of the infectious period is $1/0.25 = 4$ time units. As can be seen from Table 7.4.1, when $R_0 = 1.25$, the contact rates per unit time are $\lambda = 0.05$ and $\lambda = 0.5$, and expected durations of the infectious period are $1/0.04 = 25$ and $1/0.4 = 2.5$ times units, respectively, for Cases 1 and 2.

Table 7.4.1. Values of Parameters Giving the Same Values of R_0.

	$R_0 = 2$	$R_0 = 1.25$
Case 1	$\lambda = 2$, $\gamma = 1$	$\lambda = 0.05$, $\gamma = 0.04$
Case 2	$\lambda = 0.5$, $\gamma = 0.25$	$\lambda = 0.5$, $\gamma = 0.4$

Presented in Table 7.4.2 are the conditional expectations and standard deviations of the waiting times to the extinction of the epidemic for the two cases in Table 7.4.1 under $R_0 = 2$ as a function of chosen values of y, the initial number of infectives in a population of size 100. The column headings, Exp1, Exp2 and SD1, SD2 symbolize the expectations and standard deviations of these waiting times for Cases 1 and 2, respectively. All numbers, which are very large, have been rounded off to three figures for ease of presentation.

Table 7.4.2. Expectations and Standard Deviations of Waiting Times to Extinction for $R_0 = 2$ as a Function of the Initial Number of Infectives y.

y	Exp1	SD1	Exp2	SD2
1	620×10^6	110×10^6	250×10^6	440×10^6
5	123×10^6	128×10^6	492×10^6	512×10^6
10	127×10^6	128×10^6	511×10^6	512×10^6
25	128×10^6	128×10^6	512×10^6	512×10^6
50	128×10^6	128×10^6	512×10^6	512×10^6
75	128×10^6	128×10^6	512×10^6	512×10^6
100	128×10^6	128×10^6	512×10^6	512×10^6

The time unit is arbitrary, but, for the sake of illustration, suppose it is a minute. There are $60 \times 24 = 1440$ minutes in a day and $365.25 \times 1440 = 525960$ minutes in a year. For $y = 25$, the expected waiting times to extinction for Cases 1 and 2 expressed in years are $128 \times 10^6/523960 = 244.29$ are $512 \times 10^6/525960 = 973.46$. Both these numbers greatly exceed expectations of life at birth in all known human populations. Therefore, for these parameter values, the model does not appear appropriate for any known human disease, except possibly for those diseases that may become endemic in a population. To make the formulation more realistic for a shorter time frame, it would be useful to introduce death from causes other than the disease in question as another absorbing state, so that persons dying from causes other than the disease in question would be accommodated in the model. Actually, many workers who have studied the SIS-process in great detail are aware of its limitations and view it as a model of an epidemic in a population of immortal individuals.

Although the model appears to be unrealistic for these parameter assignments, at least three interesting mathematical properties of the model seem to become apparent from the numbers presented in Table 7.4.2. Firstly, it appears, as one might expect, that when the initial number of infectives is small, say $y = 1$, the waiting times to extinction of the epidemic are small in relative terms but the standard deviations are relatively large, indicating there will be much variability in waiting times to extinction among realizations of the process. Secondly, for any initial number of infectives the standard deviation is the same order of magnitude as the mean, pointing to large variations in times to extinction. And thirdly, for an initial number of infectives greater than 10, the initial conditions have only a negligible impact on the expected waiting times to extinction and their standard deviations.

Table 7.4.3 contains the results of numerical experiments for Cases 1 and 2 in Table 7.4.1 when $R_0 = 1.25$. All values in this table are orders of magnitude smaller than those in Table 7.4.2 and appear to be plausible even if, for example, the time unit is a day. Observe that values of the parameters γ and λ have been chosen such that the expectations and standard deviations for Case 2 are those for Case 1 divided by 10 and rounded off to two decimal places.

Table 7.4.3. Expectations and Standard Deviations of Waiting Times to Extinction for R_0= 1.25 as a Function of the Initial Number of Infectives y.

y	Exp1	SD1	Exp2	SD2
1	346.43	920.53	34.64	92.05
5	1095.37	1431.13	109.54	143.11
10	1458.92	1515.83	145.89	151.58
25	1728.18	1534.18	172.82	153.42
50	1799.17	1534.68	179.92	153.47
75	1818.07	1534.69	181.81	153.47
100	1826.60	1534.69	182.86	153.47

Thus, in Case 1, the expected waiting times to extinction and their standard deviations are relatively large for a "small" contact rate

$\lambda = 0.05$ and "large" value expected of $1/0.04 = 25.0$ time units for the duration of the infectious period; whereas for a "larger" contact rate $\lambda = 0.5$ and a "shorter" expected duration of $1/0.4 = 2.5$ time units of the infectious period, the expectations and standard deviations are reduced by a factor of 10. Just as in Table 7.4.3, standard deviations are relatively large in relation to expectations, suggesting there is considerable variability in waiting times to extinction of the epidemic. And for $y > 10$, the initial number of infectives does not seem to have a large impact on the relative values of expectations and standard deviations of waiting times to extinction.

Other numerical experiments, not reported here due to lack of space, seem to support the conclusion that if the initial numbers of infectives are sufficiently large, they will have a small impact on the values of the expected waiting times to extinction of the epidemic and their variability. These experiments also suggest, as observed in Tables 7.4.2 and 7.4.3, that as y increases, the standard deviations of waiting times to extinction approach a constant whose value depends on the point in the parameter space. These observations seem to have some connection with results derived by Nasell[15] in connection with his work on using the quasi-stationary distribution of the SIS-process as the initial distribution of an unconditioned process.

7.5 An Overview of the Structure of Stochastic SIR Models

In stochastic models belonging to the SIR class, the evolution of epidemics with three types of individuals, susceptible, infectious, and removed, in a closed population are considered. Accordingly, for all $t \in [0, \infty)$, the random functions $X(t)$, $Y(t)$, and $Z(t)$ will be defined as follows: $X(t)$ and $Y(t)$ denote, respectively, the number of susceptible and infectious individuals in the population at time t, and $Z(t)$ denotes the number of infectious individuals that have been removed during the time interval $(0, t]$ for $t > 0$. Let the positive integer m be the size of the population. The population is closed in the sense that:

$$X(t) + Y(t) + Z(t) = m \tag{7.5.1}$$

for all $t \in [0, \infty)$, and it will be assumed that the initial conditions are $(X(0), Y(0), Z(0)) = (n, a, 0)$, where n and a are positive integers such that $n + a = m$. It is of interest to note, that if the values of any two of the random functions in Eq. (7.5.1) are known, then the third is determined. Thus, it is possible to reduce the dimension of the state space to two. However, in what follows, for sake of clarity, a state space with three dimensions will be described.

Because Eq. (7.3.1) holds for all $t \geq 0$, the state space of the process is the set of triples of non-negative integers defined for each $m \geq 2$ by

$$\mathfrak{S} = \{(x, y, z) \mid x + y + z = m\} \; . \tag{7.5.2}$$

Even for moderate values of m, the number of elements in the set $\mathfrak{S}$ can be quite large. As is well-known, if for $k \geq 2$ and $m \geq 1$, $\{x_i \mid i = 1, 2, \cdots, k\}$ is a set of non-negative integers such that

$$x_1 + x_2 + \cdots + x_k = m \; , \tag{7.5.3}$$

then this set contains

$$\binom{m + k - 1}{k - 1} \tag{7.5.4}$$

elements, which is well known as the number of terms in a multinomial expansion (see Feller[6] page 37). In particular, if $k = 3$, this general formula yields the formula,

$$r = \binom{m + 2}{2} = \frac{(m + 2)(m + 1)}{2} \tag{7.5.5}$$

for the number r of states in $\mathfrak{S}$. As m increases, the number of elements in $\mathfrak{S}$ becomes large. For example, for $m = 10$, 20, 30, 40, and 50 this number is 66, 231, 496, 861, and 1326 respectively; and for $m = 100$, this number is 5151. To analyze SIR-processes with state spaces of 200 or more states, special methods will be required.

As was the case with SIS-processes, when there are no infectious individuals in the population the epidemic terminates. Therefore,

$$\mathfrak{S}_1 = \{(x, 0, m - x) \mid x = 0, 1, 2, \cdots, m\} \tag{7.5.6}$$

is the set of $r_1 = m + 1$ absorbing states, from which it follows that the set $\mathfrak{S}_2$ of transient states contains

$$r_2 = \frac{(m + 2)(m + 1)}{2} - (m + 1) = \frac{m(m + 1)}{2} \tag{7.5.7}$$

elements. If, for example, $m = 20$, then $\mathfrak{S}_2$ has $r_2 = 231 - 21 = 210$ states. To obtain a useful ordering of the elements in $\mathfrak{S}_2$ it will be helpful to consider the set,

$$A(y) = \{(x, y, m - y - x) \mid x = 0, 1, 2, \cdots, m - y\} \tag{7.5.8}$$

defined for each number $y = 1, 2, \cdots, m$ of infectives in the population. Observe there are $m - y + 1$ states in this set and the set $A(m)$ is the singleton $\{(0, m, 0)\}$, indicating that all individuals in the population are infected. Given the definition in Eq. (7.5.8), the set of transient states may be represented as the disjoint union

$$\mathfrak{S}_2 = \bigcup_{y=1}^{m} A(y) \,. \tag{7.5.9}$$

Like the SIS-processes discussed in the preceding sections, SIR-processes are Markov jump processes in continuous time whose infinitesimal generators are determined by the following assumptions. Let the vector,

$$\mathbf{W}(t) = (X(t), Y(t), Z(t)) \tag{7.5.10}$$

represent the state of the process at time $t \in [0, \infty)$ and let $\mathbf{i}$ and $\mathbf{j}$ be elements of the state space $\mathfrak{S}$. For t, $h > 0$, with h small, and any $\mathbf{i} = (x, y, z)$ suppose there rate constants $\beta(\mathbf{i})$ and $\gamma(\mathbf{i})$ such that if $\mathbf{j} = (x - 1, y + 1, z)$, then

$$\mathbb{P}\left[\mathbf{W}(t+h) = \mathbf{j} \mid \mathbf{W}(t) = \mathbf{i}\right] = \beta(\mathbf{i})h + o(h) \,. \tag{7.5.11}$$

But, if $\mathbf{j} = (x, y - 1, z + 1)$, then

$$\mathbb{P}\left[\mathbf{W}(t+h) = \mathbf{j} \mid \mathbf{W}(t) = \mathbf{i}\right] = \gamma(\mathbf{i})h + o(h) \,, \tag{7.5.12}$$

and

$$\mathbb{P}\left[\mathbf{W}(t+h) = \mathbf{j} \mid \mathbf{W}(t) = \mathbf{i}\right] = o(h) \tag{7.5.13}$$

if $\mathbf{j} \neq (x - 1,\ y + 1,\ z)$ or $\mathbf{j} \neq (x,\ y - 1,\ z + 1)$. According to these assumptions, the number of infectives in the population either increases of decreases by one during any small time interval so that it becomes useful to describe the state space in terms of the number y of infectious individuals in the population as above. One could, however, also describe it in terms of the number x of susceptibles in the population at any time.

From now on it will be supposed that for each $y = 0, 1, 2, \cdots, m$, the states in the set $A(y)$ are arranged in lexicographic order and these sets in turn are ordered in ascending values of y. Observe that in this notation $A(0) = \mathfrak{S}_1$, the set of absorbing states. From the semi-Markov perspective, with this ordering of the state space $\mathfrak{S}$, the $r \times r$ matrix of latent risks may be represented in the partitioned form,

$$\boldsymbol{\Theta} = \begin{bmatrix} \mathbf{0} & \mathbf{0} \\ \boldsymbol{\Theta}_{21} & \boldsymbol{\Theta}_{22} \end{bmatrix}, \tag{7.5.14}$$

where $\boldsymbol{\Theta}_{21}$ is a $r_2 \times r_1$ matrix governing one-step transitions from the set $\mathfrak{S}_2$ of transient states to the set $\mathfrak{S}_1$ of absorbing states and $\boldsymbol{\Theta}_{22}$ is a $r_2 \times r_2$ matrix governing one-step transitions among transient states.

The sub-matrices of $\boldsymbol{\Theta}$ may in turn be partitioned according to the number y of infectives in the population. For transitions from the subset $A(y)$, $y \geq 1$, of transient states, let $\boldsymbol{\Theta}_{21}(y, 0)$ represent the $(m - y + 1) \times (m + 1)$ sub-matrix of latent risks governing transitions to the set $A(0)$ of absorbing states. According to the assumptions on the infinitesimal generator of the process, transitions into the set $A(0)$ are possible only from the set $A(1)$. Therefore, the $r_2 \times r_1$ sub-matrix $\boldsymbol{\Theta}_{21}$ has the partitioned form

$$\boldsymbol{\Theta}_{21} = \begin{bmatrix} \boldsymbol{\Theta}_{21}(1,0) \\ \mathbf{0} \\ \vdots \\ \mathbf{0} \end{bmatrix}. \tag{7.5.15}$$

Similarly, let $\boldsymbol{\Theta}_{22}(y, y')$ be the $(m - y + 1) \times (m - y' + 1)$ sub-matrix of latent risks governing one-step transitions from the set $A(y)$ to the set $A(y')$. According to the assumptions on the infinitesimal generator of the process, $\boldsymbol{\Theta}_{22}(y, y')$ is a zero matrix unless $y' = y - 1$

or $y' = y + 1$. Therefore, $r_2 \times r_2$ matrix $\mathbf{\Theta}_{22}$ has the partitioned form

$$\mathbf{\Theta}_{22} = \begin{bmatrix} \mathbf{0} & * & \mathbf{0} & \mathbf{0} & \cdots & \cdots & \mathbf{0} \\ * & \mathbf{0} & * & \mathbf{0} & \cdots & \cdots & \mathbf{0} \\ \mathbf{0} & * & \mathbf{0} & * & \cdots & \cdots & \mathbf{0} \\ \vdots & \vdots & \vdots & \vdots & \vdots & \vdots & \vdots \\ \mathbf{0} & \mathbf{0} & \cdots & \cdots & * & \mathbf{0} & * \\ \mathbf{0} & \mathbf{0} & \cdots & \cdots & \mathbf{0} & * & \mathbf{0} \end{bmatrix}, \tag{7.5.16}$$

where the $*$'s represent sub-matrices $\mathbf{\Theta}_{22}(y-1, y)$ and $\mathbf{\Theta}_{22}(y, y+1)$.

All the sub-matrices in the matrix $\mathbf{\Theta}$ of latent risks are sparse. To illustrate this property consider transitions from the set $A(1)$ of transient states to the set $A(0)$ of absorbing states for the case $m = 3$. In this case, an enumeration of the set $A(0)$ is:

$$A(0) = \{(0,0,3),\ (1,0,2),\ (2,0,1),\ (3,0,0)\} \tag{7.5.17}$$

and that of the set $A(1)$ is:

$$A(1) = \{(0,1,2),\ (1,1,1),\ (2,1,0)\}\ . \tag{7.5.18}$$

Let the rows and columns of the 3×4 sub-matrix $\mathbf{\Theta}_{21}(1,0)$ be indexed, respectively, by the elements of the sets $A(1)$ and $A(0)$. Then, because only the transitions

$$(0,1,2) \to (0,0,3),\ (1,1,1) \to (1,0,2) \text{ and } (2,1,0) \to (2,0,1) \tag{7.5.19}$$

can occur with positive probability, this sub-matrix has the form

$$\mathbf{\Theta}_{21}(1,0) = \begin{bmatrix} * & 0 & 0 & 0 \\ 0 & * & 0 & 0 \\ 0 & 0 & * & 0 \end{bmatrix}, \tag{7.5.20}$$

where the $*$'s are positive latent risk functions. Sparse matrices of this form will also be said to have positive principal diagonals.

To complete the illustration, consider transitions from the set of transient states $A(1)$ to the set $A(2)$. For the case $m = 3$, an enumeration of $A(2)$ is

$$A(2) = \{(0,2,1), (1,2,0)\}\ . \tag{7.5.21}$$

Let the rows and columns of the 3×2 sub-matrix $\mathbf{\Theta}_{22}(1,2)$ be indexed by the elements of the sets $A(1)$ and $A(2)$, respectively. In this case, only the transitions,

$$(1,1,1) \to (0,2,1) \text{ and } (2,1,0) \to (1,2,0) \tag{7.5.22}$$

can occur with positive probability. Therefore, the sub-matrix $\mathbf{\Theta}_{21}(1,0)$ has the form,

$$\mathbf{\Theta}_{21}(1,0) = \begin{bmatrix} 0 & 0 \\ * & 0 \\ 0 & * \end{bmatrix}, \tag{7.5.23}$$

where again the $*$'s are non-zero latent risk functions. Sparse matrices of this form will also be said to have positive sub-principal diagonals. Observe the case $m = 3$, can easily be extended to any positive integer m.

In general, for $y = 2, \cdots, m$, any transition from a state in the set $A(y)$ to a state in $A(y-1)$ will be of the form,

$$(x, y, m - y - x) \to (x, y - 1, m - (y - 1) - x) . \tag{7.5.24}$$

Because the index x remains constant for this type of transition, the sparse $(m - y + 1) \times (m - (y - 1) + 1)$ sub-matrix $\mathbf{\Theta}_{22}(y, y-1)$ will have a positive principal diagonal. Any transition from the set $A(y)$ to the set $A(y+1)$ will, for $x \geq 1$, be of the form,

$$(x, y, m - y - x) \to (x - 1, y + 1, m - y - x) . \tag{7.5.25}$$

In this case, the index x decreases by 1 and it is easy to see that the $(m - y + 1) \times (m - (y + 1) + 1)$ sparse sub-matrix $\mathbf{\Theta}_{22}(y, y+1)$ has a positive principal sub-diagonal.

To complete a formulation of a SIR-process, it will be necessary to specify forms of the latent risk functions in Eqs. (7.5.11) and (7.5.12), which can assume infinitely many forms. If $\mathbf{i} = (x, y, z)$, then widely used forms of these functions are:

$$\beta(\mathbf{i}) = \lambda p x y \tag{7.5.26}$$

$$\gamma(\mathbf{i}) = \gamma y . \tag{7.5.27}$$

Just as with a SIS-process, λ may be interpreted as the contact rate per unit time in a Poisson process, γ as a scale parameter of an exponential distribution such that $1/\gamma$ is the expected duration of the infectious period, and p as the probability of infection per contact. By using an argument similar to that in Section 7.2 for SIS-processes, it would also be possible to derive the forms of the latent risk functions in Eqs. (7.5.26) and (7.5.27) under the assumption that life cycles among individuals in the population are independent in a probabilistic sense, but the details will be left to the reader. When the latent risk functions are chosen as in Eqs. (7.5.26) and (7.5.27), the resulting SIR-process has frequently been referred to as a stochastic model for the general epidemic (see Bailey[1]).

Various other versions of SIR-processes have been proposed in the literature by choosing particular forms of the latent risk function $\beta(\mathbf{i})$ with $\gamma(\mathbf{i})$ chosen as in Eq. (7.5.27). In what follows let λ be a positive parameter. Among these forms as suggested by Neuts and Li[16] is:

$$\beta(\mathbf{i}) = \lambda x y^{\alpha} , \tag{7.5.28}$$

where $\alpha \in (0, 1]$ is a parameter measuring the degree of interaction among infectives and susceptibles. A form suggested by Saunders[19] for modeling the transmission of myxomatosis among rabbits is:

$$\beta(\mathbf{i}) = \frac{\lambda x y}{(x+y)^{\frac{1}{2}}} . \tag{7.5.29}$$

Rather than focusing attention on particular choices of the latent risk functions $\beta(\mathbf{i})$ and $\gamma(\mathbf{i})$, it seems more appropriate to develop general algorithms (some of which are described in the next section) that make it feasible to study the impact of a variety of choices of these risk functions on the behavior of the process by computer intensive methods.

There is a rather large literature on SIR-processes. Included in the more recent literature is the paper by Billard and Zhao,[3] containing a description of a method for solving the forward Kolmogorov differential equations in the time inhomogeneous case, using a triangularization scheme due to Severo. Another paper of interest is that of Gani and Purdue[7] devoted to matrix-geometric methods for a general stochastic epidemic, which is related to the semi-Markov perspective discussed in this and other chapters. Finally, the paper by Capasso[4] may be consulted for a counting process approach to SIR-processes.

7.6 Algorithms for SIR-Processes with Large State Spaces

Many distributions and quantities of interest in analyzing the evolution of an epidemic governed by an SIR-process may be computed in terms of sub-matrices of the transition matrix $\mathbf{P}$ of the embedded Markov chain. As before, $\mathbf{R}$ is a $r_2 \times r_1$ matrix of probabilities for transitions from transient states to absorbing states, and $\mathbf{Q}$ is a $r_2 \times r_2$ matrix of probabilities for transitions among transient states. As we have seen in the foregoing sections, many calculations of interest will involve computing elements of the inverse $\mathbf{M}$ of the matrix $\mathbf{I}_{r_2} - \mathbf{Q}$. But, even for populations of moderate size, the number of transient states can be very large, making it difficult, or even impossible, to compute the desired inverse matrix. For example, if population size m is 500, then the number of transient states is $r_2 = (500)(501)/2 = 125250$ and the number of absorbing states is $r_1 = 501$. Such examples clearly illustrate the need for algorithms designed to compute only those elements of $\mathbf{M}$ needed to complete a calculation. It should also be mentioned that other orderings of the states, which give rise to triangular arrays, could be useful for doing calculations for larger values of m. But the ordering described above is useful when attention is focused on the set of absorbing states, and three concrete problems have been chosen to illustrate the concepts for this ordering.

The first problem is that of finding the distribution of the final size of an epidemic. Suppose, for example, an epidemic starts in the transient state $(n, a, 0)$ with $n \geq 1$ susceptibles and $a \geq 1$ infectives such that $n + a = m$. Then, the epidemic ends when there are no infectives and the population reaches absorbing state $(X, 0, m - X)$, where the random variable X is the number of susceptibles in the population. Let the random variable U denote the number of the n initial susceptibles that were infected by the end of the epidemic. By definition, the value of U is the final size of the epidemic. It is easy to see that

$$X = n - U \,. \tag{7.6.1}$$

Therefore, to find the distribution of the final size of the epidemic one must compute the conditional probabilities for the elements of the set of absorbing states,

$$\{(n-u, 0, m-(n-u)) \mid u = 0, 1, \cdots, n\} \ , \tag{7.6.2}$$

given the initial state $(n, a, 0)$. As discussed previously, these conditional probabilities are the row in the $r_2 \times r_1$ matrix,

$$\mathbf{F} = \mathbf{MR} \tag{7.6.3}$$

of absorption probabilities corresponding to the transient state $(n, a, 0)$.

A second problem is that of finding the conditional expectation of the waiting time to the end of the epidemic, given that the process starts in the transient state $(n, a, 0)$. According to the discussion is Section 7.3 (see Eq. (7.3.19)), one needs to consider the $r_2 \times r_1$ matrix of Laplace transforms,

$$\widehat{\mathbf{f}}^{(1)}(0) = \mathbf{M}\left(\widehat{\mathbf{r}}^{(1)}(0) + \widehat{\mathbf{q}}^{(1)}(0)\mathbf{MR}\right) . \tag{7.6.4}$$

For any positive integer k, let $\mathbf{1}_k$ be a $k \times 1$ column vector. Then, because the epidemic ends when some absorbing state is reached, the desired conditional expectation is the negative of the element in the $r_2 \times 1$ column vector,

$$\widehat{\mathbf{f}}^{(1)}(0)\mathbf{1}_{r_1} = \mathbf{M}\left(\widehat{\mathbf{r}}^{(1)}(0) + \widehat{\mathbf{q}}^{(1)}(0)\mathbf{MR}\right)\mathbf{1}_{r_1} \tag{7.6.5}$$

corresponding to the transient state $(n, a, 0)$ (see Eq. (7.3.9)).

The third problem is that of finding the conditional variance of the waiting time to the end of the epidemic, given that the process starts in some transient state. As discussed in Section 7.3, to find this variance the $r_2 \times 1$ column vector,

$$\widehat{\mathbf{f}}^{(2)}(0)\mathbf{1}_{r_1} = \mathbf{M}\left(\widehat{\mathbf{r}}^{(2)}(0) + \widehat{\mathbf{q}}^{(2)}(0)\mathbf{MR} + 2\widehat{\mathbf{q}}^{(1)}(0)\widehat{\mathbf{f}}^{(1)}(0)\right)\mathbf{1}_{r_1} \tag{7.6.6}$$

of second order moments (see Eq. (7.3.10)), needs to be considered, and from this vector the element corresponding to the initial transient state $(n, a, 0)$ must be selected.

It will be noted that both Eqs. (7.6.5) and (7.6.6) contain the $r_2 \times r_1$ matrix $\mathbf{MR}$ of absorption probabilities, which satisfies the condition,

$$\mathbf{F1}_{r_1} = \mathbf{MR1}_{r_1} = \mathbf{1}_{r_2} . \tag{7.6.7}$$

Consequently, by using this condition, Eq. (7.6.5) may be written in the form,

$$\widehat{\mathbf{f}}^{(1)}(0)\mathbf{1}_{r_1} = \mathbf{M}\left(\widehat{\mathbf{r}}^{(1)}(0)\mathbf{1}_{r_1} + \widehat{\mathbf{q}}^{(1)}(0)\mathbf{1}_{r_2}\right) . \tag{7.6.8}$$

But, because of the structure of the sparse matrices $\widehat{\mathbf{r}}^{(1)}(0)$ and $\widehat{\mathbf{q}}^{(1)}(0)$ is such that each row of the $r_2 \times 1$ column vector,

$$\mathbf{G}(0) = \widehat{\mathbf{r}}^{(1)}(0)\mathbf{1}_{r_1} + \widehat{\mathbf{q}}^{(1)}(0)\mathbf{1}_{r_2} \tag{7.6.9}$$

is the sum of at most two non-zero quantities, it can be computed without enumerating the sparse matrices in question. Therefore, if the ith row of the matrix $\mathbf{M}$, say $\mathbf{M}_{(\mathbf{i})}$ could be computed without finding the entire inverse of $\mathbf{I}_{r_2} - \mathbf{Q}$, then the desired conditional expectation would be given by:

$$\nu_i = -\mathbf{M}_{(\mathbf{i})}\mathbf{G}(0) \tag{7.6.10}$$

for the initial state $\mathbf{i} = (n, a, 0)$ (see Eq. (7.3.9)). As will be shown subsequently, computer programs to compute ν_i may be written with relative ease.

Although the expectation in Eq. (7.6.10) may be computed with relative ease, the computation of the corresponding conditional variance would require substantially more computer time and may be more difficult to program. By using (7.6.7), it can be seen that an alternative representation of Eq. (7.6.6) is:

$$\widehat{\mathbf{f}}^{(2)}(0)\mathbf{1}_{r_1} = \mathbf{M}\left(\widehat{\mathbf{r}}^{(2)}(0)\mathbf{1}_{r_1} + \widehat{\mathbf{q}}^{(2)}(0)\mathbf{1}_{r_2} + 2\widehat{\mathbf{q}}^{(1)}(0)\widehat{\mathbf{f}}^{(1)}(0)\mathbf{1}_{r_1}\right) . \tag{7.6.11}$$

Just as with the first-order derivatives of Laplace transforms, the $r_2 \times 1$ column vector,

$$\widehat{\mathbf{r}}^{(2)}(0)\mathbf{1}_{r_1} + \widehat{\mathbf{q}}^{(2)}(0)\mathbf{1}_{r_2} \tag{7.6.12}$$

involving second order derivatives is such that each row is the sum of at most two non-zero quantities and may be computed with relative ease. But, to compute the $r_2 \times 1$ vector,

$$2\widehat{\mathbf{q}}^{(1)}(0)\widehat{\mathbf{f}}^{(1)}(0)\mathbf{1}_{r_1} , \tag{7.6.13}$$

all the elements of the vector in Eq. (7.6.8) will be required, which may make the calculations prohibitive for even moderate population sizes, even though it would not be necessary to enumerate the matrix $\widehat{\mathbf{q}}^{(1)}(0)$. However, as will be shown in the rest of this section, it will be feasible to carry out selected calculations for moderate values of m, the total population size.

As a first step in outlining the ideas underlying the development of some algorithms for executing the above calculations, suppose the process starts in some transient state $\mathbf{i} = (n, a, 0)$ and let

$$\boldsymbol{\pi}^{(0)} = \left\{ \pi^{(0)}(\boldsymbol{\nu}) \mid \boldsymbol{\nu} \in \mathfrak{S} \right\} \tag{7.6.14}$$

be a $1 \times r$ row vector such that $\pi^{(0)}(\boldsymbol{\nu}) = 0$ for all $\boldsymbol{\nu} \neq \mathbf{i}$ and $\pi^{(0)}(\mathbf{i}) = 1$. Given the initial distribution $\boldsymbol{\pi}^{(0)}$ of the embedded Markov chain, let the $1 \times r$ row vector $\boldsymbol{\pi}^{(k)}$ be the distribution of the chain at the kth step for $k \geq 1$. Then, the sequence of state distributions,

$$\left\{ \boldsymbol{\pi}^{(k)} \mid k = 1, 2, \cdots \right\} \tag{7.6.15}$$

may be calculated recursively according to the formula,

$$\boldsymbol{\pi}^{(k)} = \boldsymbol{\pi}^{(k-1)}\mathbf{P} , \tag{7.6.16}$$

where $\mathbf{P}$ is the $r \times r$ one-step transition matrix of the embedded Markov chain. At this juncture, it will be helpful to recall that this matrix has the partitioned form,

$$\mathbf{P} = \begin{bmatrix} \mathbf{I}_{r_1} & \mathbf{0} \\ \mathbf{R} & \mathbf{Q} \end{bmatrix} . \tag{7.6.17}$$

For every $k = 0, 1, 2, \cdots$, it will also be useful to partition the vector $\boldsymbol{\pi}^{(k)}$ into a $1 \times r_1$ sub-vector,

$$\boldsymbol{\pi}_1^{(k)} = \left\{ \pi^{(k)}(\boldsymbol{\nu}) \mid \boldsymbol{\nu} \in \mathfrak{S}_1 \right\} \tag{7.6.18}$$

for absorbing states, and a $1 \times r_2$ sub-vector,

$$\boldsymbol{\pi}_2^{(k)} = \left\{ \pi^{(k)}(\boldsymbol{\nu}) \mid \boldsymbol{\nu} \in \mathfrak{S}_2 \right\} \tag{7.6.19}$$

for transient states so that

$$\boldsymbol{\pi}^{(k)} = \left\{ \boldsymbol{\pi}_1^{(k)} \quad \boldsymbol{\pi}_2^{(k)} \right\} . \tag{7.6.20}$$

Observe that, because only those cases in which the process starts in some transient state are being considered, $\boldsymbol{\pi}_1^{(0)} = \mathbf{0}$, a zero vector.

Upon iteration of Eq. (7.6.16), it can be seen that

$$\boldsymbol{\pi}^{(k)} = \boldsymbol{\pi}^{(0)} \mathbf{P}^k \tag{7.6.21}$$

for $k \geq 1$. But, the k-th power of $\mathbf{P}$ may be represented in the form,

$$\mathbf{P}^k = \begin{bmatrix} \mathbf{I}_{r_1} & \mathbf{0} \\ \mathbf{F}^{(k)} & \mathbf{Q}^k \end{bmatrix} , \tag{7.6.22}$$

where

$$\mathbf{F}^{(k)} = \left(\sum_{\nu=0}^{k-1} \mathbf{Q}^k \right) \mathbf{R} . \tag{7.6.23}$$

Therefore, it follows that at the kth step the sub-vector of $\boldsymbol{\pi}^{(k)}$ of absorbing states is given by:

$$\boldsymbol{\pi}_1^{(k)} = \boldsymbol{\pi}_2^{(0)} \mathbf{F}^{(k)} , \tag{7.6.24}$$

and the sub-vector for transient states determined by the formula,

$$\boldsymbol{\pi}_2^{(k)} = \boldsymbol{\pi}_2^{(0)} \mathbf{Q}^k . \tag{7.6.25}$$

For most models of epidemics, it can be shown that:

$$\lim_{k \uparrow \infty} \mathbf{Q}^k = \mathbf{0} , \tag{7.6.26}$$

a $r_2 \times r_2$ zero matrix. Therefore, from Eq. (7.6.25) it can be seen that

$$\lim_{k \uparrow \infty} \boldsymbol{\pi}_2^{(k)} = \mathbf{0} , \tag{7.6.27}$$

a $1 \times r_2$ zero vector. Moreover, from Eq. (7.6.24) it follows that

$$\lim_{k\uparrow\infty} \boldsymbol{\pi}_1^{(k)} = \boldsymbol{\pi}_2^{(0)}\mathbf{F}\,, \tag{7.6.28}$$

where $\mathbf{F}$ is a $r_2 \times r_1$ matrix of absorption probabilities.

From these observations, one can conclude if the sequence

$$\left\{\boldsymbol{\pi}^{(k)} \mid k = 0, 1, 2, \cdots\right\} \tag{7.6.29}$$

of state distributions is computed for finitely many k and the sequence of sub-vectors

$$\left\{\boldsymbol{\pi}_1^{(k)} \mid k = 0, 1, 2, \cdots\right\} \tag{7.6.30}$$

for absorbing states is selected, then this sequence will converge to:

$$\boldsymbol{\pi}_2^{(0)}\mathbf{F}\,, \tag{7.6.31}$$

which is the row of the matrix $\mathbf{F}$ of absorption probabilities corresponding to the initial state $\mathbf{i} = (n, a, 0)$. Hence, by choosing k sufficiently large, the conditional distribution of the final size of the epidemic may be approximated.

Similarly, one may select the sequence

$$\left\{\boldsymbol{\pi}_2^{(k)} = \boldsymbol{\pi}_2^{(0)}\mathbf{Q}^k \mid k = 0, 1, 2, \cdots\right\} \tag{7.6.32}$$

for transient states to compute an approximation to the row of the matrix $\mathbf{M}$ corresponding to the initial state $\mathbf{i} = (n, a, 0)$. For, by summing the first $n_1 + 1$ terms of this sequence, it can be seen that

$$\sum_{k=0}^{n_1} \boldsymbol{\pi}_2^{(k)} = \boldsymbol{\pi}_2^{(0)} \left(\sum_{k=0}^{n_1} \mathbf{Q}^k\right)\,. \tag{7.6.33}$$

Therefore, if n_1 is sufficiently large, this vector sum will approximate the vector $\boldsymbol{\pi}_2^{(0)}\mathbf{M}$.

The theory just outlined is very helpful for obtaining an overview of the ideas, but is not useful for developing an algorithm for computing the sequence of the state distributions in Eq. (7.6.29), because it would entail the enumeration of large sparse matrices. To simplify the notation, from now on a state (x, y, z) of the process will be represented by the abbreviated symbol (x, y). For $y = 1, 2, \cdots, m$, let the element $p(x, y; x', y')$ of the transition matrix P of the embedded Markov represent the transition $(x, y) \to (x', y')$. For any (x, y), all these transition probabilities will be zero unless $(x', y') = (x - 1, y + 1)$, indicating that an infective has infected a susceptible, or $(x', y') = (x, y - 1)$, indicating an infective has been removed from the population. Let $\beta(x, y)$ and $\gamma(y)$ be, respectively, the latent risks for these transitions. Aside from the conditions, $\beta(0, y) = 0$ for all $y = 1, 2, \cdots, m$ and $\beta(x, 0) = 0$ for $x = 0, 1, 2, \cdots, m$, which must be satisfied, while the non-negative function $\beta(x, y)$ can be quite arbitrary. Briefly, these conditions state that if the population contains no susceptibles or infectives, then there can be no new infections. Similarly, $\gamma(y) > 0$ for $y = 1, 2, \cdots, m$, but $\gamma(0) = 0$.

For any $y = 1, 2, \cdots, m$, the conditional probability for the transition $(x, y) \to (x - 1, y + 1)$ is:

$$p(x, y; x - 1, y + 1) = \frac{\beta(x, y)}{\gamma(y) + \beta(x, y)}, \tag{7.6.34}$$

and the conditional probability for the transition $(x, y) \to (x, y - 1)$ is:

$$p(x, y; x, y - 1) = \frac{\gamma(y)}{\gamma(y) + \beta(x, y)}. \tag{7.6.35}$$

With the transition probabilities so defined, it is possible to compute the sequence of state distributions in Eq. (7.6.29) by using only those non-negative elements in the sparse matrix $\mathbf{P}$ that are necessary to perform the required calculations.

Now suppose that in step $k - 1$, for $k \geq 1$ of a recursive calculation, the $1 \times r$ vector $\boldsymbol{\pi}^{(k-1)}$ has been computed. Then, because any state in the set $A(0) = \mathfrak{S}_1$ of absorbing states can be entered in one step only from a state in the set $A(1)$ of transient states, it can be seen that the elements in the $1 \times r_1$ vector $\boldsymbol{\pi}_1^{(k)}$ for absorbing states could be calculated using the formula,

$$\pi^{(k)}(x, 0) = \pi^{(k-1)}(x, 1)\, p(x, 1; x, 0) \tag{7.6.36}$$

for $x = 0, 1, 2, \cdots, m$. Similarly, for each fixed $y = 1, 2, \cdots, m$, the elements in the $1 \times r_2$ vector $\boldsymbol{\pi}_2^{(k)}$ for transient states in the set $A(y)$ can be calculated using the formula,

$$\pi^{(k)}(x,y) = \pi^{(k-1)}(x,y+1)p(x,y+1;x,y) + \pi^{(k-1)}(x+1,y-1)p(x+1,y-1;x,y) \tag{7.6.37}$$

for $x = 0, 1, 2, \cdots, m-y$. The recursive procedure stops for some $k = n_1$ such that the vector $\boldsymbol{\pi}_2^{(k)}$ is sufficiently close to a zero vector. Neuts and Li[16] have reported good performance times for any algorithm similar to the one outlined for approximating $\boldsymbol{\pi}_2^{(0)}\mathbf{F}$ for the case $m = 1000$.

The elements of the $r_2 \times 1$ vector $\mathbf{G}(0)$ in Eq. (7.6.10) may also be described succinctly using the generic formula in Eq. (7.4.3). For moderate values of m, the algorithm just described, along with the formula in Eq. (7.3.4), could be used to compute the $r_2 \times 1$ vector in Eq. (7.6.11), but the details involved in the procedures required to compute these vectors will be left to the reader.

7.7 A Numerical Study of SIR-Processes

The matrix structures described in Section 7.5 are well-suited for writing software for the numerical implementation of SIR-processes, using interactive and array manipulating languages such as APL. It is possible, having some skill with such languages, to quickly develop programs to compute the distribution of the final size of the epidemic, as well as the expectation and standard deviation of the duration of the epidemic, if any state in the set of transient states is used as the initial state. In such straightforward implementations, however, the total population size must remain small in order to accommodate the large sparse matrices that arise. Despite this limitation on total population size, valuable information may nevertheless be obtained on the quantitative behavior of the process for populations of a single household, or of a small collection of households. In this section, the results of some illustrative computer experiments will be presented. By implementing the algorithms described in Section 7.6 in some compiled language such as C++, it would be feasible to handle larger population sizes, using a detailed looping structure not required for APL implementations.

The forms of the latent risk functions chosen for the numerical experiments presented in this section are those that have been widely used in the study of SIR-processes. The risk function for transitions of the form $(x,y) \to (x-1, y+1)$, for $x \geq 1$, indicating that a susceptible has been infected, was chosen as:

$$\beta(x,y) = \lambda pxy \; , \tag{7.7.1}$$

where $\lambda > 0$ is the expected number of contacts per unit time and p is the probability of infection per contact. For transitions of the form $(x,\ y) \to (x,\ y-1)$, denoting the removal of an infective from the population with $y \geq 1$, the latent risk function,

$$\gamma(y) = \gamma y \tag{7.7.2}$$

was used. In this case, $\gamma > 0$ may be interpreted as a scale parameter in an exponential distribution, such that $1/\gamma$ is the expected duration of the infectious period.

With these parameterizations of the latent risk functions, an SIR-process is a three-parameter model. To simplify the presentation of the numerical results, the process will be reduced to a one-parameter model by letting $\gamma = p = 1$. This means that the time unit is the expected duration of the infectious period and the probability p of infection per contact is subsumed in the parameter λ. It is also of interest to note that with these values of γ and p, $R_0 = \lambda p/\gamma = \lambda$. As in Section 7.6, let the random variable U be the final size of an epidemic and suppose the initial state is $(n, 1, 0)$, consisting of n susceptibles and one infective. The first function to be studied numerically for chosen values of λ is:

$$\mathbb{P}\left[U = u\right] = f(u; \lambda) \; , \tag{7.7.3}$$

the probability density function of U, where $u = 0, 1, 2, \cdots, n$.

Presented in Table 7.7.1 are values of the density in Eq. (7.7.3) for the indicated values of λ and the initial state $(6, 1, 0)$. For the cases $\lambda = 0.05$ and $\lambda = 0.1$, the mode of the density is at $u = 0$, indicating the event that none of the initial 6 susceptibles becomes infected is the most probable, with probabilities 0.7692 and 0.6250, respectively, for the two cases. But, for the three cases $\lambda = 0.5$, $\lambda = 1.0$ and

$\lambda = 2.0$, the density is bimodal with modes at $u = 0$ and $u = 6$. Thus, in these cases, the most likely events are that none of the initial 6 susceptibles becomes infected, or they all become infected. Even for the high value of $R_0 = \lambda = 2$, all 6 initial susceptibles become infected with probability 0.9067; while none become infected with probability 0.0769. In computer experiments not reported here, it was observed that the density had properties similar to those in Table 7.7.1 for larger values of n. Bailey[1] has presented graphs of the density under consideration based on different methods of computation and initial conditions in his treatment of the general stochastic epidemic.

Table 7.7.1. Probability Density Function of the Final Size of the Epidemic for Selected Values of λ and Initial State $(6, 1, 0)$.

u	$f(u; 0.05)$	$f(u; 0.10)$	$f(u; 0.50)$	$f(u; 1.00)$	$f(u; 2.00)$
0	0.7692	0.6250	0.2500	0.1429	0.0769
1	0.1477	0.1667	0.0612	0.0238	0.0076
2	0.0524	0.0881	0.0368	0.0105	0.0021
3	0.0206	0.0558	0.0351	0.0081	0.0011
4	0.0076	0.0361	0.0499	0.0113	0.0012
5	0.0022	0.0206	0.1117	0.0368	0.0044
6	0.0004	0.0078	0.4552	0.7665	0.9067

For larger values of n, it becomes impractical to present the densities of the final size of the epidemic in an informative tabular form for selected values of λ. It is, however, possible to glean some numerical insights into the quantitative behavior of an SIR-epidemic by considering the expectation and standard deviation of the random variables T and U, denoting, respectively, the duration and final size of the epidemic. Let SD_T and SD_U be the standard deviations of the random variables T and U. Table 7.7.2 contains values of these measures of central tendency and variation for the selected values of λ in Table 7.7.1 and the initial state $(15, 1, 0)$.

Table 7.7.2. Expectations and Standard Deviations for the Duration and Final Size of an Epidemic for Selected Values of λ and Initial State $(15, 1, 0)$.

λ	$E[T]$	SD_T	$E[U]$	SD_U
0.05	1.5550	0.8564	1.4523	2.4906
0.10	2.3012	1.4881	4.2399	5.0238
0.50	3.3839	0.5203	12.9380	5.0865
1.00	3.3736	0.7457	13.9937	3.7410
2.00	3.3751	0.9970	14.4987	2.6925

Unlike the SIS-processes that were studied in Section 7.4 in which susceptibles can be infected repeatedly by infectives, the expected durations as well as standard deviations of SIR-epidemics would be relatively small, because all infectives in the population would eventually be removed. As can be seen by inspecting the values of $E[T]$ and SD_T in Table 7.7.2, this statement seems valid. For the values of λ considered in the table, $E[T]$ is relatively small and SD_T is less than $E[T]$ in all cases. Recall that the time unit is the expected duration of the infectious period. Then, for $\lambda = 0.05$, the expected waiting time to extinction of the epidemic is 1.5550 time units; while for $\lambda = 2.0$, this expectation rises to 3.3751 time units. It should be noted, however, that it has been observed in computer experiments not reported here that the values of $E[T]$ and SD_T are quite sensitive to changes in the values of the parameters γ and λ, as well as the initial state $(n, a, 0)$.

As one would expect, the expectation $E[U]$ and standard deviation SD_U of the final size of SIR-epidemics are quite sensitive to values of λ. For example, when $\lambda = 0.05$, the expected number of the initial 15 susceptibles that would be infected is 1.4523 with a standard deviation of 2.4906, but for $\lambda = 0.5$, 1.0, and 2.0, the vast majority of the initial 15 susceptibles would be infected with expected numbers of $E[U] = 12.9380$, 13.9937, and 14.4987, respectively. That the corresponding standard deviations are smaller than the these expectations indicates the density of U is these cases are skewed to the right as observed in Table 7.7.1. In computer output not reported here, it was observed that the densities of U were bimodal for these values of λ and similar in shapes to those tabulated in Table 7.7.1.

7.8 Embedding Deterministic Models in SIS-Processes

A capability for computing Monte Carlo realizations of the stochastic processes under study can be very useful in visualizing the behavior of a process and may further augment any mathematical analysis of a model. Accordingly, the purpose of this section is to begin the description of an approach to approximating continuous time SIS-processes by discrete time Markov chains that not only provides very efficient algorithms for computing Monte Carlo realizations of the process, but also a framework that can easily be extended to the more complicated SIR-process, as well as even more general processes that arise in connection with the international HIV/AIDS epidemic. Within this framework, it is also possible to embed deterministic models in a stochastic process, as will be made clear. Quite often these deterministic models are either identical to or closely resemble models that would arise if an investigator were working strictly within a deterministic paradigm.

Let $h > 0$ be some fixed number and suppose the evolution of an SIS-process is accounted for on some discrete set of time points $S_h = \{kh \mid k = 0, 1, 2, \cdots\}$. A discrete time approximation to a process in continuous time may be constructed by considering events that may occur, given the state of the process at time kh, during the time interval $(kh, (k+1)h] = \{x \in [0, \infty) \mid kh < x \leq (k+1)h\}$. To simplify the notation, instead of using the phrase "at time kh" repeatedly, the symbol h will be dropped and replaced by "at time $t \in S_h$". With this understanding, an interval of the form $(kh,\ (k+1)h]$ may also be denoted by $(t, t+h]$, which will be useful in studying limiting cases as $h \downarrow 0$. As before, the number of susceptibles and infectives in the population at time $t \in [0, \infty)$ in a continuous time SIS-process will be denoted by $X(t)$ and $Y(t)$, respectively. But, to distinguish clearly between the random functions of the continuous time process and those of its discrete time approximation, the random functions $X_d(t)$ and $Y_d(t)$ for the discrete time process will, respectively, denote the number of susceptibles and infectives in the population at time $t \in S_h$. Again, if $m \geq 2$ is total population size, then

$$X_d(t) + Y_d(t) = m \tag{7.8.1}$$

for all $t \in S_h$.

Given a contact between an infective and a susceptible, let the conditional probability $p \in (0,1)$ denote the susceptible individual is infected and let $q = 1 - p$. In a randomly mixing population and for h sufficiently small, $Y_d(t)/m$ is the probability a susceptible contacts an infective;

$$p(t) = \frac{Y_d(t)p}{m} \tag{7.8.2}$$

is the probability per contact that a susceptible is infected during the time interval $(t, t+h]$; and $q(t) = 1 - p(t) = (X_d(t) + Y_d(t)q)/m$ is the probability a susceptible escapes infection during this time interval.

Now let the random function $C(t)$ be the number of contacts a susceptible has with infectives during the time interval $(t, t+h]$ with probability density function,

$$\mathbb{P}[C(t) = c] = f(c, t), \ c = 0, 1, 2 \cdots . \tag{7.8.3}$$

Then, assuming contacts are independent,

$$Q(t) = \sum_{c=0}^{\infty} f(c, \ t) q^c(t) \tag{7.8.4}$$

is the conditional probability a susceptible escapes infection during the time interval $(t, t+h]$, given the state $(X_d(t), Y_d(t))$ of the population at time t, and $P(t) = 1 - Q(t)$ is the conditional probability a susceptible becomes infected during this time interval.

If $G(s, t)$ is the probability generating function of $C(t)$, then from Eq. (7.8.4) it follows that

$$Q(t) = G(q(t), \ t) \ . \tag{7.8.5}$$

Moreover, if it is assumed that $C(t)$ is a Poisson process with parameter $\lambda > 0$ and stationary independent increments, then for all $t \in S_h$ the density in Eq. (7.8.3) has the form,

$$f(c; t) = \frac{e^{-\lambda h}(\lambda h)^c}{c!}, \ c = 0, 1, 2, \cdots \tag{7.8.6}$$

so that Eq. (7.8.5) becomes

$$Q(t) = G(q(t), \ t) = \exp\left[\lambda h(q(t) - 1)\right]$$

$$= \exp\left[-\lambda h p(t)\right] = \exp\left[-\lambda p h \frac{Y_d(t)}{m}\right] . \tag{7.8.7}$$

To count the number of susceptibles who are infected during the time interval $(t,\, t+h]$, for $X_d(t) \geq 1$ let $\xi_k(I)$, $k = 1, 2, \cdots, X_d(t)$, be a collection of conditionally independent and identically distributed (*c.i.i.d.*) Bernoulli indicators such that $\xi_k(I) = 1$ if the kth susceptible is infected during $(t, t+h]$ and let $\xi_k(I) = 0$ otherwise. Then, the number $X_I(t+h)$ of susceptibles who are infected during the time interval $(t, t+h]$ is given by the random sum,

$$X_I(t+h) = \sum_{k=1}^{X_d(t)} \xi_k(I) . \tag{7.8.8}$$

Hence, the number $X_E(t+h)$ of susceptibles who escape infection during this time interval is $X_E(t+h) = X_d(t) - X_I(t+h)$. As is well-known, given $X_d(t)$, the random variable $X_I(t+h)$ has a conditional binomial distribution with index $X_d(t)$ and probability $P(t) = 1 - Q(t) = 1 - \exp\left[-\lambda p h (Y_d(t)/m)\right]$. More precisely,

$$\mathbb{P}\left[X_I(t+h) = x \mid X_d(t)\right] = \binom{X_d(t)}{x} P^x(t) Q(t)^{X_d(t)-x} , \tag{7.8.9}$$

where $x = 0, 1, 2, \cdots, X_d(t)$ (see Section 6.4 for technical details).

The next step in constructing a discrete time approximation to a continuous time SIS-process is to consider the number of infectives who recover during some time interval $(t, t+h]$. Suppose the duration D_I of the infectious period of any infective has an exponential distribution with parameter $\gamma > 0$. Then, given an infective at t, the conditional probability of being infectious at time $t+h$ is:

$$q_R = \mathbb{P}\left[D_I > t+h \mid D_I > t\right]$$

$$= \frac{\mathbb{P}\left[D_I > t+h\right]}{\mathbb{P}\left[D_I > t\right]} = \exp\left[-\gamma h\right] . \tag{7.8.10}$$

Thus, $p_R = 1 - q_R = 1 - \exp\left[-\gamma h\right]$ is the conditional probability that an infective returns to the susceptible state during $(t, t+h]$.

Let the random variable $Y_R(t+h)$ be the number of infectives at t who recover, i.e., return to the susceptible state during $(t, t+h]$. For $Y_d(t) \geq 1$, let $\xi_k(R)$, $k = 1, 2, \cdots, Y_d(t)$, be a collection of *c.i.i.d.* Bernoulli indicator random variables such that $\xi_k(R) = 1$ if the kth infective recovers during $(t, t+h]$ and let $\xi_k(R) = 0$ otherwise. Then,

$$Y_R(t+h) = \sum_{k=1}^{Y_d(t)} \xi_k(R) \,. \tag{7.8.11}$$

Just as in Eq. (7.8.8), given $Y_d(t)$, the random variable $Y_R(t+h)$ has a conditional binomial distribution with index $Y_d(t)$ and probability p_R so that:

$$\mathbb{P}\left[Y_R(t+h) = y \mid Y_d(t)\right] = \binom{Y_d(t)}{y} p_R^y q_R^{Y_d(t)-y} \tag{7.8.12}$$

for $y = 0, 1, 2, \cdots, Y_d(t)$.

With these definitions of the random functions $X_I(t)$ and $Y_R(t)$, it can be seen that, given values of the random functions $X_d(t)$ and $Y_d(t)$ at $t \in S_h$, the numbers of susceptibles and infectives in the population at time $t+h \in S_h$ are determined by the recursive stochastic evolutionary equations,

$$\begin{aligned} X_d(t+h) &= X_d(t) - X_I(t+h) + Y_R(t+h) \\ Y_d(t+h) &= X_I(t+h) + Y_d(t) - Y_R(t+h) \,. \end{aligned} \tag{7.8.13}$$

Thus, given state $(X_d(t), Y_d(t))$ of the discrete time process at time $t \in S_h$, to compute Monte Carlo realizations of the process at $t+h$ it suffices to compute realizations of the pair of binomial random variables $(X_d(t+h), Y_d(t+h))$ and apply Eqs. (7.8.13). From these equations it is clear that, given numerical values of the parameters λ, p and γ and initial values $X_d(0) = n$ and $Y_d(0) = a$, samples of realizations of the process may be computed recursively for $t = h, 2h, \cdots, n_1 h$, where $n_1 > 0$ is some prescribed integer. Observe that these parameters could also be used in the construction of a continuous time SIS-process with random functions $X(t)$ and $Y(t)$.

Given $(X_d(t), Y_d(t))$, it will be assumed that the binomial random variables $X_d(t+h)$ and $Y_d(t+h)$ are conditionally independent. Under this assumption, the stochastic process consisting of the pairs of random variables $\{(X_d(t), Y_d(t) \mid t \in S_h\}$ may be formulated as a Markov chain whose stationary transition probabilities are determined by Eqs. (7.8.13) and the binomial densities in Eqs. (7.8.9) and (7.8.12), but the formal details will be left to the reader. Because the conditional law of evolution for Markov chains of this type is determined by binomial distributions, they are sometimes referred to as chain binomial models. However, these chain binomial models are not those discussed in the earlier literature of stochastic models of epidemics, where the time unit was the latent period and the infectious period was reduced to a single point in time.

With each passing year, the time required to compute Monte Carlo simulations using desktop computers is decreasing, but a need remains for structures that may be analyzed with fewer computations. One is thus lead to consider conditional expectations of the random functions in Eqs. (7.8.13), given the evolution of the process up to time $t > 0$. Let the symbol $\mathfrak{B}(t)$ stand for the phrase 'given the evolution of the process up to time t'. (Technically, $\mathfrak{B}(t)$ is a sub-σ-algebra induced by the set of random functions $\{(X_d(u), Y_d(u) \mid u \leq t\}$.) By taking conditional expectations in Eqs. (7.8.13) given $\mathfrak{B}(t)$, it follows from the binomial densities in Eqs. (7.8.9) and (7.8.12) that

$$E\left[X_d(t+h) \mid \mathfrak{B}(t)\right] = X_d(t)Q(t) + Y_d(t)p_R \tag{7.8.14}$$

$$E\left[Y_d(t+h) \mid \mathfrak{B}(t)\right] = X_d(t)P(t) + Y_d(t)q_R \,. \tag{7.8.15}$$

The unconditional expectation of the random variable $X_d(t+h)$ is:

$$E\left[X_d(t+h)\right] = E\left[E\left[X_d(t+h) \mid \mathfrak{B}(t)\right]\right] \,. \tag{7.8.16}$$

But, this expectation cannot be determined directly from Eq. (7.8.14), because $Q(t) = \exp\left[-\lambda p h(Y_d(t)/m)\right]$ is a non-linear function of the random variable $Y_d(t)$. However, if the initial values $X_d(0) = n$ and $Y_d(0) = a$ have been assigned, then the conditional expectations on the left in Eqs. (7.8.14) and (7.8.15) are determined for $t = 0$ and are unconditional expectations, because the right-hand sides of the equations are constant. Now suppose one views these values,

$$\widehat{X}_d(h) = X_d(0)Q(0) + Y_d(0)p_R \tag{7.8.17}$$

$$\widehat{Y}_d(h) = X_d(0)P(0) + Y_d(0)q_R \tag{7.8.18}$$

of the conditional expectations in Eqs. (7.8.14) and (7.8.15) as estimates of the random variables $X_d(h)$ and $Y_d(h)$. Actually, this view is often used in stochastic processes and mathematical statistics. For, if X is any random variable with a finite variance and one wishes to estimate X by some value $\widehat{X}$ such that $E[(X-\widehat{X})^2]$ is a minimum, then $\widehat{X} = E[X]$.

If one takes this process of estimation one more step and lets the symbols $\widehat{P}(h)$ and $\widehat{Q}(h)$ denote the functions $P(h)$ and $Q(h)$ evaluated at $\widehat{Y}_d(h)$, then the right-hand sides of Eqs. (7.8.17) and (7.8.18) could be used to compute $\widehat{X}_d(2h)$ and $\widehat{Y}_d(2h)$. By continuing this process recursively, one arrives at the set on non-linear difference equations,

$$\widehat{X}_d((k+1)h) = \widehat{X}_d(kh)\widehat{Q}(kh) + \widehat{Y}_d(kh)p_R \tag{7.8.19}$$

$$\widehat{Y}_d((k+1)h) = \widehat{X}_d(kh)\widehat{P}(kh) + \widehat{Y}_d(kh)q_R\,, \tag{7.8.20}$$

where $k = 0, 1, 2, \cdots$. Thus, "estimates" of the sample functions may be computed with relative ease. Moreover, these difference equations resemble a model that would arise if one were working strictly within a discrete time deterministic paradigm. From now on these non-linear difference equations will be referred to as a deterministic model embedded in a stochastic process. As will be illustrated subsequently, the procedure just described is quite general and may be used to embed deterministic models in a variety of discrete time stochastic processes.

With the non-linear difference equations in Eqs. (7.8.19) and (7.8.20), it seems natural to consider the case $h \downarrow 0$. To this end, observe that for any constant $b > 0$, $\exp[-bh] = 1-bh+o(h)$, where $o(h)/h \to 0$ as $h \downarrow 0$. Consequently, equivalent forms of these difference equations are:

$$\widehat{X}(t+h) = \widehat{X}(t)\left(1 - \lambda ph\frac{\widehat{Y}(t)}{m}\right) + \widehat{Y}(t)\gamma h + o(h) \tag{7.8.21}$$

$$\widehat{Y}(t+h) = \widehat{X}(t)\lambda ph\frac{\widehat{Y}(t)}{m} + \widehat{Y}(t)\gamma h + o(h)\,. \tag{7.8.22}$$

Observe the subscript "d" has been dropped in anticipation of a passage to continuous time. After some algebraic rearrangements, divisions by h, and passages to the limit as $h \downarrow 0$, the following differential equations

$$\frac{d\widehat{X}(t)}{dt} = -\lambda p \frac{\widehat{X}(t)\widehat{Y}(t)}{m} + \gamma\widehat{Y}(t) \tag{7.8.23}$$

$$\frac{d\widehat{Y}(t)}{dt} = \lambda p \frac{\widehat{X}(t)\widehat{Y}(t)}{m} - \gamma\widehat{Y}(t) \tag{7.8.24}$$

arise. An equivalent and useful form of Eq. (7.8.24) is:

$$\frac{d\widehat{Y}(t)}{dt} = \left(\frac{R_0\widehat{X}(t)}{m} - 1\right)\gamma\widehat{Y}(t)\,, \tag{7.8.25}$$

where $R_0 = \lambda p/\gamma$, a threshold parameter for a CMJ-process determined by the parameters γ, λ, and p.

From this equation, it can be seen that, according to the embedded deterministic model, whether the number of infectives in the population increases or decreases depends not only on R_0 but also on $f(t) = \widehat{X}(t)/m$, the fraction of the population that are susceptible. Thus, if $R_0 f(t) > 1$, then the number of infectives is increasing; if $R_0 f(t) < 1$, then this number is decreasing; and if $R_0 f(t) = 1$, then there is no change in this number. If the fraction $f(0) = n/m$ is near one, then initially R_0 plays a decisive role in the behavior of Eq. (7.8.25). These observations suggest that a somewhat sharper view of the role played by R_0 in the evolution of the process may be gained by also considering the embedded deterministic model along with the stochastic model.

Indeed, historically, in most discussions of SIS-processes, a set of deterministic differential equations, essentially equivalent to those above, serve as a point of departure and a stochastic SIS-model is usually introduced as an extension of a deterministic system. In this section, however, this historical process has been reversed and it has been shown how a deterministic model may be embedded in a stochastic process by the procedure just outlined. Actually, by extending these techniques, it is also possible to relax some of the very restrictive conditions used in the formulation of an SIS-process. For example, attention need not be restricted to the case where the infectious period has an exponential distribution determined by a constant risk function γ; distributions with non-constant risk functions can instead be incorporated into a model. To analyze such models effectively from a practical perspective, however, the use of computer intensive methods, including Monte Carlo simulation, is basic. In a later section, these methods will be discussed in more detail along with a brief treatment of SIR-processes. An interesting numerical and theoretical study of a logistic SIS-process and some of its extensions has been reported by Jacquez and Simon.[8]

7.9 Embedding Deterministic Models in SIR-Processes

In this section the principles of approximating stochastic processes in continuous time by a discrete time process, as outlined in the preceding section, will be extended to the SIR-processes presented in Section 7.5. Attention will also be given to assessing the performance of a deterministic model embedded in a stochastic process as a measure of central tendency for the sample functions of the process by Monte Carlo simulation. To this end, let the random functions $X(t)$ and $Y(t)$ denote, respectively, the number of susceptibles and infectives in the population at time $t \in [0, \infty)$ and let the random function $Z(t)$ denote the number infectives who have been removed during the time interval $(0, t]$, $t > 0$. As before, it will be assumed that the population is closed and of size $m \geq 2$ so that for all $t \in [0, \infty)$,

$$X(t) + Y(t) + Z(t) = m \; . \tag{7.9.1}$$

Just as in Section 7.8, for a given set S_h of discrete time points, let $X_d(t)$, $Y_d(t)$, and $Z_d(t)$ denote the corresponding random functions for the discrete time approximation to the process in continuous time. These random functions also satisfy Eq. (7.9.1) for all $t \in S_h$. For every $t \in S_h$, let the random functions $X_I(t+h)$ be the number of susceptibles $X_d(t)$ at t who are infected during the time interval $(t, t+h]$. It will assumed that, given $X_d(t)$, the conditional distribution of the random variable $X_I(t+h)$ is binomial with index $X_d(t)$ and probability $P(t)$. In symbols, $X_I(t+h) \sim CB(X_d(t), P(t))$. Various forms of the probability $P(t)$ will be considered subsequently and $Q(t) = 1 - P(t)$ by definition. Similarly, let the random function $Y_R(t+h)$ be the number of infectives $Y_d(t)$ at $t \in S_h$ who have been removed during the time interval $(t, t+h]$. It will be assumed that $Y_R(t+h) \sim CB(Y_d(t), p_R)$, where the probability p_R will be specified subsequently and $q_R = 1 - p_R$. Another assumption basic to the construction of the model is that, given $X_d(t)$ and $Y_d(t)$, the random variables $X_I(t+h)$ and $Y_R(t+h)$ are conditionally independent.

For a discrete time SIR-process, the recursive stochastic evolutionary equations take a simple form, given these definitions of the random functions $X_I(t+h)$ and $Y_R(t+h)$. For, let $(X_d(t), Y_d(t), Z_d(t))$ be the state of the population at time $t \in S_h$. Then, the state of the population at time $t+h$ is given by the equations,

$$
\begin{aligned}
X_d(t+h) &= X_d(t) - X_I(t+h) \\
Y_d(t+h) &= X_I(t+h) + Y_d(t) - Y_R(t+h) \\
Z_d(t+h) &= Z_d(t) + Y_R(t+h) \ .
\end{aligned}
\tag{7.9.2}
$$

By using the techniques outlined in Section 7.8, it can be shown that the deterministic model embedded in the discrete time stochastic process takes the form,

$$
\begin{aligned}
\widehat{X}((k+1)h) &= \widehat{X}(kh)\widehat{Q}(kh) \\
\widehat{Y}((k+1)h) &= \widehat{X}(kh)\widehat{P}(kh) + \widehat{Y}(kh)q_R \\
\widehat{Z}((k+1)h) &= \widehat{Z}(kh) + \widehat{Y}(kh)p_R \ ,
\end{aligned}
\tag{7.9.3}
$$

for $k = 0, 1, 2, \cdots$. For any assigned initial state $(n, a, 0)$ such that $n + a = m$, Monte Carlo realizations of the discrete time process may be computed recursively from Eqs. (7.9.2) and the corresponding trajectory for the embedded deterministic model may be computed recursively using Eqs. (7.9.3). Observe that even for large values of m, which would make the use of large sparse matrices prohibitive, this discrete time system could be used to obtain results using computer intensive methods.

The probability $P(t)$ may be chosen in various ways, depending on the situation being considered. If, for example, it is assumed that, given the state $(X_d(t), Y_d(t), Z_d(t))$ of the population at time t, a susceptible makes contact with infectives according to a Poisson process with parameter $Y_d(t)\lambda$, and each contact results in an infection with probability $p \in (0,1)$. Then, by using probability generating functions as in Section 7.8, it can be shown that the conditional probability any susceptible at t escapes infection during the time interval $(t, t+h]$ is:

$$Q(t) = \exp\left[-Y_d(t)\lambda ph\right] \tag{7.9.4}$$

so that $P(t) = 1 - \exp[-Y_d(t)\lambda ph]$ for all $t \in S_h$.

On the other hand, if it is assumed that mixing among susceptibles and infectives is such that $Y_d(t)/(X_d(t) + Y_d(t))$ is the probability a susceptible contacts an infective during $(t,\ t+h]$, then for $X_d(t) + Y_d(t) \neq 0$ and $X_d(t) \geq 1$,

$$p(t) = \frac{Y_d(t)p}{X_d(t) + Y_d(t)} \tag{7.9.5}$$

is the conditional probability that a susceptible is infected per contact with an infective during $(t,\ t+h]$, and $q(t) = 1-p(t)$ is the probability of escaping infection. If one now assumes that a susceptible makes contacts with infectives according to a Poisson process with parameter λ and uses probability generating functions as in Section 7.8, then

$$Q(t) = \exp\left[-\frac{-\lambda phY_d(t)}{X_d(t) + Y_d(t)}\right] \tag{7.9.6}$$

is the conditional probability that a susceptible escapes infection during $(t, t+h]$ for all $t \in S_h$ and $P(t) = 1 - Q(t)$.

With regard to the duration of the infectious period, just as in Section 7.8, it will assumed that the duration D_I of this period has an exponential distribution with scale parameter $\gamma > 0$. Under this assumption, for every $t \in S_h$, the conditional probability an infective is removed from the population during any time interval $(t, t+h]$ is $p_R = 1 - \exp[-\gamma h]$ and by definition $q_R = \exp[-\gamma h]$. If one uses the form of the function $Q(t)$ in Eq. (7.9.4) and then proceeds as in Section 7.8, then as $h \downarrow 0$ in Eq. (7.9.3) the differential equations,

$$\frac{d\widehat{X}(t)}{dt} = -\widehat{X}(t)\widehat{Y}(t)\lambda p$$

$$\frac{d\widehat{Y}(t)}{dt} = \widehat{X}(t)\widehat{Y}(t)\lambda p - \gamma\widehat{Y}(t)$$

$$\frac{d\widehat{Z}(t)}{dt} = \gamma\widehat{Y}(t) \tag{7.9.7}$$

arise. But, if one uses the form of $Q(t)$ in Eq. (7.9.6), then as $h \downarrow 0$ in Eq. (7.9.3), this assumption gives rise to the differential equations,

$$\frac{d\widehat{X}(t)}{dt} = -\frac{\widehat{X}(t)\widehat{Y}(t)\lambda p}{\widehat{X}(t)+\widehat{Y}(t)}$$

$$\frac{d\widehat{Y}(t)}{dt} = \frac{\widehat{X}(t)\widehat{Y}(t)\lambda p}{\widehat{X}(t)+\widehat{Y}(t)} - \gamma\widehat{Y}(t)$$

$$\frac{d\widehat{Z}(t)}{dt} = \gamma\widehat{Y}(t)\,. \tag{7.9.8}$$

Differential equations of this form have been used by many authors, but by using a stochastic process as a starting point in their derivation, it can be seen that the parameters γ, λ, and p have clear probabilistic interpretations.

For deterministic models, threshold conditions may be derived by manipulating a differential equation governing the evolution of infectives in a population. As before, let $R_0 = \lambda p/\gamma$ be the threshold parameter for a CMJ-process determined by the parameters γ, λ, and p. Then, the middle differential equation in Eq. (7.9.7) may be represented in the form,

$$\frac{d\widehat{Y}(t)}{dt} = \left(R_0\widehat{X}(t) - 1\right)\gamma\widehat{Y}(t)\,; \tag{7.9.9}$$

whereas that in Eq. (7.9.8) takes the form,

$$\frac{d\widehat{Y}(t)}{dt} = \left(\frac{R_0\widehat{X}(t)}{\widehat{X}(t)+\widehat{Y}(t)} - 1\right)\gamma\widehat{Y}(t)\,. \tag{7.9.10}$$

When the initial state of the population is $(n, a, 0)$, then initially, $R_0 n$ is a threshold parameter for Eq. (7.9.9) and $R_0 n/(n+a)$ is a threshold parameter for Eq. (7.9.10). These parameters clearly illustrate the effects of initial conditions on the behavior of a deterministic system. For in (7.9.9), the function $\widehat{Y}(t)$ increases or decreases according to whether $R_0 n > 1$ or $R_0 n < 1$. An identical statement holds for the threshold parameter $R_0 n/(n+a)$ for Eq. (7.9.10), but in this case the fraction $n/(n+a)$ of susceptibles in the initial population plays a significant role.

The last topic to be considered in this section is that of assessing whether the trajectories of a deterministic model embedded in a stochastic process are good measures of central tendency for the sample functions of the process for the case of a discrete time model. Let $W(t)$ be some random function of a discrete time process defined on a set S_h of discrete time points. As was illustrated in Section 7.8, when the laws of evolution of a Markov chain depend on non-linear functions of the sample functions, it is often difficult to derive useful formulas for $\mu(t) = E[W(t)]$, the mean function of $W(t)$, in terms of the parameters of the process. Suppose a deterministic model is embedded in the process and $\widehat{W}(t)$ is the value of the trajectory at $t \in S_h$ computed using this model. One approach to assessing whether $\widehat{W}(t)$ is a good measure of central tendency for the random function $W(t)$ is to compare $\mu(t)$ and $\widehat{W}(t)$ on some finite set of time points $S_h(n_1) = \{t \mid t = 0, h, 2h, \cdots, n_1 h\}$, where n_1 is some preassigned positive integer. One could also compare $\widehat{W}(t)$ with the median function $m(t)$ of $W(t)$, but deriving useful formulas for this function may also be very difficult.

Fortunately, the method of Monte Carlo simulation provides a useful approach to not only assessing whether $\widehat{W}(t)$ is a good measure of central tendency but also provides insights into the variability among realizations of the random function $W(t)$. Suppose, for example, n_2 independently and identically distributed realizations of the random function $W(t)$ are computed for every $t \in S_h(n_1)$. Let $W_i(t)$ be the ith sample at t, for $i = 1, 2, \cdots, n_2$. Then, as is well-known, the sample mean function,

$$\overline{W}_{n_2}(t) = \frac{1}{n_2} \sum_{i=1}^{n_2} W_i(t) \tag{7.9.11}$$

is an unbiased estimator of the mean function $\mu(t)$ in the sense that $E[\overline{W}_{n_2}(t)] = \mu(t)$, and by the strong law of large numbers, it follows that $\overline{W}_{n_2}(t) \to \mu(t)$ as $n_2 \to \infty$ with probability one for all $t \in S_h(n_2)$. One could also compute $\widehat{m}(t)$, an estimate of the median function $m(t)$, at every $t \in S_h(n_1)$ from the Monte Carlo sample of size n_2. Furthermore, the extreme value statistics,

$$\begin{aligned} U_1(t) &= \min\{W_i(t) \mid i = 1, 2, \cdots, n_2\} \\ U_2(t) &= \max\{W_i(t) \mid i = 1, 2, \cdots, n_2\} \end{aligned} \tag{7.9.12}$$

could also be computed for every $t \in S_h(n_1)$.

Finally, to assess whether the trajectory $\{\widehat{W}(t) \mid t \in S_h(n_1)\}$ of the embedded deterministic model is a good measure of central tendency for the sample functions of the process, the set of points

$$\{(U_1(t), U_2(t), \overline{W}_{n_2}(t), \widehat{m}(t), \widehat{W}(t)) \mid t \in S_h(n_1)\} \tag{7.9.13}$$

of dimension five could be plotted simultaneously to provide visual judgements as to where the trajectory of the embedded deterministic model stands in relation to the trajectories of the Monte Carlo statistics.

The Monte Carlo method just described has been used by Mode et al.[13,14] in studying discrete time stochastic models of HIV/AIDS epidemics. Similar techniques have been used extensively by Tan and his colleagues (see for example Tan and Byers[20]). Kurtz[11] has presented limit theorems describing the convergence of sequences of Markov jump processes to differential equations. Specific examples of such convergence have been given by Kryscio and Lefèvre[10] and Jacquez and Simon[8] in their study of a logistic SIS-process. It should be mentioned that the method of embedding a deterministic model in a stochastic process as described in this and the preceding section involves no limit theorems and is, therefore, different from the approach of Kurtz. An extensive and thorough mathematical treatment of several classes of SIS and SIR deterministic models has been given by Capasso,[5] but throughout this book deterministic models will be considered only in conjunction with stochastic formulations as exemplified by the results in this and the preceding section.

In an interesting study of an SIS-process, West and Thompson[21] have reported the results of simulation experiments using the methods under discussion. They found that the time taken to compute a sample of Monte Carlo realizations of a discrete time approximation to the continuous time process was much less than if algorithms simulating the continuous time process were used. Moreover, a graphic comparison of the two methods of simulation showed that the results did not differ significantly. The random function that was the focus of attention of these authors was the fraction of susceptibles in the population at any time.

7.10 Convergence of Discrete Time Models

As discussed in Sections 7.8 and 7.9, suppose a discrete time approximation to some process in continuous time is defined on some lattice $S_h = \{kh \mid k = 0, 1, 2, \cdots\}$ of points, where $h > 0$. A question that naturally arises is: if $h \downarrow 0$, then in what sense will this discrete time process converge to the process in continuous time? No attempt will be made to answer this question in a complete mathematical sense. Rather it will be shown that if one views a Markov jump process in continuous time from a semi-Markov perspective, then the one-step transition function of the discrete time process will converge to that of one in continuous time as $h \downarrow 0$. Although the argument presented in what follows is quite general, for the sake of concreteness, it will be presented in terms of one of the SIR-processes discussed in Section 7.9.

For $x \geq 1$ and $y \geq 1$, suppose at some time t the continuous time SIR-process is in state (x, y, z). Then, the version of this process to be considered is the case where transition $\mathbf{i} = (x, y, z) \rightarrow (x-1, y+1, z)$ has the latent risk function $\beta(x, y, z) = xy\lambda p$, and further, the transition $(x, y, z) \rightarrow (x, y-1, z+1)$ has the latent risk function $y\gamma$, where γ and λ are positive constants and $p \in (0, 1)$. From a semi-Markov perspective, given that a transition occurs, the conditional probabilities of these transitions are:

$$\pi(\mathbf{i}, \mathbf{j}) = \frac{xy\lambda p}{xy\lambda p + y\gamma}, \tag{7.10.1}$$

if $\mathbf{j} = (x-1, y+1, z)$, and

$$\pi(\mathbf{i},\mathbf{j}) = \frac{y\gamma}{xy\lambda p + y\gamma} , \tag{7.10.2}$$

if $\mathbf{j} = (x, y-1, z+1)$. Further, for $t \in [0, \infty)$, the sojourn time in state $\mathbf{i}$ has an exponential distribution with distribution function

$$A(\mathbf{i}, t) = 1 - \exp\left[-\left(xy\lambda p + y\gamma\right) t\right] . \tag{7.10.3}$$

Therefore, according to the discussion in Section 3.7, given that the process enters state $\mathbf{i}$ at time 0, the conditional probability that there is a jump to state $\mathbf{j} \in \{(x-1, y+1, z), (x, y-1, z+1)\}$ during the time interval $(0, t]$, $t > 0$, is:

$$A(\mathbf{i},\mathbf{j},t) = A(\mathbf{i},t)\pi(\mathbf{i},\mathbf{j}) . \tag{7.10.4}$$

Let $A^{(h)}(\mathbf{i},\mathbf{j},t)$ be the corresponding function for the discrete time process defined on the lattice S_h. It will be shown that this process converges to the one in continuous time in the sense that for any $t \in (0, \infty)$,

$$\lim_{h \downarrow 0} A^{(h)}(\mathbf{i},\mathbf{j},t) = A(\mathbf{i},\mathbf{j},t) . \tag{7.10.5}$$

In the discrete time approximation to the process in continuous time, for any $t \in S_h$ and state $\mathbf{i} = (x,\, y,\, z)$, the conditional probability of a susceptible escaping infection during the time interval $(t, t+h]$ is $Q(t) = \exp[-y\lambda ph]$, so that $P(t) = 1 - \exp[-y\lambda ph]$ is the conditional probability of infection per susceptible during this time interval. Let the random function $X_I(t+h)$ be the number of susceptibles infected during $(t, t+h]$. Then, by assumption $X_I(t+h) \sim CB(x, P(t))$. Similarly, in the discrete time process, $q_R = \exp[-\gamma h]$ is the conditional probability that an infective at t is not removed from the population during the time interval $(t, t+h]$, and $p_R = 1 - \exp[-\gamma h]$ is the conditional probability of removal. As in the previous sections, let the random function $Y_R(t+h)$ denote the number of infectives that were removed during the time interval. Then, by assumption, $Y_R(t+h) \sim CB(y, p_R)$. It is further assumed that, given the state $\mathbf{i} = (x, y, z)$ of the population at time t, the random variables $X_I(t+h)$ and $Y_I(t+h)$ are conditionally independent.

With these assumptions in force, if the discrete time process is in state $\mathbf{i} = (x, y, z)$ at time $t \in S_h$, then

$$\mathbb{P}\left[X_I(t+h) = 0, Y_R(t+h) = 0 \mid \mathbf{i}\right] = Q^x(t) q_R^y =$$

$$\exp\left[-\left(xy\lambda p + y\gamma\right) h\right] = 1 - \left(xy\lambda p + y\gamma\right) h + o(h) \tag{7.10.6}$$

is the conditional probability of no jump occurring during the time interval $(t, t+h]$. The conditional probability that one susceptible is infected and no infective is removed during this time interval is:

$$\mathbb{P}\left[X_I(t+h) = 1, Y_R(t+h) = 0 \mid \mathbf{i}\right] =$$

$$\binom{x}{1} P(t) Q^{x-1}(t) q_R^y = xy\lambda ph + o(h)\,. \tag{7.10.7}$$

Similarly, the conditional probability that no susceptibles are infected and one infective is removed during this time interval is:

$$\mathbb{P}\left[X_I(t+h) = 0, Y_R(t+h) = 1 \mid \mathbf{i}\right] =$$

$$Q^x(t) \binom{y}{1} p_R q_R^{y-1} = y\gamma h + o(h)\,. \tag{7.10.8}$$

By adding Eqs. (7.10.6) through (7.10.8), it can be seen that:

$$\sum_{\nu_1, \nu_2} \mathbb{P}\left[X_I(t+h) = \nu_1, Y_R(t+h) = \nu_2 \mid \mathbf{i}\right] = 1 + o(h)\;, \tag{7.10.9}$$

where the sum extends over the set $\{(\nu_1, \nu_2) \mid (0,0), (1,0), (0,1)\}$. Thus, as $h \downarrow 0$, the probability mass associated with this sum goes to one. Given that $\mathbf{i} = (x, y, z)$ is the state of the discrete time process at time t and a jump occurs in during $(t, t+h]$,

$$\pi^{(h)}(\mathbf{i}, \mathbf{j}) = \frac{xy\lambda ph + o(h)}{\left(xy\lambda p + \gamma\right) h + o(h)} \tag{7.10.10}$$

is the conditional probability of a jump to state $\mathbf{j} = (x - 1, y + 1, z)$.

Further,

$$\pi^{(h)}(\mathbf{i},\mathbf{j}) = \frac{y\gamma h + o(h)}{(xy\lambda p + \gamma)\, h + o(h)} \tag{7.10.11}$$

is the conditional probability of a jump to state $\mathbf{j} = (x, y-1, z+1)$. It is clear that these probabilities approach those in Eqs. (7.10.1) and (7.10.2) as $h \downarrow 0$.

Now let $t \in (0, \infty)$. Then, for any $h > 0$, there is a positive integer k such that $t \in (kh, (k+1)h]$. According to Eq. (7.10.6), if the discrete time process enters state $\mathbf{i}$ at time 0, then $\exp[-(xy\lambda p + y\gamma)kh]$ is the probability the process is still in this state after k time intervals of length h. Therefore,

$$A^{(h)}(\mathbf{i}, kh) = 1 - \exp\left[-\left(xy\lambda p + y\gamma\right) kh\right] \tag{7.10.12}$$

is the conditional probability that a jump occurs during the time interval $(0, kh]$. But, as $h \downarrow 0$, the integer k may be chosen such that $t - kh$ can be made arbitrarily small. Hence, the distribution function in Eq. (7.10.12) converges to that in Eq. (7.10.3) as $h \downarrow 0$ and Eq. (7.10.5) follows, because the exponential function $\exp[-t]$ is continuous for $t \in (0, \infty)$.

7.11 References

1. N. T. J. Bailey, *The Mathematical Theory of Infectious Diseases and Its Applications,* 2nd ed., Charles Griffin and Company Limited, London, 1975.
2. N. G. Becker, *Analysis of Infectious Disease Data,* Chapman and Hall, London, New York, 1989.
3. L. Billard and Z. Zhao, Three-Stage Stochastic Epidemic Model: An Application to AIDS, *Mathematical Biosciences* **107:** 431-449, 1991.
4. V. Capasso, A Counting Processes Approach for Age-Dependent Epidemic Systems, *Lecture Notes in Biomathematics* **86:** 118-128, J. P. Gabriel, C. Lefèvre and P. Picard (eds.), *Stochastic Processes in Epidemic Theory,* Springer-Verlag, Berlin, New York, Tokyo, 1990.
5. V. Capasso, *Lecture Notes in Biomathematics* **97:** *Mathematical Structures of Epidemic Systems,* Springer-Verlag, Berlin, New York, Tokyo, 1993.

6. W. Feller, *An Introduction to Probability Theory and Its Applications, I,* 3rd ed., John Wiley and Sons, Inc., New York, London, 1968.
7. J. Gani and P. Purdue, Matrix-Geometric Methods for the General Stochastic Epidemic, *IMA Journal of Mathematics Applied in Medicine and Biology* **1:** 333-342, 1984.
8. J. A. Jacquez and C. P. Simon, The Stochastic SI Model with Recruitment and Deaths I. Comparison with the Closed SIS Model, *Mathematical Biosciences* **117:** 77-125, 1993.
9. W. O. Kermack and A. G. McKendrick, A Contribution to the Mathematical Theory of Epidemics, *Proceedings of the Royal Society of London Series* A **115:** 700-721, 1927.
10. R. J. Kryscio and C. Lefèvre, On the Extinction of the S-I-S Stochastic Logistic Epidemic, *Journal of Applied Probability* **27:** 685-694, 1989.
11. T. G. Kurtz, Limit Theorems for Sequences of Jump Markov Processes Approximating Ordinary Differential Processes, *Journal of Applied Probability* **8:** 344-356, 1971.
12. C. Lefèvre, Stochastic Epidemic Models for S-I-R Infectious Diseases: A Brief Survey of General Theory, *Lecture Notes in Biomathematics* **86:** 1-12, J. P. Gabriel, C, Lefèvre and P. Picard (eds.), *Stochastic Processes in Epidemic Theory,* Springer-Verlag, Berlin, New York, Tokyo, 1990.
13. C. J. Mode, H. E. Gollwitzer and N. Herrmann, A Methodological Study of a Stochastic Model of an AIDS Epidemic, *Mathematical Biosciences* **92:** 201-229, 1989.
14. C. J. Mode, H. E. Gollwitzer, M. A. Salsburg and C. K. Sleeman, A Methodological Study of a Nonlinear Stochastic Model of an AIDS Epidemic with Recruitment, *IMA Journal of Mathematics Applied in Medicine and Biology* **6:** 179-203, 1989.
15. I. Nasell, The Quasi-Stationary Distribution of the Closed Endemic SIS Model, *Advances in Applied Probability* **28:** 895-932, 1996.
16. M. F. Neuts and J. M. Li, An Algorithmic Study of SIR Stochastic Epidemic Models, *Lecture Notes in Statistics* **114**: 295, C. C. Heyde, Y. V. Prohorov, R. Pyke, and S. T. Rachev (eds.), *Athens Conference on Applied Probability and Time Series, I, Applied Probability,* Springer-Verlag, Berlin, New York, Tokyo, 1995.
17. R. H. Norden, On the Distribution of the Time to Extinction in the Stochastic Logistic Population Model, *Advances in Applied Probability* **14:** 687-708, 1982.
18. R. Ross, An Application of the Theory of Probabilities to the Study

of a priori Pathometry I, *Proceedings of the Royal Society of London Series* A **92:** 204-230, 1916.

19. I. W. Saunders, A Model for Myxomatosis, *Mathematical Biosciences* **42:** 116-122, 1980.
20. W. Y. Tan and R. H. Byers, Jr., A Stochastic Model of the HIV Epidemic and HIV Infection Distribution in a Homosexual Population, *Mathematical Biosciences* **113:** 115-143, 1993.
21. R. W. West and J. R. Thompson, Models for the Simple Epidemic, *Mathematical Biosciences* **141:** 29-39, 1997.

Chapter 8
THRESHOLD PARAMETERS FOR MULTI-TYPE BRANCHING PROCESSES

8.1 Introduction

In Chapter 6, we saw that the early stages of an epidemic could be approximated by one-type CMJ-branching processes, which provided a useful framework for definitions and derivations of formulas for threshold parameters. Furthermore, in our study of SIS and SIR processes in Chapter 7, we saw that threshold parameters for CMJ-processes - which also appeared in differential equations embedded in these classes of stochastic processes - were very useful in studying threshold behaviors of these deterministic models. Accordingly, the purpose of this chapter is to develop and apply some models of multi-type branching processes in the search for threshold parameters for the behavior of epidemics in their early stages. The general framework for our analysis will be analogous to that in Chapter 6 in that discrete time multi-type BGW-processes embedded in continuous time multi-type CMJ-processes will be the principal tools used in the construction of threshold parameters. For the most part, this chapter contains a collection of ideas and illustrative examples rather than the results of computer intensive experiments.

When the concept of type is introduced into a formulation, it is possible to conceive of many more subclasses in multi-type branching processes than in processes with one type. Consequently, in this chapter, attention will be restricted to the so-called irreducible case, which will be defined in the next section. Unlike some of the early applications of branching processes in genetics, where the concept of type corresponded to well-defined ideas, such as genotype and phenotype, when choosing a multi-type branching process formulation as an approximation to the early stages of an epidemic, defining the concept of type in a useful way, as we will see, is not always straightforward. Indeed, it will be shown by examples that the concept of type is very much dependent not only on the causal agent of the disease, but also on the environment and structure of the population in which the epidemic occurs. When, for example, the causal organism of an epidemic has alternate hosts, as is the case for the plague and malaria, it becomes necessary to digress from the mathematical discussion and present some basic biological knowledge of the pathogen and its hosts.

8.2 Overview of the Structure of Multi-Type CMJ-Processes

The ideas underlying multi-type CMJ-processes are similar to those outlined in Section 6.2 for one-type processes, except that the concept of type, which may assume many forms, plays a basic role. As an aid to motivating the results of this section, it will be useful to give an example of the concept of type, when a model for an epidemic of a sexually transmitted disease is formulated within the framework of a multi-type CMJ-process. For example, suppose infections are transmitted only through heterosexual contacts. Then, an infection is said to be of type 1 if an infected male infects a susceptible female. Similarly, an infection of type 2 occurs if an infected female infects a susceptible male. The set of all males (females) infected by an infected female (male) throughout her (his) infectious period will constitute a generation of her (his) offspring. As a first approximation, suppose the spread of infections in a heterosexual population is modeled as a discrete time two-type BGW-process with time corresponding to generations. For any generation, let m_{12} be the expected total number of susceptible males infected by an infective female throughout her infectious period, and define the expectation m_{21} similarly for females infected by infective males. Then, the matrix,

$$\mathfrak{M} = \begin{bmatrix} 0 & m_{12} \\ m_{21} & 0 \end{bmatrix} \tag{8.2.1}$$

of offspring means, which plays a fundamental role in the theory of a two-type BGW-process, is irreducible and periodic. Some results for multi-type BGW-processes with irreducible periodic matrices of offspring means, along with references, may be found in Mode[16] (see Chapter 2).

A multi-type BGW-process may always be embedded in a continuous time multi-type CMJ-process and the above example illustrates that the structure of the process must be sufficiently general to accommodate a periodic matrix for the embedded BGW-process. A square irreducible non-negative matrix $\mathfrak{M}$ is said to be positively regular if there is a positive integer n such that all elements in the matrix $\mathfrak{M}^n$ are positive. Observe that periodic non-negative matrices are not positively regular. Even though the theory in Mode[16] (see Chapter 3), for a multi-type CMJ-process was developed for the case where the matrix $\mathfrak{M}$ was irreducible and positively regular, it may, fortunately, be extended to the case where this matrix is irreducible and periodic.

Because the concept of type may take various forms, depending on the infectious disease being considered, those facets of the general theory of multi-type CMJ-processes to be used in this section will be described for the case of $m \geq 2$ types of infection. Consider an individual who is infected at $t = 0$ with an infection of type i, and for $t > 0$ let the integer-valued random function $N_{ij}(t)$ be the number of individuals infected by this infective during $(0, t]$ with infections of type j. In a subsequent section, a method rooted in the theory of semi-Markov processes in continuous time for constructing examples of these random functions will be outlined, but such constructions will not exhaust the possibilities. It will be assumed that the expectations,

$$m_{ij}(t) = E\left[N_{ij}(t)\right] \tag{8.2.2}$$

are finite for all $t > 0$ and that the monotone limits

$$m_{ij} = \lim_{t\uparrow\infty} m_{ij}(t) \tag{8.2.3}$$

are also finite for all $i, j = 1, 2, \cdots, m$. The limits in Eq. (8.2.3) determine the $m \times m$ matrix $\mathfrak{M} = (m_{ij})$ of offspring means for the embedded multi-type BGW-process.

To accommodate the evolution of the process in continuous time, let the integer-valued random function $Z_j(t)$ represent the number of infected individuals in the population with infections of type

$j = 1, 2, \cdots, m$ at time $t > 0$. Then, in an epidemic emanating from a single infective of type i at $t = 0$, the conditional expected number of infectives of type j at $t > 0$ is given by:

$$M_{ij}(t) = E_i [Z_j(t)] \ . \tag{8.2.4}$$

It can be shown that under rather general conditions, the expectations in Eq. (8.2.4) are finite for all $t > 0$. The $m \times m$ matrix $\widehat{\mathbf{m}}(\lambda) = (\widehat{m}_{ij}(\lambda))$ of Laplace-Stieltjes transforms,

$$\widehat{m}_{ij}(\lambda) = \int_0^\infty e^{-\lambda t} m_{ij}(dt) \ , \tag{8.2.5}$$

which converge for all $\lambda \geq 0$ in the examples considered in this book, will play an important role in defining a threshold parameter for the process in continuous time, and the equation,

$$\mathfrak{M} = \widehat{\mathbf{m}}(0) \tag{8.2.6}$$

connects the matrix of offspring means for the embedded multi-type BGW-process with the matrix of Laplace-Stieltjes transforms in (8.2.5).

As an aid to deducing the behavior of the expectation functions in Eq. (8.2.4) as $t \uparrow \infty$, it will be useful to derive a system of renewal-type integral equations. To this end, for $t \in [0, \infty)$ let $G_i(t)$ denote the distribution function of the infectious period for an infective of type i. Then, because a new line of descent begins with the infection of each susceptible, for $t > 0$ and $i, j = 1, 2, \cdots, m$, a renewal argument yields the system,

$$M_{ij}(t) = \delta_{ij} (1 - G_i(t)) + \sum_{\nu=1}^{m} \int_0^t m_{i\nu}(du) M_{\nu j}(t-u) du \tag{8.2.7}$$

of renewal-type integral equations, where δ_{ij} is the Kronecker delta. To cast this system in a useful matrix form, define $m \times m$ matrices by $\mathbf{M}(t) = (M_{ij}(t))$ and $\mathbf{D}(t) = (\delta_{ij}(t)(1 - G_i(t)))$, a diagonal matrix. The integral Eqs. (8.2.7) may be written in the compact form,

$$\mathbf{M}(t) = \mathbf{D}(t) + \int_0^t \mathbf{m}(du) \mathbf{M}(t-u) \ . \tag{8.2.8}$$

For $\lambda > 0$ sufficiently large, it can be shown that the Laplace transforms,

$$\widehat{M_{ij}}(\lambda) = \int_0^\infty e^{-\lambda t} M_{ij}(t) dt \tag{8.2.9}$$

converge for all pairs (i, j). Accordingly, define $m \times m$ matrices by $\widehat{\mathbf{M}}(\lambda) = (\widehat{M_{ij}}(\lambda))$ and $\widehat{\mathbf{D}}(\lambda)$, a diagonal matrix of Laplace transforms of the matrix $\mathbf{D}(t)$ and let $\mathbf{I}_m$ be an identity matrix. Then, a passage to Laplace transforms in Eq. (8.2.8) yields the linear equation,

$$\widehat{\mathbf{M}}(\lambda) = \widehat{\mathbf{D}}(\lambda) + \widehat{\mathbf{m}}(\lambda)\widehat{\mathbf{M}}(\lambda) \tag{8.2.10}$$

for the matrix $\widehat{\mathbf{M}}(\lambda)$ with the solution,

$$\widehat{\mathbf{M}}(\lambda) = (\mathbf{I}_m - \widehat{\mathbf{m}}(\lambda))^{-1} \widehat{\mathbf{D}}(\lambda) = \frac{\widehat{\mathbf{B}}(\lambda)\widehat{\mathbf{D}}(\lambda)}{\det(\mathbf{I}_m - \widehat{\mathbf{m}}(\lambda))}, \tag{8.2.11}$$

where $\widehat{\mathbf{B}}(\lambda)$ is the adjoint of the matrix $\mathbf{I}_m - \widehat{\mathbf{m}}(\lambda)$. From Eq. (8.2.11), one can see that the behavior of the expectation functions as $t \uparrow \infty$ is associated with the roots of the determinantal equation

$$\Delta(\lambda) = \det(\mathbf{I}_m - \widehat{\mathbf{m}}(\lambda)) = 0\,. \tag{8.2.12}$$

Although a limit theorem in Mode[16] Chapter 3, describing the behavior of the mean functions in Eq. (8.2.4) as $t \uparrow \infty$, used the condition that the matrix $\widehat{\mathbf{m}}(\lambda)$ be positively regular for all $\lambda \geq 0$ (because it seemed to cover most cases of interest at the time), it would actually have sufficed to require that this matrix be irreducible and non-negative for all $\lambda \geq 0$. That many of the results of this chapter concerning multi-type CMJ-processes would also hold for the case where the matrix $\widehat{\mathbf{m}}(\lambda)$ is irreducible and non-negative for $\lambda \geq 0$ can be seen by reading an extensive account of the Perron-Frobenius theory of irreducible non-negative matrices in the classic book by Gantmacher[12] (see Chapter XIII). One result concerns a root $\lambda = \alpha$ of Eq. (8.2.12). If the Perron-Frobenius root of the matrix $\widehat{\mathbf{m}}(0) = \mathfrak{M}$ is greater that one, then there exists a simple real root r of Eq. (8.2.12) such that $r > 0$ and if $\lambda = \sigma + i\tau$ is any other root of this equation, then $\sigma < r$. The root r may be viewed as a threshold parameter in the sense that, under rather general conditions, it can be shown that there are positive constants c_{ij} and $\beta < r$ such that

$$M_{ij}(t) = c_{ij}e^{rt} + O(e^{\beta t}) \tag{8.2.13}$$

holds for all $i, j = 1, 2, \cdots, m$. Thus, in the long run, an epidemic of any type of infection would grow exponentially at rate r per unit time, and the parameter r will be referred to as the intrinsic growth rate of the epidemic.

Among the objectives of this chapter is the derivation of formulas for ρ_{pf}, the Perron-Frobenius root of the matrix $\mathfrak{M}$. But, when the model passes certain levels of complexity, as will be illustrated by examples, it will be necessary to use numerical algorithms for finding values of ρ_{pf}. The quantity ρ_{pf} is a threshold parameter in the sense that it can be shown that if $\rho_{pf} \leq 1$, then the epidemic becomes extinct with probability one. But, if $\rho_{pf} > 1$, then there is a positive probability of extinction depending on the type of the initial individual; however, on the set of non-extinction, the epidemic grows without bound. If $\rho_{pf} \geq 1$, then $r \geq 0$, but if $\rho_{pf} < 1$, then there may exist a root $r < 0$ of Eq. (8.2.12). Although it has not been proven, it is interesting to conjecture that Eq. (8.2.13) would continue to hold so that $r < 0$ could be interpreted as the rate of extinction of the epidemic in continuous time.

Finding numerical values of the roots of Eq. (8.2.12) can be difficult. It is thus of interest to consider alternative approaches to calculating r, the intrinsic growth rate of an epidemic. Let $\rho_{pf}(\lambda)$ be the Perron-Frobenius root of the matrix and suppose an efficient algorithm for finding numerical values of the eigenvalues of the matrix as a function of λ is available. Rather than solving Eq. (8.2.12) directly for r, an equivalent and alternative way of proceeding is to use the bisection method to search for a value of $\lambda = r$ such that $\rho_{pf}(r) = 1$. This method has been found to work quite well when $\rho_{pf}(0) > 1$.

8.3 A Class of Multi-Type Life Cycle Models

In the preceding section, for an individual who is infected at $t = 0$ with an infection of type $i = 1, 2, \cdots, m$, the integer-valued random function $N_{ij}(t)$ was defined for $t > 0$ as the number of susceptible individuals infected by this infective during $(0, t]$ with infections of type $j = 1, 2, \cdots, m$. There are many approaches to developing models for the collection $i = 1, 2, \cdots, m$,

$$\mathbf{N}_i(t) = (N_{ij}(t) \mid j = 1, 2, \cdots, m) \tag{8.3.1}$$

of random functions taking values in the set $\mathbb{N}^{(m)}$ of m-dimensional vectors of non-negative integers. The purpose of this section is to outline an extension of the approach described in Section 6.2 for the one-type case. To this end, with each type $i = 1, 2, \cdots, m$, there is associated a life history $\mathcal{H}_i = (T_i, \mathbf{K}_i)$, where T_i is a scalar-valued random variable with range $[0, \infty)$ denoting the length of the infectious period and $\mathbf{K}_i$ is a vector-valued process taking values in the set $\mathbb{N}^{(m)}$. The components of this vector-valued process are:

$$\mathbf{K}_i(t) = (K_{ij}(t) \mid j = 1, 2, \cdots, m) \ , \tag{8.3.2}$$

where, for $t > 0$, $K_{ij}(t)$ denotes the potential number of susceptibles infected with infections of type j during $(0, t]$ by an individual of type i infected at $t = 0$. As in Section 6.2, it will be assumed that for each i, the random variable T_i and the $\mathbf{K}_i$-process are independent.

For $t \in [0, \infty)$, let

$$G_i(t) = \mathbb{P}\left[T_i \leq t\right] \tag{8.3.3}$$

be the distribution function of the random variable T_i, where it is assumed that $G_i(0) = 0$ and $G_i(t) \to 1$ as $t \to \infty$ for all $i = 1, 2, \cdots, m$. In all models considered in this chapter, these distribution functions will have *p.d.f.*'s continuous on $(0, \infty)$ denoted by $g_i(t)$. Another function that will play a basic role is the m-dimensional probability generating function (*p.g.f.*) of the $\mathbf{K}_i$-process. Let $\mathbf{s} = (s_j \mid j = 1, 2, \cdots, m)$ be a m-dimensional vector such that $s_j \in [0, 1]$ for all $j = 1, 2, \cdots, m$. From now on, for any integer $m \geq 1$, the notation $\mathbf{s} \in [0, 1]^{(m)}$ will be used to express this condition succinctly. Then, $f_i(\mathbf{s},t)$, the *p.g.f.* of the $\mathbf{K}_i$-process, is defined by:

$$f_i(\mathbf{s},t) = E\left[\prod_{j=1}^{m} s_j^{K_{ij}(t)}\right] \tag{8.3.4}$$

for all $i = 1, 2, \cdots, m$ and $t \in [0, \infty)$.

Just as in Section 6.2, the vector-valued $\mathbf{K}_i$-process continues until it is stopped at the end of the infectious period. To take this stoppage into account, the vector-valued $\mathbf{N}_i$-process in Eq. (8.3.1) will be defined as follows. Fix $t \in (0, \infty)$. If $T_i > t$, then

$$\mathbf{N}_i(t) = \mathbf{K}_i(t) \ . \tag{8.3.5}$$

for all $i = 1, 2, \cdots, m$. But, if $T_i \leq t$, then

$$\mathbf{N}_i(t) = \mathbf{K}_i(T_i) \ . \tag{8.3.6}$$

for all $i = 1, 2, \cdots, m$. For $\mathbf{s} \in [0, 1]^{(m)}$ and $t \in [0, \infty)$, the *p.g.f.* of the $\mathbf{N}_i$-process is defined by

$$h_i(\mathbf{s},t) = E\left[\prod_{j=1}^{m} s_j^{N_{ij}(t)}\right] \ . \tag{8.3.7}$$

By using an argument similar to that used in the derivation of Eq. (8.3.6), it can be shown that the integral equations,

$$h_i(\mathbf{s},t) = (1 - G_i(t))\, f_i(\mathbf{s},t) + \int_0^t f_i(\mathbf{s},x) g_i(x) dx \ , \tag{8.3.8}$$

where $i = 1, 2, \cdots, m$, provide connections among the functions just defined. For $t \in [0, \infty)$, $i = 1, 2, \cdots, m$, and $j = 1, 2, \cdots, m$, let

$$\nu_{ij}(t) = E\left[K_{ij}(t)\right] \tag{8.3.9}$$

be the expectation functions of the $\mathbf{K}_i$-process, and let $m_{ij}(t)$ be the expectation functions of the $\mathbf{N}$-process (see Eq. (8.2.2)). Then, by using a procedure similar to that used in the derivation of Eq. (8.3.8), it can be shown that:

$$m_{ij}(t) = (1 - G_i(t))\, \nu_{ij}(t) + \int_0^t \nu_{ij}(x) g_i(x) dx \tag{8.3.10}$$

holds for all $i, j = 1, 2, \cdots, m$.

Just as in the one-type case, continuous density functions defined for $t \in (0, \infty)$:

$$b_{ij}(t) = \frac{d\nu_{ij}(t)}{dt} \tag{8.3.11}$$

of the expectation functions of the **K**-process will play a basic role in deriving formulas for threshold parameters for CMJ-processes in continuous time. An integration by parts in Eq. (8.3.10) leads to the equations,

$$m_{ij}(t) = \int_0^t b_{ij}(x)(1 - G_i(x))dx , \tag{8.3.12}$$

which hold for all $i, j = 1, 2, \cdots, m$, $t \in (0, \infty)$, and express the expectation functions of the **N**-process in terms of the densities in Eq. (8.3.11). For the class of life cycle models under consideration, the Laplace-Stieltjes transforms in Eq. (8.2.5) take the form,

$$\widehat{m}_{ij}(\lambda) = \int_0^\infty e^{-\lambda t} m_{ij}(dt) = \int_0^\infty e^{-\lambda t} b_{ij}(t)(1 - G_i(t))dt , \tag{8.3.13}$$

which, by assumption, converge for all $\lambda \in [0, \infty)$.

For those models in which the density functions in Eq. (8.3.11) are constant, formulas for threshold parameters and procedures for calculating them may be quite tractable. For example, suppose that for each type $i = 1, 2, \cdot \cdot \cdot, m$, an infective who was infected at time $t = 0$ with an infection of type i, contacts susceptibles during the interval $(0, t]$, $t > 0$, according to a Poisson process $C_i(t)$ with positive parameter κ_i. Then, for $j = 1, 2, \cdot \cdot \cdot, m$, let $p_{ij} \geq 0$ be the conditional probability per contact that an infective of type i infects a susceptible with a type j infection. To cover the case where a susceptible may escape infection when contacting an infective, let $p_{i,m+1}$ denote the conditional probability a susceptible escapes infection per contact with an infective of type i. It will be assumed that the condition,

$$\sum_{j=1}^{m+1} p_{ij} = 1 \tag{8.3.14}$$

holds for all $i = 1, 2, \cdot \cdot \cdot, m$. A plausible rationale for choosing these conditional probabilities will be discussed subsequently.

As a first step in extending the K-process defined in Section 6.4 from the one-dimensional to the multi-dimensional case, for each i, let $\boldsymbol{\eta}_i = (\eta_{ij} \mid j = 1, 2, \cdots, m+1)$ be a vector of Bernoulli indicators such that:

$$\sum_{j=1}^{m+1} \eta_{ij} = 1 \ , \tag{8.3.15}$$

$\eta_{ij} = 1$ if an infective of type i infects a susceptible with an infection of type j, and $\eta_{ij} = 0$ otherwise. Then,

$$\mathbb{P}\left[\eta_{ij} = 1\right] = p_{ij} \tag{8.3.16}$$

and, by definition, for $\mathbf{s} \in [0,1]^{(m+1)}$ the *p.g.f.* of the random vector $\boldsymbol{\eta}_i$ is:

$$E\left[\prod_{j=1}^{m+1} s_j\right] = \sum_{j=1}^{m+1} p_{ij} s_j \ . \tag{8.3.17}$$

Now, given $C_i(t)$, let $\boldsymbol{\eta}_i^{(\nu)}$, $\nu = 1, 2, \cdots, C_i(t)$, be a collection of conditionally independent and identically distributed copies of the random vector $\boldsymbol{\eta}_i$. Then, for each i and $C_i(t) > 0$, the $\mathbf{K}_i$-process is defined as the random sum,

$$\mathbf{K}_i(t) = \sum_{\nu=1}^{C_i(t)} \boldsymbol{\eta}_i^{(\nu)} \tag{8.3.18}$$

and $\mathbf{K}_i(t) = \mathbf{0}$, a zero vector, if $C_i(t) = 0$. Actually, the $\mathbf{K}_i$-process in Eq. (8.3.2) is the first m components of the vector-valued process defined in Eq. (8.3.18). From Eq. (8.3.17), it can be seen that the conditional *p.g.f.* of the $\mathbf{K}_i$-process, given $C_i(t)$, is:

$$E\left[\prod_{j=1}^{m+1} s_j^{K_{ih}(t)} \mid C_i(t)\right] = \left(\sum_{j=1}^{m+1} p_{ij} s_j\right)^{C_i(t)} \ . \tag{8.3.19}$$

Because the C_i-process is Poisson with parameter κ_i, by using condition in Eq. (8.3.16) it follows that the unconditional *p.g.f.* of the $\mathbf{K}_i$-process is:

$$E\left[\left(\sum_{j=1}^{m+1} p_{ij}s_j\right)^{C_i(t)}\right] = \prod_{j=1}^{m+1} \exp\left[\kappa_i p_{ij} t(s_j - 1)\right] . \tag{8.3.20}$$

In particular, the *p.g.f.* in Eq. (8.3.4) is the marginal *p.g.f.* for the first m components of that in Eq. (8.3.20), which may be derived by setting $s_{m+1} = 1$ in Eq. (8.3.20). Thus, for $\mathbf{s} \in [0,1]^{(m)}$ the *p.g.f.* in Eq. (8.3.4) takes the form,

$$f_I(\mathbf{s},t) = \prod_{j=1}^{m} \exp\left[\kappa_i p_{ij} t(s_j - 1)\right] . \tag{8.3.21}$$

Therefore, in this case, the random functions in the vector of Eq. (8.3.2) are independent Poisson processes with parameters $\kappa_i p_{ij}$ and expectations $\nu_{ij}(t) = \kappa_i p_{ij} t$ so that the densities in Eq. (8.3.11) are the constants,

$$b_{ij}(t) = \kappa_i p_{ij} \tag{8.3.22}$$

for all $i, j = 1, 2, \cdots, m$.

When these densities are constant, then the expectation function in Eq. (8.3.12) takes the form,

$$m_{ij}(t) = \kappa_i p_{ij} \int_0^t (1 - G_i(x))\, dx \ , \tag{8.3.23}$$

and by letting $t \uparrow \infty$, it can be seen that the elements of the matrix $\mathfrak{M} = (m_{ij})$ of offspring means for the embedded BGW-process have the form:

$$m_{ij} = \mu_i \kappa_i p_{ij}, \tag{8.3.24}$$

where

$$\mu_i = \int_0^\infty (1 - G_i(x))\, dx \tag{8.3.25}$$

is the expected length of the infectious period for an infective of type i. Analogously, from the formula for R_0 in Eq. (6.5.4), some authors label the expectation of the form in Eq. (8.3.24) as R_{0ij}. But, for the case where the matrix $\mathfrak{M}$ is irreducible, the threshold parameter for a CMJ-process in continuous time is the Perron-Frobenius root of the matrix $\mathfrak{M}$.

As a first step in deriving formulas for calculating r, the intrinsic growth rate of the epidemic, it is of interest to set down a formulas for the Laplace-Stieltjes transforms in Eq. (8.2.5) for the case of constant densities. From Eq. (8.3.24), it can be seen that for $\lambda > 0$ and all $i, j = 1, 2, \cdots, m$ these transforms take the form,

$$\widehat{m}_{ij}(\lambda) = \int_0^\infty e^{-\lambda t} m_{ij}(dt) = \kappa_i p_{ij} \left(\frac{1 - \widehat{g}_i(\lambda)}{\lambda} \right) , \tag{8.3.26}$$

where $\widehat{g}_i(\lambda)$ is the Laplace transform of $g_i(t)$, the *p.d.f.* of the infectious period of the ith type. Just as in Chapter 6, it will be of interest to calculate values of extinction probability as a means of judging the likelihoods of minor or major epidemics. To this end, it is necessary to consider the m-dimensional vector-valued random variable,

$$\mathbf{N}_i = (N_{i1}, N_{i2}, \cdots, N_{im}) = \lim_{t \uparrow \infty} \mathbf{N}_i(t) , \tag{8.3.27}$$

representing the total number of susceptibles with various types of infections infected by an infective of type $i = 1, 2, \cdots, m$ by the end of the infectious period. By letting $t \uparrow \infty$ in Eq. (8.3.8), it can be seen that the *p.g.f.*'s of these random variables are determined by the equations,

$$h_i(\mathbf{s}) = \int_0^\infty f_i(\mathbf{s}, t) g_i(t) dt \tag{8.3.28}$$

for $i = 1, 2, \cdots, m$. Given that an epidemic begins with one infective of type i, let q_i denote the conditional probability that it becomes extinct, and let $\mathbf{q} = (q_1, q_2, \cdots, q_m)$ be a vector of these probabilities. Then, just as in the case of one-type BGW-processes, it can be shown that these probabilities satisfy the equations,

$$q_i = h_i(\mathbf{q}) , \tag{8.3.29}$$

where $i = 1, 2, \cdots, m$. Even when the density functions are constants, these formula may take on a variety of explicit forms, depending on the choice of the distributions for the lengths of the infectious periods. In subsequent sections of this chapter, these formulas will be explored in more detail for various choices of distributions.

8.4 Threshold Parameters for Two-Type Systems

Before proceeding to more complex systems, it will be useful as a didactic exercise to illustrate the concepts set forth in the previous section by some simple algebra for two-type systems, under the assumption of constant infection rate densities. Throughout this section, it will be assumed that for $i = 1, 2$ the length of the infectious period follows an exponential distribution with parameter $\gamma_i > 0$ and *p.d.f.*:

$$g_i(t) = \gamma_i \exp\left[-\gamma_i t\right], \ t \in [0, \infty) . \tag{8.4.1}$$

Under this assumption, the elements m_{ij} of the matrix $\mathfrak{M}$ of expectations for the embedded BGW-process (see Eq. (8.2.4)), have the simple form,

$$m_{ij} = \frac{\kappa_i p_{ij}}{\gamma_i} . \tag{8.4.2}$$

Similarly, the matrix of Laplace-Stieltjes transforms with elements determined by Eq. (8.3.27) has the form,

$$\widehat{\mathbf{m}}(\lambda) = \begin{bmatrix} \dfrac{\kappa_1 p_{11}}{\gamma_1 + \lambda} & \dfrac{\kappa_1 p_{12}}{\gamma_1 + \lambda} \\ \\ \dfrac{\kappa_2 p_{21}}{\gamma_2 + \lambda} & \dfrac{\kappa_2 p_{22}}{\gamma_2 + \lambda} \end{bmatrix} . \tag{8.4.3}$$

Even though the two-type case is a simple system, it may be interpreted in many ways, but in this section, only two interpretations will be considered. Suppose, for example, one is studying a sexually transmitted disease in a human population and that infective females infect only susceptible males and infective males infect only susceptible females. Let types 1 and 2, respectively, denote females and males. Then, the matrix of transforms in Eq. (8.4.3) has the cyclic form,

$$\widehat{\mathbf{m}}(\lambda) = \begin{bmatrix} 0 & \dfrac{\kappa_1 p_{12}}{\gamma_1 + \lambda} \\ \\ \dfrac{\kappa_2 p_{21}}{\gamma_2 + \lambda} & 0 \end{bmatrix} , \tag{8.4.4}$$

with the Perron-Frobenius root

$$\rho_{pf}(\lambda) = \left(\left(\frac{\kappa_1 p_{12}}{\gamma_1 + \lambda} \right) \left(\frac{\kappa_2 p_{21}}{\gamma_2 + \lambda} \right) \right)^{\frac{1}{2}} . \tag{8.4.5}$$

Therefore, the threshold parameter for the system is:

$$\rho_{pf} = \rho_{pf}(0) = \left(\left(\frac{\kappa_1 p_{12}}{\gamma_1}\right)\left(\frac{\kappa_2 p_{21}}{\gamma_2}\right)\right)^{\frac{1}{2}}. \tag{8.4.6}$$

The intrinsic growth rate r of the epidemic is the appropriate root of the equation $\rho_{pf}(\lambda) = 1$, and, with the help of MAPLE, it can be shown that:

$$r = -\frac{1}{2}\gamma_1 - \frac{1}{2}\gamma_2 + \frac{1}{2}\sqrt{\left((\gamma_1 - \gamma_2)^2 + 4\gamma_1\gamma_2\rho_{pf}^2\right)}. \tag{8.4.7}$$

That this formula is the appropriate root of the equation $\rho_{pf}(\lambda) = 1$ can easily be checked. For, it can be shown that if $\rho_{pf} < 1$, then $r < 0$; if $\rho_{pf} > 1$, then $r > 0$; but, if $\rho_{pf} = 1$, then $r = 0$. Just as in the one-type case, the threshold parameter ρ_{pf} in Eq. (8.4.6) is sensitive to the expected lengths $\mu_i = 1/\gamma_i$, $i = 1, 2$, of infectious periods. Thus, for fixed values of the other parameters and sufficiently small values of γ_1 and γ_2 corresponding to large expected durations of infectious periods, threshold values such that $\rho_{pf} > 1$ may result.

There are other examples of two-type systems in which all the elements of the matrix $\mathfrak{M}$ may be positive. The specific example to be considered is that of bubonic plague, an infectious disease affecting over one hundred types of animals, including rats and humans. This disease is caused by the bacterium *Yersinia pestis,* which is carried by the rat flea, *Xenopsylla cheopsis.* Only adult flea females transmit the bacteria among animal hosts by drinking blood that contains the bacteria, and the bacteria in turn multiply in the flea's gut. When a flea carrying the bacteria bites another susceptible animal, it regurgitates the infected blood into the host and infects the host with the bacteria. It has been reported that a single bacterium is sufficient to cause infection. Whenever rats and humans live in close proximity to one another, together with fleas as a vector of the causal agent, four types of transmission may occur; namely, rat to rat, rat to human, human to rat, and human to human.

Bubonic plague is also known as the black death and epidemics of the disease have had a profound effect on European history. Among the notable epidemics in Europe are the Plague of Justinian 558 AD, and that in 14th century Europe, resulting in a decrease in human population estimated at about 25% in some countries. More recent epidemics in Europe have occurred in Austria in 1711, and in the Balkans from 1770 to 1772. In some parts of the world, the disease still exists in animal populations and outbreaks in humans occur from to time to time, for example, that in Surat, India in 1994.

To formulate a model within the framework of a two-type CMJ-process, let humans be type 1 and rats type 2. Then, there are four transmission types $\{(i,j) \mid i,j = 1,2\}$ to consider. For example, $(1,1)$ denotes the transmission of bacteria from human to human. Because the rate of contact may depend on the type of transmission, let κ_{ij} be the contact rate per unit time for a transmission of type (i,j) and let p_{ij} be the probability of infection per contact of this type. By using procedures similar to those in Section 8.3, one may conclude that the density of the Poissonian process for transmission type (i,j) is the constant $\kappa_{ij}p_{ij}$, and to simplify the notation let $a_{ij} = \kappa_{ij}p_{ij}$. Of course, if the a's were defined as $a_{ij} = \kappa_i p_{ij}$ as in Eq. (8.4.2) the results that follow would be applicable.

Because the output of the symbolic package MAPLE is easier to read and comprehend when the input does not involve ratios, it will be helpful to define R_0-values for each type (i,j) of transmission by the formula,

$$R_{ij} = \frac{a_{ij}}{\gamma_i} \,. \tag{8.4.8}$$

In this notation, the matrix $\mathfrak{M}$ may be expressed in the form,

$$\mathfrak{M} = \begin{bmatrix} R_{11} & R_{12} \\ R_{21} & R_{22} \end{bmatrix} . \tag{8.4.9}$$

Therefore, the threshold parameter for this process is:

$$\rho_{pf} = \frac{1}{2}\left(R_{11} + R_{22} + \sqrt{\left((R_{11} - R_{22})^2 + 4R_{12}R_{21} \right)} \right) . \tag{8.4.10}$$

As a first step in deriving a formula for the intrinsic growth rate of the epidemic, observe that each element of the matrix $\widehat{\mathbf{m}}(\lambda)$ has the form,

$$\widehat{m}_{ij}(\lambda) = \frac{a_{ij}}{\gamma_i + \lambda} \,. \tag{8.4.11}$$

Furthermore, by applying the formula in Eq. (8.4.10), it can be seen that the Perron-Frobenius root of the matrix $\widehat{\mathbf{m}}(\lambda)$ is:

$$\rho_{pf}(\lambda) = \frac{1}{2}\left(\frac{a_{11}}{\gamma_1+\lambda} + \frac{a_{22}}{\gamma_2+\lambda} + \sqrt{\zeta(\lambda)}\right) , \tag{8.4.12}$$

where

$$\zeta(\lambda) = \left(\frac{a_{11}}{\gamma_1+\lambda} - \frac{a_{22}}{\gamma_2+\lambda}\right)^2 + 4\left(\frac{a_{12}}{\gamma_1+\lambda}\right)\left(\frac{a_{21}}{\gamma_2+\lambda}\right) .$$

With the help of MAPLE, the equation $\rho_{pf}(\lambda) = 1$ may be solved symbolically to yield a formula for r, the intrinsic growth rate of the epidemic. To ease the notation, let

$$\xi = (\gamma_1-\gamma_2)^2 + (a_{11}-a_{22})^2 + 2(a_{11}(\gamma_2-\gamma_1) + a_{22}(\gamma_1-\gamma_2)) + 4a_{12}a_{21} . \tag{8.4.13}$$

Then, r may be expressed in the succinct form,

$$r = \frac{1}{2}(-\gamma_1 - \gamma_2 + a_{11} + a_{22} + \sqrt{\xi}) . \tag{8.4.14}$$

As it should, when $a_{11} = a_{22} = 0$, this formula reduces to the algebraic form of that in Eq. (8.4.7).

Turning next to extinction probabilities, when the lengths of the infectious periods follow exponential distributions and the vector-valued **K**-processes are Poissonian with independent components, the *p.g.f.* in Eq. (8.3.28) takes the form,

$$\begin{aligned} h_i(s_1,s_2) &= \frac{\gamma_i}{\gamma_i + a_{i1}(1-s_1) + a_{i2}(1-s_2)} \\ &= \frac{1}{1+R_{i1}(1-s_1)+R_{i2}(1-s_2)} \end{aligned} \tag{8.4.15}$$

for $i = 1, 2$. In particular, for the case of a sexually transmitted disease among heterosexuals in a human population when $R_{11} = R_{22} = 0$, the *p.g.f.*'s for females and males depend on only one variable and have the respective forms,

$$h_1(s) = \frac{1}{1+R_{12}(1-s)} \tag{8.4.16}$$

$$h_2(s) = \frac{1}{1 + R_{21}(1-s)} \; . \tag{8.4.17}$$

Given that an epidemic begins with an infected female, let q_1 be the conditional probability that it becomes extinct and let q_2 denote the corresponding probability for an epidemic beginning with an infected male. Then, because a new line of descent begins with the infection of either a susceptible female or male, by using chains of reasoning similar to the one-type case, it can be shown that the extinction probabilities satisfy the equations,

$$q_1 = h_1(q_2) \tag{8.4.18}$$

$$q_2 = h_2(q_1) \; . \tag{8.4.19}$$

Therefore, the probabilities q_1 and q_2 are the appropriate roots of:

$$s_1 = h_1(h_2(s_1)) \tag{8.4.20}$$

$$s_2 = h_2(h_1(s_2)) \; . \tag{8.4.21}$$

With the help of MAPLE, it can be shown that the appropriate roots of these equations are:

$$q_1 = \frac{R_{21} + 1}{R_{21} + R_{12}R_{21}} \tag{8.4.22}$$

$$q_2 = \frac{R_{12} + 1}{R_{12} + R_{12}R_{21}} \; . \tag{8.4.23}$$

When the threshold parameter satisfies the condition,

$$\rho_{pf} = \sqrt{R_{12}R_{21}} > 1, \tag{8.4.24}$$

then, as they should, the extinction probabilities satisfy $0 < q_i < 1$ for $i = 1, 2$.

For the case where the matrix $\mathfrak{M}$ is positively regular, useful and simple formulas for the extinction probabilities are difficult to derive, even with the help of MAPLE. However, when the threshold parameter satisfies the condition $\rho_{pf} > 1$, then, given numerical values of all the parameters of the system, the vector $\mathbf{q} = (q_1, q_2)$ may be calculated recursively. For $\mathbf{s} = (s_1, s_2)$, let

$$\mathbf{h}(\mathbf{s}) = (h_1(\mathbf{s}), h_2(\mathbf{s})) \tag{8.4.25}$$

be a vector of $p.g.f.$'s of the form defined in Eq. (8.4.15). Then, as in the one-type case, the vector $\mathbf{q}$ is a solution of the vector equation,

$$\mathbf{s} = \mathbf{h}(\mathbf{s}) \ . \tag{8.4.26}$$

To solve this equation numerically, define a sequence of vectors by:

$$\mathbf{q}^{(1)} = \mathbf{h}(\mathbf{0}) \tag{8.4.27}$$

$$\mathbf{q}^{(n+1)} = \mathbf{h}(\mathbf{q}^{(n)}) \tag{8.4.28}$$

for $n \geq 1$. Then, it can be shown that:

$$\mathbf{q} = \lim_{n\uparrow\infty} \mathbf{q}^{(n)} \ . \tag{8.4.29}$$

In many cases, convergence is quite rapid, so this recursive procedure provides a practical way of calculating extinction probabilities. It can also be shown that this procedure will yield values such that $0 < q_i < 1$ for $i = 1, 2$.

A simple case arises for the model of a sexually transmitted disease in a heterosexual population of humans if the distributions of the infectious periods in females and males are the same, so that it is the case that $\gamma_1 = \gamma_2 = \gamma > 0$. Then, the formula in Eq. (8.4.7) for the intrinsic growth rate of the epidemic takes the simple form,

$$r = \gamma(\rho_{pf} - 1) = \frac{\rho_{pf} - 1}{\mu} \ , \tag{8.4.30}$$

where μ is the expected length of the infectious period. Observe that this formula is similar to that for the one-type case in Eq. (6.5.13). For some choices of parameter values, it can be shown that although the probabilities that the epidemic becomes extinct are quite high, the intrinsic growth rate can be quite high, suggesting that an epidemic evolving from one or two infectives either becomes extinct with a high probability or grows explosively.

For example, suppose that $R_{12} = 1.05$ and $R_{21} = 1.25$. Then, $\rho_{pf} = 1.14560$, $q_1 = 0.87805$, $q_2 = 0.86772$, and the intrinsic growth rate is $r = 0.14564\gamma$. Now suppose the parameters of the system vary in such a way that R_{12} and R_{21} are constant. Under this supposition, if the time unit is the expected duration of the infectious period so that $\gamma = 1$, then, given that the epidemic does not become extinct, the eventual growth rate per unit time would be 14.564%. On the other hand, if the expected duration of the infectious period is $\mu = 1/2$ time unit, then this percentage becomes $2 \times (14.564) = 29.128\%$.

8.5 On the Parameterization of Contact Probabilities

In a sense, this section is a digression from the principal theme of this chapter. Nevertheless, the ideas outlined below will be useful in subsequent sections of this and later chapters. In the foregoing section, types corresponded to females and males for sexually transmitted diseases, or to rats and humans for bubonic plague. But, as one moves to systems with greater heterogeneity, the problem of constructing contact probabilities arises. Suppose, for example, an insect vector of some disease may occupy $m \geq 1$ environmental niches and human hosts live in $n \geq 1$ communities such as villages. A basic problem in formulating models of contact probabilities is that of constructing a bivariate distribution, describing the probabilities for contacts of type (i, j) among insects from the ith niche with humans from the jth community, where $i = 1, 2, \cdots, m$, and $j = 1, 2, \cdots, n$. The problem of constructing such probabilities may be stated as follows: Given the relative frequencies of the various types of vectors and hosts at the beginning of a time interval, construct a bivariate probability density function $p(i, j)$ for observing contacts of type (i, j) between insects from niche i and hosts from community j. Ideally, the construction should be sufficiently general to include random as well as various schemes of assortative mixing.

Mathematically, the problem reduces to constructing a joint distribution function determined by its marginals. Thus, given two distribution functions $F(x)$ and $G(y)$ of the random variables X and Y, the problem is to construct a bivariate distribution function $H(x, y)$ such that $F(x)$ and $G(y)$ are the marginal distribution functions. Among the authors who have discussed the literature on this problem are Mardia,[15] Whitt,[20] and Johnson and Kotz.[14] For the class of problems under consideration, it will suffice to restrict our attention to the case in which the random variables X and Y have finite variances. In this case, it is well-known that the distribution function that minimizes the correlation between X and Y is:

$$H_0(x,y) = \max(0, F(x) + G(y) - 1) \ , \tag{8.5.1}$$

and the distribution function that maximizes the correlation between X and Y is:

$$H_1(x,y) = \min(F(x), G(y)) \ . \tag{8.5.2}$$

These results are frequently attributed to Hoeffding and Frechet. From a substantive point of view, a positive correlation near one would correspond to positive assortative mixing; while a negative correlation near minus one would represent the case of "opposites" tend to attract, i.e., negative assortative mixing.

Another class of bivariate distribution functions with the marginals $F(x)$ and $G(y)$ is that determined by the Farlie-Morgenstern formula,

$$H_2(x,y) = F(x)G(y)\left[1 + \alpha(1 - F(x))(1 - G(y))\right] \ , \tag{8.5.3}$$

where α is a parameter such that $|\alpha| \leq 1$. Observe that when $\alpha = 0$, the random variables X and Y are independent and the cases $\alpha = 1$ and $\alpha = -1$ correspond, respectively, to positive and negative correlations of the random variables X and Y. Therefore, by varying the parameter α over the interval $[-1, 1]$, various mixing schemes could be considered.

A limitation of the Farlie-Morgenstern class of distributions, however, is that the correlation ρ of the random variables X and Y is necessarily rather low. For example, for the case in which F and G are the uniform distribution function on the interval $[0, 1]$, it can be shown that $|\rho| \leq 1/3$; moreover, numerical experiments with other marginals suggest that the Farlie-Morgenstern system by itself would be insufficient to characterize various systems of assortative mixing in which one would expect values of ρ such that $|\rho| \geq 1/3$. One is thus led to consider mixtures of the three distribution functions described above to obtain higher levels of correlation. Let θ_0 and θ_1 be numbers such that $0 \leq \theta_0 \leq 1$, $0 \leq \theta_1 \leq 1$, $0 \leq \theta_0 + \theta_1 \leq 1$, and let $\theta_2 = 1 - \theta_0 - \theta_1$. Then, the mixture

$$H(x,y) = \theta_0 H_0(x,y) + \theta_1 H_1(x,y) + \theta_2 H_2(x,y) \ , \tag{8.5.4}$$

is a bivariate distribution function with marginals $F(x)$ and $G(y)$.

By varying the three parameters θ_0, θ_1, and α, it will be possible to create a variety of mixing systems, including random and various schemes of assortative mixing. For example, if $\theta_2 = 1$ and $\alpha = 0$, a random mixing system would result, but if $\theta_1 = 0.95$, $\theta_2 = 0.05$ and $\alpha = 1$, then the mixing system could be classified as positive assortative. It should be mentioned that the scheme set forth in Eq. (8.5.4) is one of many distributions determined by its marginals. Additional material of interest may be found in Dall'Aglio et al.[8] Further, note that the set

$$\{< \theta_1, \theta_2, \alpha >| \, 0 < \theta_1 < 1, 0 < \theta_2 < 1, 0 < \theta_1 + \theta_2 < 1, -1 \leq \alpha \leq 1\} \tag{8.5.5}$$

will be referred to as the parameter space $\boldsymbol{\Theta}$ of the mixing model.

Given the values of the three parameters, the probability $p(i,j)$ for a contact of type (i,j) may be computed as follows: At the beginning of an epidemic, let the $H > 0$ be the total number of human hosts and let $V > 0$ be the total number of insect vectors. Among these totals, let V_i be the number of insects in niche i and let H_j be the number of hosts in community j. Then, the relative frequencies of insects in niche i is $v_i = V_i/V$ and the relative frequency of hosts in community j is $h_j = H_j/H$. The distribution function corresponding to these frequencies for insects is:

$$F(i) = \sum_{k=1}^{i} v_k \text{ for } i = 0, 1, \cdots, m \,, \tag{8.5.6}$$

where, by definition, $F(0) = 0$. A distribution function for hosts denoted by $G(j)$, $j = 1, 2, \cdots, n$, may be defined similarly. By letting these distribution functions play the roles of the marginal distribution functions $F(x)$ and $G(y)$ going into the construction of the bivariate distribution function Eq. (8.5.4), the *p.d.f.* $p(i,j)$ may be computed using the formula,

$$p(i,j) = H(i,j) - H(i-1,j) - H(i,j-1) + H(i-1,j-1) \,, \tag{8.5.7}$$

where, by definition, $H(t; i, j) = 0$ if either $i \leq 0$ or $j \leq 0$.

Given the bivariate *p.d.f.* in Eq. (8.5.7), the probability that a host contacts an insect from niche i is, by definition, the marginal *p.d.f.*:

$$p_1(i) = \sum_{j=1}^{n} p(i,j) \ , \tag{8.5.8}$$

defined for $i = 1, 2, \cdots, m$. Similarly, the probability that an insect contacts a host from community j is, by definition, the marginal *p.d.f.*:

$$p_2(j) = \sum_{i=1}^{m} p(i,j) \ , \tag{8.5.9}$$

defined for $j = 1, 2, \cdots, n$. Therefore, the conditional probability that an insect from niche $i = 1, 2, \cdots, m$ contacts a host in community j is:

$$p(j \mid i) = \frac{p(i,j)}{p_1(i)} \ , \tag{8.5.10}$$

provided that $p_1(i) \neq 0$. Similarly, for $p_2(j) \neq 0$, given a host in community $j = 1, 2, \cdots, n$, the conditional probability of a contact with an insect from niche i is:

$$p(i \mid j) = \frac{p(i,j)}{p_2(j)} \ . \tag{8.5.11}$$

As we shall see, such conditional probabilities will be useful in the next section.

8.6 Threshold Parameters for Malaria

According the US National Institute of Allergy and Infectious Diseases (NIAID), four species of malaria parasite cause disease in humans, namely, *Plasmodium vivax, P. malariae, P. falciparum*, and *P. ovale.* Of these four parasites, *P. falciparum* is the most common and causes the most deaths. It has been estimated by the World Health Organization (WHO) that each year 300 to 500 million people develop malaria and 1.5 to 3 million, mostly children, die from the disease. More than 90% of the cases occur in countries of tropical Africa and more than 6% occur in India, Brazil, Sri Lanka, Afghanistan, Vietnam, and Columbia.

The parasite has a complex life cycle and spends most of its life in the red blood cells of humans. Parasites are transmitted by female mosquitos, who ingest them while feeding on an infected person's blood and then inject them when biting another person. Upon entering the human host, the parasite invades a liver cell, assumes a new form, and most make copies of themselves. The infected liver cell eventually ruptures and releases parasites into the bloodstream where they infect red blood cells. Most parasites continue to reproduce within the blood cells, which eventually die and release parasites, which in turn infect other cells. While in the blood cells, parasites develop into female and male forms, and when these cells are ingested by a mosquito, they burst and release sexual forms of the parasite. Within the mosquito, the two sexual forms merge to create an oocyst, which, after maturing, ruptures and releases thousands of parasites that migrate to the salivary glands for the mosquito's next bite. At the present time, malaria can be treated by drugs and vaccines which remain under development. However, treatment with drugs and the development of vaccines are both complicated by genetic diversity in immune responses to malaria parasites among humans, as well as genetic diversity among the cells of the parasite, which differ in their ability to invade human cells and cause disease.

As a first step toward developing a multi-type CMJ-branching process approximation to the early stages of an epidemic of malaria within the framework outlined in Section 8.3, suppose mosquitos live in $m \geq 1$ environmental niches and humans live in $n \geq 1$ habitats. Among the mosquitos, let $v_i > 0$ be the fraction who live in the ith niche, and among the humans, let $h_j > 0$ be the fraction who live in the jth habitat. It will be assumed that these fractions are constant and satisfy the conditions,

$$\sum_{i=1}^{m} v_i = 1 \tag{8.6.1}$$

$$\sum_{j=1}^{n} h_j = 1 \ . \tag{8.6.2}$$

By using the procedure outlined in Section 8.6 (see Eqs. (8.5.10) and

(8.5.11)), given these frequencies and a point in the three-dimensional parameter space $\mathbf{\Theta}$, one can then calculate the conditional probability $p(j \mid i)$ that a mosquito from the ith environmental niche contacts (bites) a human from the jth habitat. Similarly, given a host in habitat j, the conditional probability $p(i \mid j)$ he or she is contacted (bitten) by mosquito from niche i could be calculated.

At some risk of over-simplification, but for the sake of illustration, suppose some vaccine has been developed and is effective in a certain fraction of people. Among the humans in habitat j, let $p_I(j)$ be the fraction who have been immunized against malarial parasites by the vaccine and let $p_S(j)$ be the fraction who remain susceptible. It will be assumed that $p_I(j) + p_S(j) = 1$ for all $j = 1, 2, \cdots, n$. Also suppose, for the sake of simplicity, that when a susceptible host is bitten by an infected mosquito, the host is infected with probability one. To initiate an epidemic, it will be supposed that a small number of infective mosquitos and hosts are introduced into the system, and that an epidemic evolves from this small number of initial infectives.

Given that a mosquito from niche i is infected by an infective host at time $t = 0$, let the random function $K_{ij}(t)$ denote the number of susceptible hosts in habitat j infected by this mosquito during the time interval $(0, t]$, $t > 0$. Now suppose that mosquitos make contacts with human hosts according to a Poisson process with contact rate κ_{12} per unit time. The conditional probability that an infective mosquito from niche i contacts and infects a susceptible host in habitat j is $p(j \mid i)p_S(j)$. Therefore, by the reasoning of the previous sections, it can be shown that $K_{ij}(t)$ is a Poissonian process with *p.g.f.* :

$$f_{ij}(s_j, t) = \exp\left[\kappa_{12} p(j \mid i) p_S(j) t \left(s_j - 1\right)\right] \tag{8.6.3}$$

for $i = 1, 2, \cdots, m$, and $j = 1, 2, \cdots, n$. Moreover, for each fixed i, it can be shown that the processes $\{K_{i1}(t), \cdots, K_{in}(t)\}$ are independent. Let $\mathbf{s} = (s_1, s_2, \cdots, s_n)$ be a vector in $[0, 1]^{(n)}$. Then, the *p.g.f.* of this vector of random functions is:

$$f_i(\mathbf{s}, t) = \prod_{j=1}^{n} f_{ij}(s_j, t) = \exp\left[\kappa_{12} t \sum_{j=1}^{n} p(j \mid i) p_S(j) \left(s_j - 1\right)\right] \tag{8.6.4}$$

for $i = 1, 2, \cdots, m$.

Similarly, suppose a host in habitat j is infected by an infectious mosquito at time $t = 0$ and let the random function $K_{ji}(t)$ denote the potential number of mosquitos from niche i infected by this host during $(0, t]$, $t > 0$. By assumption, humans have contact with mosquitos according to a Poisson process with rate κ_{21} per unit time. Then, by following the chain of reasoning outlined above, for every $j = 1, 2, \cdots, m$, it can be shown that the vector $\{K_{j1}(t), \cdots, K_{jm}(t)\}$ of processes has the *p.g.f.* :

$$f_j(\mathbf{s},t) = \exp\left[\kappa_{21} t \sum_{i=1}^{m} p(i \mid j)(s_i - 1)\right], \tag{8.6.5}$$

where in this case $\mathbf{s}$ is a vector in $[0,1]^{(m)}$. In Eq. (8.6.5), it has been tacitly assumed that at the beginning of the epidemic, the fraction of susceptible mosquitos in the insect population in each niche is virtually one.

To complete the formulation of the model, what remains is to specify distributions for the infectious periods in mosquitos and humans. In the case of mosquitos, this period would correspond to the life span of the insect. Let the indices 1 and 2, respectively, denote mosquitos and human hosts. Tractable and interesting results may be obtained if the gamma type *p.d.f.*'s:

$$g_\nu(t) = \frac{\beta^{\alpha_\nu}}{\Gamma(\alpha_\nu)} t^{\alpha_\nu - 1} \exp[-\beta_\nu t], \ t \in (0, \infty) \tag{8.6.6}$$

are chosen for distributions of the infectious periods of insects, $\nu = 1$, and human hosts, $\nu = 2$. According to these choices of distributions, the expected length of an infectious period is α_ν / β_ν for $\nu = 1, 2$.

For the system under consideration, the threshold parameter is determined by the elements of two matrices of non-negative conditional expectations. Let $\mathfrak{M}_{12}$ be a $m \times n$ matrix defined by:

$$\mathfrak{M}_{12} = (m_{ij} \mid i = 1, 2, \cdots, m; \ j = 1, 2, \cdots, n), \tag{8.6.7}$$

where m_{ij} is the expected number of human hosts in habitat j infected by a mosquito from niche i during its infectious period. Similarly, let m_{ji} denote the number of mosquitos in niche i infected by a host from habitat j during his or her infectious period, and let $\mathfrak{M}_{21}$ denote a $n \times m$ matrix with these elements. Then, the $(m+n) \times (m+n)$ expectation matrix $\mathfrak{M}$ of the BGW-process embedded in the multi-type CMJ-process has the cyclic form,

$$\mathfrak{M} = \begin{bmatrix} \mathbf{0} & \mathfrak{M}_{12} \\ \mathfrak{M}_{21} & \mathbf{0} \end{bmatrix}, \tag{8.6.8}$$

and the threshold parameter of the system is the Perron-Frobenius root ρ_{pf} of the matrix $\mathfrak{M}$. When expressed in terms of the parameters of the system, the elements of the matrix $\mathfrak{M}_{12}$ have the form,

$$m_{ij} = \kappa_{12} p(j \mid i) p_S(j) \frac{\alpha_1}{\beta_1} \tag{8.6.9}$$

for $i = 1, 2, \cdots, m$, and $j = 1, 2, \cdots, n$. But, for $j = 1, 2, \cdots, n$, and $i = 1, 2, \cdots, m$, the elements of the matrix $\mathfrak{M}_{21}$ have the form,

$$m_{ji} = \kappa_{21} p(i \mid j) \frac{\alpha_2}{\beta_2}\,. \tag{8.6.10}$$

To develop algorithms for calculating the intrinsic growth rate of the epidemic, it will be necessary to consider a specific case of the $(m+n) \times (m+n)$ matrix $\widehat{\mathbf{m}}(\lambda)$ of Laplace-Stieltjes transforms defined for $\lambda \geq 0$, which has a partitioned form as in Eq. (8.6.8) with sub-matrices $\widehat{\mathbf{m}}_{12}(\lambda)$ and $\widehat{\mathbf{m}}_{21}(\lambda)$. The Laplace transform of a gamma-type density of the form in Eq. (8.6.6) has the tractable form,

$$\widehat{g}_\nu(\lambda) = \left(\frac{\beta_\nu}{\beta_\nu + \lambda} \right)^{\alpha_\nu} \tag{8.6.11}$$

for $\nu = 1, 2$. Given this functional form, the elements of the matrix $\widehat{\mathbf{m}}_{12}(\lambda)$ would be determined by the formula

$$\widehat{m}_{ij}(\lambda) = \kappa_{12} p(j \mid i) p_S(j) \left(\frac{1 - \widehat{g}_1(\lambda)}{\lambda} \right) \tag{8.6.12}$$

for $i = 1, 2, \cdots, m$, and $j = 1, 2, \cdots, n$, while the elements of the matrix $\widehat{\mathbf{m}}_{21}(\lambda)$ would be determined by the formula,

$$\widehat{m}_{ji}(\lambda) = \kappa_{21} p(i \mid j) \left(\frac{1 - \widehat{g}_2(\lambda)}{\lambda} \right) \tag{8.6.13}$$

for $j = 1, 2, \cdots, n$, and $i = 1, 2, \cdots, m$. Software could then be written to compute the values of the matrix $\widehat{\mathbf{m}}(\lambda)$ as a function of λ, whenever numerical values for the parameters of the system are specified. Furthermore, given a computer program to find eigenvalues of the matrix $\widehat{\mathbf{m}}(\lambda)$, one could compute the Perron-Frobenius root $\rho_{pf}(\lambda)$ of the matrix as a function of λ. The bisection method could then be used to find a value of $\lambda = r$, such that $\rho_{pf}(r) = 1$, to determine the intrinsic growth rate r of the epidemic.

The last topic to be considered in this section is that of extinction probabilities. Let $\mathbf{s}_1 = (s_i \mid i = 1, 2, \cdots, m)$ be a vector in $[0,1]^{(m)}$, and let $\mathbf{s}_2 = (s_j \mid j = 1, 2, \cdots)$ be a vector in $[0,1]^{(n)}$. Then, it follows from Eqs. (8.6.4) and (8.6.11) that for an infectious mosquito in niche i, the *p.g.f.* of the distribution of the numbers of humans in each of the n habitats infected by this insect at the end of its infectious period is determined by the formula,

$$h_{1i}(\mathbf{s}_2) = \int_0^\infty f_i(\mathbf{s}_2,t)g_1(t)dt$$

$$= \left(\frac{\beta_1}{\beta_1 + \kappa_{12} \sum_{j=1}^{n} p(j \mid i) p_S(j) (1 - s_j)} \right)^{\alpha_1} \tag{8.6.14}$$

for $i = 1, 2, \cdots, m$. Similarly, for an infectious human in habitat j the *p.g.f.* of the number insects in the m niches infected by this human at the end of his infectious period is given by the formula,

$$h_{2j}(\mathbf{s}_1) = \left(\frac{\beta_2}{\beta_2 + \kappa_{21} \sum_{i=1}^{m} p(i \mid j) (1 - s_i)} \right)^{\alpha_2} \tag{8.6.15}$$

for $j = 1, 2, \cdots, n$. Both these *p.g.f.*'s are those for a multi-dimensional discrete distribution on vectors of non-negative integers known as the negative multinomial distribution.

Now, for $\mathbf{s}_2 \in [0,1]^{(n)}$, define a m-dimensional vector of *p.g.f.*'s $\mathbf{h}_1(\mathbf{s}_2) = (h_{1i}(\mathbf{s}_2) \mid i = 1, 2, \cdots, m)$, and for $\mathbf{s}_1 \in [0,1]^{(m)}$, define a n-dimensional vector of *p.g.f.*'s $\mathbf{h}_2(\mathbf{s}_1) = (h_{2j}(\mathbf{s}_2) \mid j = 1, 2, \cdots, n)$. Given that an epidemic begins with an infectious insect in niche $i = 1, 2, \cdots, m$, let q_{1i} be the conditional probability the epidemic becomes extinct, and define the conditional probability q_{2j} similarly for an epidemic that begins with an infectious host in habitat $j = 1, 2, \cdots, n$. Further, let $\mathbf{q}_1 = (q_{1i} \mid i = 1, 2, \cdots, m)$ and $\mathbf{q}_2 = (q_{2j} \mid j = 1, 2, \cdots, n)$ be vectors of these probabilities. Then, just as in the simple case of a sexually transmitted disease in humans as in Section 8.4, it can be shown that these vectors of extinction probabilities are a solution of the equations,

$$\mathbf{s}_1 = \mathbf{h}_1(\mathbf{h}_2(\mathbf{s}_1)) \tag{8.6.16}$$

$$\mathbf{s}_2 = \mathbf{h}_2(\mathbf{h}_1(\mathbf{s}_2)) \; . \tag{8.6.17}$$

In the cyclic multi-type case under consideration, the classification of threshold conditions for vectors of extinction probabilities as solutions of Eqs. (8.6.16) and (8.6.17) is more complex than that for the single type case (see **Theorem 6.2.1**), for there are many possibilities. Nevertheless, there is a case that gives rise to an interesting extension of this theorem to the cyclic multi-dimensional case. Observe that the compound function $\mathbf{h}_1(\mathbf{h}_2(\mathbf{s}_1))$ may be viewed as a vector of *p.g.f.*'s for the offspring distributions of a m-dimensional multi-type BGW-process. It can also be shown that the $m \times m$ matrix of expectations for these offspring distributions is $\mathfrak{M}_{11} = \mathfrak{M}_{12}\,\mathfrak{M}_{21}$. Similarly, the $n \times n$ matrix of expectations for a n-dimensional BGW-process determined by the vector $\mathbf{h}_2(\mathbf{h}_1(\mathbf{s}_2))$ of compound *p.g.f.*'s is $\mathfrak{M}_{22} = \mathfrak{M}_{21}\mathfrak{M}_{21}$. Some definite statements, which are straightforward extensions of the general results in Section 1.7 of Mode,[16] may be made for the case where both the matrices $\mathfrak{M}_{11}$ and $\mathfrak{M}_{22}$ are positively regular.

Let ρ_{1pf} and ρ_{2pf} be the Perron-Frobenius roots of the matrices $\mathfrak{M}_{11}$ and $\mathfrak{M}_{22}$, respectively, and let $\mathbf{1}_m$ be a vector of ones of some dimension $m \geq 1$. When the relations $<$ or $=$ are used with two vectors, it means that the corresponding elements of each vector satisfy these relations. The four threshold conditions to be considered are: (1) if $\rho_{1pf} > 1$ and $\rho_{2pf} > 1$, then $\mathbf{q}_1 < \mathbf{1}_m$ and $\mathbf{q}_2 < \mathbf{1}_n$; (2) if $\rho_{1pf} > 1$ and $\rho_{2pf} \leq 1$, then $\mathbf{q}_1 < \mathbf{1}_m$ and $\mathbf{q}_2 = \mathbf{1}_n$, (3) if $\rho_{1pf} \leq 1$ and $\rho_{2pf} > 1$, then $\mathbf{q}_1 = \mathbf{1}_m$ and $\mathbf{q}_2 < \mathbf{1}_n$, and (4) if $\rho_{1pf} \leq 1$ and $\rho_{2pf} \leq 1$, then $\mathbf{q}_1 = \mathbf{1}_m$ and $\mathbf{q}_2 = \mathbf{1}_n$. The vectors $\mathbf{q}_1$ and $\mathbf{q}_2$ are minimal solutions of Eqs. (8.6.16) and (8.6.17) in the sense described in Mode,[16] and just as in the one-type case, recursive procedures may be developed to compute them.

From the biological point of view, it is interesting to note that whether an epidemic becomes extinct with probability one could depend on whether it starts with an infected insect or human. From the mathematical point of view, it may be possible to condense these four statements. Let $\sigma(\mathbf{A})$ be the spectrum, the set of eigenvalues, of any square matrix $\mathbf{A}$. Observe that the matrices $\mathfrak{M}_{11}$ and $\mathfrak{M}_{22}$ are sub-matrices of $\mathfrak{M}^2$ (see Eq. (8.6.8)). Therefore, it is the case that $\sigma(\mathfrak{M}_{11}) \cup \sigma(\mathfrak{M}_{22}) = \{\lambda^2 \mid \lambda \in \sigma(\mathfrak{M})\}$. For example, if the Perron-Frobenius root ρ_{pf} of $\mathfrak{M}$ satisfies the condition $\rho_{pf} \leq 1$, then $\rho_{1pf} \leq 1$ and $\rho_{2pf} \leq 1$.

When m and n are relatively small, the system will depend on only a few parameters so that computer experiments designed to explore the behavior of the model in chosen regions of the parameter space can be carried out with relative ease. For example, if $m = n = 2$, then the system will depend on seven basic parameters, namely the frequency v_1 of niche 1 for mosquitos; the frequency h_1 of habitat 1 for the host population, three parameters for the contact model outlined in Section 8.5; and the two rate constants κ_{12} and κ_{21}. To assess the effects of a vaccine as expressed by the fractions $p_S(j)$, $j = 1, 2$ per habitat of those in the population who remain susceptible, an investigator may wish to calculate threshold parameters for selected combinations of the seven basic parameters. The model outlined in this section was motivated by the interesting papers of Dye and Hasibeder[10] and Hasibeder.[13] Further interesting results, based on stochastic models, which deal with the long-term behavior of a malaria epidemic, may be found in Nasell[19] and the references cited therein.

8.7 Epidemics in a Community of Households

In recent years, a number of authors have applied ideas from branching processes in an effort to develop frameworks for the calculation of threshold parameters for the spread of communicable diseases among a community of households. Among these authors are Becker et al.,[5] Becker and Dietz,[6] and Becker and Hall.[7] In this field of activity, a major contribution of epidemic models has been the determination of critical levels of immunity, the minimum fraction of persons in a community that need to be immunized so as to prevent epidemics, and persistent endemic infection. In this section, it will be shown, by illustrative examples, that such models may be fruitfully formulated within the framework of multi-type CMJ-processes. In particular, a variant of the life cycle structure set forth in Section 8.3 will be utilized.

Consider a community of H households and among these let $H(n,s)$ be the number with n members, s of whom are susceptible. Then, by definition, the distribution of households is:

$$h(n,s) = \frac{H(n,s)}{H} , \tag{8.7.1}$$

where $n = 1, 2, \cdots, N$, for each n, $s = 0, 1, 2, \cdots, n$, and N is some arbitrary positive integer. The number of households of size n is:

$$H(n) = \sum_{s=0}^{n} H(n,s) . \tag{8.7.2}$$

Therefore, the total number of persons in the community is:

$$T_P = \sum_{n=1}^{N} nH(n) . \tag{8.7.3}$$

It will be assumed that infection spreads in a community by contacts among persons from different households as well as persons within households. If a person in the community is chosen at random, then:

$$g(n,s) = \frac{nH(n,s)}{T_P} \tag{8.7.4}$$

is the probability that he or she comes from a household with n members, s of whom are susceptible, where $n = 1, 2, \cdots, N$, and where $s = 0, 1, 2 \cdots, n$. There is an interesting and useful connection between the *p.d.f.*'s in Eqs. (8.7.1) and (8.7.4). The marginal *p.d.f.* for household size is:

$$h_1(n) = \sum_{s=0}^{n} h(n,s) , \tag{8.7.5}$$

and, by definition, the mean household size in the community is:

$$\mu_H = \sum_{n=1}^{N} n h_1(n) = \frac{T_P}{H} \,. \tag{8.7.6}$$

Therefore, it follows from Eqs. (8.7.1) and (8.7.4) that the densities are related according to the formula,

$$g(n, s) = \frac{n h(n, s)}{\mu_H} \,. \tag{8.7.7}$$

Other measures associated with the distribution of households will also be of interest and will prove useful in what follows. The variance of household size in the community is:

$$\sigma_H^2 = \sum_{n=1}^{n} (n - \mu_H)^2 \, h_1(n) \,. \tag{8.7.8}$$

By definition, the marginal *p.d.f.* for susceptibles among households is:

$$h_2(s) = \sum_{n=s}^{N} h(n, s) \tag{8.7.9}$$

for $s = 0, 1, 2, \cdots, N$, and the mean and variance of this distribution are:

$$\mu_S = \sum_{s=0}^{N} s h_2(s) \,, \tag{8.7.10}$$

and

$$\sigma_S^2 = \sum_{s=0}^{N} (s - \mu_S)^2 \, h_2(s) \,. \tag{8.7.11}$$

In what follows, it will be assumed that in a large community the distribution $g(n, s)$ does not change significantly during the early stages of an epidemic.

A crucial step in formulating a model within the framework of a multi-type branching process is that of defining the concept of type based on some useful classification of individuals in a population.

Individuals in a population may be classified in many ways, but, in this section, only one illustrative example will be considered. Suppose, for example, that individuals are classified according to the type of household in which they reside. In this case, an individual will be said to be of type $\tau = (n, s)$ if he or she is a member of a household with n members, s of whom are susceptible. According to this classification, any person in the community is a member of the set of types:

$$\mathfrak{T}_P = \{\tau = (n, s) \mid n = 1, 2, \cdots, N;\ s = 0, 1, 2, \cdots, n\}\ . \tag{8.7.12}$$

Knowing the number of elements in a set of types is also a crucial step in formulating a multi-type branching process. To determine the number of elements in the set in Eq. (8.7.12), observe that for each n the number of possible values of s is $n + 1$. Therefore, the number of elements in the set $\mathfrak{T}_P$ is:

$$\sum_{n=1}^{N} (n + 1) = \frac{N\,(N + 3)}{2}\ . \tag{8.7.13}$$

If infectives are classified according to the type of household in which they reside when infected, then infectives can emanate only from those households in which there is as least one susceptible. Therefore, the set of types of infectives in the population is the subset:

$$\mathfrak{T}_I = \{\tau = (n, s) \mid n = 1, 2, \cdots, N;\ s = 1, 2, \cdots, n\} \tag{8.7.14}$$

of $\mathfrak{T}_P$. Whether a particular classification of infectives is useful in formulating a branching process depends, in part, on the number of elements in the set $\mathfrak{T}_I$. For, if this number is too large, then the expectation matrix $\mathfrak{M}$ of the embedded BGW-process may be so large that useful results would be very difficult to obtain. It is can be seen that the number of elements in the set $\mathfrak{T}_I$ is:

$$m = \sum_{n=1}^{N} n = \frac{N\,(N + 1)}{2} \tag{8.7.15}$$

From this formula it is clear that for moderate values of N, the maximum household size in a community, the resulting values of m

will yield matrices $\mathfrak{M}$ that can be managed on many computer platforms. If, for example, $N = 10$, then $m = 55$, and if $N = 15$, then $m = 120$. In many communities households of sizes 10 to 15 would be very rare. Thus, in this age of computers with increasing speed and memory capacities, this choice of classification of infectious individuals in a community can lead to models that can be usefully implemented on computers, and is, therefore, worthy of further consideration.

As a first step toward formulating a model for the spread of infections in a community, suppose infectives have contact with members of a community outside their households according to a Poisson process with rate κ_C per unit time. Furthermore, suppose the probability of infection per contact for a susceptible having contact with an infective is p. Under the assumption that members of the community have contact outside their households at random, $g(n,s)sp/n$ is the probability that any type of infective contacts and infects a susceptible of type $\tau = (n,s)$ outside his or her household. Given that an infective of type τ_1 at $t = 0$, let the random function $K_C(\tau_1, \tau_2; t)$ denote the number of susceptibles outside his or her household of type τ_2 infected by this infective during the time interval $(0, t]$, $t > 0$. If one works within the structure outlined in Section 8.3, then, when $\tau_2 = (n,s)$, it follows that this random function follows a Poisson distribution with expectation,

$$\nu_C(\tau_1, \tau_2; t) = E\left[K_C(\tau_1, \tau_2; t)\right] = \frac{\kappa_C g(n,s)spt}{n} \tag{8.7.16}$$

for every $\tau_1 \in \mathfrak{T}_I$.

When a newly infected individual of type $\tau_1 = (n,s)$, $s \geq 1$, is infected at $t = 0$, then $s - 1$ susceptibles remain in the household following his or her infection. Let the random function $K_H(\tau_1; t)$ denote the number infected during the time interval $(0, t]$, $t > 0$. Suppose the waiting time to infection for each of these susceptibles follows an exponential distribution with parameter $\beta_H > 0$; moreover, suppose these waiting times are independent. Then, it can be shown that $K_H(\tau_1; t)$ has a binomial distribution with index $s - 1$ and probability,

$$F_H(t) = 1 - e^{-\beta_H t} \tag{8.7.17}$$

so that its expectation is:

$$\nu_H(\tau_1; t) = E\left[K_H(\tau_1; t)\right] = (s-1)\, F_H(t)\ . \tag{8.7.18}$$

It is interesting to observe that the density of this expectation is the non-constant function

$$b_H(\tau_1;t) = \frac{d\nu_H(\tau_1;t)}{dt} = (s-1)\,\beta_H e^{-\beta_H t}\ , \tag{8.7.19}$$

defined for $t \geq 0$.

To complete the formulation of the model for the spread of infections in a community, suppose the infectious period of each infective follows an exponential distribution with parameter $\gamma > 0$. For this model, denote the elements of the $m \times m$ matrix $\mathfrak{M}$ of expectations for the embedded BGW- process by $m(\tau_1, \tau_2)$. Then, for any $\tau_1 \in \mathfrak{T}_I$ and $\tau_2 = (n, s) \neq \tau_1$, it follows from Eqs. (8.7.16) and (8.3.12) that:

$$m(\tau_1,\tau_2) = \frac{\kappa_C g(n,s)sp}{n}\int_0^\infty e^{-\gamma t}dt = \frac{\kappa_C g(n,s)sp}{n\gamma}\ . \tag{8.7.20}$$

But, if $\tau_1 = \tau_2 = (n, s)$, then, by using Eq. (8.7.19), it can be shown that:

$$m(\tau_1,\tau_1) = \frac{\kappa_C g(n,s)sp}{n\gamma} + \frac{(s-1)\,\beta_H}{\beta_H+\gamma}\ . \tag{8.7.21}$$

It will be instructive to set down the structure of the matrix $\mathfrak{M}$ for selected small values of N, the maximum size of households in a community. To simplify the notation, let

$$a_{ns} = \frac{\kappa_C g(n,s)sp}{n\gamma} \tag{8.7.22}$$

and

$$b_s = \frac{(s-1)\,\beta_H}{\beta_H+\gamma} \tag{8.7.23}$$

for $s = 1, 2, \cdots, N$. Then, for the case $N = 2$, the matrix $\mathfrak{M}$ has the form,

$$\mathfrak{M} = \begin{bmatrix} a_{11} & a_{21} & a_{22} \\ a_{11} & a_{21} & a_{22} \\ a_{11} & a_{21} & a_{22}+b_1 \end{bmatrix}\ . \tag{8.7.24}$$

And, for the case $N = 3$, this matrix has the form,

$$\mathfrak{M} = \begin{bmatrix} a_{11} & a_{21} & a_{22} & a_{31} & a_{32} & a_{33} \\ a_{11} & a_{21} & a_{22} & a_{31} & a_{32} & a_{33} \\ a_{11} & a_{21} & a_{22}+b_1 & a_{31} & a_{32} & a_{33} \\ a_{11} & a_{21} & a_{22} & a_{31} & a_{32} & a_{33} \\ a_{11} & a_{21} & a_{22} & a_{31} & a_{32}+b_1 & a_{33} \\ a_{11} & a_{21} & a_{22} & a_{31} & a_{32} & a_{33}+b_2 \end{bmatrix} . \tag{8.7.25}$$

From an inspection of the matrix in Eq. (8.7.24), it can be seen that its rank is two, and, with the help of MAPLE, it can be shown that the characteristic polynomial of the matrix is

$$X\left(a_{11}b_1 + a_{21}b_1 - (a_{11} + a_{21} + a_{22} + b_1)X + X^2\right) . \tag{8.7.26}$$

Therefore, the threshold parameter in this case will be the appropriate root of a polynomial of degree two and can easily be written down from Eq. (8.7.26). Similarly, from an inspection of the matrix in Eq. (8.7.25), it can be seen that its rank is three, and it can be shown that the Perron-Frobenius root of the matrix is the appropriate root of a third degree polynomial, whose coefficients are rather complicated functions of the elements of the matrix. Because of this complexity, no attempt will be made to present these coefficients here.

In general, one is led to conjecture that the Perron-Frobenius root of the matrix $\mathfrak{M}$ for N, an arbitrary positive integer, is the appropriate root of a polynomial of degree N, but the details will be left to the reader. For those who prefer computer intensive numerical investigations to complex algebra, it would be relatively straightforward to write software that calls a library routine to compute the Perron-Frobenius roots as functions of selected points in the parameter space of the model. By also writing software that reflects various vaccination strategies in the distribution $\{g(\tau) \mid \tau \in \mathfrak{T}_P\}$, the efficacy of alternative strategies could be studied by computer intensive methods. Just as in the foregoing sections, procedures for calculating extinction probabilities and the intrinsic growth rate of the epidemic could be derived, but again the details will be left to the reader as a research exercise.

8.8 Highly Infectious Diseases in a Community of Households

As illustrated in the foregoing sections, when formulating a model of an epidemic within the framework of a branching process, the definition of type plays a basic role. Consider a highly infectious disease in a community of households, and suppose that when a susceptible in a household is infected, all other susceptibles in the household are infected by the end of the infectious period of the initial infective. A model of this type has been considered by Becker and Dietz,[6] who used the following classification of infectious individuals. A newly infected individual will be said to be of type s if there are s susceptibles remaining in his or her household just after his or her infection, where $s = 0, 1, 2, \cdots, N-1$, and N is the maximum size of a household. Apart from this classification of infectives, all other ingredients of the model remain the same as those defined in Section 8.7 except that the probability that a susceptible becomes infected per contact with an infective is $p = 1$.

To simplify the notation, let $\mu_I = \kappa_C/\gamma$ be the expected number of susceptibles in the community infected by an infectious individual outside his or her household by the end of his or her infectious period. Then, in a community in which individuals outside households mix at random, the expected number of infectives of type $s-1$ produced by an infective outside his or her household is given by:

$$m_s = \mu_I \sum_{n=s}^{N} g(n,s)\frac{s}{n} = \frac{\mu_I}{\mu_H} \sum_{n=s}^{N} sh(n,s) = \frac{\mu_I}{\mu_H} sh_2(s) \,, \tag{8.8.1}$$

(see Eqs. (8.7.7) and (8.7.9)), for $s = 1, 2, \cdots, N$. Because in his or her household the initial infective, by assumption, infects all other members of the household by the end of the infectious period, all his or her "offspring" are of type 0. It follows, therefore, that the $N \times N$ matrix $\mathfrak{M}$ of expectations for the embedded BGW-process has a very special form. For example, when $N = 4$, this matrix is of rank two and has the form,

$$\mathfrak{M} = \begin{bmatrix} m_1 & m_2 & m_3 & m_4 \\ m_1+1 & m_2 & m_3 & m_4 \\ m_1+2 & m_2 & m_3 & m_4 \\ m_1+3 & m_2 & m_3 & m_4 \end{bmatrix} . \tag{8.8.2}$$

With the help of MAPLE, it is easy to show that the characteristic polynomial of this matrix is:

$$X^2\left(X^2 - (m_4 + m_3 + m_2 + m_1)X - m_2 - 2m_3 - 3m_4\right) \tag{8.8.3}$$

By mathematical induction on N, it can be shown that for arbitrary N the characteristic polynomial of the matrix $\mathfrak{M}$ with rank two has the form

$$(-X)^{N-2}\left[X^2 - \left(\sum_{s=1}^{N} m_s\right)X - \sum_{s=1}^{N}(s-1)m_s\right] . \tag{8.8.4}$$

But, from Eq. (8.8.1) it can be seen that:

$$\sum_{s=1}^{N} m_s = \frac{\mu_I \mu_S}{\mu_H} \tag{8.8.5}$$

and

$$\sum_{s=1}^{N} s m_s = \frac{\mu_I}{\mu_H}\left(\mu_S^2 + \sigma_S^2\right) = \frac{\mu_I \mu_S^2}{\mu_H} a_S , \tag{8.8.6}$$

where, by definition, $a_S = 1 + \sigma_S^2/\mu_S^2$. Observe that this function depends only on σ_S/μ_S, the coefficient of variation of susceptibles among households.

After some further algebraic manipulation, it can be shown from Eq. (8.8.4) that the threshold parameter for the spread of infections among individuals in the community is:

$$\rho_I = \frac{\mu_I \mu_S}{2\mu_H}\left[1 + \left(1 + \frac{4\mu_H}{\mu_I \mu_S}\left(\mu_S a_s - 1\right)\right)^{\frac{1}{2}}\right] . \tag{8.8.7}$$

This threshold parameter is of particular interest, because it allows for the presence of immune individuals in the community as reflected in the household distribution. Some authors define a threshold parameter, which is a generalization of R_0 in the one-type processes, for the case where all members of the community are susceptible, but, from a theoretical point of view, there is no compelling need to restrict the concept of a threshold parameter to this very special case. If all the members of the community are susceptible, then $\mu_S = \mu_H$ and $\sigma_S = \sigma_H$, so that Eq. (8.8.7) takes the form,

$$\rho_{I0} = \frac{\mu_I}{2}\left[1 + \left(1 + \frac{4\left(\mu_H a_H - 1\right)}{\mu_I}\right)^{\frac{1}{2}}\right] . \tag{8.8.8}$$

As it should, when each household consists of only one individual so that $\mu_H = a_H = 1$, then

$$\rho_{I0} = \mu_I = R_0 , \tag{8.8.9}$$

the threshold parameter for a one-type CMJ-process. It is interesting to note from Eq. (8.8.8) that if the product $\mu_H a_H$ is sufficiently large, then it may be the case that $\rho_{I0} > 1$ even though $\mu_I = R_0 < 1$. This observation suggests that the household structure can play a crucial role as to whether an epidemic spreads or dies out in a community. For example, if the concept of household were extended to include the presence of large mixing groups, such as schools, then $\mu_H a_H$ could be large.

An epidemic of a highly infectious disease in a community may also be viewed from the perspective of the spread of the disease from household to household. Under the assumption an initial infective eventually infects all susceptibles in his or her household by the end of his or her infectious period, it will be useful to classify households by the number of initial susceptibles. Thus, a household will be said to be of type i if it initially contains i susceptibles, where $i = 1, 2, \cdots, N$. If one ignores the problem of formulating a model for the evolution of the epidemic within a household in continuous time, then the $N \times N$ matrix $\mathfrak{M}$ of expectations for the embedded BGW- process has a very simple form and can be derived using a simple argument.

Let the random variable ξ_j denote the number of susceptibles infected in households of type j by any infectious individual by the end of his or her infectious period. For a household of type i, let $\xi_j(\nu)$, $\nu = 1, 2, \cdots, i$, be *i.i.d.* copies of ξ_j. Then, the total number of households of type j infected by members of households of type i is given by the random variable,

$$N_{ij} = \sum_{\nu=1}^{i} \xi_j(\nu) \tag{8.8.10}$$

for $i, j = 1, 2, \cdots, N$. For every $\nu = 1, 2, \cdots, i$, $E[\xi_j(\nu)] = m_j$. Therefore, the ij-th element in the matrix $\mathfrak{M}$ has the form,

$$m_{ij} = E\left[N_{ij}\right] = im_j\ . \tag{8.8.11}$$

In particular, if $N = 3$, then this matrix has the form,

$$\mathfrak{M} = \begin{bmatrix} m_1 & m_2 & m_3 \\ 2m_1 & 2m_2 & 2m_3 \\ 3m_1 & 3m_2 & 3m_3 \end{bmatrix}, \tag{8.8.12}$$

and is of rank one.

In general, for N an arbitrary positive integer, it can be shown that the characteristic polynomial of the rank one matrix $\mathfrak{M}$ may be represented in the form,

$$(-X)^{N-1}\left(\sum_{s=1}^{N} sm_s - X\right)\ . \tag{8.8.13}$$

From this result, it is easy to see that the threshold parameter for the spread of the epidemic among households is

$$\rho_H = \sum_{s=1}^{N} sm_s = \frac{\mu_I \mu_S^2}{\mu_H} a_S\ , \tag{8.8.14}$$

(see Eq. (8.8.6)). Observe that the threshold parameters ρ_I and ρ_H may be expressed as functions of each other, but the details will be left to the reader as a research exercise.

To illustrate how these threshold parameters may be useful in testing the efficacy of alternative strategies for vaccinating members of a community, suppose, for the sake of simplicity, that all members of the community are susceptible and let $h(n)$, $n = 1, 2, \cdots, N$, be the distribution of household size. Furthermore, suppose according to Strategy 1 all members of each household are vaccinated. As is often the case, also suppose that the vaccine is not completely effective so that with probability $v \in (0,1)$ a susceptible is immune after vaccination and with probability $1-v$ he or she remains susceptible. If it is assumed that the success of vaccinations among a household of susceptibles of size n can be modeled as independent Bernoulli trials, then the distribution of household types (n, s) following vaccination would be given by:

$$h^{(1)}(n,s) = h(n)\binom{n}{s}(1-v)^s\, v^{n-s}\,, \tag{8.8.15}$$

for $n = 1, 2, \cdots, N$, and $s = 0, 1, 2, \cdots, n$. If, however, a household of size n was selected with probability w_n according to strategy 2, then the distribution of household types would take the form,

$$h^{(2)}(n,s) = h(n)\left[1 - w_n + w_n\binom{n}{s}(1-v)^s\, v^{n-s}\right]. \tag{8.8.16}$$

It is clear that these distributions could be used to calculate values of the threshold parameters ρ_I and ρ_H and thereby assess the efficacy of the two alternative strategies in computer intensive experiments, but the details will not be pursued here.

Other vaccination strategies for those cases where households contain immune and susceptible individuals would, evidently, lead to more complex mixtures of distributions than those in Eqs. (8.8.15) and (8.8.16). The papers by Becker and his colleagues cited above may be consulted for further details on vaccination strategies as well as for models of epidemics in households. Related work on stochastic models of epidemics in communities of households, based on branching processes, may be found in the recent papers of Ball[2] and Ball et al.[3] A volume of papers edited by D. Mollison[18] also contains papers relevant to epidemics in a community of households. In particular, the paper of Dietz[9] contains an appendix on vaccine-preventable disease issues amenable to modeling. Although threshold parameters are useful and interesting, relying solely on one set of calculated values in formulating a public health policy could be misleading. In this connection, numerical projections of an epidemic, involving Monte Carlo and deterministic methods, would be very helpful in understanding more fully the implications of a set of values for threshold parameters. A presentation of procedures for projections based on discrete time approximations to continuous time one-type CMJ-processes may be found in Mode.[17] In subsequent chapters, these issues will be explored more thoroughly by computer intensive experiments.

8.9 References

1. R. M. Anderson and R. M. May, *Infectious Diseases of Humans - Dynamics and Control,* Oxford University Press, Oxford, New York, Tokyo, 1992.
2. F. Ball, The Threshold Behavior of Stochastic Epidemics Among a Population Divided Into Households, *Lecture Notes in Statistics* **114:** 253-266, C. C. Heyde, Y. V. Prohorov, R. Pyke and S. T. Rachov (eds.), *Athens Conference on Applied Probability and Time Series, I, Applied Probability,* Springer-Verlag, Berlin, New York, Tokyo, 1995.
3. F. Ball, D. Mollison and G. Scalia-Tomba, Epidemics with Two Levels of Mixing, *Annals of Applied Probability* **7:** 46-89, 1997.
4. R. Bartoszynski, On a Certain Model of an Epidemic, *Applications Mathematicae* **XIII(2):** 139-151, 1975.
5. N. G. Becker, A. Bahrampour and K. Dietz, Threshold Parameters for Epidemics in Different Community Settings, *Mathematical Biosciences* **129:** 189-208, 1995.
6. N. G. Becker and K. Dietz, The Effect of Household Distribution on Transmission and Control of Highly Infectious Diseases, *Mathematical Biosciences* **127:** 207-219, 1995.
7. N. G. Becker and R. Hall, Immunization Levels for Preventing Epidemic in a Community of Households Made up of Individuals of Various Types, *Mathematical Biosciences* **132:** 205-216, 1996.
8. G. Dall'Aglio, S. Kotz and G. Salinetti (eds.), *Advances in Probability Distributions with Given Marginals - Beyond Copulas,* Kluwer Academic Publishers, Dordrecht, Boston, London, 1991.
9. K. Dietz, Some Problems in the Theory of Infectious Disease Transmission and Control, D. Mollison, (ed.), *Epidemic Models: Their Structure and Relation to Data,* Cambridge University Press, 1995, pp. 3-16.

10. C. Dye and G. Hasibeder, Population Dynamics of Mosquito-Borne Disease: Effects of Flies Which Bite Some People More Frequently Than Others, *Transactions of The Royal Society of Tropical Medicine and Hygiene* **80:** 69-79, 1986.

11. W. Feller, *An Introduction to Probability Theory and Its Applications, I,* 3rd ed., John Wiley and Sons, Inc., New York, London, 1968.

12. F. R. Gantmacher, *The Theory of Matrices, II,* Chelsea Publishing Company, New York, 1960.

13. G. Hasibeder, Population Dynamics of Mosquito-borne Disease: Persistence in a Completely Heterogeneous Environment, *Theoretical Population Biology* **33:** 31-53, 1988.

14. N. L. Johnson and S. Kotz, *Distributions in Statistics - Continuous Multivariate Distributions,* Wiley, New York, 1972.

15. K. V. Mardia, *Families of Bivariate Distributions*, Griffen's Statistical Monographs, Hafner, Darien, Connecticut, 1976.

16. C. J. Mode, *Multitype Branching Processes - Theory and Applications,* American Elsevier, New York, 1971.

17. C. J. Mode, *Stochastic Processes in Demography and Their Computer Implementation,* Springer-Verlag, Berlin, 1985.

18. D. Mollison, (ed.), *Epidemic Models: Their Structure and Relation to Data,* Cambridge University Press, 1995.

19. I. Nasell, On the Quasi-Stationary Distribution of the Ross Malaria Model, *Mathematical Biosciences* **107:** 187-207, 1991.

20. W. Whitt, Bivariate Distributions with Given Marginals, *Annals of Statistics* **4:** 1280-1289, 1976.

Chapter 9
COMPUTER INTENSIVE METHODS FOR THE MULTI-TYPE CASE

9.1 Introduction

As in Chapter 8, the framework of continuous time CMJ-processes will form the basis for the definition, derivation and computation of threshold parameters. But, unlike the ideas and results of Chapter 8, which were based on the class of life cycle models outlined in Section 8.3, the life cycle models to be constructed in this chapter will be approached from a different point of view, which is more suitable for modeling diseases with stages such as HIV/AIDS. Furthermore, rather than deriving special formulas, as was often emphasized in Chapter 8, greater attention will be focused on the structure of the process and computer intensive methods, because as models increase in complexity it is frequently the case that useful and informative explicit formulas, expressing threshold parameters as functions of the parameters of the model, cannot be derived. With the help of specially written software, however, it is often possible to gain insight into the properties of complex models through computer intensive experimentation as will be demonstrated by examples.

According to estimates published by the World Health Organization on the worldwide HIV/AIDS epidemic, heterosexual male-female sexual intercourse accounts for more than 70% of adult HIV infections; whereas, the more widely publicized epidemic among homo-bisexual men in the developed countries accounts for only 5% to 10% of HIV infections. Epidemics of HIV/AIDS among heterosexuals occur most extensively in sub-Saharan Africa, south Asia, and southeast Asia. A fundamental facet of epidemics of sexually transmitted diseases in heterosexual populations is the formation and dissolution of partnerships, within which sexual contacts occur. Consequently, this chapter will focus on the formulation and numerical analysis of stochastic partnership models, a class of models that has been given relatively little attention in the literature on mathematical models of the international HIV/AIDS epidemic.

9.2 A Simple Semi-Markovian Partnership Model

Consider some infectious disease with two stages, not infected and infected, caused by some agent that may be transmitted only through heterosexual contact, and suppose the life cycle of a newly infected female is considered with respect to the following set of states for a semi-Markov process. The set $\mathfrak{S}_{f1}$ of absorbing states contains one state defined as F_1-infected female dead. The set $\mathfrak{S}_{f2}$ of transient states contains $F_2 = < 1 >$-single infected female; $F_3 = < 1,0 >$-infected female in partnership with a noninfected male; and $F_4 = < 1,1 >$-infected female in partnership with a male infected by her. Because from the perspective of a branching process, the infectious period of a female begins when she is infected by an infected male partner, it will be necessary to include another transient state $F_5 =< 1,1 >$, indicating that a newly infected female was infected by her male partner. Observe that as long as this infected female is in state F_5, she is not at risk of infecting other males, but as soon as the single state F_2 is entered she becomes eligible to seek a new male partner. In the branching process approximation to the early stages of the epidemic, it will be assumed that all new male partners of an infected female are not infected.

Similarly, the set $\mathfrak{S}_{m1}$ of absorbing states for males contains the single state M_1-infected male dead and the set $\mathfrak{S}_{m2}$ of transient state contains the following four states: $M_2 = < 1 >$-single infected male; $M_3 = < 0,1 >$-noninfected female in partnership with infected male; $M_4 = < 1,1 >$-infected male in partnership with a female infected by him; and $M_5 = < 1,1 >$-a newly infected male who was infected by his female partner.

The constant latent risks, governing transitions among these states will be defined in terms of the following rate constants. Positive death rates per unit time for uninfected females will be denoted by μ_{f0} with an incremental rate of μ_{f1} when a female becomes infected, so that $\mu_f = \mu_{f0}+\mu_{f1}$ is the death rate for infected females. The corresponding death rates for males are μ_{m0}, μ_{m1}, and μ_m. The positive constants ρ and σ will represent, respectively, the rates of partnership formation and separation per unit time. Because a sexual contact between an infective and her (his) uninfected partner may not lead to an infection, two probabilities of infection per sexual contact will be introduced into the model. Let q_f be the probability that an infected female infects her uninfected male partner per sexual contact, and define the probability q_m similarly for infected males.

After a partnership is formed, it will be assumed that waiting times among sexual contacts are independent and identically distributed exponential random variables with a common parameter $\beta > 0$. Therefore, if a partnership is formed at $t = 0$, then the random function $C(t)$, representing the number of sexual contacts during the time interval $(0, t]$, for $t > 0$, has a Poisson distribution with parameter βt. Let T be a latent random variable denoting the waiting time for an infected female to infect her uninfected male partner, given that infection did not occur on the first sexual contact. Then, under the assumption of conditional independence,

$$P\left[T > t \mid C(t) = c\right] = (1 - q_f)^c \tag{9.2.1}$$

is the conditional probability that an infection occurs sometime after t. Because $C(t)$ has a Poisson distribution with parameter βt, the unconditional probability of T exceeding t is:

$$P\left[T > t\right] = \exp\left[-\beta t\right] \sum_{c=0}^{\infty} \frac{(\beta t(1 - q_f))^c}{c!} = \exp\left[-\beta q_f t\right] \ , \tag{9.2.2}$$

from which it follows that the random variable T has an exponential distribution with parameter βq_f. The constant latent risk function for the transition, $< 1, 0 > \to < 1, 1 >_f$, representing the case an infected female infected her uninfected male partner, will, therefore, be assigned as βq_f. Similarly, the transition $< 0, 1 > \to < 1, 1 >$, for the case an infected male infects his uninfected female partner, will be assigned the latent risk function βq_m. It should be mentioned in passing that the assumption of constancy of infection per sexual contact may, in the future, have to be modified (see for example Jewell[2] for empirical evidence that such probabilities may not be constant for the case of HIV disease).

Given the above definitions of latent risks, the 5×5 matrix of latent risks for infected females takes the form,

$$\boldsymbol{\Theta}_f = \begin{bmatrix} 0 & 0 & 0 & 0 & 0 \\ \mu_f & 0 & \rho(1-q_f) & \rho q_f & 0 \\ \mu_f & \mu_{m0}+\sigma & 0 & \beta q_f & 0 \\ \mu_f & \mu_m+\sigma & 0 & 0 & 0 \\ \mu_f & \mu_m+\sigma & 0 & 0 & 0 \end{bmatrix} \tag{9.2.3}$$

and that for infected males takes the form,

$$\boldsymbol{\Theta}_m = \begin{bmatrix} 0 & 0 & 0 & 0 & 0 \\ \mu_m & 0 & \rho(1-q_m) & \rho q_m & 0 \\ \mu_m & \mu_{f0}+\sigma & 0 & \beta q_m & 0 \\ \mu_m & \mu_f+\sigma & 0 & 0 & 0 \\ \mu_m & \mu_f+\sigma & 0 & 0 & 0 \end{bmatrix}. \tag{9.2.4}$$

Observe that the elements $\rho(1-q_f)$ and ρq_f in the matrix $\boldsymbol{\Theta}_f$ are, respectively, the risks that an uninfected male escapes infection or is infected by his female partner on first contact. It is also of interest to observe that $\boldsymbol{\Theta}_f$ is a matrix of latent risks for a reducible semi-Markov process; for when an infected female exits from state F_5, the initial state, she never returns to that state and the number of males she infects prior to her death is the number of visits to state F_4. Similar comments hold for the matrix of latent risks $\boldsymbol{\Theta}_m$ for infected males. In the model under consideration, it has also tacitly been assumed that once a female or male is infected, she or he remains infectious throughout the remainder of her or his life span.

Before proceeding to the further development of the model, it will be instructive to identify the distribution functions $G_i(t)$ for the life span of an infectious individual of type $i = 1, 2$ (see integral Eqs. (8.2.7) for the mean functions of a general two-type CMJ-process).

For the case of females evolving according to the semi-Markov process outlined above, let $f_{f,5,1}(t)$ be the *p.d.f.* of the waiting time to absorption in state 1, given that a female is infected at time $t = 0$, and let $F_{f,5,1}(t)$ be the corresponding distribution function defined for $t \in [0, \infty)$. Then, if infected females are designated as infectives of type 1, the distribution function of the infectious period would be chosen as $G_1(t) = F_{f,5,1}(t)$. Similarly, for infected males, the distribution functions of the infectious period would be chosen as $G_2(t) = F_{m,5,1}(t)$. In principle, formulas for the Laplace transforms for these absorption densities may be derived and inverted to obtain $G_1(t)$ and $G_2(t)$ as functions of $t \in [0, \infty)$ (see Eq. (3.8.8)), but this exercise will not be undertaken here.

The next step in constructing a branching process approximation to the early stages of an epidemic would be that of defining the random function $N_{ij}(t)$, the number of susceptibles with type j infections who were infected during the time interval $(0, t]$, $t > 0$, by an infective of type i infected at time $t = 0$, a step that will be undertaken in the next section.

9.3 Linking the Simple Life Cycle Model to a Branching Process

As a first step in linking the life cycle model to the branching process, let the random function $N_{f,5,4}(t)$ for the life cycle model denote the number of times an infected female visits state F_4 during the time interval $(0, t]$, $t > 0$, given that state F_5 was entered at $t = 0$. A similar random function $N_{m,5,4}(t)$ may be defined for infected males. Every visit of an infected female to state F_4 signals that she has infected another susceptible male. By definition, an infection of type 1 occurs when a susceptible female is infected by her infectious male partner, and an infection of type 2 occurs when a susceptible male is infected by his infectious female partner. Therefore, in the branching process, the random function $N_{12}(t)$, denoting the number of susceptible males infected during the time interval $(0, t]$ by a female infected at $t = 0$, is identified by letting $N_{12}(t) = N_{f,5,4}(t)$. Similarly, for a susceptible male infected at $t = 0$, let the random function $N_{21}(t)$ in the branching process denote the number of susceptible females infected by this male during the time interval $(0,t]$; then this random function is identified by letting $N_{21}(t) = N_{m,5,4}(t)$. It is interesting to note that, unlike the formulation discussed in Section 8.3, the random variables T_1 and $N_{12}(t)$ are not independent, where T_1 is the life span of a female after she becomes infected. Among other things, it is this property that differentiates the life cycle models developed is this chapter from those of Chapter 8.

With these definitions of type, it is easy to establish links between risk functions of the life cycle processes defined in Section 9.2 and the 2×2 matrix of expectations,

$$\mathfrak{M} = \begin{bmatrix} 0 & m_{12} \\ m_{21} & 0 \end{bmatrix} \tag{9.3.1}$$

for a BGW-process embedded in a two-type CMJ-process. Recall that $m_{12} = \lim_{t\uparrow\infty} E[N_{12}(t)]$ and m_{21} is defined similarly. If $\mathbf{\Theta}_f = (\theta_{f,i,j})$ is the matrix of latent risks for the semi-Markov process for females and $\mathbf{P}_f = (p_{f,i,j})$ is the transition matrix of the embedded Markov chain, then the elements of $\mathbf{P}_f$ are given by:

$$p_{f,i,j} = \frac{\theta_{f,i,j}}{\theta_{f,i,\cdot}} , \tag{9.3.2}$$

where $\theta_{f,i,\cdot} = \sum_j \theta_{f,i,j} \neq 0$. Moreover, the matrix $\mathbf{P}_f$ may be represented in the partitioned form,

$$\mathbf{P}_f = \begin{bmatrix} 1 & \mathbf{0} \\ \mathbf{R}_f & \mathbf{Q}_f \end{bmatrix} , \tag{9.3.3}$$

where the matrix $\mathbf{R}_f$ is 4×1 and the matrix $\mathbf{Q}_f$ is 4×4.

Given that an infected female is in transient state $i \in \mathfrak{S}_{f2}$ at $t = 0$, let $m_{f,i,j}$ be the conditional expectation of the number of visits to transient state $j \in \mathfrak{S}_2$ prior to her death. Then, the 4×4 matrix of these expectations is given by:

$$\mathbf{M}_f = (m_{f,i,j} \mid i \in \mathfrak{S}_{f2},\ j \in \mathfrak{S}_{f2}) = \left(\mathbf{I}_4 - \mathbf{Q}_f\right)^{-1} . \tag{9.3.4}$$

Thus, given that a female is in state F_5 at $t = 0$,

$$m_{12} = m_{f,5,4} \tag{9.3.5}$$

is the expected number of visits to state F_4, i.e., male partners infected, prior to her death. Let the 4×4 matrix $\mathbf{M}_m = (m_{m,i,j})$ be defined similarly for infected males. Then, for an infected male in state M_5 at $t = 0$,

$$m_{21} = m_{m,5,4} \tag{9.3.6}$$

is the expected number of female partners infected prior to his death. When the matrix of expectations for the embedded BGW-process is of the form in Eq. (9.3.1), then a threshold parameter of interest is its Perron-Frobenius root which has the form,

$$\rho_{pf} = (m_{12}m_{21})^{\frac{1}{2}} \ . \tag{9.3.7}$$

From the computational perspective, this formula is of interest in its own right, because it can be computed repeatedly with relative ease in computer intensive experiments.

However, for the simple process under consideration it is feasible to derive relatively simple formulas expressing the functions $m_{ij}(t)$ in Eq. (8.2.2), as well as the Laplace-Stieltjes transforms in $\widehat{m}_{ij}(\lambda)$ (see Eq. (8.2.5)), in terms of the parameters of the model. Whenever this is practical, an alternative formula for ρ_{pf} may be derived, which will not only eliminate the need for inverting matrices but also provide a practical way of computing the intrinsic positive growth rate r of the epidemic, whenever it exists, along with extinction probabilities for the continuous time CMJ-branching process. Consider a single female in state F_2 at $t = 0$ and let $f_{f,2,4}(t)$ be the density of the waiting time to first entrance into state F_4, signaling that a male partner has been infected. There are two cases to consider; namely, either state F_4 is entered for the first time without returning to the single state or there is a return to the single state F_2 before state F_4 is entered.

Let $g_{f,2,4}(t)$ be the density of the waiting time to first entrance into state F_4 without a return to state F_2 and let $\mathbf{a}_f(t) = (a_{f,i,j}(t))$ be the 5×5 matrix of one-step transition densities for females. Then, by a renewal argument, it can be shown that:

$$g_{f,2,4}(t) = a_{f,2,4}(t) + \int_0^t a_{f,2,3}(s)a_{f,3,4}(t-s)ds \text{ for } t > 0 \ . \tag{9.3.8}$$

Given that the process is in state F_2 at $t = 0$, let $f_{f,2,2}(t)$ be the density of the first return time to state F_2 without a visit to state F_4. Then,

$$f_{f,2,2}(t) = \int_0^t a_{f,2,3}(s)a_{f,3,2}(t-s)ds \text{ for } t > 0 . \tag{9.3.9}$$

And, by another renewal argument, it follows that the function $f_{f,2,4}(t)$ satisfies the renewal type integral equation,

$$f_{f,2,4}(t) = g_{f,2,4}(t) + \int_0^t f_{f,2,2}(s)f_{f,2,4}(t-s)ds \text{ for } t > 0 . \tag{9.3.10}$$

Every return to state F_4 signals the event that another male has been infected by the infected female prior to her death and successive returns to this state may be described by a renewal process. Accordingly, let $f_{f,4,4}(t)$ be the density of the first return time to state F_4, given that the process is in state F_4 at $t = 0$. Then,

$$f_{f,4,4}(t) = \int_0^t a_{f,4,2}(s)f_{f,2,4}(t-s)ds \text{ for } t > 0 . \tag{9.3.11}$$

And, the distribution function corresponding to this density is:

$$F_{f,4,4}(t) = \int_0^t f_{f,4,4}(s)ds \text{ for } t > 0 . \tag{9.3.12}$$

Let the random function $N_{f,4,4}(t)$ be the number of returns to state F_4 during the time interval $(0,t]$ for $t > 0$, given that the process is in state F_4 at $t = 0$.

To determine the distribution of this random function, the n-fold convolution of the distribution function in Eq. (9.3.12) with itself will be needed. Accordingly, for $t \geq 0$, let $F_{f,4,4}^{(0)}(t) = 1$, and for $n \geq 1$ let $F_{f,4,4}^{(n)}(t)$ be the n-fold convolution of the distribution function in Eq. (9.3.12) with itself. Then, by well-known results from renewal theory, it follows that the distribution of the random function $N_{f,4,4}(t)$ is:

$$h_{f,4,4}^{(n)}(t) = P\left[N_{f,4,4}(t) = n\right] = F_{f,4,4}^{(n)}(t) - F_{f,4,4}^{(n+1)}(t) \tag{9.3.13}$$

for $n = 0, 1, 2, \cdots$, and $t > 0$. Furthermore, the mean function corresponding to this distribution is given by the series,

$$E\left[N_{f,4,4}(t)\right] = \sum_{n=1}^{\infty} F_{f,4,4}^{(n)}(t) , \tag{9.3.14}$$

which converges for all $t \geq 0$.

From the perspective of the branching process, a female is at risk of infecting males as soon as she is infected by her male partner, symbolized by entrance into state F_5. Thus, one is led to consider

$$f_{f,5,4}(t) = \int_0^t a_{f,5,2}(s) f_{f,2,4}(t-s) ds \text{ for } t > 0 , \tag{9.3.15}$$

the density of the waiting time to first entrance into state F_4, signaling the infected female has infected her first male partner after leaving state F_5. Let the random function $N_{f,4,4}^{(m)}(t)$ be the number of males infected by this female during the time interval $(0, t]$ for $t > 0$, given that state F_4 was entered at $t = 0$. Then, for $t \geq 0$,

$$N_{f,4,4}^{(m)}(t) = 1 + N_{f,4,4}(t) \tag{9.3.16}$$

and its expectation is

$$m_{f,4,4}(t) = \sum_{n=0}^{\infty} F_{f,4,4}^{(n)}(t) . \tag{9.3.17}$$

Given that a female in state F_5 is infected at $t = 0$, let the random function $N_{t,5,4}(t)$ denote the number of susceptible males infected by this female during the time interval $(0, t]$, $t > 0$. As mentioned above, this function provides a link to a continuous two-type CMJ-process by letting $N_{12}(t) = N_{t,5,4}(t)$ with expectation $m_{12}(t)$. By another renewal argument, it follows that this expectation is given by:

$$m_{12}(t) = m_{f,5,4}(t) = \int_0^t f_{f,5,4}(s) m_{f,4,4}(t-s) ds . \tag{9.3.18}$$

By a completely analogous argument, one could derive a formula for the expected number $E[N_{21}(t)] = m_{21}(t) = m_{m,5,4}(t)$ of females infected by a male during $(0, t]$ for $t > 0$, given that state M_5 was entered at $t = 0$.

For the simple model under consideration, the Laplace-Stieltjes transform in Eq. (8.2.5) for females infecting males takes the form,

$$\widehat{m}_{12}(\lambda) = \int_0^\infty e^{-\lambda t} m_{12}(dt) = \int_0^\infty e^{-\lambda t} m_{f,5,4}(dt) = \frac{\widehat{f}_{f,5,4}(\lambda)}{1 - \widehat{F}_{f,4,4}(\lambda)} , \tag{9.3.19}$$

where $\widehat{f}_{f,5,4}(\lambda)$ is the Laplace transform of the function $f_{f,5,4}(t)$, and $\widehat{F}_{f,4,4}(\lambda)$ is the Laplace-Stieltjes transform of the distribution function $F_{f,4,4}(t)$, $\lambda \geq 0$, and $t \geq 0$. By passing to Laplace transforms in all the above convolution integrals, it would be possible to express the transform in Eq. (9.3.19) in terms on the parameters of the system. It is of interest to note that the component transforms making up these formulas would have the simple form,

$$\widehat{a}_{f,i,j}(\lambda) = \frac{\theta_{f,i,j}}{\theta_{f,i,\cdot} + \lambda} , \tag{9.3.20}$$

for $i \neq j$. A similar formula for the transform $\widehat{m}_{21}(\lambda)$ corresponding to males infecting females may be written down, but the details will be omitted. At this juncture, it is also of interest to observe that the above derivation would remain valid for other types of Laplace transforms than those in Eq. (9.3.20). For example, the above derivation would remain valid if the sojourn times in transient states were mixtures of gamma type distributions.

In terms of the above derivation, the Perron-Frobenius root of the 2×2 matrix $\widehat{\mathbf{m}}(\lambda)$ of Laplace-Stieltjes transforms is:

$$\rho_{pf}(\lambda) = (\widehat{m}_{12}(\lambda)\widehat{m}_{21}(\lambda))^{\frac{1}{2}} . \tag{9.3.21}$$

Observe that $\rho_{pf}(0) = \rho_{pf}$, the root in Eq. (9.3.1). When $\rho_{pf} > 1$, the parameter r, the intrinsic growth rate of the epidemic, may be found by elementary numerical searches for values of λ such that $\rho_{pf}(\lambda) = 1$ as will be shown by examples in a subsequent section. But even for the simple model under consideration, finding negative values of r when $\rho_{pf} < 1$ can be a delicate problem, because searches for values of r must be restricted to values of λ such all Laplace transforms in Eq. (9.3.10) are positive.

All the results on threshold parameters presented so far provide indicators as to the behavior of the process in the long run, but it is also of interest to provide some information as to the evolution of the process in continuous time $t \in [0, \infty)$. One approach to providing such information is to compute the means $M_{ij}(t)$ in Eq. (8.2.7) as functions of $t \in [0, \infty)$, an operation that would entail finding numerical solutions to systems of renewal type integral equations. To find such numerical solutions, it would be necessary to compute numerical values of the expectations $m_{ij}(t)$ for $t \in [0, \infty)$.

As can be seen for Eq. (9.3.20), the Laplace-Stieltjes transforms of these functions have a relatively simple algebraic form, which in principle could be inverted to find explicit formulas for $m_{12}(t)$ and $m_{21}(t)$. Moreover, explicit formulas for these functions would involve linear combinations of exponentials with perhaps polynomials in t as coefficients, but their derivation would entail much tedious algebra.

An alternative approach to the problem would be that of using a software package such as MAPLE with a capability of doing computer algebra. Within such a package, programs could be written to derive Laplace-Stieltjes transforms of all functions of interest, which, in turn, could be symbolically inverted and then numerically evaluated, thus bypassing the need for complicated explicit formulas. Indeed, from the computational and computer programming points of view, it is easier to work with the structure of a model rather than with special formulas. The book, Char et al.,[1] may be consulted for further detail on the MAPLE programming language.

9.4 Extinction Probabilities for the Simple Life Cycle Model

Let q_1 and q_2, respectively, be the conditional probabilities that an epidemic becomes extinct, given that it starts with either one infected female or male at $t = 0$. When $\rho_{pf} > 1$, these probabilities may be positive and less than one, but if $\rho_{pf} \leq 1$, then it can be shown that under rather general conditions $q_1 = q_2 = 1$. It is, therefore, of interest to develop methods for calculating q_1 and q_2 as functions of the parameters of the model when $\rho_{pf} > 1$. Fortunately, for the simple model under consideration, these probabilities may be calculated with relative ease.

Given that the process starts in state F_5 at $t = 0$, the probability that state F_4 is visited at least once prior to the death of an infected female is:

$$\varphi_{f,5,4} = \lim_{t \uparrow \infty} \int_0^t f_{f,5,4}(s)ds = \widehat{f}_{f,5,4}(0)\,. \tag{9.4.1}$$

Similarly, if the process is in state F_4 at $t = 0$, then

$$\varphi_{f,4,4} = \lim_{t \uparrow \infty} F_{f,4,4}(t) = \widehat{F}_{f,4,4}(0) \tag{9.4.2}$$

is the conditional probability the process returns to state F_4 at least once prior to the death of the female. If state F_4 is visited at least once, then the total number of males infected by a female is given by the random variable,

$$N_{f,4,4}^{(m)} = \lim_{t \uparrow \infty} N_{f,4,4}^{(m)}(t)\ . \tag{9.4.3}$$

Furthermore, by letting $t \uparrow \infty$ in Eq. (9.3.13), it follows that

$$P\left[N_{f,4,4}^{(m)} = n\right] = (1 - \varphi_{f,4,4})\varphi_{f,4,4}^{n-1} \tag{9.4.4}$$

for $n = 1, 2, 3, \cdots$.

Given that the process starts in state F_5 at $t = 0$, let the random variable $N_{f,5,4}^{(m)}$ be the total number of males infected by a female prior to her death. If state F_4 is not visited at least once prior to the death of the female, then $N_{f,5,4}^{(m)} = 0$ with probability $g_{f,5,4}(0) = 1 - \varphi_{f,5,4}$, but for $N_{f,5,4}^{(m)} = n \geq 1$

$$P\left[N_{f,5,4}^{(m)} = n\right] = g_{f,5,4}(n) = \varphi_{f,5,4}(1 - \varphi_{f,4,4})\varphi_{f,4,4}^{n-1} \tag{9.4.5}$$

Therefore, for $| s | \leq 1$, the probability generating function of the random variable $N_{f,5,4}^{(m)}$ takes the form,

$$G_{f,5,4}^{(m)}(s) = \sum_{n=0}^{\infty} g_{f,5,4}(n)s^n = 1 - \varphi_{f,5,4} + \frac{\varphi_{f,5,4}(1 - \varphi_{f,4,4})s}{1 - \varphi_{f,4,4}s} \tag{9.4.6}$$

A similar formula for $G^{(f)}_{m,5,4}(s)$, the probability generating function of the random variable $N^{(f)}_{m,5,4}$, representing the total number of females infected by a male who was in state M_5 at $t = 0$, may be derived by substituting the subscript m for f throughout.

Because females infect males, and males in turn infect females, it follows from well-known results from branching processes that the extinction probabilities satisfy the system of equations,

$$q_1 = G^{(m)}_{f,5,4}(q_2) \tag{9.4.7}$$

and

$$q_2 = G^{(f)}_{m,5,4}(q_1)\ . \tag{9.4.8}$$

Equivalently, it follows that q_1 and q_2 satisfy the equations:

$$s_1 = G^{(m)}_{f,5,4}(G^{(f)}_{m,5,4}(s_1)) \tag{9.4.9}$$

and

$$s_2 = G^{(f)}_{m,5,4}(G^{(m)}_{f,5,4}(s_2))\ . \tag{9.4.10}$$

Just as in the simple BGW-process by using well-known properties of probability generating functions, it can be shown using these equations that if $\rho_{pf} \leq 1$, then $q_1 = q_2 = 1$, but if $\rho_{pf} > 1$, then q_1 and q_2 are the smallest roots of Eqs. (9.4.9) and (9.4.10) such that $0 < q_1 < 1$ and $0 < q_2 < 1$.

Values of extinction probabilities may be computed numerically in at least two ways. One way is to define a sequence $\{q_1(n), q_2(n)\}$ recursively by putting $q_1(0) = G^{(m)}_{f,5,4}(0)$ and $q_2(0) = G^{(f)}_{m,5,4}(0)$ and for $n \geq 1$ let

$$q_1(n) = G^{(m)}_{f,5,4}(q_2(n-1)) \tag{9.4.11}$$

and

$$q_2(n) = G^{(f)}_{M,5,4}(q_1(n-1))\ . \tag{9.4.12}$$

It can be shown that the sequence $\{q_1(n), q_2(n)\}$ is monotone increasing in each element and converges to the limit $\{q_1, q_2\}$ when $\rho_{pf} > 1$. An alternative method is to solve Eqs. (9.4.9) and (9.4.10) algebraically. For example, a solution of Eq. (9.4.9) such that $s_1 \neq 1$ is:

$$s_1 = \frac{1 - \varphi_{f,4,4} + \varphi_{f,4,4}\varphi_{m,5,4} - \varphi_{f,5,4}\varphi_{m,5,4}}{\varphi_{m,4,4} - \varphi_{f,4,4}\varphi_{m,4,4} + \varphi_{f,4,4}\varphi_{m,5,4}} \tag{9.4.13}$$

A similar formula for a root s_2 of Eq. (9.4.10) may be written down. If $\rho_{pf} > 1$, $0 < |s_1| < 1$, and $0 < |s_2| < 1$, then $q_1 = |s_1|$ and $q_2 = |s_2|$. As a check on the numerical accuracy of the calculations, it is often useful to compute q_1 and q_2 recursively as well as by the application of formulas of the form in Eq. (9.4.13).

9.5 Computation of Threshold Parameters for the Simple Model

Because the formation and dissolution of partnerships is the central focus of the simple model for an epidemic of some sexually transmitted disease, it is natural to ask what impact waiting times among partnerships and the durations of partnerships have on such threshold parameters as the Perron-Frobenius root of the expectation matrix in Eqs. (9.3.1) (see Eq. (9.3.7)). To obtain some answers to this question, the following parameter values were chosen for the simple model. It was assumed that for non-infected females, the expectation of life following the initiation of sexual activity was 60 years, which led to choosing μ_{f0} as 1/60. When a female becomes infected with HIV, it was assumed that, in the absence of other competing risks, her expectation of life was 12 years so that $\mu_{f1} = 1/12$. The corresponding expectations for males were chosen as 55 and 12 years.

Following the formation of a partnership, it was assumed that sexual contacts occurred on the average of twice a week, giving rise to the value for β of about 104 contacts per year. The probability that an infected male infected a susceptible female partner per contact was chosen as $q_m = 1/100 = 0.01$. It is interesting to note that this value is greater than the values for the heterosexual transmission of HIV reported by Longini et al.,[3] which were about $1/200 = 0.005$. Even though the model and software allow for assigning different values to q_f, the probability an infected female infects her non-infected male partner per contact, in these experiments it was also assumed that $q_f = 0.01$. The rationale for choosing these values of q_f and q_m was to insure finding values of the Perron-Frobenius roots in the interval $[2, 5]$, which suggests that an epidemic would spread rapidly in a population. In the absence of other competing risks, $1/\sigma$ is the expected duration of a partnership and $1/\rho$ is the expected waiting time among partnerships. Values of ρ and σ were determined by choosing $1/\sigma$ and $1/\rho$ as 1/12, 1, 2, 4, 6, $\cdots$, 20 years in all possible combinations. The Perron-Frobenius root ρ_{pf} was then computed as a function of ρ and σ for all possible pairs $< \rho, \sigma >$ in the set,

$$\{(\rho,\sigma) \mid 1/\rho = 1/12, 1, 2, 4, \cdots, 20;\ 1/\sigma = 1/12, 1, 2, 4, \cdots, 20\}. \tag{9.5.1}$$

Thus, a total of $12 \times 12 = 144$ values of ρ_{pf} were calculated, some of which are reported in Table 9.5.1. The programming language used to carry out the numerical results presented in this and the next section was APL*Plus III, a user-friendly version of APL that operates under Microsoft Windows.

Table 9.5.1. Values of the Threshold Parameter ρ_{pf} for Pairs of Values of $< 1/\rho, 1/\sigma >$ Expressed in Years.

$1/\rho\backslash 1/\sigma$	1/12	1	2	4	6	8	10
1/12	5.254	4.683	3.399	3.356	1.913	1.669	1.514
1	0.805	2.380	2.151	1.710	1.462	1.310	1.208
2	0.418	1.549	1.536	0.902	0.825	0.768	0.727
4	0.213	0.912	0.977	0.902	0.825	0.768	0.727
6	0.143	0.646	0.716	0.685	0.639	0.602	0.575
8	0.108	0.501	0.565	0.533	0.522	0.495	0.475
10	0.086	0.408	0.467	0.463	0.441	0.421	0.405

As an aid to interpreting Table 9.5.1, note that the first row of the table contains values of $1/\sigma$, the expected durations of partnership, expressed in years, in the absence of other competing risks. Similarly, the first column of the table contains the values of $1/\rho$, the expected waiting times among partnerships expressed in years, while the body of the table contains the $7 \times 7 = 49$ values of ρ_{pf}, corresponding to the pairs $< 1/\rho, 1/\sigma >$. It is of interest to note that when $1/\rho = 1/12 = 8.3333 \times 10^{-2}$ of a year or one month, then $\rho_{pf} > 1$ for all expected durations of partnership. This indicates that for these pairs of values of $< 1/\rho, 1/\sigma >$ the epidemic could become established in the population with a positive probability depending on the type of the initial individual. It is also of interest to note from the table that for all values of $1/\rho \geq 4$, the Perron-Frobenius root satisfies the condition, $\rho_{pf} < 1$, for all listed values of $1/\sigma$ so that for these pairs of values of $< 1/\rho, 1/\sigma >$ the epidemic would die out eventually with probability one.

As one would expect, values of threshold parameter ρ_{pf} are not only very sensitive to the parameters ρ and σ, governing the formation and dissolution of partnerships, but also to values of $q_f = q_m$, the probabilities of infection per sexual contact. To demonstrate this sensitivity, values of ρ_{pf} were calculated for a population in which there is a rapid exchange of sexual partners as shown in Table 9.5.2.

Table 9.5.2. Values of Threshold Parameter for Selected Values of $q_f = q_m$.

$(1/\rho, 1/\sigma)$	$q_f = 0.010$	$q_f = 0.005$	$q_f = 0.001$
$(1/52, 1/52)$	7.590	3.832	0.773
$(1/52, 1/12)$	8.565	4.458	0.922
$(1/12, 1/52)$	2.844	1.436	0.290
$(1/12, 1/12)$	5.254	2.735	0.566

To interpret this table, observe that when the waiting time among partnerships is on average one week, 1/52, and the duration of each partnership is also one week on the average, then the threshold parameter of the process is $\rho_{pf} = 7.59$, which suggests that an epidemic would rapidly become established in the population. As the value of q_f decreases in the table so does the value of ρ_{pf} as one would expect. Observe that for all values of the pair $(1/\rho, 1/\sigma)$ in the table, the epidemic would not become established in the population when $q_f = 0.001$.

In a branching process, however, the condition $\rho_{pf} > 1$ only signals the possibility that an epidemic will become established in a population, but provides no information as to the conditional probability that it will die out or spread, given the type of the initial individual. Moreover, just knowing that $\rho_{pf} > 1$ yields no information regarding the intrinsic growth rate of the epidemic other than r must be positive. Therefore, in the next section, attention will be given to calculating values of the extinction probabilities and intrinsic growths rates of an epidemic.

9.6 Extinction Probabilities and Intrinsic Growth Rates

Presented in Table 9.6.1 are calculated values of ρ_{pf}, q_1, q_2 and r, the intrinsic growth rate of an epidemic given that extinction does not occur, corresponding to selected values of the pair $(1/\rho, 1/\sigma)$. The extinction probabilities q_1 and q_2 were calculated by applying the recursive formulas in Eqs. (9.4.11) and (9.4.12) for 50 iterations as well as formulas of the type in Eq. (9.4.13). Whenever the values of s_1 and s_2 calculated according to these formulas were such that $|s_1| < 1$ and $|s_2| < 1$, then the values of the recursive procedure converged to $|s_1|$ and $|s_2|$ in all cases presented in the table, indicating these values were indeed the extinction probabilities q_1 and q_2. A bisection method was applied to formula (9.3.21) for $\rho_{pf}(\lambda)$ to find values of $r = \lambda$ such that $\rho_{pf}(r) = 1$. Apart from variations in the parameters ρ and σ, all other parameters of the model had the same values as those in the preceding section.

Table 9.6.1. Extinction Probabilities and Intrinsic Growth Rates of an Epidemic for Selected Values of $< 1/\rho, 1/\sigma >$ Expressed in Years.

$< 1/\rho, 1/\sigma >$	ρ_{pf}	q_1	q_2	r
$<1/12,1>$	4.68293	0.24208	0.24426	0.30628
$<1/12,1.25>$	4.26259	0.56597	0.56735	0.27166
$<1/12,1.50>$	3.91953	0.89513	0.89549	0.24386
$<1,1>$	2.38004	0.45351	0.45615	0.11604
$<1,1.25>$	2.43766	0.80901	0.80996	0.11186

By way of interpreting the values in the table, observe that according to the second row, if, in the absence of other competing risks, the expected waiting times among partnerships is $1/\rho = 1/12$ of a year or one month and the expected duration of waiting times among partnerships is $1/\sigma = 1$ year, then the probabilities that the epidemic becomes extinct are $q_1 = 0.24208$ and $q_2 = 0.24426$, given that the epidemic starts with an infected female or male, respectively.

For such a population, the epidemic would grow at the rapid rate of $r = 0.30628$ or 30.626% per year, given that it does not become extinct. As one might expect, the longer the latent expected durations of partnership, i.e. values of $1/\sigma$ in the table, the greater the probabilities of extinction. For example, for the pairs of values $(1/12, 1.50)$ and $(1, 1.25)$, the extinction probabilities exceed 0.8 so that for such populations the epidemic would become extinct over 80 percent of the time. But, if the epidemic does not become extinct, then the annual intrinsic growth rates of the epidemic would exceed 10% and 20%, respectively, for these two cases. These rapid rates of annual increase suggest, therefore, that in the partnership model under consideration, there will be high probabilities that an epidemic started by either an infected female or male in a large population of susceptibles will quite often become extinct with a probability substantially greater than zero, but, given that the epidemic does not become extinct, it will tend to spread explosively in the population.

9.7 A Partnership Model for the Sexual Transmission of HIV

As with many infectious diseases that may be sexually transmitted, HIV/AIDS has several stages which are characterized by $CD4^+$ counts, as discussed in a previous chapter. For the sake of simplicity, only four stages of the disease will be considered in the partnership model of a HIV/AIDS epidemic in a heterosexual population to be described in this section. To fix ideas, in stage 1 an individual is infected but not seropositive, in stage 2 an individual is seropositive but not symptomatic, in stage 3 an individual is symptomatic, and in stage 4 there is a diagnosis of full-blown AIDS. In compliance with epidemiological evidence, it will be assumed that the probability per sexual contact that an infected male or female infects his or her susceptible partner depends on the stage of the disease. Accordingly, let q_{fi} be the probability per sexual contact that an infected female in stage i of the disease infects her susceptible male partner, define the probability q_{mi} similarly for infected males, and let $\mathbf{q}_f$ and $\mathbf{q}_m$ be vectors of these probabilities.

Evolution through the four stages of HIV disease will assumed to be linear for both females and males and governed by a continuous time Markov process with four states. Accordingly, let γ_{fi} be a positive parameter in a latent exponential distribution governing the length of stay of a female in stage $i = 1, 2, 3, 4$ of the disease and define the parameter γ_{mi} similarly for infected males. Deaths due to AIDS are taken into account by exits from stage 4. To accommodate susceptible non-infected females or males, the symbol 0 will be used for notational convenience to designate a susceptible individual and will henceforth, for the sake of brevity, be referred to as state 0. Similarly, to simplify the terminology, stages of the disease will henceforth be referred to as states.

In this formulation, the background risks of female and male deaths also depend on the state of an individual; thus, the parameters μ_{fi} for $i = 0, 1, 2, 3, 4$, are the background risks of death for females in state i and μ_{mi} for $i = 0, 1, 2, 3, 4$, are defined similarly for males. The positive parameters ρ and σ are defined as the latent rates of partnership formation and dissolution respectively. In principle, more parameters could be introduced to accommodate dependence on states of HIV disease for both females and males, as well as different rates of partnership formation for females and males, but, for the sake of simplicity, attention will be confined to these two parameters. Just as in the simple model discussed in the previous sections, after a partnership is formed, it will be assumed that waiting times among sexual contacts are independent and identically distributed exponential random variables with a common parameter $\beta > 0$. Therefore, if a partnership is formed at $t = 0$, then the random function $C(t)$, representing the number of sexual contacts during the time interval $(0, t]$, for $t > 0$, has a Poisson distribution with parameter βt.

From the perspective of linking a partnership model, governing the evolution of an epidemic caused by a sexually transmitted disease, to a multi-type CMJ-process, a "birth" occurs when either a non-infected female or male is infected by an infected partner. As a first step toward formulating a model, consider a female who has just been infected by her male partner and the set of states for a semi-Markov process, labeled as the $\mathbf{S}_{f,1}$-process, describing her evolution up to the time this partnership dissolves. For this process, the set $\mathfrak{S}_{f,1,1}$ of five absorbing states will be chosen as: (d)-infected female dead and (i)-

a single female in state $i = 1, 2, 3, 4$, of HIV disease. Whenever an infected female is in a single state, she is at risk of acquiring a non-infected male partner and infecting him; thus, entrance into a single state signals the beginning of another semi-Markov process, governing the possibility of infecting other males. This will be discussed subsequently and will be labeled as the $\mathbf{S}_{f,2}$-process.

A partnership will be said to be of type (i, j) if the female and male are in states i and j, respectively. Because the evolution of the process is dependent on the states of HIV disease for both a female and male, the set $\mathfrak{S}_{f,1,2}$ of transient states for the $\mathbf{S}_{f,1}$-process will be chosen as follows: The set $\mathbf{F}_{1,i}$ of types of partnerships such that the female is in state $i = 1, 2, 3, 4$, of HIV disease is $\mathbf{F}_{1,i} = \{(i, j) \mid j = 1, 2, 3, 4\}$, and the set of all transient states will be chosen as

$$\mathfrak{S}_{f,1,2} = \bigcup_{i=1}^{4} \mathbf{F}_{1,i} \tag{9.7.1}$$

arranged in lexicographic order. The state space $\mathfrak{S}_{f,1} = \mathfrak{S}_{f,1,1} \cup \mathfrak{S}_{f,1,2}$ for the $\mathbf{S}_{f,1}$-process thus contains 21 states altogether.

The state space for the $\mathbf{S}_{f,2}$-process contains the following 25 states. The set of absorbing states $\mathfrak{S}_{f,2,1}$ consists of one state, $(d)_f$, infected female dead, and the set $\mathfrak{S}_{f,2,2}$ of transient states contains the set $\mathfrak{S}_{f,1,s} = \{(i)_f \mid i = 1, 2, 3, 4\}$ of single females by state of HIV disease as well as a set of partnership types. Let $\mathbf{F}_{2,i} = \{(i, j) \mid j = 0, 1, 2, 3, 4\}$ be the set of partnership types such that the female is state $i =$ 1,2,3,4 of HIV disease. Observe that the partnership type $< i, 0 >$ indicates that a female in state i of HIV disease is in partnership with a susceptible male. Given these definitions, the set of transient states for the $\mathbf{S}_{f,2}$-process will be chosen as

$$\mathfrak{S}_{f,2,2} = \mathfrak{S}_{f,1,s} \cup \bigcup_{i=1}^{4} \mathbf{F}_{2,i} \ , \tag{9.7.2}$$

where the partnership types are again arranged in lexicographic order.

There are also corresponding processes, labeled $\mathbf{S}_{m,1}$ and $\mathbf{S}_{m,2}$, for a male who has just been infected by his female partner. The symbol $(d)_m$ will represent a dead male and for $i = 1, 2, 3, 4$, $< i >_m$will stand for a single male in state i of HIV disease. For the $\mathbf{S}_{m,1}$-process, $\mathbf{M}_{1,j} = \{(i,j) \mid i = 1,2,3,4\}$ will be the set of partnership types such that the male is in state $j = 1,2,3,4$, of HIV disease. And, for the $\mathbf{S}_{m,2}$-process, $\mathbf{M}_{2,j} = \{(i,j) \mid i = 0,1,2,3,4\}$ is the set of partnership types such that the male is in state $j = 1,2,3,4$, of HIV disease. Given these definitions, the state spaces $\mathfrak{S}_{m,1}$ and $\mathfrak{S}_{m,2}$ for the processes $\mathbf{S}_{m,1}$ and $\mathbf{S}_{m,2}$ may be defined just as above, but in these cases it should be remembered that partnership types are ordered by the state of HIV disease of the male.

9.8 Latent Risks for the Partnership Model of HIV/AIDS

Although the partnership model just described is rather complex, it is fortunate that the matrices of latent risks are sparse and have simple forms. The 21×21 matrix of latent risks for the $\mathbf{S}_{f,1}$-process may be represented in the partitioned form:

$$\boldsymbol{\Theta}_{f,1} = \begin{bmatrix} \mathbf{0} & \mathbf{0} \\ \boldsymbol{\Theta}_{1,1,0} & \boldsymbol{\Theta}_{1,1,1} \end{bmatrix} . \tag{9.8.1}$$

The 16×5 matrix $\boldsymbol{\Theta}_{1,1,0}$ may in turn be represented in the partitioned form:

$$\boldsymbol{\Theta}_{1,1,0} = \begin{bmatrix} \boldsymbol{\Theta}_{1,1,0}(1) \\ \boldsymbol{\Theta}_{1,1,0}(2) \\ \boldsymbol{\Theta}_{1,1,0}(3) \\ \boldsymbol{\Theta}_{1,1,0}(4) \end{bmatrix} . \tag{9.8.2}$$

Each of the 4×5 sub-matrices in this matrix also has a simple form. For example, the matrix $\boldsymbol{\Theta}_{1,1,0}(1)$ corresponding the set $\mathbf{F}_{1,1}$ of partnerships such that the female is in state 1 of HIV disease has the form:

$$\boldsymbol{\Theta}_{1,1,0}(1) = \begin{bmatrix} \mu_{f1} & \mu_{m1} + \sigma & 0 & 0 & 0 \\ \mu_{f1} & \mu_{m2} + \sigma & 0 & 0 & 0 \\ \mu_{f1} & \mu_{m3} + \sigma & 0 & 0 & 0 \\ \mu_{f1} & \mu_{m4} + \sigma & 0 & 0 & 0 \end{bmatrix} . \tag{9.8.3}$$

Observe that the first column is the risk of a transition to state $(d)_f$, indicating that a female member of a partnership in state 1 of HIV disease has died. Similarly, the second column of the matrix contains the risks that a female in state 1 of the disease returns to the single state by either the death of a male partner or the dissolution of the partnership for other reasons. In general, the submatrix $\boldsymbol{\Theta}_{1,1,0}(i)$ has the element μ_{fi} in the first column and the second column in $\boldsymbol{\Theta}_{1,1,0}(1)$ is moved to the column corresponding to the her state of HIV disease when a female in partnership enters a single state.

The 16×16 submatrix $\boldsymbol{\Theta}_{1,1}$ in (9.8.1) may partitioned into 4×4 sub-matrices and has the form:

$$\boldsymbol{\Theta}_{1,1,1} = \begin{bmatrix} \boldsymbol{\Theta}_{1,1,1}(1,1) & \boldsymbol{\Theta}_{1,1,1}(1,2) & \mathbf{0} & \mathbf{0} \\ \mathbf{0} & \boldsymbol{\Theta}_{1,1,1}(2,2) & \boldsymbol{\Theta}_{1,1,1}(2,3) & \mathbf{0} \\ \mathbf{0} & \mathbf{0} & \boldsymbol{\Theta}_{1,1,1}(3,3) & \boldsymbol{\Theta}_{1,1,1}(3,4) \\ \mathbf{0} & \mathbf{0} & \mathbf{0} & \boldsymbol{\Theta}_{1,1,1}(4,4) \end{bmatrix} . \tag{9.8.4}$$

Each of the 4×4 of the non-zero sub-matrices in turn has a simple form. For $i = 1,2,3,4,$

$$\boldsymbol{\Theta}_{1,1,1}(i,i) = \begin{bmatrix} 0 & \gamma_{m1} & 0 & 0 \\ 0 & 0 & \gamma_{m2} & 0 \\ 0 & 0 & 0 & \gamma_{m3} \\ 0 & 0 & 0 & 0 \end{bmatrix} , \tag{9.8.5}$$

indicating for a female in a fixed state i of HIV disease, there is a transition in the type of partnership only if the male partner advances to the next state of HIV disease. Analogously, for $i = 1,2,3$, the matrix of latent risks for the female member of the partnership to advance to the next state of HIV has the diagonal form:

$$\boldsymbol{\Theta}_{1,1,1}(i,i+1) = \begin{bmatrix} \gamma_{fi} & 0 & 0 & 0 \\ 0 & \gamma_{fi} & 0 & 0 \\ 0 & 0 & \gamma_{fi} & 0 \\ 0 & 0 & 0 & \gamma_{fi} \end{bmatrix} . \tag{9.8.6}$$

For the $\mathbf{S}_{f,2}$-process the 25×25 matrix of latent risks may be represented in the partitioned form:

$$\boldsymbol{\Theta}_{f,2} = \begin{bmatrix} \mathbf{0} & \mathbf{0} & \mathbf{0} \\ \boldsymbol{\Theta}_{2,1,0} & \boldsymbol{\Theta}_{2,1,1} & \boldsymbol{\Theta}_{2,1,2} \\ \boldsymbol{\Theta}_{2,2,0} & \boldsymbol{\Theta}_{2,2,1} & \boldsymbol{\Theta}_{2,2,2} \end{bmatrix} , \tag{9.8.7}$$

where $\mathbf{\Theta}_{2,1,0}$ is a 4×1 column vector with elements μ_{fi} for $i = 1, 2, 3, 4$, the female death rates by state of HIV disease. The 4×4 submatrix $\mathbf{\Theta}_{2,1,1}$, containing transition rates among states of HIV disease for single females, has the form:

$$\mathbf{\Theta}_{2,1,1} = \begin{bmatrix} 0 & \gamma_{f1} & 0 & 0 \\ 0 & 0 & \gamma_{f2} & 0 \\ 0 & 0 & 0 & \gamma_{f3} \\ 0 & 0 & 0 & 0 \end{bmatrix} . \tag{9.8.8}$$

And the 4×20 submatrix $\mathbf{\Theta}_{2,1,2}$ has the quasi-diagonal form:

$$\mathbf{\Theta}_{2,1,2} = \begin{bmatrix} \mathbf{\Theta}_{2,1,2}(1,1) & \mathbf{0} & \mathbf{0} & \mathbf{0} \\ \mathbf{0} & \mathbf{\Theta}_{2,1,2}(2,2) & \mathbf{0} & \mathbf{0} \\ \mathbf{0} & \mathbf{0} & \mathbf{\Theta}_{2,1,2}(3,3) & \mathbf{0} \\ \mathbf{0} & \mathbf{0} & \mathbf{0} & \mathbf{\Theta}_{2,1,2}4,4) \end{bmatrix} , \tag{9.8.9}$$

where for $i = 1, 2, 3, 4$, $\mathbf{\Theta}_{2,1,2}(i,i) = (\rho(1 - q_{fi}), \rho q_{fi}, 0, 0, 0)$, a 1×5 vector of rates governing the entrance of a female into partnership by state of HIV disease of the male partner.

With regard to the last row of the partitioned matrix $\mathbf{\Theta}_{f,2}$, the 20×1 matrix $\mathbf{\Theta}_{2,2,0}$, containing death rates for females in partnership by states, has the partitioned form:

$$\mathbf{\Theta}_{2,2,0} = \begin{bmatrix} \mu_{f1}\mathbf{1}_4 \\ \mu_{f2}\mathbf{1}_4 \\ \mu_{f3}\mathbf{1}_4 \\ \mu_{f4}\mathbf{1}_4 \end{bmatrix} . \tag{9.8.10}$$

where $\mathbf{1}_4$ is a 4×1 vector of ones. The 20×4 matrix $\mathbf{\Theta}_{2,2,1}$, containing rates for the transition of females in partnerships to single states by states of HIV disease, has the partitioned form:

$$\mathbf{\Theta}_{2,2,1} = \begin{bmatrix} \mathbf{\Theta}_{2,2,1}(1,1) & \mathbf{0} & \mathbf{0} & \mathbf{0} \\ \mathbf{0} & \mathbf{\Theta}_{2,2,1}(2,2) & \mathbf{0} & \mathbf{0} \\ \mathbf{0} & \mathbf{0} & \mathbf{\Theta}_{2,2,1}(3,3) & \mathbf{0} \\ \mathbf{0} & \mathbf{0} & \mathbf{0} & \mathbf{\Theta}_{2,2,1}(4,4) \end{bmatrix} , \tag{9.8.11}$$

where for $i = 1, 2, 3, 4$,

$$\mathbf{\Theta}_{2,2,1}(i,i) = \begin{bmatrix} \mu_{m0} + \sigma \\ \mu_{m1} + \sigma \\ \mu_{m2} + \sigma \\ \mu_{m3} + \sigma \\ \mu_{m4} + \sigma \end{bmatrix}. \tag{9.8.12}$$

Finally, the 20×20 matrix $\mathbf{\Theta}_{2,2,2}$, containing rates of transitions among states of HIV disease for females and males in partnership has the partitioned form:

$$\mathbf{\Theta}_{2,2,2} = \begin{bmatrix} \mathbf{\Theta}_{2,2,2}(1,1) & \mathbf{\Theta}_{2,2,2}(1,2) & \mathbf{0} & \mathbf{0} \\ \mathbf{0} & \mathbf{\Theta}_{2,2,2}(2,2) & \mathbf{\Theta}_{2,2,2}(2,3) & \mathbf{0} \\ \mathbf{0} & \mathbf{0} & \mathbf{\Theta}_{2,2,2}(3,3) & \mathbf{\Theta}_{2,2,2}(3,4) \\ \mathbf{0} & \mathbf{0} & \mathbf{0} & \mathbf{\Theta}_{2,2,2}(4,4) \end{bmatrix}. \tag{9.8.13}$$

The 5×5 non-zero matrices on the principal diagonal have the form:

$$\mathbf{\Theta}_{2,2,2}(i,i) = \begin{bmatrix} 0 & \beta q_{fi} & 0 & 0 & 0 \\ 0 & 0 & \gamma_{m1} & 0 & 0 \\ 0 & 0 & 0 & \gamma_{m2} & 0 \\ 0 & 0 & 0 & 0 & \gamma_{m3} \\ 0 & 0 & 0 & 0 & 0 \end{bmatrix}, \tag{9.8.14}$$

for $i = 1, 2, 3, 4$ and the non-zero off-diagonal matrices have the diagonal form:

$$\mathbf{\Theta}_{2,2,2}(i,i+1) = diag(\gamma_{fi}, \gamma_{fi}, \gamma_{fi}, \gamma_{fi}) \tag{9.8.15}$$

for $i = 1, 2, 3$.

When partnerships types are ordered according to the state of HIV disease of the male partner as described above, the matrices $\mathbf{\Theta}_{m,1}$ and $\mathbf{\Theta}_{m,2}$, corresponding to the $\mathbf{S}_{m,1}$ and $\mathbf{S}_{m,2}$ processes, have the same forms as those just described. To construct these matrices, it suffices to replace every rate pertaining to a transition of a female to the corresponding one for a male, and, whenever a male rate occurs, change it to the same rate for a female.

9.9 Linking the Partnership Model to a Branching Process

A first step in linking the partnership model just described to a multi-type branching process is that of defining infection types for females and males, which are used to identify lines of "descent". When a transition of the form $(0, j) \rightarrow (1, j)$ occurs in the $\mathbf{S}_{m,2}$-process, indicating that a male in state j of HIV disease has infected his susceptible female partner, a potential line of descent begins with this infected female who will be said to be of type $(1, j)$. And, when the transition $(i, 0) \rightarrow (i, 1)$ occurs in the $\mathbf{S}_{f,2}$-process, a potential line of descent begins with this infected male, who will be said to be of type $(i, 1)$. Thus, the branching process generated by the partnership model of HIV/AIDS will have eight types of individuals. Let $\mathcal{T}_f = \{(1, j) \mid j = 1, 2, 3, 4\}$ be the set of infection types for females and let $\mathcal{T}_m = \{(i, 1) \mid i = 1, 2, 3, 4\}$ be the set of infection types for males.

Given that a female is of type $\tau_f \in \mathcal{T}_f$, let $\mathfrak{m}_{\tau_f, \tau_m}$, $\tau_m \in \mathcal{T}_m$ be the expected number of male partners she infects prior to her death, and define the conditional expectation m_{τ_m, τ_f} similarly for infected males of type τ_m. The 8×8 matrix $\mathfrak{M}$ of expectations for the 8-type BGW-process embedded in the CMJ-process contains two 4×4 matrices:

$$\mathfrak{M}_{1,2} = \left(\mathfrak{m}_{\tau_f, \tau_m} \mid \tau_f \in \mathcal{T}_f,\ \tau_m \in \mathcal{T}_m \right) \tag{9.9.1}$$

$$\mathfrak{M}_{2,1} = \left(\mathfrak{m}_{\tau_m, \tau_f} \mid \tau_m \in \mathcal{T}_m,\ \tau_f \in \mathcal{T}_f \right) , \tag{9.9.2}$$

representing males infected by females and females infected by males. Therefore, the 8×8 matrix $\mathfrak{M}$ has the cyclic partitioned form,

$$\mathfrak{M} = \begin{bmatrix} \mathbf{0} & \mathfrak{M}_{1,2} \\ \mathfrak{M}_{2,1} & \mathbf{0} \end{bmatrix} . \tag{9.9.3}$$

To calculate the threshold parameter ρ_{pf}, the Perron-Frobenius root of the matrix $\mathfrak{M}$, it will be necessary to describe algorithms for calculating the matrices $\mathfrak{M}_{1,2}$ and $\mathfrak{M}_{2,1}$ in terms of the parameters of the system. Let $\mathbf{P}_{f,1}$ be the 21×21 matrix for the embedded Markov chain in the $\mathbf{S}_{f,1}$-process, let $\mathbf{R}_{f,1}$ be the 16×5 matrix of probabilities governing transitions from transient states to absorbing states, let $\mathbf{Q}_{f,1}$ be 16×16 matrix of probabilities governing transitions among transient states, and let $\mathbf{M}_{f,1} = (\mathbf{I}_{16} - \mathbf{Q}_{f,1})^{-1}$ be the 16×16 matrix of expectations. Then, as is well-known from the theory of absorbing Markov chains, the 16×5 matrix:

$$\mathbf{A}_{f,1} = \mathbf{M}_{f,1}\mathbf{R}_{f,1} \tag{9.9.4}$$

contains the conditional probabilities $a_{i,j}$, that if a process starts in some transient state $i \in \mathfrak{S}_{f,1,2}$, then $a_{i,j}$ is the probability the process terminates in absorbing state $j \in \mathfrak{S}_{f,1,1}$.

The $\mathcal{S}_{f,2}$-process begins when the $\mathcal{S}_{f,1}$- process terminates in some single state $\mathfrak{S}_{f,1,s} = \{(i)_f \mid i = 1, 2, 3, 4\}$. Consequently, the 4×4 submatrix of $\mathbf{A}_{f,1}$,

$$\Xi_{f,1} = (a_{i,j} \mid i \in \mathcal{T}_f, j \in \mathfrak{S}_{f,1,s}) \tag{9.9.5}$$

constitutes a set of initial probabilities for the $\mathcal{S}_{f,2}$-process. Let $\mathbf{P}_{f,2}$ be the 25×25 matrix of transition probabilities for the Markov chain embedded in the $\mathcal{S}_{f,2}$-process, let $\mathbf{M}_{f,2} = (\mathbf{I}_{24} - \mathbf{Q}_{f,2})^{-1}$ be the corresponding 24×24 matrix of expectations, and consider the 4×4 submatrix $\mathbf{\Psi}_{f,2}$ of $\mathbf{M}_{f,2}$ defined by

$$\mathbf{\Psi}_{f,2} = (m_{f,2,i,j} \mid i \in \mathfrak{S}_{f,1,s}, j \in \mathcal{T}_m) \ . \tag{9.9.6}$$

Then, the matrix $\mathfrak{M}_{1,2}$ is given by

$$\mathfrak{M}_{1,2} = \Xi_{f,1}\mathbf{\Psi}_{f,2} \ . \tag{9.9.7}$$

By letting the $\mathcal{S}_{m,1}$ and $\mathcal{S}_{m,2}$ processes play the same roles as the $\mathcal{S}_{f,1}$ and $\mathcal{S}_{f,2}$ processes as outlined above, a similar procedure may be used to calculate the matrix $\mathfrak{M}_{2,1}$.

In principle, all the calculations just outlined could be done to compute the 8×8 matrix $\widehat{\mathbf{m}}(\lambda)$ as functions of λ, the variable in Laplace-Stieltjes transforms (see Eq. (8.2.5)). Furthermore, for each λ such that all Laplace transforms $\widehat{a}_{ij}(\lambda)$ are positive, it would be possible, in principle, to find $\rho_{pf}(\lambda)$, the Perron-Frobenius root of the matrix $\widehat{\mathbf{m}}(\lambda)$. By doing these calculations repeatedly, it would also be possible, in principle, to find r, the intrinsic growth rate of an epidemic, by searching for a value of $\lambda = r$ such that $\rho_{pf}(r) = 1$. However, given the size of the matrices that must be inverted repeatedly for the HIV/AIDS model under consideration, finding r could take a considerable amount of computer time. Moreover, writing the software to carry out such an exercise could also be technically challenging, which leads one to ask whether another approach might be more fruitful.

Another approach to exploring the properties of the HIV/AIDS model under consideration would be to write the software required to compute the mean functions $M_{ij}(t)$ in Eq. (8.2.7), as numerical solutions of systems of renewal type integral equations as functions of $t \geq 0$. Such software would be relatively easy to write, particularly for discrete time formulations, and, in the long run would be more informative, since it would provide a methodology for studying the properties of the model as functions of $t \geq 0$.

A description of the algorithms needed to develop such software, along with numerous demographic applications of one type CMJ-process in discrete time, may be found in Mode.[5] By using techniques illustrated in that book, it appears that it would be feasible to compute not only the intrinsic growth rate r of an epidemic, without finding any Perron-Frobenius roots of the matrix $\widehat{\mathbf{m}}(\lambda)$, but also a number of other quantities of epidemiological interest as functions of the parameters of the model and as functions of time $t \geq 0$. Unlike the simple partnership model introduced in foregoing sections, the computation of extinction probabilities of the epidemic appears to be very difficult for the HIV/AIDS model with stages accommodating the formation and dissolution of partnerships.

9.10 Some Numerical Experiments with the HIV Model

A rationale for choosing values of mortality parameters was based on the observation that if μ is the parameter in a latent exponential life span distribution, then $1/\mu$ is the expected latent life span. Thus, to reflect higher risks of death when infected with HIV, the reciprocals of the female mortality parameters μ_{fi}, for $i = 1, 2, 3$, and 4, were chosen as $60, 15, 15, 15$, and 5 years, respectively; similarly, the reciprocals of the mortality parameters for males were chosen as $55, 15, 15, 15$, and 5 years. The parameter β was again chosen as about 104 contacts per year or an average of about two sexual contacts per week; the vector

$\mathbf{q}_m$, giving the probability per contact that an infected male infects his susceptible female partner as a function of the stage of HIV disease was chosen as $\mathbf{q}_m = < 0.005, 0.0025, 0.0025, 0.005 >$. Observe that the probability of infection for stages 2 and 3 of the disease is half that of that for stages 1 and 4, simulating the so-called bathtub effect and reflecting the idea that these probabilities depend on the concentration of free virus particles in the body fluids. The factor of one-half, however, is arbitrary. For the sake of simplicity, the corresponding vector $\mathbf{q}_f$ for infected females was equated to $\mathbf{q}_m$, even though the model and the software allow for different values for infected females and males.

Values of the parameters γ_{fi}, governing the durations of stay in the four stages of HIV disease, $i = 1, 2, 3$, and 4, were chosen as the estimates reported by Longini et al.[3] expressed in years. The corresponding values of the parameters γ_{mi} for $i = 1, 2, 3$, and 4 for males were assigned the same values as those for females, even though the model and the software may accommodate different values for females and males. Values of ρ and σ were determined by choosing $1/\sigma$ and $1/\rho$ as $1/12, 1, 2, 4, 6, \cdots, 20$ years in all possible combinations. The Perron-Frobenius root ρ_{pf} of the 8×8 matrix in Eq. (9.9.3) was then computed as a function of ρ and σ for all possible pairs $< \rho, \sigma >$, yielding $12 \times 12 = 144$ values. It is of interest to note in passing that the amount of time required to compute these 144 values was about 20 seconds on the desktop computer used to do the calculations. In carrying out these calculations, 144 16×16 and 24×24 matrices were inverted along with numerous matrix multiplications. Not too many years ago executing this number calculations on a desktop computer within a few seconds would have been nearly inconceivable.

Because of space limitations, only 49 of the 144 values of ρ_{pf} described above are presented in Table 9.10.1, where all values have been rounded to two decimal places. Observe that the columns of the table correspond to values of $1/\sigma$, the expected latent durations of partnership in the sense of the model of competing risks described in a preceding section, while the rows of the table correspond to the values of $1/\rho$, the expected latent waiting times among partnerships. As can be seen from the values presented in the table, ρ_{pf} appears to be more sensitive to values of ρ than those of σ. For example, only the first two rows of the table corresponding to those values of ρ such the $1/\rho = 1/12$, a month, and 1 year resulted in values of $\rho_{pf} > 1$, indicating that an epidemic would become established in a population with positive probability, i.e. the branching process would be supercritical.

Although it was not shown in the table, for $\rho = 12$, it turned out that the branching process would be supercritical for all values of σ such that $1/12 \leq 1/\sigma \leq 16$ and would become subcritical for some values of $1/\sigma > 16$ years, indicating that the epidemic would die out eventually with probability one. For $\rho = 1$ in row two of the table, it can be seen that the branching process would be supercritical only for $1/\sigma = 1$, 2, and 4 but critical, $\rho_{pf} = 1.00$, for $1/\sigma = 6$. It is interesting to note that all other values of ρ_{pf} in the table are less than one so that in all these cases the epidemic would die out eventually with probability one.

Table 9.10.1. Perron-Frobenius Roots for Selected Values of $1/\rho$ and $1/\sigma$ Expressed in Years.

$1/\rho \backslash 1/\sigma$	1/12	1	2	4	6	8	10
1/12	1.70	2.22	1.90	1.54	1.35	1.24	1.16
1	0.26	1.07	1.15	1.08	1.00	0.94	0.90
2	0.13	0.69	0.80	0.81	0.77	0.74	0.72
4	0.07	0.40	0.50	0.54	0.53	0.52	0.51
6	0.05	0.28	0.36	0.40	0.41	0.40	0.40
8	0.03	0.22	0.29	0.32	0.33	0.33	0.32
10	0.03	0.18	0.24	0.27	0.27	0.27	0.27

As mentioned in a previous section, the computations just described entail the inversion of many 24×24 matrices, giving rise to questions regarding their numerical reliability. Presented in Table 9.10.2 is a subset of the set of 144 condition numbers of some of the 24×24 matrices that were inverted in the above operations to compute Perron-Frobenius roots. As can be seen from the table, these numbers range from a high of 221.6 to a low of about 11.0. As a rule of thumb, condition numbers in the range 10^6 to 10^8 are indications that an inverse of a matrix may not be numerically reliable. Because all condition numbers in the table are relatively small, there is good evidence that the computation of the inverses of these matrices were indeed numerically reliable. When inverting rather large matrices as those under consideration, it is recommended that a sample of condition numbers be routinely inspected to assure the numerical quality of the inverses.

Table 9.10.2. Condition Numbers of 24×24 Matrices for Selected Values of $1/\rho$ and $1/\sigma$ Expressed in Years.

$1/\rho \backslash 1/\sigma$	1/12	1	2	4	6	8	10
1/12	221.6	53.4	37.5	28.6	25.4	23.7	22.7
1	41.0	30.8	26.3	22.4	20.8	19.9	19.3
2	25.8	23.4	21.6	19.5	18.4	17.7	17.3
4	17.7	18.0	17.5	16.6	16.1	15.7	15.4
6	14.9	15.8	15.6	15.2	14.8	14.6	14.4
8	13.5	14.6	14.6	14.3	14.1	13.9	13.8
10	12.7	13.8	13.9	13.7	13.6	13.5	13.4

Mention should also be made of the fact that the system is very sensitive to changes in the parameter values. For, in a computer experiment not reported here, the vectors $\mathbf{q}_f$ and $\mathbf{q}_m$ were set equal to the constant value 0.005, which led to values of ρ_{pf} of greater magnitude than those reported in Table 9.10.1 with many more supercritical cases. Such experiments demonstrate that a condition of nonconstancy of the elements of these vectors, particularly when the probability of infection per contact is lower in some stages of the disease than others, can have a significant impact on whether an epidemic becomes established in a population with positive probability.

To further demonstrate the dependence of ρ_{pf} on values of the constant vectors $\mathbf{q}_f$ and $\mathbf{q}_m$, as well as the parameters ρ and σ, another set of illustrative values of the threshold parameter are presented in Table 9.10.3 at selected values of the constant q_f in the vectors $\mathbf{q}_f$ and $\mathbf{q}_m$. In particular, the values of ρ and σ were chosen such that the waiting times among partnerships as well as the expected durations of partnership were short as would be the case in a highly promiscuous population of heterosexuals.

Table 9.10.3. Values of Threshold Parameter for Selected Values of $q_f = q_m$.

$(1/\rho, 1/\sigma)$	$q_f = 0.010$	$q_f = 0.005$	$q_f = 0.001$
$(1/52, 1/52)$	6.716	3.386	0.682
$(1/52, 1/12)$	7.951	4.116	0.847
$(1/12, 1/52)$	2.470	1.246	0.251
$(1/12, 1/12)$	4.700	2.437	0.502

It is interesting to note that in these experiments, the largest values of the threshold parameter ρ_{pf} were obtained when the latent expected waiting times among partnerships were one week, $1/52$ of a year, and the latent expected durations of partnership were one month, $1/12$ of a year, see the second row of the table. Also note that the branching process would be subcritical in populations characterized by the parameters values in the column of the table corresponding to the value $q_f = 0.001$, indicating that in such populations the epidemic would become extinct with probability one.

It has been documented that there are several strains of HIV-1, the form the virus being considered in the calculations presented in this section. Moreover, it seems plausible that some strains may have a longer incubation period than others, and therefore, it is of interest to conduct a computer experiment in which the expected length of this period is greater than that used in the experiments described above. To test the impact of a longer incubation period on the threshold parameter of the branching process, it was assumed that the expected length of the duration of stay in stage 1 of the disease was then $1/0.3 = 3.3333$ years instead of 2.4 months as assumed in the previous experiments. The values of all other parameters of the model were the same as those used in the experiment, whose results are displayed in Table 9.10.1, and the results of this experiment are presented in Table 9.10.4.

Table 9.10.4. Perron-Frobenius Roots for Longer Expected Time in Stage 1 for Selected Values of $1/\rho$ and $1/\sigma$ Expressed in Years.

$1/\rho \backslash 1\sigma$	1/12	1	2	4	6	8	10
1/12	2.13	2.89	2.52	2.05	1.80	1.64	1.54
1	0.32	1.40	1.52	1.43	1.33	1.25	1.19
2	0.17	0.89	1.06	1.08	1.03	0.99	0.96
4	0.09	0.52	0.66	0.72	0.72	0.70	0.69
6	0.06	0.37	0.48	0.54	0.55	0.54	0.53
8	0.04	0.28	0.38	0.43	0.44	0.44	0.44
10	0.03	0.23	0.31	0.36	0.37	0.37	0.37

By comparing this table with Table 9.10.1, it can be seen that if the numbers in these tables were presented as a three-dimensional surfaces, the shapes of the two surfaces would be much the same, but the magnitudes of the threshold parameters in the second experiment would be greater. Such comparative experiments provide numerical evidence that the expected length of the incubation period of HIV can have a significant impact on the threshold parameter of an epidemic. Indeed, in promiscuous populations, values of the threshold parameter are sensitive to all parameters of the model, including the parameter β, the expected number of sexual contacts per unit time, as has been shown in experiments not presented here. From the point of view of public health intervention strategies, it appears that the parameters of the model that are most controllable are the probabilities of infection per contact, which could be influenced by the use of condoms distributed by public health workers or by their availability for purchase through commercial channels.

9.11 Stochasticity and the Development of Major Epidemics

In Chapter 8 and in the foregoing sections of this chapter, attention has been focused on the derivation of methods for calculating values of threshold parameters with a view towards providing insights as to whether a major or minor epidemic would occur. If $\rho_{pf} \leq 1$, then a minor epidemic would occur, but, if $\rho_{pf} > 1$, then a major epidemic would occur. For one-type CMJ-processes, some attention was given to the derivation of the distribution of the total size of an epidemic when $R_0 \leq 1$ in Section 6.6. But, at this juncture in time, little seems to have been done on extending the results of Section 6.6 to the multi-type case, because of analytic and numerical difficulties. However, as has been illustrated by numerical examples in a preceding section of this chapter on two-type CMJ-processes in continuous time, when $\rho_{pf} > 1$, the probability that an epidemic becomes extinct can exceed 0.5. A question that naturally arises is: what can one say about the size of an epidemic in those cases where extinction does not occur? Among the useful experimental approaches to obtaining answers to such questions is to write computer software to compute and statistically summarize samples of Monte Carlo realizations of the process and thus obtain information on its evolutionary behavior.

The writing of software to compute Monte Carlo realizations of multi-type CMJ-processes in continuous time can be a time consuming task, which forces an investigator to make choices as to where to expend time and limited resources. Some algorithms for one-type CMJ-processes in discrete time, which are approximations to processes in continuous time may be found in Mode[5] and could be used as a starting point for the development of such software. A limitation of any formulation of an epidemic model as a branching process, however, is that it will not accommodate "interactions" among individuals in a population. Consequently, a decision was made to focus efforts on developing and writing software for a related class of nonlinear stochastic processes that are extensions of multi-type CMJ-processes and accommodate such interactions among individuals in a population. Such models will be developed in the subsequent chapters, but to obtain partial answers to the question raised above, attention will be focused on the results of some Monte Carlo simulations of one-type BGW-processes embedded in CMJ-processes. When considering the experimental results that follow, the reader should keep in mind the caveat that they seem most plausible for diseases with short infectious periods, i.e., short generation times or that are highly contagious so that an epidemic would develop in a population of susceptibles within a few generations of the embedded branching process.

In the examples of one-type CMJ-processes considered in Section 6.5 (see Eq. (6.5.9)), the random variable N, denoting number of susceptibles infected by each infective by the end of the infectious period for the embedded BGW-process, followed a geometric distribution with *p.d.f.*,

$$P[N = n] = pq^n \, , \tag{9.11.1}$$

where $n = 0, 1, 2, \cdots$, $p = 1/(R_0 + 1)$ and $q = R_0/(R_0 + 1)$. This is a particularly interesting and simple case to study, because the parameter p is a function of the threshold parameter R_0. During the course of the Monte Carlo experiments, it was also observed that the evolutionary behavior of the process was very sensitive to the functional form of the *p.d.f.* of N. To demonstrate this sensitivity, the case where N followed a Poisson distribution with parameter R_0 was also considered. Under this assumption, the *p.d.f.* of N had the form:

$$P[N = n] = \exp[-R_0] \frac{R_0^n}{n!} \, , \tag{9.11.2}$$

where $n = 0, 1, 2, \cdots$. In the tables that follow, these "offspring" distributions will be referred succinctly as geometric and Poisson variation.

In all Monte Carlo simulation experiments reported in this section, 100 generations of the embedded BGW-process were considered and 500 realizations of the process computed to generate 500×101 arrays. For 100 generations of an epidemic to occur, the length of the expected infectious period would need to be short or the disease highly contagious. In all cases, it was assumed that the 500 realizations of the epidemic evolved from one infective introduced into a large population of susceptibles. Thus, the first column of the array consisted of the initial infective and the remaining columns represented the 100 generations. The simulated data were statistically summarized by computing the minimum, maximum, and mean of the 500 realizations for each generation, i.e. columns, as outlined in Section 7.9. To gain further insight into the extreme values of the process, indicating the possible occurrence of major epidemics, the 99% quantiles were also computed for each generation. Finally, the empirical probabilities of extinction by generation were also computed. Three supercritical values of R_0 were considered in these illustrative experiments; namely,

$R_0 = 1.01$, $R_0 = 1.05$ and $R_0 = 1.1$. As one would expect, the evolutionary behavior of BGW-processes generated by either geometric or Poisson variation were very sensitive to values of R_0. For example, when $R_0 = 2$ epidemics would tend to develop explosively in a population of susceptibles.

The result of the experiments for geometric and Poisson variation, respectively, are shown in Tables 9.11.1 and 9.11.2 at selected generations for the case $R_0 = 1.01$. From these tables, it can be seen that geometric variation produced larger extreme values and means for each of the displayed generation than did Poisson variation. For example, for the case of geometric variation, in generation 100 the maximum size of the simulated epidemics was 431 as compared to 262 for Poisson variation. The corresponding 99% quantiles at generation 100 were 85 and 93, respectively, which suggests that epidemics of these sizes would occur less than one percent of the time. For the case of geometric variation, the theoretical probability of extinction is $q = 1/1.01 = 0.9901$ and for the Poisson case, this probability had the value $q = 0.9802$. As they should, it appears that the estimated probabilities by generation in these tables were converging to these theoretical values. From these experiments one reaches the conclusion that although the probability of an epidemic becoming extinct is high, whenever an epidemic seeded by a few infectives develops in a susceptible population, "major" epidemics may sometimes occur, particularly for the case of geometric variation.

Table 9.11.1. Geometric Variation with $R_0 = 1.01$.

Generation	Min	Mean	Max	Quan-0.99	Prob-Exct.
0	1	1	1	1	0.000
5	0	1.080	22	13	0.832
25	0	1.798	152	50	0.946
50	0	2.472	230	105	0.972
75	0	3.394	386	115	0.978
100	0	3.526	431	85	0.980

Table 9.11.2. Poisson Variation with $R_0 = 1.01$.

Generation	Min	Mean	Max	Quan-0.99	Prob-Exct.
0	1	1	1	1	0.000
5	0	0.904	14	11	0.738
25	0	0.820	67	26	0.950
50	0	1.336	120	37	0.964
75	0	1.968	215	76	0.974
100	0	2.376	262	93	0.978

The results of the simulation experiments for the case $R_0 = 1.05$ are presented in Tables 9.11.3 and 9.11.4. For the case of geometric variation, the probability that the epidemic becomes extinct is given by $q = 1/1.05 = 0.952380$, while that for Poisson variation is $q = 0.906298$. It is interesting to observe that even though the probability of extinction of the epidemic is higher for geometric rather than Poisson variation, whenever a major epidemic occurs more susceptibles are infected in the geometric case than in the Poisson case. At 50 generations, for example, a mean of 16.59 susceptibles would be infected in the geometric case, but for the Poisson case the mean is 9.54. When $R_0 = 1.05$, the differences in the extreme value statistics for geometric and Poisson variation are much greater than they are for the case $R_0 = 1.01$. Observe that for the geometric case, the maximum value statistic at generation 100 was 8663 compared to 4947 for the Poisson case.

Table 9.11.3. Geometric Variation with R_0= 1.05.

Generation	Min	Mean	Max	Quan-0.99	Prob-Exct.
0	1	1	1	1	0.000
5	0	1.198	27	17	0.802
25	0	4.238	140	120	0.924
50	0	16.590	822	489	0.944
75	0	56.540	2529	1682	0.946
100	0	196.234	8663	5825	0.946

Table 9.11.4. Poisson Variation with R_0 = 1.05.

Generation	Min	Mean	Max	Quan-0.99	Prob-Exct.
0	1	1	1	1	0.000
5	0	1.160	21	11	0.710
25	0	3.530	149	59	0.874
50	0	9.540	472	232	0.906
75	0	32.082	1480	832	0.912
100	0	111.364	4947	2518	0.916

Tables 9.11.5 and 9.11.6 contain the results of the Monte Carlo experiments for the case $R_0 = 1.1$ and clearly demonstrate that the evolutionary development of a major epidemic in a large population of susceptibles seeded by one infective is very sensitive to the value of R_0. For, when $R_0 = 1.1$, the probability of extinction in the geometric case is $q = 1/1.1 = 0.90909$, while that for the Poisson case is given by $q = 0.82386$. Thus, even though the probability of extinction is again greater in the geometric rather than in the Poisson case, whenever a major epidemic occurs, the divergence between the extreme value statistics for the number of susceptibles infected in the geometric and Poisson cases is greater than when $R_0 = 1.05$.

Observe, for example, that at 100 generations the extreme value statistic for geometric variation was 500903, but that for Poisson variation was 322154. By the law of large numbers, the mean of 500 independent observations of the process in generation n is an unbiased and consistent estimate of R_0^n, the expected size of a population in generation n evolving according to a BGW-process. When $n = 100$ and $R_0 = 1.1$, this expectation is $(1.1)^{100} = 13781$. It is interesting to observe that, although a sample size of 500 is quite large, the estimates of 13781 differ significantly from each other and from the theoretical value. Such observations underscore the importance of stochastic variation, stochasticity, in the develop of major epidemics evolving from one infective.

Table 9.11.5. Geometric Variation with $\mathbf{R_0 = 1.1}$.

Generation	Min	Mean	Max	Quan-0.99	Prob-Exct.
0	1	1	1	1	0
5	0	1.658	26	19	0.784
25	0	9.594	373	214	0.902
50	0	96.538	3970	2280	0.908
75	0	1042.122	44469	24262	0.908
100	0	11359.854	500903	257594	0.908

Table 9.11.6. Poisson Variation with $\mathbf{R_0 = 1.1}$.

Generation	Min	Mean	Max	Quan-0.99	Prob-Exct.
0	1	1	1	1	0
5	0	1.588	18	13	0.638
25	0	12.070	210	167	0.808
50	0	132.734	2729	11806	0.820
75	0	1421.778	29462	21070	0.820
100	0	15456.066	322154	223164	0.820

9.12 On Controlling an Epidemic

In Section 9.11 the occurrence and the establishment of major epidemics seeded by one infective in a large population of susceptibles was studied by conducting Monte Carlo simulation experiments with a BGW-process for selected values of R_0. After an epidemic has been established in a population, a question that arises is: what control measures need to be taken so as to reduce R_0 to a value less than one? Alternatively, one may ask: if the value of R_0 can be controlled, then what values less than one would lead to the extinction of the epidemic within a few generations if an infective were introduced into a large population of susceptibles? When R_0 for an epidemic model is specified by the special formula $R_0 = \lambda p \mu$, where λ is the contact rate per unit time, p is the probability of infection per contact, and μ is the expected length of the infectious period, then any public health measures that would reduce the value of any or all three parameters would lessen the value of R_0. In this section, the results of some Monte Carlo simulation experiments will be reported for selected values of $R_0 < 1$.

If the initial number of infectives in a large population of susceptibles is X_0, then the expected number of infectives in the nth generation is $X_0 R_0^n$ when the epidemic evolves according to a BGW-process. When X_0 is large, this expectation may decrease rather slowly even if $R_0 < 1$. As one would expect, and as was confirmed in several Monte Carlo simulation experiments not reported here, one could expect the extinction of the epidemic within a few generations only for values of the threshold parameter such that $0 < R_0 < 0.5$. Tables 9.12.1 and 9.12.2 contain summaries, respectively, of the results for two illustrative Monte Carlo simulation experiments for geometric and Poisson variation when $R_0 = 0.25$. In both these experiments, the initial number of infectives was chosen as $X_0 = 100$, the sample size was 500 realizations, and the length of all samples was 100 generations.

Table 9.12.1. Geometric Variation with $\mathbf{R_0 = 0.25}$.

Generation	Min	Mean	Max	Quan-0.99	Prob-Exct.
0	100	100	100	100	0.000
1	11	25.340	40	38	0.000
5	0	0.090	3	2	0.926
10	0	0.002	1	0	0.988
11	0	0	0	0	1.000
12	0	0	0	0	1.000

Table 9.12.2. Poisson Variation with $\mathbf{R_0= 0.25}$.

Generation	Min	Mean	Max	Quan-0.99	Prob-Exct.
0	100	100	100	100	0.000
1	14	25.066	42	37	0.000
5	0	0.094	4	2	0.930
10	0	0.004	2	0	0.998
11	0	0.002	1	0	0.998
12	0	0	0	0	1.000

As can be seen from an inspection of these tables, the evolution of the epidemic was much the same for geometric and Poisson variation. For the case of geometric variation, the epidemic had become extinct by the 11th generation, and in the Poisson case extinction occurred in the 12th generation. In results not presented here for the case $R_0 = 0.5$, the epidemic had become extinct in the 17th and 18th generations, respectively, for geometric and Poisson variation. Of course, the larger the value of X_0, the longer would be the waiting time to the extinction of an epidemic, but the results of these Monte Carlo experiments suggest that if public health interventions can result in values of R_0 sufficiently small, then substantial levels of control of an epidemic may be achieved. On the other hand, in Monte Carlo experiments with $R_0 = 0.95$ and $X_0 = 100$, the epidemic was not extinct for either geometric or Poisson variation after 100 generations with 500 realization samples. Thus, unless control measures can reduce R_0 to sufficiently small values, say in the interval $(0, 0.25]$, epidemics may persist in populations for long periods of time.

9.13 References

1. B. W. Char, K. O. Geddes, G. H. Gonnet, B. Leong, M. B. Monagan and S. M. Watt. *MAPLE V Language Reference Manual*, Springer-Verlag, Berlin, New York, 1991.
2. N. P. Jewell and S. C. Shiboski, Statistical Analysis of HIV Infectivity Based on Partner Studies, *Biometrics* **46:** 1133-1150, 1990.
3. I. M. Longini, Jr., W. S. Clark, L. M. Haber and R. Horsburgh, Jr., The Stages of HIV Infection: Waiting Times and Infection Transmission Probabilities, *Lecture Notes in Biomathematics* **83:** 111-137, C. Castillo-Chavez (ed.), *Mathematical and Statistical Approaches in AIDS Epidemiology,* Springer-Verlag, Berlin, New York, Tokyo, 1989.
4. C. J. Mode, *Multitype Branching Processes - Theory and Applications,* American Elsevier, New York, 1971.
5. C. J. Mode, *Stochastic Processes in Demography and Their Computer Implementation,* Springer-Verlag, Berlin, 1985.

Chapter 10
NON-LINEAR STOCHASTIC MODELS IN HOMOSEXUAL POPULATIONS

10.1 Introduction

As has been demonstrated in Chapters 6, 7, 8, and 9, branching process approximations to the early stages of epidemics of sexually transmitted diseases, as well as other types of diseases, can be very useful in deriving formulas for threshold parameters, which have been symbolized by many authors in terms of the generic symbol R_0. Even though work within a branching process framework can yield useful and interesting results, it is widely recognized that this framework is not sufficiently rich to accommodate various types of interactions among individuals in a population that may contribute significantly to the evolution of an epidemic. Among these interactions for the case of sexually transmitted diseases is a conscious selection of sexual partners that may, in the case of diseases with several infectious stages, depend on the stage of the person. For example, a susceptible person may avoid sexual contact with a person known to be infected, and infected persons in similar stages of a disease may have a tendency to select each other as sexual partners as suggested by anecdotal evidence that people infected with HIV may have a tendency to select sexual partners according to similar $CD4^+$ counts. It has also been documented that individuals of a population may be partitioned into behavioral classes defined by the number of sexual partners per unit time (see Laumann et al.[7]). Therefore, it seems plausible that conscious selection of sexual partners may also occur by behavioral class. That is, persons with desires for many sexual partners are more likely to have sexual contacts with persons having similar desires; whereas those who desire fewer sexual partners are likely to have sexual contacts with persons who desire fewer contacts. Accordingly, in this chapter, non-linear stochastic models with capabilities for accommodating such interactions among persons in a population will be formulated and analyzed by computer intensive methods.

The material presented in this chapter is related to several papers that appeared in the recent literature on stochastic models of HIV/AIDS epidemics in populations of homosexual men, which were designed to expedite computer intensive experimentation. Among these papers are those by Tan and his colleagues, Tan and Byers,[21] Tan[20,19] and Tan and Xi.[22] These authors sometimes refer to their work under the heading of chain multinomial models. Two earlier papers which also belong to this genre are those of Mode et al.[14,15] More recently, stochastic models of this type have been fit to actual data on an HIV/AIDS epidemic in Sleeman and Mode.[17,18] Due to space limitations in most research journals, however, it has not been feasible to present a more complete account of the mathematical structure forming the basis for these stochastic models.

Accordingly, the original goal of this chapter was to present a more complete account of this basis, which would be useful for people wishing to learn more about these models. But, as the work proceeded, new algorithmic approaches to formulating stochastic models in this class were uncovered, particularly with respect to a more complete use of latent risk functions and competing risks to accommodate transitions among stages of a disease. This use of competing risks in turn led to explicit connections between the stochastic process and systems of non-linear differential equations embedded in the process, which became very useful in the search for threshold conditions for the stochastic process. Consequently, most of the mathematical results, as well as the software described in this chapter, are new.

10.2 Types of Individuals and Contact Structures

A fundamental problem underlying the formulation of stochastic models accommodating interactions among individuals in a population is the formulation of probabilistic models of contact structures, which in turn depend on a set of types used to partition a population according to behavioral classes and stages of a disease. For example, consider a population with $m \geq 1$ behavioral classes defined in terms of the expected number of sexual partners per unit time and a disease with $n \geq 1$ infectious stages. Then, the set of types of individuals in the population could be chosen as:

$$\Upsilon = \{\tau = (i, j) \mid i = 1, 2, \cdots, m;\ j = 0, 1, 2, \cdots, n\} \ , \tag{10.2.1}$$

where i denotes the behavioral class of an individual and j the state of the person with respect to disease. By definition, $j = 0$ denotes a susceptible person, and $j = 1, 2, \cdots, n$, a person in stage j of a disease.

By necessity, any computer implementation of a model must be on some discrete time scale, and, accordingly, let

$$t \in S_h = \{t = kh \mid k = 0, 1, 2, \cdots\} \ , \tag{10.2.2}$$

be the time lattice under consideration, where $h > 0$. At time $t \in S_h$, let the random function $X(t; \tau)$ denote the number of persons of type $\tau \in \Upsilon$ in the population. A fundamental random function, going into the formulation of models of contact structures, is the frequency of an individual of type τ is the population at time t, which is defined by:

$$U(t; \tau) = \frac{X(t; \tau)}{\sum_{\tau' \in \Upsilon} X(t; \tau')} \ , \tag{10.2.3}$$

provided that $X(t; \tau) > 0$ for some $\tau \in \Upsilon$.

To formalize the idea that sexual partners may be chosen according to preferences influenced by behavioral class and state with respect to disease, the concept of acceptance probabilities will be introduced. If a person is of type τ_1, let $\alpha(\tau_1, \tau_2)$ denote the conditional probability that a person of type τ_2 is acceptable as a sexual partner. Formulas for these acceptance probabilities may be chosen in many ways, but for the sake of simplicity, suppose the indices i and j are expressed in terms of some numerical scale. Then, if $\tau_1 = (i_1, j_2)$ and $\tau_2 = (i_2, j_2)$, the functions $\alpha(\tau_1, \tau_2)$ will be chosen as:

$$\alpha(\tau_1, \tau_2) = \exp\left[- \left(\beta_1 \mid i_1 - i_2 \mid + \beta_2 \mid j_1 - j_2 \mid\right)\right] \ , \tag{10.2.4}$$

where $\beta_1 \geq 0$ and $\beta_2 \geq 0$ are parameters to be chosen. Observe that if $\beta_1 = \beta_2 = 0$, then $\alpha(\tau_1, \tau_2) = 1$ for all pairs (τ_1, τ_2), which, as will be shown, corresponds to random assortment with respect to behavioral class and state of disease. Furthermore, it can be seen that the larger the values of β_1 and β_2, the greater the conditional probability that a person of type τ_1 will find a person of a similar type τ_2 acceptable as a sexual partner.

Given a person of type τ_1 at time t, let $\gamma(t; \tau_1, \tau_2)$ be the conditional probability that a person of type τ_1 has contact with a potential sexual partner of type τ_2 during the time interval $(t, t+h]$. By the law of total probability,

$$\sum_{\tau' \in \Upsilon} U(t; \tau')\alpha(\tau_1, \tau') \tag{10.2.5}$$

is the probability that a person of type τ_1 at time t has contact with some person as a potential sexual partner during the time interval $(t, t+h]$. Therefore, by an application of Bayes' theorem,

$$\gamma(t; \tau_1, \tau_2) = \frac{U(t; \tau_2)\alpha(\tau_1, \tau_2)}{\sum_{\tau' \in \Upsilon} U(t; \tau')\alpha(\tau_1, \tau')} \,. \tag{10.2.6}$$

Observe that for all $\tau_1 \in \Upsilon$ and $t \in S_h$ the condition

$$\sum_{\tau_2 \in \Upsilon} \gamma(t; \tau_1, \tau_2) = 1 \tag{10.2.7}$$

is satisfied. Furthermore, if $\beta_1 = \beta_2 = 0$ so that $\alpha(\tau_1, \tau_2) = 1$ for all pairs (τ_1, τ_2), then Eq. (10.2.6) becomes

$$\gamma(t; \tau_1, \tau_2) = U(t; \tau_2) \,, \tag{10.2.8}$$

which, by definition, is random assortment.

For each $\tau_1 \in \Upsilon$ and $t \in S_h$, let

$$\mathbf{\Gamma}(t; \tau_1) = (\gamma(t; \tau_1, \tau_2) \mid \tau_2 \in \Upsilon) \tag{10.2.9}$$

be a vector of contact probabilities for a person of type τ_1. Next let the random function $Z(t; \tau_1, \tau_2)$ denote the number of persons of type τ_1 at time t who seek potential partners of type τ_2 during the time interval $(t, t+h]$, and let

$$\mathbf{Z}(t;\tau_1) = (Z(t;\tau_1,\tau_2) \mid \tau_2 \in \Upsilon) \tag{10.2.10}$$

denote a vector of these random functions. Then, it will assumed that, given $X(t;\tau_1)$, the conditional distribution of this random vector is multinomial with index $X(t;\tau_1)$ and probability vector $\mathbf{\Gamma}(t;\tau_1)$. In symbols,

$$\mathbf{Z}(t;\tau_1) \sim CMultinom\,(X(t;\tau_1), \mathbf{\Gamma}(t;\tau_1)) \ . \tag{10.2.11}$$

According to the formulation under consideration, members of a population make contacts or mix, during any time interval $(t, t+h]$, according to the multinomial distribution in Eq. (10.2.11). Such mixing may, or may not, result in the formation of partnerships, containing pairs of individuals within which sexual contacts may occur. It seems reasonable to suppose, however, that during any time interval, there would be some maximum number of potential partnerships of type (τ_1, τ_2), with one member of type $\tau_1 \in \Upsilon$ and the other of type $\tau_2 \in \Upsilon$, that could be formed. Let the random function $N(t;\tau_1,\tau_2)$ denote the maximum potential number of pairs of partnerships that may be formed during any time interval $(t, t+h]$. Because the total number of individuals of type τ_1 in partnerships of type (τ_1, τ_2) for some $\tau_2 \in \Upsilon$ cannot exceed $X(t;\tau_1)$, it follows that the inequality,

$$\sum_{\tau_2 \in \Upsilon} N(t;\tau_1,\tau_2) \leq X(t;\tau_1) \tag{10.2.12}$$

must be satisfied with probability one for all $\tau_1 \in \Upsilon$. Similarly, the inequality,

$$\sum_{\tau_1 \in \Upsilon} N(t;\tau_1,\tau_2) \leq X(t;\tau_2) \tag{10.2.13}$$

must hold with probability one for all $\tau_2 \in \Upsilon$.

Evidently, the random function $N(t;\tau_1,\tau_2)$ may be chosen in a number of ways, but in the models considered in this chapter it will be chosen as follows. If $\tau_1 \neq \tau_2$, then

$$N(t;\tau_1,\tau_2) = \min\,(Z(t;\tau_1,\tau_2), Z(t;\tau_2,\tau_1)) \ . \tag{10.2.14}$$

But, if $\tau_1 = \tau_2$, then

$$N(t; \tau_1, \tau_1) = \left[\frac{Z(t; \tau_1, \tau_1)}{2}\right], \tag{10.2.15}$$

where $[\cdot]$ stands for the greatest integer function. The rationale for the choice of the random function in Eq. (10.2.14) seems clear and that for Eq. (10.2.15) is the following. If there are $Z(t; \tau_1, \tau_1)$ persons of type τ_1 who seek partners of the same type τ_1 during the time interval $(t, t+h]$, then, for the case $Z(t; \tau_1, \tau_1)$ is even, the total number of partnership pairs that may be formed is $Z(t; \tau_1, \tau_1)/2$; but, if $Z(t; \tau_1, \tau_1)$ is odd, then one person may be without a partner. It can easily be checked that when the random function $N(t; \tau_1, \tau_2)$ is chosen as in Eqs. (10.2.14) and (10.2.15), then the inequalities in Eqs. (10.2.12) and (10.2.13) will be satisfied with probability one.

Many authors, particularly those working within deterministic paradigms, have required that balance equations of the form

$$\gamma(t; \tau_1, \tau_2) X(t; \tau_1) = \gamma(t; \tau_2, \tau_1) X(t; \tau_2) \tag{10.2.16}$$

be satisfied for all $t \in S_h$ and pairs (τ_1, τ_2). The rationale for imposing such balance conditions in deterministic formulations seems clear, but they may impose unnecessary constraints on the parameter space underlying a model. However, in the stochastic formulation under consideration, such balance conditions are not needed.

10.3 Probabilities of Susceptibles Being Infected

Given a susceptible person of type $\tau_1 = (i_1, 0)$ at time t, let $\rho(t; \tau_1, \tau_2)$ denote the conditional probability that this person has a sexual partner of type τ_2 during the time interval $(t, t+h]$. According to one's point of view, this probability may be chosen in various ways. One approach to choosing this probability is to suppose that the mixing and search for potential sexual partners induces this conditional probability according to the frequency interpretation of probability. Under this view, this conditional probability would be chosen as:

$$\rho(t; \tau_1, \tau_2) = \frac{N(t; \tau_1, \tau_2)}{\sum_{\tau' \in \Upsilon} N(t; \tau_1, \tau')} \tag{10.3.1}$$

for all τ_1 and τ_2, whenever the ratio is well-defined. An alternative point of view for choosing this conditional probability will be discussed subsequently.

However the conditional probability $\rho(t;\tau_1,\tau_2)$ is chosen, the behavioral classes to which individuals belong will be characterized in terms of the expected number of sexual partners per unit time and the expected number of sexual contacts per partner. Accordingly, let $\lambda(i)$ denote the expected number of sexual partners a person belonging to class $i = 1,2,\cdots,m$, has per unit time, and assume the number of partners follows a Poisson process with parameter $\lambda(i)$ so that $\lambda(i)h$ is the expected number of sexual partners during the time interval. Similarly, suppose the number of sexual contacts per partner follows a Poisson process with parameter $\eta(i)$ for class i so that during the time interval $(t,t+h]$ the expected number of sexual contacts per partner is $(1+\eta(i))h$. Observe that by definition, a person is not a sexual partner unless at least one contact occurs during any time interval.

Let $q(j)$ be the probability that a susceptible person is infected per sexual contact when his partner is in state $j = 1,2,\cdots,n$, with respect to disease, and let $p(j) = 1-q(j)$ be the probability of escaping infection per contact. By definition, $q(0) = 0$, because a non-infected partner cannot transmit an infectious agent to his susceptible partner. Then, under the assumption that the number of sexual contacts per partner during the time interval $(t,t+h]$ occur according to a Poisson process with support $c = 1,2,\cdots$, the conditional probability that a susceptible person of type $\tau_1 = (i_1,0)$ at time t escapes infection during $(t,t+h]$ when his sexual partner is of type $\tau_2 = (i_2,j_2)$ is given by:

$$\begin{aligned} p(t;\tau_1,\tau_2) &= \exp\left[-\eta(i_1)h\right]\sum_{c=1}^{\infty}\frac{(\eta(i_1)h)^{c-1}}{(c-1)!}(p(j_2))^c \\ &= p(j_2)\exp\left[-\eta(i_1)hq(j_2)\right] . \end{aligned} \tag{10.3.2}$$

By the law of total probability,

$$P_{par}(t;\tau_1) = \sum_{\tau_2\in\Upsilon}\rho(t;\tau_1,\tau_2)p(t;\tau_1,\tau_2) \tag{10.3.3}$$

is the conditional probability that a susceptible person of type τ_1 at time t escapes infection per sexual partner during the time interval

$(t, t+h]$. Thus,

$$Q_{par}(t;\tau_1) = 1 - P_{par}(t;\tau_1) \tag{10.3.4}$$

is the conditional probability that a susceptible person of type τ_1 becomes infected during $(t, t+h]$.

But, the number of sexual partners a person of type $\tau_1 = (i_1, 0)$ has during the time interval $(t, t+h]$, by assumption, follows a Poisson distribution with parameter $\lambda(i_1)$ and support $x = 0, 1, 2, \cdots$. Therefore,

$$\begin{aligned} P(t;\tau_1) &= \exp\left[-\lambda(i_1)h\right] \sum_{x=0}^{\infty} \frac{(\lambda(i_1)h)^x}{x!} (P_{par}(t;\tau_1))^x \\ &= \exp\left[-\lambda(i_1)hQ_{par}(t;\tau_1)\right] \end{aligned} \tag{10.3.5}$$

is the conditional probability that a person of type τ_1 at time t escapes infection from all sexual partners during $(t, t+h]$. Therefore, by taking all possible sexual partners into account,

$$Q(t;\tau_1) = 1 - P(t;\tau_1) = \lambda(i_1)Q_{par}(t;\tau_1)h + o(h) \tag{10.3.6}$$

is the conditional probability that a susceptible of type τ_1 becomes infected during $(t, t+h]$. This result justifies using the expression

$$\lambda(i_1)Q_{par}(t;\tau_1) \tag{10.3.7}$$

as the latent risk for a susceptible of type τ_1 being infected during the time interval $(t, t+h]$ in semi-Markovian models for the life cycles of individuals that will be developed in the next section.

Another choice for the conditional probability $\rho(t;\tau_1,\tau_2)$ would be the contact probability $\gamma(t;\tau_1,\tau_2)$ defined in a previous section (see Eq. (10.2.6)). But, it should be noted that this choice would not take into account restrictions of the type in Eqs. (10.2.12) and (10.2.13), arising in the formation of partnership pairs. As will be shown subsequently, if this approach is used, then the form of the embedded system of differential equations will be simplified by avoiding problems of non-differentiability that arise in connection with Jacobian matrices when investigating the stability of equilibrium points of differential equations.

10.4 Semi-Markovian Processes as Models for Life Cycles

Unlike most models formulated within a deterministic paradigm, where attention is often focused on the population as a whole, in many stochastic formulations of population dynamics, particularly in branching processes, life cycle models for individuals are basic components of the system. Moreover, from life cycle models for individuals, one may proceed to components of the system describing the population as a whole. As has been illustrated in previous chapters, state spaces and corresponding matrices of latent risks are some of the basic tools underlying the construction of semi-Markovian processes.

Every life cycle ends with the death of an individual. Consequently, the set of absorbing states for the life cycle model for individuals will be chosen as

$$\mathfrak{S}_1 = \{E_1, E_2\} \ , \tag{10.4.1}$$

where E_1 denotes death from a cause other than disease and E_2 death caused by the disease under consideration. The transient states $\mathfrak{S}_2$ for the life cycle model will be chosen as the set of ordered pairs,

$$\mathfrak{S}_2 = \{(i,j) \mid i = 1, 2, \cdots, m;\ j = 0, 1, 2, \cdots, n\} \ , \tag{10.4.2}$$

where i denotes the behavioral class and j the state with respect to disease. Observe that the set of transient states is merely the set Υ of types of individuals defined before. Altogether, the state space of the process $\mathfrak{S} = \mathfrak{S}_1 \cup \mathfrak{S}_2$ contains $2 + m(n+1)$ states. From now on the elements of the set $\mathfrak{S}_2$ of transient states will be arranged in lexicographic order.

The $(2 + m(n+1)) \times (2 + m(n+1))$ matrix of latent risks $\boldsymbol{\Theta} = (\theta_{ij})$ may be represented in the partitioned form,

$$\boldsymbol{\Theta} = \begin{bmatrix} \mathbf{0}_{11} & \mathbf{0}_{12} \\ \boldsymbol{\Theta}_{21} & \boldsymbol{\Theta}_{22} \end{bmatrix} , \tag{10.4.3}$$

where $\mathbf{0}_{11}$ is a 2×2 zero matrix and $\mathbf{0}_{12}$ is a $2 \times m(n+1)$ zero matrix, indicating transitions from absorbing states are impossible. Further, the $(m(n+1)) \times 2$ matrix $\boldsymbol{\Theta}_{21}$ governs transitions from transient states to absorbing states and the $(m(n+1)) \times (m(n+1))$ matrix $\boldsymbol{\Theta}_{22}$ governs transitions among transient states. As we will see, some of the elements of $\boldsymbol{\Theta}$ may be functions of $t \in S_h$.

Before proceeding to the general case, it will be helpful to set down the form of the sub-matrices $\boldsymbol{\Theta}_{21}$ and $\boldsymbol{\Theta}_{22}$ for the case of two behavioral classes, $m = 2$, and one stage of disease, $n = 1$. In this case, the 4×2 sub-matrix $\boldsymbol{\Theta}_{21}$ of latent risks, governing transitions from the set of four transient states,

$$\mathfrak{S}_2 = \{(1,0),(1,1),(2,0),(2,1)\} \tag{10.4.4}$$

into the set $\mathfrak{S}_2 = \{E_1, E_2\}$ of absorbing states has the form,

$$\boldsymbol{\Theta}_{21} = \begin{bmatrix} \mu_0 & 0 \\ \mu_0 & \mu_1 \\ \mu_0 & 0 \\ \mu_0 & \mu_1 \end{bmatrix}, \tag{10.4.5}$$

where μ_0 is the risk of death for a susceptible person and μ_1 is an incremental risk of death for a person in stage 1 of the disease.

As an aid to describing the structure of the sub-matrix $\boldsymbol{\Theta}_{22}$, governing transitions among transient states, consider subsets of transient states $A(1)$ and $A(2)$ defined by:

$$A(i) = \{(i,0),(i,1)\} \tag{10.4.6}$$

for $i = 1, 2$. Then, the 4×4 matrix $\boldsymbol{\Theta}_{22}$ may be represented in the partitioned form,

$$\boldsymbol{\Theta}_{22} = \begin{bmatrix} \boldsymbol{\Theta}_{22}(1,1) & \boldsymbol{\Theta}_{22}(1,2) \\ \boldsymbol{\Theta}_{22}(2,1) & \boldsymbol{\Theta}_{22}(2,2) \end{bmatrix} \tag{10.4.7}$$

of 2×2 sub-matrices. For example, the 2×2 sub-matrix $\boldsymbol{\Theta}_{22}(1,1)$ of latent risks governs transitions from states in the set $A(1)$ into itself; while the 2×2 sub-matrix $\boldsymbol{\Theta}_{22}(1,2)$ of latent risks governs transitions from states in the set $A(1)$ to states in the set $A(2)$, i.e., changes in behavioral classes during any time interval. In this case, transitions among behavioral classes will be accommodated by introducing the 2×2 matrix of latent risks,

$$\boldsymbol{\Psi} = \begin{bmatrix} 0 & \psi_{12} \\ \psi_{21} & 0 \end{bmatrix}, \tag{10.4.8}$$

governing transitions among classes 1 and 2.

Let $\tau_1 = (1,0)$ stand for a susceptible person in behavioral class 1. Then, the 2×2 sub-matrix $\mathbf{\Theta}_{22}(1,1)$ has the form

$$\mathbf{\Theta}_{22}(1,1) = \begin{bmatrix} 0 & \lambda(1)Q_{par}(t;\tau_1) \\ 0 & 0 \end{bmatrix}, \tag{10.4.9}$$

(see Eq. (10.3.7) for the definition of the latent risk functions governing the infection of susceptibles during any time interval $(t, t+h]$). Observe that according to the second row of this matrix, transitions from the infected state 1 to the susceptible state 0 are, by assumption, impossible in the formulation under consideration. As one can see from Eq. (10.4.9), the matrix $\mathbf{\Theta}_{22}(1,1)$ is actually a function of $t \in S_h$. Thus, a more precise definition of the latent risks is that they are conditional on the evolution of the process up to time t during the time interval $(t, t+h]$.

Because transitions among the sets $A(1)$ and $A(2)$ of transient states represent changes in behavioral classes during any time interval $(t, t+h]$, the sub-matrix $\mathbf{\Theta}_{22}(1,2)$ of risks, governing transitions from behavioral class 1 to 2, has the form,

$$\mathbf{\Theta}_{22}(1,2) = \begin{bmatrix} \psi_{12} & 0 \\ 0 & \psi_{12} \end{bmatrix}; \tag{10.4.10}$$

while the sub-matrix governing transitions from class 2 to 1 has the form,

$$\mathbf{\Theta}_{22}(2,1) = \begin{bmatrix} \psi_{21} & 0 \\ 0 & \psi_{21} \end{bmatrix}. \tag{10.4.11}$$

If $n = 2$ stages of disease were considered and transitions among the stages of the disease were allowed, then the 2×2 matrix of latent risks,

$$\mathbf{\Gamma} = \begin{bmatrix} 0 & \gamma_{12} \\ \gamma_{21} & 0 \end{bmatrix}, \tag{10.4.12}$$

governing transitions among the stages of a disease would be introduced. One could then proceed to construct the matrices $\mathbf{\Theta}_{21}$ and $\mathbf{\Theta}_{22}$ along lines similar to those outlined above, but rather than pursuing this route, it is more expeditious from the point of view of writing software to proceed to the general case of $m \geq 2$ behavioral classes and $n \geq 2$ stages of a disease.

To this end, let $\mathbf{1}_{n+1}$ be a $(n+1)\times 1$ column vector with constant element 1 and let $\boldsymbol{\mu}_d$ be a $(n+1) \times 1$ vector with the elements,

$$\boldsymbol{\mu}_d = \begin{bmatrix} 0 \\ \mu_1 \\ \vdots \\ \mu_n \end{bmatrix} , \tag{10.4.13}$$

where μ_i, $i = 1, 2, \cdots, n$, is an incremental risk of death for a person in stage i of disease. Given these definitions, the $m(n+1) \times 2$ matrix $\boldsymbol{\Theta}_{21}$ of latent risks, governing transitions from the set of transient states to the set of absorbing states, may be represented in the partitioned form,

$$\boldsymbol{\Theta}_{21} = \begin{bmatrix} \mu_0 \mathbf{1}_{n+1} & \boldsymbol{\mu}_d \\ \mu_0 \mathbf{1}_{n+1} & \boldsymbol{\mu}_d \\ \vdots & \vdots \\ \mu_0 \mathbf{1}_{n+1} & \boldsymbol{\mu}_d \end{bmatrix} . \tag{10.4.14}$$

In the general case, $\boldsymbol{\Psi} = (\psi_{ij})$ is a $m \times m$ matrix of latent risks, governing transitions among behavioral classes, and $\boldsymbol{\Gamma} = (\gamma_{ij})$ is a $n \times n$ matrix of risks, governing transitions among stages of disease. Just as in the simple case outlined above, the $m(n+1)\times$ $m(n+1)$ sub-matrix $\boldsymbol{\Theta}_{22}$ may be represented in the partitioned form,

$$\boldsymbol{\Theta}_{22} = (\boldsymbol{\Theta}_{22}(i,j) \mid i,j = 1, 2, \cdots, m) , \tag{10.4.15}$$

where each sub-matrix $\boldsymbol{\Theta}_{22}(i,j)$ is of order $(n+1) \times (n+1)$. Further, let $\tau(i) = (i, 0)$ denote a susceptible person in class i and define a $1 \times n$ row vector $\boldsymbol{\Phi}(i)$ by

$$\boldsymbol{\Phi}(i) = (\lambda(i) Q_{par}(t; \tau(i), 0, \cdots, 0)) \tag{10.4.16}$$

for $i = 1, 2, \cdots, m$.

Then, because within each risk class the sub-matrices $\boldsymbol{\Theta}_{22}(i,i)$ on the quasi-diagonal of $\boldsymbol{\Theta}_{22}$ contain latent risks that govern transitions among states of disease, these $(n+1) \times (n+1)$ matrices have the partitioned form,

$$\boldsymbol{\Theta}_{22}(i,i) = \begin{bmatrix} 0 & \boldsymbol{\Phi}(i) \\ \mathbf{0}_n & \boldsymbol{\Gamma} \end{bmatrix} \tag{10.4.17}$$

for $i = 1, 2, \cdots, m$, where $\mathbf{0}_n$ is a $n \times 1$ vector of zeros. All sub-matrices of $\boldsymbol{\Theta}_{22}$ off the quasi-diagonal contain those latent risks, governing transitions among behavioral classes. Just as in the simple case outlined above, these matrices have a simple diagonal form. For, let $\mathbf{I}_{n+1}$ be an identity matrix of order $n+1$. Then, if $i \neq j$,

$$\boldsymbol{\Theta}_{22}(i,j) = diag(\psi_{ij}) = \psi_{ij}\mathbf{I}_{n+1} \,. \tag{10.4.18}$$

In passing, it should be mentioned that the structured matrices just described are very helpful in writing software to handle the book keeping aspects of computer experiments such as sorting data by types of individuals in Monte Carlo simulation experiments.

10.5 Stochastic Evolutionary Equations for the Population

Having outlined the structure of the semi-Markovian processes describing the life cycles of individuals in the population, the next step in the formulation of the model is to proceed to the evolution of the population as a whole, using the latent risks described in the previous section. Because, as just illustrated, some latent risks may depend on $t \in S_h$, from now on all latent risks will carry the argument t, even though most of them will be constant. Suppose at some time t a matrix $\boldsymbol{\Theta}(t) = (\theta(t; \tau_1, \tau_2))$ has been specified for some number $m \geq 1$ of behavioral classes and $n \geq 1$ stages of disease. For every t, it will be assumed that this matrix is constant on the interval $(t, t+h]$. By definition, for every transient state $\tau_1 \in \mathfrak{S}_2$, the total risk function on this interval is:

$$\theta(t; \tau_1) = \sum_{\tau_2 \in \mathfrak{S}} \theta(t; \tau_1, \tau_2) \,. \tag{10.5.1}$$

Whenever the risk functions are constant on the time interval $(t, t+h]$, it can be shown, by appealing to the classical theory of competing risks, that, given an individual is in state $\tau_1 \in \mathfrak{S}_2$ at time t, the conditional probability $\pi(t;\tau_1,\tau_1)$ that he is still in this state at time $t+h$ is:

$$\pi(t;\tau_1,\tau_1) = \exp\left[-\theta(t;\tau_1)h\right] . \tag{10.5.2}$$

Therefore, the conditional probability of a jump to some other state during this time interval is $1-\exp\left[-\theta(t;\tau_1)h\right]$. Consequently, another appeal to the theory of competing risks leads to the conclusion that, given an individual in transient state τ_1 at time t,

$$\pi(t;\tau_1,\tau_2) = \left(1-\exp\left[-\theta(t;\tau_1)h\right]\right)\frac{\theta(t;\tau_1,\tau_2)}{\theta(t;\tau_1)} \tag{10.5.3}$$

is the conditional probability of a jump to some state $\tau_2 \in \mathfrak{S}$ such that $\tau_2 \neq \tau_1$ during the time interval $(t, t+h]$. As they should, for every $\tau_1 \in \mathfrak{S}_2$ and $t \in S_h$, these conditional probabilities satisfy the condition,

$$\sum_{\tau_2\in\mathfrak{S}} \pi(t;\tau_1,\tau_2) = 1 . \tag{10.5.4}$$

For every $\tau_1 \in \mathfrak{S}_2$ and $t \in S_h$, let

$$\mathbf{\Pi}(t;\tau_1) = (\pi(t;\tau_1,\tau_2) \mid \tau_2 \in \mathfrak{S}) \tag{10.5.5}$$

be a vector of these conditional probabilities.

Given there are $X(t;\tau_1)$ persons of type $\tau_1 \in \mathfrak{S}_2$ in the population at time t, let the random function $X_T(t+h;\tau_1,\tau_2)$ denote the number of persons that undergo the transition $\tau_1 \to \tau_2$ during $(t, t+h]$. And, let

$$\mathbf{X}_T(t+h;\tau_1) = (X_T(t;\tau_1,\tau_2) \mid \tau_2 \in \mathfrak{S}) \tag{10.5.6}$$

be a vector of these random functions. It will be assumed that for every τ_1, given $X(t;\tau_1)$, this random vector has a conditional multinomial distribution with index $X(t;\tau_1)$ and probability vector $\mathbf{\Pi}(t;\tau_1)$. In symbols,

$$\mathbf{X}_T(t+h;\tau_1) \sim CMultinom\left(X(t;\tau_1), \mathbf{\Pi}(t;\tau_1)\right) \tag{10.5.7}$$

for every $\tau_1 \in \mathfrak{S}_2$.

To accommodate recruits entering the population, let $\varphi(\tau)$ be the probability that a recruit of type $\tau \in \mathfrak{S}_2$ enters the population during $(t, t+h]$. It will be assumed that these probabilities constitute a proper probability distribution so the condition,

$$\sum_{\tau \in \mathfrak{S}_2} \varphi(\tau) = 1 \tag{10.5.8}$$

is satisfied. The number of recruits of type τ entering the population during $(t, t+h]$ will be denoted by the random function $X_R(t+h;\tau)$. If it is assumed that recruits enter the population according to a Poisson process at rate μ_r per unit time, then it can be shown that the random function $X_R(t+h;\tau)$ has a conditional Poisson distribution with parameter $\mu_r\varphi(\tau)h$. In symbols,

$$X_R(t+h;\tau) \sim CPois\left(\mu_r\varphi(\tau)h\right) . \tag{10.5.9}$$

For the one-sex model of a homosexual population under consideration, the stochastic evolutionary equations for computing Monte Carlo realizations of the process have a simple form. For, let the random function $X(t+h;\tau_1)$ be the number of persons of type $\tau_1 \in \mathfrak{S}_2$ in the population at time $t+h$, given the collection of random functions,

$$\{X(t;\tau) \mid \tau \in \mathfrak{S}_2\} \tag{10.5.10}$$

at time t. Then,

$$X(t+h;\tau_1) = X_R(t+h;\tau_1) + \sum_{\tau \in \mathfrak{S}_2} X_T(t+h;\tau,\tau_1) \tag{10.5.11}$$

for all $\tau_1 \in \mathfrak{S}_2$.

It is often useful to account for deaths in the software. In this connection, for any $\tau_d \in \mathfrak{S}_1$, the number of deaths of type τ_d occurring during the time interval $(t, t+h]$ is given by the random function,

$$X_D(t+h;\tau_d) = \sum_{\tau \in \mathfrak{S}_2} X_T(t+h;\tau,\tau_d) . \tag{10.5.12}$$

Another useful statistic to take into account in the software is the incidence of new infections during any time interval $(t, t+h]$. For a susceptible person of type $\tau_1(i) = (i, 0)$, the transition represented by

$\tau_1(i) \to \tau_2(i) = (i,1)$ indicates that a person in behavioral class i, where $i = 1, 2, \cdots, m$, has been infected. Therefore, the incidence of new infections during this time interval is given by the random function,

$$X_{INC}(t+h) = \sum_{i=1}^{m} X_T(t+h; \tau_1(i), \tau_2(i)) . \tag{10.5.13}$$

From the foregoing, it may be seen that the principal component of the software needed to compute Monte Carlo realizations of the process is a program for computing realizations of a multinomial random vector. For this reason, models of the type under consideration are sometimes referred to as chain multinomial models. Many statistical software packages contain programs to simulate realizations of multinomial random vectors, but, if such a program is not readily available, it is not difficult to write one. The software needed to statistically summarize the simulated realizations of the population process is, however, more complex and difficult to write than that for simulating realizations of a multinomial random vector. But, the task of writing such software may be simplified if an array manipulating language such as APL is used.

10.6 Embedded Non-linear Difference Equations

Even though the evolution of an epidemic in a real population is subject to much variation and uncertainty, deterministic models tend to dominate the literature. It is, therefore, of interest to make connections between stochastic and deterministic formulations along lines similar to those outlined in Chapter 3. A question that naturally arises is in what sense is a trajectory computed according to a deterministic model a measure of central tendency for the sample functions of a stochastic process? A commonly used measure of central tendency of any random variable is an expectation or conditional expectation.

Accordingly, let $\mathfrak{B}(t)$ denote a σ-sub-algebra in a probability space underlying the process induced by the sample functions of the process up to time t. Then, for every $\tau_1 \in \mathfrak{S}_2$, from Eq. (10.5.11) it can be seen that given $\mathfrak{B}(t)$, the conditional expectation of the random function $X(t+h;\tau_1)$ is:

$$E\left[X(t+h;\tau_1)\mid \mathfrak{B}(t)\right] = \mu_r\varphi(\tau_1)h + \sum_{\tau\in\mathfrak{S}_2} X(t;\tau)\pi(t;\tau,\tau_1)\,. \quad (10.6.1)$$

In general, the conditional probability $\pi(t;\tau,\tau_1)$ will be a non-linear function of the sample functions of the process at t and is thus a random variable so that the expectation of $X(t;\tau)\pi(t;\tau,\tau_1)$ cannot be expressed in elementary terms. Consequently, the operation of taking expectations in Eq. (10.6.1) to obtain unconditional expectations will not yield useful results. However, if initial conditions $\{X(0;\tau_1)\mid \tau_1\in\mathfrak{S}_2\}$ are specified, then $\pi(0;\tau,\tau_1)$ will be known for all pairs (τ,τ_1) and thus the conditional expectation,

$$\widehat{X}(h;\tau_1) = E\left[X(h;\tau_1)\mid \mathfrak{B}(t)\right] \quad (10.6.2)$$

may be determined for all $\tau_1\in\mathfrak{S}_2$. And, given these values, all the π-functions may be estimated by:

$$\widehat{\pi}(h;\tau;\tau_1)\,, \quad (10.6.3)$$

and thus $X(2h;\tau_1)$ may be estimated by:

$$\widehat{X}(2h;\tau_1) = \mu_r\varphi(\tau_1)h + \sum_{\tau\in\mathfrak{S}_2} \widehat{X}(h;\tau)\widehat{\pi}(h;\tau,\tau_1) \quad (10.6.4)$$

for all $\tau_1\in\mathfrak{S}_2$.

In general, if the values $\{\widehat{X}(t,\tau_1)\mid \tau_1\in\mathfrak{S}_2\}$ are known, then all the conditional π-probabilities may be estimated and one obtains a set of non-linear difference equations,

$$\widehat{X}(t+h;\tau_1) = \mu_r\varphi(\tau_1)h + \sum_{\tau\in\mathfrak{S}_2} \widehat{X}(t;\tau)\widehat{\pi}(t;\tau,\tau_1) \quad (10.6.5)$$

for $\tau_1\in\mathfrak{S}_2$. It is clear that these equations may be evaluated recursively for all $t\in S_h$, given a set of numerically specified initial conditions. Similarly, for every $\tau_d\in\mathfrak{S}_1$, the number of deaths of type τ_d occurring in the time interval $(t,t+h]$ would be estimated by:

$$\widehat{X}_D(t+h;\tau_d) = \sum_{\tau\in\mathfrak{S}_2} \widehat{X}(t;\tau)\widehat{\pi}(t;\tau,\tau_d)\,. \quad (10.6.6)$$

for all $t \in S_h$. In a similar vein, according to the embedded non-linear difference equations, the incidence of infections during $(t, t+h]$ would be estimated by:

$$\widehat{X}_{INC}(t+h) = \sum_{i=1}^{m} \widehat{X}(t; \tau_1(i))\widehat{\pi}(t; \tau_1(i), \tau_2(i)) , \tag{10.6.7}$$

where $\tau_1(i) = (i, 0)$ and $\tau_2(i) = (i, 1)$.

There are at least two advantages to embedding non-linear difference equations in the stochastic population process. First of all, the procedure just outlined provides a systematic approach to finding connections between a stochastic formulation and a set of deterministic equations that may arise if an investigator were working solely within a deterministic paradigm. A second reason is that non-linear difference equations are easier to implement and require much less computer time, because only one trajectory needs to be computed rather than a sample of trajectories that is required in the execution of Monte Carlo simulation experiments. As will be shown by examples, however, if an investigator were to confine his or her attention to trajectories computed according to a deterministic model, then his or her conclusions may, in fact, be quite misleading when compared with a statistically summarized sample of Monte Carlo realizations of a population process, particularly when there is a positive probability that an epidemic will become extinct.

To further expedite a mathematical analysis of the embedded deterministic equations, it will be helpful to cast Eqs. (10.6.5) in vector-matrix form. To this end, let $h = 1$ and define a $m(n+1) \times m(n+1)$ matrix of estimates of transition probabilities for the population process by

$$\widehat{\mathbf{\Pi}}_{22}(t) = (\widehat{\pi}(t; \tau_1, \tau_2) \mid \tau_1 \in \mathfrak{S}_2, \tau_2 \in \mathfrak{S}_2) \tag{10.6.8}$$

for all $t \in S_h$. To make the notation consistent with that in the next section, vectors with a prime will stand for row vectors; while those without a prime will denote column vectors. Thus, let

$$\mathbf{R}' = (\mu_r \varphi(\tau_1) \mid \tau_1 \in \mathfrak{S}_2) \tag{10.6.9}$$

and

$$\widehat{\mathbf{X}}'(t) = \left(\widehat{X}(t; \tau_1) \mid \tau_1 \in \mathfrak{S}_2\right) \tag{10.6.10}$$

for $t \in S_h$ be $1 \times m(n+1)$ row vectors. Then, Eqs. (10.6.5) may be written in the compact vector-matrix form

$$\widehat{\mathbf{X}}'(t+1) = \mathbf{R}' + \widehat{\mathbf{X}}'(t)\widehat{\mathbf{\Pi}}_{22}(t) \tag{10.6.11}$$

for $t \in S_h$.

Let $\widehat{\mathbf{X}}'(0)$ denote the preassigned initial vector. Then,

$$\widehat{\mathbf{X}}'(1) = \mathbf{R}' + \widehat{\mathbf{X}}'(0)\widehat{\mathbf{\Pi}}_{22}(0) , \tag{10.6.12}$$

and by another iteration, it can be seen that

$$\widehat{\mathbf{X}}'(2) = \mathbf{R}'\left(\mathbf{I}_{m(n+1)} + \widehat{\mathbf{\Pi}}_{22}(1)\right) + \widehat{\mathbf{X}}'(0)\widehat{\mathbf{\Pi}}_{22}(0)\widehat{\mathbf{\Pi}}_{22}(1) , \tag{10.6.13}$$

where $\mathbf{I}_{m(n+1)}$ is a $m(n+1) \times m(n+1)$ identity matrix. In general, by continuing this iterative procedure, for any $t \geq 2$, it can be shown that

$$\begin{aligned}\widehat{\mathbf{X}}'(t) = \mathbf{R}'(\mathbf{I}_{m(n+1)} &+ \widehat{\mathbf{\Pi}}_{22}(t-1) + \widehat{\mathbf{\Pi}}_{22}(t-2)\widehat{\mathbf{\Pi}}_{22}(t-1) + \cdots \\ &+ \prod_{\nu=1}^{t-1} \widehat{\mathbf{\Pi}}_{22}(\nu)) + \widehat{\mathbf{X}}'(0)\prod_{\nu=0}^{t-1} \widehat{\mathbf{\Pi}}_{22}(\nu) .\end{aligned} \tag{10.6.14}$$

From this result, it can be seen that a necessary condition for the vector $\widehat{\mathbf{X}}'(t)$ to become independent of the initial vector $\widehat{\mathbf{X}}'(0)$ as $t \uparrow \infty$ is that

$$\lim_{t\uparrow\infty} \prod_{\nu=0}^{t-1} \widehat{\mathbf{\Pi}}_{22}(\nu) = \mathbf{0}_{m(n+1)} \, . \tag{10.6.15}$$

a $m(n+1) \times m(n+1)$ zero matrix.

In computer experiments, it is often of interest to consider the case that one infective is introduced into a population of susceptibles that have been evolving according to the above deterministic model. When there are no infectives in the population and all recruits are susceptible, then it can be seen by inspection of the system that the transition matrix in Eq. (10.6.8) is constant, say $\mathbf{\Pi}_{22}$. In this case, Eq. (10.6.14) becomes

$$\widehat{\mathbf{X}}'(t) = \mathbf{R}'\left(\mathbf{I}_{m(n+1)} + \mathbf{\Pi}_{22} + \mathbf{\Pi}_{22}^2 + \cdots + \mathbf{\Pi}_{22}^{t-1}\right) + \widehat{\mathbf{X}}'(0)\mathbf{\Pi}_{22}^t . \tag{10.6.16}$$

The matrix $\mathbf{\Pi}_{22}$ may actually be viewed as that for transitions among transient states in a time homogeneous Markov chain with a finite state space and two absorbing states. As has been demonstrated in previous chapters, under general conditions, it can be shown that such matrices have the property

$$\lim_{t\uparrow\infty} \mathbf{\Pi}_{22}^{t} = \mathbf{0}_{m(n+1)} \,. \tag{10.6.17}$$

Therefore, in this case the vector in Eq. (10.6.16) has a limit as $t \uparrow \infty$ independent of initial conditions, which is given by

$$\lim_{t\uparrow\infty} \widehat{\mathbf{X}}'(t) = \mathbf{R}' \left(\mathbf{I}_{m(n+1)} - \mathbf{\Pi}_{22}\right)^{-1} \,. \tag{10.6.18}$$

For those computer experiments in which one infective is introduced into a population of susceptibles that are assumed to have been evolving according to the above deterministic model, the vector in Eq. (10.6.18) may be chosen as the initial vector.

10.7 Embedded Non-linear Differential Equations

The non-linear difference equations discussed in Section 10.6 may be viewed as discrete time approximations to differential equations in continuous time, and as $h \downarrow 0$ one would expect that a set of differential equations would arise. From the analytic point of view, differential equations may be easier to handle than difference equations, and, moreover, their analysis could be helpful in deriving threshold conditions for the stochastic process. From the definitions of the π-conditional probabilities in Section 10.5, it follows that for all $\tau \in \mathfrak{S}_2$,

$$\widehat{\pi}(t;\tau,\tau) = 1 - \widehat{\theta}(t;\tau)h + o(h) \,, \tag{10.7.1}$$

where $\widehat{\theta}(t;\tau)$ is an estimate of the total risk function $\theta(t;\tau)$ and it is the case that $o(h)/h \to 0$ as $h \downarrow 0$. Similarly, if $\tau \neq \tau_1$, then

$$\widehat{\pi}(t;\tau,\tau_1) = \widehat{\theta}(t;\tau,\tau_1)h + o(h) \,. \tag{10.7.2}$$

From these relationships, it follows that the non-linear difference equations in Eq. (10.6.5) may be represented as:

$$\widehat{X}(t+h;\tau_1) = \mu_r\varphi(\tau_1)h + \widehat{X}(t;\tau_1)\left(1 - \widehat{\theta}(t;\tau_1)h\right)$$

$$+ \sum_{\tau \neq \tau_1} \widehat{X}(t;\tau)\widehat{\theta}(t;\tau,\tau_1)h + o(h) \tag{10.7.3}$$

for every $\tau_1 \in \mathfrak{S}_2$. Thus, by transposing terms and forming the ratios,

$$\frac{\widehat{X}(t+h;\tau_1) - \widehat{X}(t;\tau_1)}{h} \tag{10.7.4}$$

and letting $h \downarrow 0$, one arrives at the system of embedded differential equations,

$$\frac{d\widehat{X}(t;\tau_1)}{dt} = \mu_r \varphi(\tau_1) - \widehat{X}(t;\tau_1)\widehat{\theta}(t;\tau_1) + \sum_{\tau \neq \tau_1} \widehat{X}(t;\tau,\tau_1)\,, \tag{10.7.5}$$

which hold for all $t \in [0, \infty)$ and $\tau_1 \in \mathfrak{S}_2$.

To analyze these equations further, it will be useful to represent them in a canonical vector-matrix notation. To this end, define a square matrix $\widehat{\Xi}(t)$ whose transpose is given by:

$$\widehat{\Xi}'(t) = \widehat{\mathbf{\Theta}}_{22}(t) - diag\left(\widehat{\theta}(t;\tau_1) \mid \tau_1 \in \mathfrak{S}_2\right) . \tag{10.7.6}$$

Observe that the matrix $\widehat{\Xi}(t)$ contains the negatives of the total risk functions on its principal diagonal (see Eq. (10.5.1)). From now on $'$ will stand for the transpose of a matrix. And let $\widehat{\mathbf{X}}(t)$ and $\mathbf{R}$ be column versions of the row vectors defined in Section 10.6. Then, the above differential equations may be represented in the succinct form,

$$\frac{d\widehat{\mathbf{X}}(t)}{dt} = \mathbf{R} + \widehat{\Xi}(t)\widehat{\mathbf{X}}(t) . \tag{10.7.7}$$

As will be shown by examples in the next section, there is a constant square matrix $\mathbf{A}$ and a square matrix $\widehat{\mathbf{W}}(t)$ of non-linear terms involving sexual contacts such that:

$$\widehat{\Xi}(t) = \mathbf{A} + \widehat{\mathbf{W}}(t) . \tag{10.7.8}$$

Therefore, the embedded non-linear differential equations take the form,

$$\frac{d\widehat{\mathbf{X}}(t)}{dt} = \mathbf{R} + \mathbf{A}\widehat{\mathbf{X}}(t) + \widehat{\mathbf{W}}(t)\widehat{\mathbf{X}}(t) , \tag{10.7.9}$$

with $\widehat{\mathbf{X}}(0)$ as the initial vector.

To integrate this system, consider the general inhomogeneous system of the form,

$$\frac{d\mathbf{x}(t)}{dt} = \mathbf{A}\mathbf{x}(t) + \mathbf{g}(t) \tag{10.7.10}$$

for $t \in [0, \infty)$, where $\mathbf{x}(t)$ and $\mathbf{g}(t)$ are finite dimensional column vectors of functions and $\mathbf{A}$ is a square matrix of constants. Then, consider the transformation,

$$\mathbf{y}(t) = e^{-\mathbf{A}t}\mathbf{x}(t) . \tag{10.7.11}$$

Upon differentiation one can see that:

$$\frac{d\mathbf{y}(t)}{dt} = -\mathbf{A}e^{-\mathbf{A}t}\mathbf{x}(t) + e^{-\mathbf{A}t}\frac{d\mathbf{x}(t)}{dt}$$

$$= -\mathbf{A}e^{-\mathbf{A}t}\mathbf{x}(t) + e^{-\mathbf{A}t}\left(\mathbf{A}\mathbf{x}(t) + \mathbf{g}(t)\right) = e^{-\mathbf{A}t}\mathbf{g}(t) , \tag{10.7.12}$$

because the matrix $\mathbf{A}$ commutes with the exponential matrix $e^{-\mathbf{A}t}$. If $\mathbf{x}(0)$ is the initial vector for the system in Eq. (10.7.10), then from Eq. (10.7.11) it follows that $\mathbf{y}(0) = \mathbf{x}(0)$ so that by integrating Eq. (10.7.12) it can be seen that:

$$\mathbf{y}(t) = \mathbf{x}(0) + \int_0^t e^{-\mathbf{A}s}\mathbf{g}(s)ds . \tag{10.7.13}$$

Thus, from Eq. (10.7.11) it may be concluded that $t > 0$,

$$\mathbf{x}(t) = e^{\mathbf{A}t}\mathbf{x}(0) + \int_0^t e^{\mathbf{A}s}\mathbf{g}(t-s)ds . \tag{10.7.14}$$

Finally, by applying this general result to Eq. (10.7.9) with

$$\mathbf{g}(t) = \mathbf{R} + \widehat{\mathbf{W}}(t)\widehat{\mathbf{X}}(t) , \tag{10.7.15}$$

it follows that for $t > 0$,

$$\widehat{\mathbf{X}}(t) = e^{\mathbf{A}t}\widehat{\mathbf{X}}(0) + \int_0^t e^{\mathbf{A}s}\mathbf{R}ds + \int_0^t e^{\mathbf{A}s}\widehat{\mathbf{W}}(t-s)\widehat{\mathbf{X}}(t-s)ds . \tag{10.7.16}$$

From this integral representation of $\widehat{\mathbf{X}}(t)$, it can be seen that the eigenvalues of the matrix $\mathbf{A}$ will play a basic role in determining the behavior of the embedded differential equations as $t \uparrow \infty$. In particular, if the eigenvalues of $\mathbf{A}$ have negative real parts, then the initial conditions "wear off" in the sense that:

$$\lim_{t \uparrow \infty} e^{\mathbf{A}t} \widehat{\mathbf{X}}(0) = \mathbf{0}_{m(n+1)} , \tag{10.7.17}$$

a zero column vector of dimension $m(n+1)$, for every initial vector $\widehat{\mathbf{X}}(0)$. Observe that one immediate advantage to considering the embedded differential equations is that the deduction of Eq. (10.7.17) involves a much simpler argument than would have been required to deduce the same result from the general form of the solution to the discrete non-linear difference equations in Eq. (10.6.13).

For the case where the initial population contains no infectives and no infective recruits enter the population subsequently, the matrix $\widehat{\mathbf{W}}(t)$ is a zero matrix for all $t \geq 0$. In this case, the solution of the embedded differential equations has the simple vector-matrix representation,

$$\widehat{\mathbf{X}}(t) = e^{\mathbf{A}t} \widehat{\mathbf{X}}(0) + \int_0^t e^{\mathbf{A}s} \mathbf{R} ds . \tag{10.7.18}$$

If the matrix $\mathbf{A}$ is also non-singular, then integration yields the symbolic formula,

$$\widehat{\mathbf{X}}(t) = e^{\mathbf{A}t} \widehat{\mathbf{X}}(0) + \mathbf{A}^{-1} e^{\mathbf{A}t} \mathbf{R} - \mathbf{A}^{-1} \mathbf{R} , \tag{10.7.19}$$

which, with the help of such symbolic software packages as MAPLE, may be evaluated numerically at chosen points $t \in [0, \infty)$.

10.8 Examples of Coefficient Matrices

As a first step toward the goal of exploring some properties of the differential equations in Eq. (10.7.9), it will be of interest to give some examples of the coefficients matrices $\mathbf{A}$ and $\widehat{\mathbf{W}}(t)$ in this system of equations. One of the simplest cases to explore is that of $m = 2$ two behavioral classes and $n = 1$ one stage of disease. In this case, there are four types of persons; namely, $\tau_1 = (1, 0)$, $\tau_2 = (1, 1), \tau_3 = (2, 0)$, and $\tau_4 = (2, 1)$, and the rates of transition among the two behavioral classes may be represented in the 2×2 matrix,

$$\mathbf{\Psi} = \begin{bmatrix} 0 & \psi_{12} \\ \psi_{21} & 0 \end{bmatrix}. \tag{10.8.1}$$

Furthermore, if one applies the formula in Eq. (10.7.6), then it can be seen that the transpose of the matrix $\mathbf{A}$ has the form,

$$\mathbf{A}' = \begin{bmatrix} a_{11} & 0 & \psi_{12} & 0 \\ 0 & a_{22} & 0 & \psi_{12} \\ \psi_{21} & 0 & a_{33} & 0 \\ 0 & \psi_{21} & 0 & a_{44} \end{bmatrix}, \tag{10.8.2}$$

where $a_{11} = -(\mu_0+\psi_{12})$, $a_{22} = -(\mu_0+\mu_1+\psi_{12})$, $a_{33} = -(\mu_0+\psi_{21})$, and $a_{44} = -(\mu_0 + \mu_1 + \psi_{21})$. Similarly, it can be shown that the transpose the matrix $\widehat{\mathbf{W}}(t)$ has the form,

$$\widehat{\mathbf{W}}'(t) = \begin{bmatrix} w_{11} & w_{12} & 0 & 0 \\ 0 & 0 & 0 & 0 \\ 0 & 0 & w_{33} & w_{34} \\ 0 & 0 & 0 & 0 \end{bmatrix}, \tag{10.8.3}$$

where it is the case that $w_{11} = -\lambda(1)\hat{Q}_{par}(t;\tau_1)$, $w_{12} = \lambda(1)\hat{Q}_{par}(t;\tau_1)$, $w_{33} = -\lambda(2)\hat{Q}_{par}(t;\tau_3)$, and $w_{34} = \lambda(2)\hat{Q}_{par}(t;\tau_3)$. Observe that all the non-diagonal elements of the matrix $\mathbf{A}$ are non-negative; while elements on the principal diagonal will be negative if at least one of the parameters are positive. Also observe that the row sums of the matrix in Eq. (10.8.3) are zero. Even for more complicated cases, the $\widehat{\mathbf{W}}$ matrix would have a similar form, but from now on in this section no further illustrative examples of this matrix will be exhibited.

Some authors (see Capasso[2]) refer to matrices having the form of Eq. (10.8.2) with negative elements on the principal diagonal and non-negative elements elsewhere as quasi-monotone. Because these matrices arise quite frequently, some basic theorems about them appear in classical books such as Gantmacher.[3] Among these theorems, which may be deduced easily from the Perron-Frobenius theory of matrices with non-negative elements, is one which states that if a matrix $\mathbf{A}$ is

$n \times n$ quasi-monotone, then there is a real simple eigenvalue λ_0 such that if λ_i is any eigenvalue of $\mathbf{A}$, then for all $i = 1, 2, \cdots, n$,

$$\mathrm{Re}\,(\lambda_i) \leq \lambda_0 \,. \tag{10.8.4}$$

As we saw in Section 10.7, if all the eigenvalues of the matrix $\mathbf{A} = (a_{ij})$ have negative real parts, i.e., it is stable, then the effects of the initial conditions "wear off" (see Eq. (10.7.17)). Necessary and sufficient conditions for a quasi-monotone matrix to be stable may be expressed in terms of conditions on its principal minors. Let

$$\begin{aligned}
\Delta_1 &= a_{11}\,, \\
\Delta_2 &= \det \begin{bmatrix} a_{11} & a_{12} \\ a_{21} & a_{22} \end{bmatrix}, \\
\Delta_3 &= \det \begin{bmatrix} a_{11} & a_{12} & a_{13} \\ a_{21} & a_{22} & a_{23} \\ a_{31} & a_{32} & a_{33} \end{bmatrix}, \\
&\ \ \vdots \\
\Delta_n &= \det \mathbf{A}\,.
\end{aligned} \tag{10.8.5}$$

Then, the eigenvalues of $\mathbf{A}$ have negative real parts if, and only if,

$$\Delta_1 < 0,\ \Delta_2 > 0, \cdots, (-1)^n\,\Delta_n > 0\,. \tag{10.8.6}$$

For a proof of this result see Gantmacher.[3] With MAPLE, these conditions may be easily checked, if $\mathbf{A}$ is not too large. In some cases one can derive symbolic forms for the eigenvalues of a matrix. For example, the symbolic form of the eigenvalues of the matrix in Eq. (10.8.2) are:

$$\begin{aligned}
\lambda_1 &= -\mu_0 \\
\lambda_2 &= -(\mu_0 + \mu_1) \\
\lambda_3 &= -(\mu_0 + \psi_{21} + \psi_{12}) \\
\lambda_4 &= -(\mu_0 + \mu_1 + \psi_{21} + \psi_{12})\,.
\end{aligned} \tag{10.8.7}$$

Because $\mu_0 > 0$, by assumption and all other parameters are non-negative, it can be seen that all eigenvalues of the matrix in Eq. (10.8.2) are negative so that the matrix $\mathbf{A}$ is stable in this case for all points in the parameter space. The dominant eigenvalue is $\lambda_0 = -\mu_0$, which is of substantive interest because it depends only on the basic mortality parameter μ_0.

Another illustrative case of interest is that for $m = 2$ behavioral classes and $n = 2$ stages of disease. In this case, the $\mathbf{A}$-matrix is 6×6 and the negative of its diagonal elements have the form,

$$\begin{aligned}
\theta_1^* &= \mu_0 + \psi_{12} \\
\theta_2 &= \mu_0 + \mu_1 + \psi_{12} + \gamma_{12} \\
\theta_3 &= \mu_0 + \mu_2 + \psi_{12} + \gamma_{21} \\
\theta_4^* &= \mu_0 + \psi_{21} \\
\theta_5 &= \mu_0 + \mu_1 + \psi_{21} + \gamma_{12} \\
\theta_6 &= \mu_0 + \mu_2 + \psi_{21} + \gamma_{21} \,.
\end{aligned} \tag{10.8.8}$$

As an aid to understanding the derivation of the expressions, observe that for $i = 2, 3, 5, 6$, θ_i is the total risk function and θ_1^* and θ_4^* are the total risk functions minus the nonlinear terms for sexual contacts. Recall that the γ's are elements of the matrix,

$$\mathbf{\Gamma} = \begin{bmatrix} 0 & \gamma_{12} \\ \gamma_{21} & 0 \end{bmatrix}, \tag{10.8.9}$$

governing transitions among the two stages of the disease.

For this case, the transpose of the matrix $\mathbf{A}$ has the form,

$$\mathbf{A}' = \begin{bmatrix}
-\theta_1^* & 0 & 0 & \psi_{12} & 0 & 0 \\
0 & -\theta_2 & \gamma_{12} & 0 & \psi_{12} & 0 \\
0 & \gamma_{21} & -\theta_3 & 0 & 0 & \psi_{12} \\
\psi_{21} & 0 & 0 & -\theta_4^* & 0 & 0 \\
0 & \psi_{21} & 0 & 0 & -\theta_5 & \gamma_{12} \\
0 & 0 & \psi_{21} & 0 & \gamma_{21} & -\theta_6
\end{bmatrix}. \tag{10.8.10}$$

The symbolic forms of the eigenvalues of this matrix are, for the most part, too cumbersome to be printed, but it is feasible to apply the determinantal criteria in Eq. (10.8.6) to determine whether the matrix is stable at all points in the parameter space. It is easy to see that $\Delta_1 < 0$ and $\Delta_2 > 0$ at all points in the parameter space, and, with the help of MAPLE, it can be shown that the determinantal criteria in Eq. (10.8.6) are indeed satisfied for all points in the parameter space. Therefore, it may be concluded that the matrix **A** is stable at all points in the parameter space. Another observation of interest is that $-\mu_0$ is also an eigenvalue of this matrix.

For more general cases with $m \geq 2$ behavioral classes and $n \geq 2$ stages of disease, the **A**-matrix may indeed be quite large. However, some insights into the nature of more general cases may be obtained by the considering the case of $m = 1$ behavioral class and $n = 4$ stages of disease. The **Γ**-matrix, governing transitions among stages of the disease, would be 4×4 for this version of the model, but the details will be omitted. For this case, the negatives of the diagonal elements of the **A**-matrix have the form,

$$\begin{aligned} \theta_1^* &= \mu_0 \\ \theta_2 &= \mu_0 + \mu_1 + \gamma_{12} \\ \theta_3 &= \mu_0 + \mu_2 + \gamma_{21} + \gamma_{23} \\ \theta_4 &= \mu_0 + \mu_3 + \gamma_{32} + \gamma_{34} \\ \theta_5 &= \mu_0 + \mu_4 + \gamma_{43} \,. \end{aligned} \tag{10.8.11}$$

And, the transpose of the 5×5 matrix **A** has the form,

$$\mathbf{A}' = \begin{bmatrix} -\theta_1^* & 0 & 0 & 0 & 0 \\ 0 & -\theta_2 & \gamma_{12} & 0 & 0 \\ 0 & \gamma_{21} & -\theta_3 & \gamma_{23} & 0 \\ 0 & 0 & \gamma_{32} & -\theta_4 & \gamma_{34} \\ 0 & 0 & 0 & \gamma_{43} & -\theta_5 \end{bmatrix} . \tag{10.8.12}$$

The matrix in Eq. (10.8.12) is an example of a matrix that may be represented in a partitioned quasi-diagonal form, which will simplify determining whether it is a stable matrix at all points in the parameter space. To see this, let $\mathbf{A}_{11} = (-\theta_1^*)$ be a one by one matrix; define a 4×4 matrix $\mathbf{A}_{22}$ by:

$$\mathbf{A}_{22} = \begin{bmatrix} -\theta_2 & \gamma_{12} & 0 & 0 \\ \gamma_{21} & -\theta_3 & \gamma_{23} & 0 \\ 0 & \gamma_{32} & -\theta_4 & \gamma_{34} \\ 0 & 0 & \gamma_{43} & -\theta_5 \end{bmatrix}, \tag{10.8.13}$$

and let $\mathbf{0}_4$ be a 4×1 vector of zeros. Then, Eq. (10.8.12) may be represented in the quasi-diagonal partitioned form,

$$\mathbf{A}' = \begin{bmatrix} \mathbf{A}_{11} & \mathbf{0}_4' \\ \mathbf{0}_4 & \mathbf{A}_{22} \end{bmatrix}. \tag{10.8.14}$$

From this form, it can be seen immediately that $-\mu_0$ is an eigenvalue of $\mathbf{A}$, and to prove that this matrix is stable for all points in the parameter space, it suffices to prove that the 4×4 matrix $\mathbf{A}_{22}$ is stable. For this matrix, it can be seen that $\Delta_1 = -\theta_2 < 0$, and with the help of MAPLE, it can be shown that

$$\Delta_2 = \mu_0^2 + \mu_0\mu_2 + \mu_0\gamma_{21} + \mu_0\gamma_{23} + \mu_1\mu_0 + \mu_1\mu_2 + \mu_1\gamma_{21} + \mu_1\gamma_{23} + \gamma_{12}\mu_0 + \gamma_{12}\mu_2 + \gamma_{12}\gamma_{23}\,. \tag{10.8.15}$$

From this symbolic form, it is clear that $\Delta_2 > 0$ for all points in the parameter space. Even though the symbolic forms of the determinants Δ_3 and Δ_4 contain too many terms to print on a page, from inspection it may be concluded that $\Delta_3 < 0$ and $\Delta_4 > 0$ at all points in the parameter space. Thus, the matrix $\mathbf{A}$ is also stable in this case.

For some points in the parameter space, the matrix in Eq. (10.8.12) has a simple upper triangular form. For example, if it is assumed that the transitions among the four stages of a disease are in only one direction, $1 \to 2 \to 3 \to 4$, then $\gamma_{21} = \gamma_{32} = \gamma_{43} = 0$, so that the matrix in Eq. (10.8.12) has a simple upper triangular form,

$$\mathbf{A}' = \begin{bmatrix} -\theta_1^* & 0 & 0 & 0 & 0 \\ 0 & -\theta_2 & \gamma_{12} & 0 & 0 \\ 0 & 0 & -\theta_3 & \gamma_{23} & 0 \\ 0 & 0 & 0 & -\theta_4 & \gamma_{34} \\ 0 & 0 & 0 & 0 & -\theta_5 \end{bmatrix}. \tag{10.8.16}$$

It is easy to see that for this matrix $\lambda_0 = \lambda_1 = -\mu_0$ is the dominant eigenvalue; moreover, the other eigenvalues are real and are given by $\lambda_i = -\theta_i$ for $i = 2, 3, 4, 5$. More generally, if transitions among behavioral classes and stages of disease can occur only in one direction, then the **A**-matrix will have a triangular form and its eigenvalues will be those negative elements on the principal diagonal, and, therefore, all such matrices will be stable. But, if these transitions may occur in any direction, then the **A**-matrix will not have a triangular form and each case will have to be tested for stability.

In the general case of $m \geq 1$ behavioral classes and $n \geq 1$ stages of disease, the $m(n+1) \times m(n+1)$ matrix **A** will have a more complicated structure. Therefore, if one attempts to verify by symbolic methods that the determinantal conditions in Eq. (10.8.6) hold at all points in the parameter space, one is faced with a complexity barrier in that the resulting algebraic expression is neither readable nor printable. Fortunately, if one adapts the practical strategy of testing the stability of the matrix **A** only at those points in the parameter space of interest, then it would a relatively easy task to write computer programs to compute the eigenvalues of **A** and test whether all real parts are indeed negative. For the most part, this is the strategy that will followed in the remaining sections of this chapter.

10.9 On the Stability of Stationary Points

When working with a deterministic model specified in terms of a system of ordinary nonlinear differential equations, a commonly followed strategy underlying a theoretical investigation is to deduce as many properties of the solutions of the system as possible without solving it symbolically or numerically. This is the strategy that will be followed in this section, but, as we will see, for the multi-parameter systems under consideration, it will be necessary to resort to numerical methods in order to obtain practical results of interest. The first step in the investigation is to write the system of differential equations in Eq. (10.7.9) in a more notationally succinct form that is amenable to analysis by suppressing the argument t.

To this end, let

$$\mathbf{x} = (x_\tau \mid \tau \in \boldsymbol{\Upsilon}) \tag{10.9.1}$$

denote a $m(n+1) \times 1$ column vector, where x_τ is the number of type $\tau \in \boldsymbol{\Upsilon}$ in the population at any time, and let

$$\mathbf{V}(\mathbf{x}) = \widehat{\mathbf{W}}(t)\widehat{\mathbf{X}}(t) \tag{10.9.2}$$

denote a $m(n+1) \times 1$ column vector to emphasize that in this section attention will be focused on the vector $\mathbf{x}$ rather than the variable t. Then, the differential equations in Eq. (10.7.9) may be represented in the compact notational form,

$$\frac{d\mathbf{x}}{dt} = \mathbf{R} + \mathbf{A}\mathbf{x} + \mathbf{V}(\mathbf{x}) \, . \tag{10.9.3}$$

Before proceeding with the analysis, it will be helpful to inspect the structure of the $m(n+1) \times 1$ vector $\mathbf{V}(\mathbf{x})$. By way of illustration, for the case $m = 3$ this vector may be conveniently represented in the partitioned form,

$$\mathbf{V}(\mathbf{x}) = \begin{pmatrix} \mathbf{V}_1(\mathbf{x}) \\ \mathbf{V}_2(\mathbf{x}) \\ \mathbf{V}_3(\mathbf{x}) \end{pmatrix} , \tag{10.9.4}$$

where $\mathbf{V}_i(\mathbf{x})$ is a $(n+1) \times 1$ vector for the ith behavioral class, $i = 1, 2, 3$. To describe the general structure of the vector $\mathbf{V}_i(\mathbf{x})$ for the ith behavioral class, consider the function $\lambda(1)\widehat{Q}_{par}(t;\tau_1)$ occurring in the $\mathbf{W}$-matrix of Eq. (10.8.3), and recall that $\lambda(1)$ is the λ-parameter for behavioral class 1; $\tau_1 = (1,0)$ is a susceptible in class 1; and $\widehat{Q}_{par}(t;\tau_1)$ is the probability that this susceptible is infected, during a small time interval $(t, t+h]$, evaluated at the vector $\mathbf{x}$.

In general, for any susceptible $\tau_1 = (i,0)$, let $\lambda(\tau_1)$ denote the λ-parameter for that behavioral class, and, to simplify the notation and emphasize that the focus of attention is the vector $\mathbf{x}$, define a function $g(\tau_1, \mathbf{x})$ by:

$$g(\tau_1, \mathbf{x}) = \lambda(\tau_1)\widehat{Q}_{par}(t;\tau_1) \, . \tag{10.9.5}$$

Then, from an inspection of the **W**-matrix in Eq. (10.8.3), it can be seen that, for the ith behavioral class, the vector $\mathbf{V}_i(\mathbf{x})$ has the form,

$$\mathbf{V}_i(\mathbf{x}) = \begin{pmatrix} -x_{\tau_1} g(\tau_1, \mathbf{x}) \\ x_{\tau_1} g(\tau_1, \mathbf{x}) \\ \mathbf{0}_{(n-1),1} \end{pmatrix}, \tag{10.9.6}$$

where $\mathbf{0}_{(n-1),1}$ is a $(n-1)\times 1$ vector of zeros for $i = 1, 2, \cdots, m$. Observe that for the case $n = 1$, $\mathbf{V}_i(\mathbf{x})$ is a 2×1 vector and $\mathbf{0}_{(n-1),1}$ is empty.

As an aid to understanding the notation, it will be helpful to consider the simple case $m = 1$ behavioral class and $n = 1$ stage of disease. In this case, the susceptible type is $\tau = 0$, the infectious type is $\tau = 1$, and the transpose of the vector $\mathbf{x}$ has the form $\mathbf{x}' = (x_0, x_1)$. Furthermore, the vectors and matrix in Eq. (10.9.3) have the forms,

$$\mathbf{R} = \mu_r \begin{pmatrix} \varphi(0) \\ \varphi(1) \end{pmatrix}, \tag{10.9.7}$$

$$\mathbf{A} = \begin{pmatrix} -\mu_0 & 0 \\ 0 & -(\mu_0 + \mu_1) \end{pmatrix}, \tag{10.9.8}$$

$$\mathbf{V}(\mathbf{x}) = \begin{pmatrix} -x_0 g(0, \mathbf{x}) \\ x_0 g(0, \mathbf{x}) \end{pmatrix}. \tag{10.9.9}$$

Although more complex cases can be described symbolically in terms of the parameters of the model, it is cumbersome to write them down. However, from the computational point of view, this complexity is not necessarily a barrier to progress if a general notation can be devised so that all the matrices and vectors can be represented numerically in an unambiguous way.

A first step in devising such a notation is to define classes of types that clearly distinguish susceptibles and infectives. Let the symbol $\Upsilon_{iS} = ((i, 0))$ denote the set of susceptible types in behavioral class i and let the symbol,

$$\Upsilon_{iI} = ((i, j) \mid j = 1, 2, \cdots, n) \tag{10.9.10}$$

denote the set of infectious types in behavioral class i. Then, the set of susceptible types is:

$$\Upsilon_S = \bigcup_{i=1}^{m} \Upsilon_{iS}, \tag{10.9.11}$$

and the set of infectious types is:

$$\Upsilon_I = \bigcup_{i=1}^{m} \Upsilon_{iI} \,. \tag{10.9.12}$$

It is clear that $\Upsilon = \Upsilon_S \cup \Upsilon_I$.

Because population numbers are always non-negative, the population state space for the differential equations in Eq. (10.9.3) is the set,

$$\mathfrak{P} = (\mathbf{x} \mid x_\tau \geq 0, \ \tau \in \Upsilon) \tag{10.9.13}$$

of $m(n+1)$-dimensional vectors of non-negative real numbers. Of particular interest is the subset of $\mathfrak{P}$ such that the population contains no infectious individuals. In symbols, this subset is:

$$\mathfrak{P}_S = (\mathbf{x} \in \mathfrak{P} \mid x_\tau = 0 \text{ for all } \tau \in \Upsilon_I) \,. \tag{10.9.14}$$

The complementary set,

$$\mathfrak{P}_I = \mathfrak{P}_S^c \tag{10.9.15}$$

is the subset of $\mathfrak{P}$ such that the population contains as least one infectious individual. When there are no infectious individuals in the population, the probability that a susceptible becomes infected is zero, so that for all $\mathbf{x} \in \mathfrak{P}_S$,

$$\mathbf{V}(\mathbf{x}) = \mathbf{0}_{m(n+1)} \,. \tag{10.9.16}$$

In Chapters 6, 8, and 9, attention was devoted to extending the concept of the threshold parameter R_0 to stochastic models of epidemics that could be approximated by simple or multi-type branching processes in the early stages of an epidemic, when a few infectious individuals were introduced into a large population of susceptibles. Such approximations can, however, be questioned, particularly for those models in which contacts among types of individuals in a population may not occur at random as in the class of models under consideration.

On the other hand, for the present model, one can imagine a population of susceptibles evolving over a long period of time in which all the recruits entering the population are also susceptibles. Under this assumption, the vector for recruits would take the form,

$$\mathbf{R}_S = (\mu_r \varphi(\tau) \mid \varphi(\tau) = 0 \text{ for all } \tau \in \Upsilon_I) \ , \tag{10.9.17}$$

and the set of differential equations governing the evolution of the population takes the linear form,

$$\frac{d\mathbf{x}}{dt} = \mathbf{R}_S + \mathbf{A}\mathbf{x} \,. \tag{10.9.18}$$

When the matrix $\mathbf{A}$ is stable (see Eq. (10.7.19)), then as $t \uparrow \infty$ the vector $\mathbf{x}$ would converge to an equilibrium vector $\widehat{\mathbf{x}} \in \mathfrak{P}_S$ satisfying the linear equation,

$$\mathbf{R}_S + \mathbf{A}\widehat{\mathbf{x}} = \mathbf{0}_{m(n+1)} \,. \tag{10.9.19}$$

If the matrix $\mathbf{A}$ is non-singular, then

$$\widehat{\mathbf{x}} = -\mathbf{A}^{-1}\mathbf{R}_S \,. \tag{10.9.20}$$

Thus, the equilibrium vector $\widehat{\mathbf{x}}$ may be easily computed, provided the matrix $\mathbf{A}$ is not too large. Observe this formula for $\widehat{\mathbf{x}}$ is the same as that which would arise in the limit as $t \uparrow \infty$ in Eq. (10.7.19).

Now suppose a small number of infectives is introduced into a population of susceptibles that has been evolving for a long period of time according to the model under discussion. A question that naturally arises is under what conditions, expressed in terms of points in the parameter space, will the number of infectious individuals either grow to significant numbers in the population or decline to insignificant numbers. Ideally, one would like to find conditions such that eventually the population vector $\mathbf{x}$ stays in the set $\mathfrak{P}_S$, indicating there are no infectives in the population. As we shall see, some answers to this question may be obtained by investigating the stability of the vector $\widehat{\mathbf{x}}$.

Before setting up the machinery to investigate the stability of the vector $\widehat{\mathbf{x}}$ in the general case, it will be helpful to pause to display a symbolic form of this vector for the case $m = 2$ behavioral classes and $n = 1$ stage of disease. For this case, the transpose of the matrix $\mathbf{A}$ is given in Eq. (10.8.2) and the vector $\mathbf{R}_S$ has the form,

$$\mathbf{R}_S = \mu_r \begin{pmatrix} \varphi(1,0) \\ 0 \\ \varphi(2,0) \\ 0 \end{pmatrix} , \tag{10.9.21}$$

where $\varphi(1,0) + \varphi(2,0) = 1$. With the help of MAPLE, it can be shown that the symbolic form of the vector $\widehat{\mathbf{x}}$ in this case is:

$$\widehat{\mathbf{x}} = \mu_r \begin{pmatrix} \frac{\mu_0 + \psi_{21}}{(\mu_0 + \psi_{21} + \psi_{12})\,\mu_0}\varphi_{10} + \frac{\psi_{21}}{(\mu_0 + \psi_{21} + \psi_{12})\,\mu_0}\varphi_{20} \\ 0 \\ \frac{\psi_{12}}{(\mu_0 + \psi_{21} + \psi_{12})\,\mu_0}\varphi_{10} + \frac{\mu_0 + \psi_{12}}{(\mu_0 + \psi_{21} + \psi_{12})\,\mu_0}\varphi_{20} \\ 0 \end{pmatrix} . \tag{10.9.22}$$

For the general case, however, the symbolic form of the vector $\widehat{\mathbf{x}} \in \mathfrak{P}_S$ is too cumbersome to print on a page, but it is not difficult to process numerically.

As a first step in proving an overview of a framework for investigating the stability of the vector $\widehat{\mathbf{x}}$, it will be necessary to consider the Jacobian matrix of the vector-valued function on the right-hand side of the differential equations in Eq. (10.9.3). To this end, suppose that for every susceptible type $\tau_1 \in \Upsilon_S$, the function $g(\tau_1, \mathbf{x})$ in Eq. (10.9.5) is a differentiable function of $\mathbf{x} \in \mathfrak{P}$ in a neighborhood of $\widehat{\mathbf{x}} \in \mathfrak{P}_S$. Then, from an inspection of Eq. (10.9.3), it can be seen that the Jacobian matrix of the system is:

$$\mathbf{J}(\mathbf{x}) = \mathbf{A} + \mathbf{J}_{\mathbf{V}}(\mathbf{x}) , \tag{10.9.23}$$

where $\mathbf{J}_{\mathbf{V}}(\mathbf{x})$ is the $m(n+1) \times m(n+1)$ Jacobian matrix of the vector $\mathbf{V}(\mathbf{x})$. Observe that from this result, it is clear that the stability of the matrix $\mathbf{A}$ will play a role in investigating the stability of the vector $\widehat{\mathbf{x}}$.

As an aid to giving an overview of the structure of the matrix $\mathbf{J}_{\mathbf{V}}(\mathbf{x})$, it will also be useful to consider a form of the vector $\mathbf{x}$ partitioned according to behavioral class. Denote the set of types in the ith behavioral class by $\Upsilon_i = \Upsilon_{iS} \cup \Upsilon_{iI}$, and let

$$\mathbf{x}_i = (x_\tau \mid \tau \in \Upsilon_i) \tag{10.9.24}$$

denote a $(n+1) \times 1$ column vector for $i = 1, 2, \cdots, m$. Then, the $m(n+1) \times 1$ column vector $\mathbf{x}$ may be represented in a partitioned form such that the vector $\mathbf{x}(i)$ occurs in the ith partition. For example, if $m = 3$, then

$$\mathbf{x} = \begin{pmatrix} \mathbf{x}_1 \\ \mathbf{x}_2 \\ \mathbf{x}_3 \end{pmatrix} . \tag{10.9.25}$$

Given this partition of the vector $\mathbf{x}$, the matrix $\mathbf{J_V}(\mathbf{x})$ may also be represented in the partitioned form,

$$\mathbf{J_V}(\mathbf{x}) = (\mathbf{J}_{ij}(\mathbf{x}) \mid i, j = 1, 2, \cdots, m) \ , \tag{10.9.26}$$

where $\mathbf{J}_{ij}(\mathbf{x})$ is a $(n+1) \times (n+1)$ matrix of partial derivatives.

From an inspection of the form of the vector $\mathbf{V}_i(\mathbf{x})$ in Eq. (10.9.6) for the ith behavioral class, it can be seen that most of these derivatives will be zero so that it suffices to consider the partial derivatives of the function,

$$h(\tau_1, \mathbf{x}) = x_{\tau_1} g(\tau_1, \mathbf{x}) \tag{10.9.27}$$

for a susceptible type $\tau_1 \in \Upsilon_{iS}$. For $\tau_1 \in \Upsilon_{iS}$, let

$$\mathbf{K}_{ij}(\mathbf{x}) = \left(\frac{\partial h(\tau_1, \mathbf{x})}{\partial x_\tau} \mid \tau \in \Upsilon_j \right) \tag{10.9.28}$$

denote a $1 \times (n+1)$ row vector of partial derivatives. Therefore, for $i, j = 1, 2, \cdots, m$, the sub-matrix $\mathbf{J}_{ij}(\mathbf{x})$ has the partitioned form

$$\mathbf{J}_{ij}(\mathbf{x}) = \begin{pmatrix} -\mathbf{K}_{ij}(\mathbf{x}) \\ \mathbf{K}_{ij}(\mathbf{x}) \\ \mathbf{0}_{(n-1),(n+1)} \end{pmatrix} , \tag{10.9.29}$$

where $\mathbf{0}_{(n-1),(n+1)}$ is a $(n-1) \times (n+1)$ zero matrix.

In studies of epidemics of HIV/AIDS, it is of interest to consider the case of $m = 3$ behavioral classes and $n = 4$ stages of disease. For this case, the Jacobian matrix $\mathbf{J}(\mathbf{x})$ would be 15×15 and difficult to represent in symbolic form. But, as illustrated in Chapter 8, computing numerical versions of the eigenvalues of matrices of this order can be done with relative ease on modern desktop computers.

10.10 Jacobian Matrices in a Simple Case

As can be seen from an inspection of the general results in the preceding section, the forms of the partial derivatives in the Jacobian matrix $\mathbf{J_V}(\mathbf{x})$ will depend on the functional forms of the conditional probability $Q_{par}(t;\tau,\mathbf{x})$ that a susceptible $\tau \in \Upsilon_S$ is infected during a small time interval $(t, t+h]$ (see Section 10.3) for a derivation of a formula for these probabilities. From now on, the argument t will be dropped in $Q_{par}(t;\tau,\mathbf{x})$ as well as other functions to emphasize that attention is being focused on the vector $\mathbf{x}$. An assumption underlying the derivation of the general results in Section 10.9 was that the function $Q_{par}(\tau,\mathbf{x})$ was differentiable in a neighborhood of a stationary point $\widehat{\mathbf{x}} \in \mathfrak{P}_S$. As can be seen from inspection, the function $\min(x,y)$ is not differentiable at all points $(x,y) \in \{(x,y) \mid x,y \geq 0\}$; and, because the conditional probability $\rho(\tau_1,\tau_2,\mathbf{x})$ that a susceptible of type $\tau_1 \in \Upsilon_S$ has a person of type τ_2 as a sexual partner during a time interval $(t,t+h]$ (see Eq. (10.3.1)), is defined in terms of the function $\min(x,y)$, it follows from Eqs. (10.3.3) and (10.3.4) that the function $Q_{par}(\tau,\mathbf{x})$ may not be differentiable at all points $\mathbf{x} \in \mathfrak{P}$ of interest.

Among the strategies for coping with this technical difficulty is to ignore the restrictions on the random functions of the process imposed by partnership pairs, which are embodied in the function $\rho(\tau_1,\tau_2,\mathbf{x})$, and choose this function directly as the contact probability $\gamma(\tau_1,\tau_2,\mathbf{x})$ defined in Section 10.2 (see Eq. (10.2.6)), as suggested in the closing paragraph of Section 10.3. To express the function $\gamma(\tau_1,\tau_2,\mathbf{x})$ in a form amenable to differentiation, it will be useful to write the acceptance probabilities $\alpha(\tau_1,\tau_2)$ in a succinct vector notation. Let

$$\boldsymbol{\beta} = \begin{pmatrix} \beta_1 \\ \beta_2 \end{pmatrix} \tag{10.10.1}$$

be a 2×1 column vector of non-negative parameters, interpret any type $\boldsymbol{\tau} = (i,j)$ as a 1×2 row vector, and let $|\boldsymbol{\tau}|$ denote a 1×2 row vector $|\boldsymbol{\tau}| = (|i|, |j|)$. Then, the acceptance probabilities in Eq. (10.2.4) may be represented in the succinct form,

$$\alpha(\tau_1,\tau_2) = e^{-|\tau_1-\tau_2|\beta}\,. \tag{10.10.2}$$

Furthermore, it will also be helpful to define the function,

$$T(\tau_1, \mathbf{x}) = \sum_{\tau \in \Upsilon} x_\tau e^{-|\tau_1 - \tau|\beta} \tag{10.10.3}$$

for all types $\tau_1 \in \Upsilon$ and all vectors $\mathbf{x} \in \mathfrak{P}$ such that $\mathbf{x} \neq \mathbf{0}$. Then, the contact probability in Eq. (10.2.6) takes the simple form,

$$\gamma(\tau_1, \tau_2, \mathbf{x}) = \frac{x_{\tau_2} e^{-|\tau_1 - \tau_2|\beta}}{T(\tau_1, \mathbf{x})} \,. \tag{10.10.4}$$

Because the embedded differential equations were derived from the nonlinear difference equations in Section 10.6 by passing to the limit as $h \downarrow 0$, it follows from Eq. (10.3.2) that the probability $p(\tau_1, \tau_2)$ a susceptible of type τ_1 escapes infection when his sexual partner is of type $\tau_2 = (i_1, j_2)$ is $p(\tau_1, \tau_2) = p(j_2)$. From now on, to simplify the notation, write the probability $p(j_2)$ as $p(\tau_2)$. Then, the escape probability in Eq. (10.3.3) for a susceptible of type τ_1 takes the form,

$$P_{par}(\tau_1, \mathbf{x}) = \sum_{\tau_2 \in \Upsilon} \gamma(\tau_1, \tau_2, \mathbf{x}) p(\tau_2) \,. \tag{10.10.5}$$

As in Section 10.3, let $q(\tau_2) = 1 - p(\tau_2)$ be the probability that a susceptible becomes infected per sexual contact when his partner is of type τ_2. Then, it can be seen that:

$$Q_{par}(\tau_1, \mathbf{x}) = 1 - P_{par}(\tau_1, \mathbf{x}) = \frac{\sum_{\tau_2 \in \Upsilon_I} x_{\tau_2} e^{-|\tau_1 - \tau_2|\beta} q(\tau_2)}{T(\tau_1, \mathbf{x})} \tag{10.10.6}$$

is the probability that a susceptible of type τ_1 is infected during any small time interval. This form of the function $Q_{par}(\tau_1, \mathbf{x})$ is clearly differentiable at all points $\mathbf{x} \in \mathfrak{P}$ except the point $\mathbf{x} = \mathbf{0}$.

The next step is to derive formulas for the elements of the Jacobian matrix $\mathbf{J_V}(\mathbf{x})$. To this end, observe that the function in $h(\tau_1, \mathbf{x})$ in (10.9.27) now has the form,

$$h(\tau_1, \mathbf{x}) = x_{\tau_1} \lambda(\tau_1) \left(\frac{\sum_{\tau_2 \in \Upsilon_I} x_{\tau_2} e^{-|\tau_1 - \tau_2|\beta} q(\tau_2)}{T(\tau_1, \mathbf{x})} \right) \,. \tag{10.10.7}$$

From an inspection of this form, it can be seen that for all $\mathbf{x} \in \mathfrak{P}_S$ and $\tau \in \Upsilon_S$,

$$\frac{\partial h(\tau_1, \mathbf{x})}{\partial x_\tau} = 0 \,. \tag{10.10.8}$$

But, if $\tau \in \Upsilon_I$, then

$$\frac{\partial h(\tau_1, \mathbf{x})}{\partial x_\tau} = \frac{x_{\tau_1}\lambda(\tau_1)e^{-|\tau_1 - \tau|\beta} q(\tau_2)}{T(\tau_1, \mathbf{x})} \tag{10.10.9}$$

for all $\mathbf{x} \in \mathfrak{P}_S$. Therefore, for $\tau_1 \in \Upsilon_{iS}$, the vector $\mathbf{K}_{ij}(\mathbf{x})$ in Eq. (10.9.28) at the stationary point $\widehat{\mathbf{x}} \in \mathfrak{P}_S$ has the form,

$$\mathbf{K}_{ij}(\widehat{\mathbf{x}}) = \left(0, \frac{\widehat{x}_{\tau_1}\lambda(\tau_1)e^{-|\tau_1 - \tau|\beta} q(\tau)}{T(\tau_1, \widehat{\mathbf{x}})} \mid \tau \in \Upsilon_{jI}\right) . \tag{10.10.10}$$

By using this general result, it can be seen that it would be relatively easy to write software such that for any numerical specification of the parameters of the model, the eigenvalues of the Jacobian matrix,

$$\mathbf{J}(\mathbf{x}) = \mathbf{A} + \mathbf{J}_{\mathbf{V}}(\mathbf{x}) \tag{10.10.11}$$

could be computed at $\mathbf{x} = \widehat{\mathbf{x}} \in \mathfrak{P}_S$, a stationary vector of the embedded differential equations in Eq. (10.9.18), and a decision could be made, by checking the signs of the real parts, as to whether the point $\widehat{\mathbf{x}}$ was indeed stable.

For the case where there is only $m = 1$ behavioral class, then the matrix $\mathbf{J}(\mathbf{x})$ takes a particularly simple form. For, if $m = 1$, then $T(\tau_1, \widehat{\mathbf{x}}) = \widehat{x}_{\tau_1}$. For the case of one stage, $n = 1$, for example, there are two types $\tau = 0, 1$ and the Jacobian matrix has the simple symbolic triangular form,

$$\mathbf{J}(\widehat{\mathbf{x}}) = \begin{pmatrix} -\mu_0 & -\lambda(1)e^{-\beta_2}q(1) \\ 0 & \lambda(1)e^{-\beta_2}q(1) - \mu_0 - \mu_1 \end{pmatrix} , \tag{10.10.12}$$

with eigenvalues $\lambda_1 = -\mu_0$ and $\lambda_2 = \lambda(1)e^{-\beta_2}q(1) - \mu_0 - \mu_1$. Thus, this matrix is stable only at those points in the parameter space such that:

$$\lambda(1)e^{-\beta_2}q(1) - \mu_0 - \mu_1 < 0 \,. \tag{10.10.13}$$

For the case $m = 1$ and $n = 2$ stages of disease, there are three types $\tau = 0, 1, 2$, and the Jacobian matrix has the form,

$$\mathbf{J}(\widehat{\mathbf{x}}) = \begin{pmatrix} j_{11} & j_{12} & j_{13} \\ 0 & j_{22} & j_{23} \\ 0 & j_{32} & j_{33} \end{pmatrix} . \tag{10.10.14}$$

where $j_{11} = -\mu_0$, $j_{12} = -\lambda(1)e^{-\beta_2}q(1)$ and $j_{13} = -\lambda(1)e^{-2\beta_2}q(2)$; where $j_{22} = \lambda(1)e^{-\beta_2}q(1) - \mu_0 - \mu_1 - \gamma_{12}$ and $j_{23} = \lambda(1)e^{-2\beta_2}q(2) - \gamma_{21}$; and finally, where $j_{32} = \gamma_{12}$ and $j_{33} = -\mu_0 - \mu_2 - \gamma_{21}$.

Although it is not immediately apparent, by visual inspection, at what points in the parameter space all the eigenvalues of this matrix have negative real parts, conditions could be derived under which the matrix $\mathbf{J}(\widehat{\mathbf{x}})$ is stable. However, this strategy will not be pursued; rather, we shall close this section with the following observation.

The condition $\boldsymbol{\beta} = \mathbf{0}$ corresponds to the case of selecting sexual partners at random among the set of types Υ in the population; while large values of both parameters in the vector $\boldsymbol{\beta}$ corresponds to the case where the selection of sexual partners of like types occurs with high probability, i.e., the selection of sexual partners is highly assortative. From Eq. (10.10.10), it can be seen that

$$\lim_{\boldsymbol{\beta}\uparrow\infty} \mathbf{K}_{ij}(\widehat{\mathbf{x}}) = \mathbf{0}_{1,(n+1)} , \tag{10.10.15}$$

where $\boldsymbol{\beta} \uparrow \infty$ denotes that both elements in the vector $\boldsymbol{\beta}$ approach ∞. From this observation, it follows from Eq. (10.10.11) that:

$$\lim_{\boldsymbol{\beta}\uparrow\infty} \mathbf{J}(\widehat{\mathbf{x}}) = \mathbf{A} . \tag{10.10.16}$$

This observation suggests that when the selection of sexual partners is highly assortative, then the stability of the matrix $\mathbf{A}$ will play a basic role in determining whether a stationary point $\widehat{\mathbf{x}} \in \mathfrak{P}_S$ is stable.

10.11 Jacobian Matrices in a More Complex Case

In this section a procedure will be developed for deriving formulas for the elements of the Jacobian matrix $\mathbf{J_V}(\mathbf{x})$, when the infection probability $Q_{par}(\tau, \mathbf{x})$ is calculated using the formulas presented in Section

10.3. A first step in this procedure is to consider a version of the probability $\rho(\tau_1, \tau_2, \mathbf{x})$ in Eq. (10.3.1) for the embedded differential equations set forth in Section 10.7. In Section 10.10, working with the probability directly was avoided, because of differentiability problems with the function $\min(x, y)$. A way around these problems is to approximate the function $\min(x, y)$ with a differential function. In this connection, consider a function $\eta_\theta(x, y)$ defined by:

$$\eta_\theta(x, y) = \frac{xy2^{\frac{1}{\theta}}}{(x^\theta + y^\theta)^{\frac{1}{\theta}}} \tag{10.11.1}$$

for $\theta > 0$, $x > 0$, and $y > 0$.

If $x < y$, then it can be seen that:

$$\eta_\theta(x, y) = x\left(\frac{2}{1 + \left(\frac{x}{y}\right)^\theta}\right)^{\frac{1}{\theta}} . \tag{10.11.2}$$

And, in general, by interchanging x and y, it can be seen that the formula,

$$\eta_\theta(x, y) = \min(x, y)\left(\frac{2}{1 + \left(\frac{\min(x, y)}{\max(x, y)}\right)^\theta}\right)^{\frac{1}{\theta}} \tag{10.11.3}$$

is valid for all $x > 0$ and $y > 0$. It can also be seen that:

$$\lim_{\theta \uparrow \infty} \eta_\theta(x, y) = \min(x, y) \tag{10.11.4}$$

for all $x > 0$ and $y > 0$. Hence, for θ sufficiently large, the differentiable function in Eq. (10.11.1) will be a good approximation to the function $\min(x, y)$. It should be mentioned that more general versions of the function in Eq. (10.11.1) have been considered by Hadeler[5] in connection with models of pair formation.

In the embedded deterministic differential equations, each of the functions $N(\tau_1, \tau_2, \mathbf{x})$ and $N(\tau_1, \tau_1, \mathbf{x})$ defined in Eqs. (10.2.14) and (10.2.15) will be computed in terms of estimates of the expectations of the random variables in the vector,

$$\mathbf{Z}(t; \tau_1) = (Z(t; \tau_1, \tau_2) \mid \tau_2 \in \Upsilon) \tag{10.11.5}$$

which follows a multinomial distribution (see Eqs. (10.2.10) and (10.2.11)). In the notation of Section 10.10, these expectations have the form,

$$x_{\tau_1} \gamma(\tau_1, \tau_2, \mathbf{x}) \, . \tag{10.11.6}$$

In the embedded differential equations, the functions in Eqs. (10.2.14) and (10.2.15) would, therefore, be approximated by:

$$N(\tau_1, \tau_2, \mathbf{x}) = \eta_\theta(x_{\tau_1} \gamma(\tau_1, \tau_2, \mathbf{x}), x_{\tau_2} \gamma(\tau_2, \tau_1, \mathbf{x})) \, , \tag{10.11.7}$$

if $\tau_1 \neq \tau_2$, and by:

$$N(\tau_1, \tau_1, \mathbf{x}) = \frac{x_{\tau_1} \gamma(\tau_1, \tau_1, \mathbf{x})}{2} \, , \tag{10.11.8}$$

if $\tau_1 = \tau_2$.

From Eq. (10.10.4), it can be seen that

$$x_{\tau_1} \gamma(\tau_1, \tau_2, \mathbf{x}) = \frac{x_{\tau_1} x_{\tau_2} e^{-|\tau_1 - \tau_2| \beta}}{T(\tau_1, \mathbf{x})} \, , \tag{10.11.9}$$

where $T(\tau_1, \mathbf{x})$ is defined in Eq. (10.10.3). Similarly, by interchanging τ_1 and τ_2, it can be seen that:

$$x_{\tau_2} \gamma(\tau_2, \tau_1, \mathbf{x}) = \frac{x_{\tau_2} x_{\tau_1} e^{-|\tau_2 - \tau_1| \beta}}{T(\tau_2, \mathbf{x})} \, . \tag{10.11.10}$$

A key observation to make at this point is to observe that even if $\tau_1 \neq \tau_2$, the numerators in (10.11.9) and (10.11.10) are equal.

Instead of substituting the formulas in Eqs. (10.11.9) and (10.11.10) directly for x and y in Eq. (10.11.1), some cumbersome algebra can be avoided if x/y_1 and x/y_2 are substituted into Eq. (10.11.1) to obtain the expression:

$$\eta_\theta\left(\frac{x}{y_1},\frac{x}{y_2}\right)=\frac{x}{y_1}\left(\frac{2}{1+\left(\frac{y_2}{y_1}\right)^\theta}\right)^{\frac{1}{\theta}}, \tag{10.11.11}$$

after some algebraic reductions. Then, by letting x be the common numerator in Eqs. (10.11.9) and (10.11.10), $y_1 = T(\tau_1, \mathbf{x})$, $y_2 = T(\tau_2, \mathbf{x})$, and the formula in Eq. (10.11.7) takes the explicit form,

$$N(\tau_1,\tau_2,\mathbf{x}) =\frac{x_{\tau_1}x_{\tau_2}e^{-|\tau_1-\tau_2|\beta}}{T(\tau_1,\mathbf{x})}\left(\frac{2}{1+\left(\frac{T(\tau_2,\mathbf{x})}{T(\tau_1,\mathbf{x})}\right)^\theta}\right)^{\frac{1}{\theta}}, \tag{10.11.12}$$

for $\tau_1 \neq \tau_2$. And, Eq. (10.11.8) becomes

$$N(\tau_1,\tau_1,\mathbf{x}) =\frac{x_{\tau_1}^2}{2T(\tau_1,\mathbf{x})}. \tag{10.11.13}$$

To further simplify the writing of formulas in what follows, let

$$f_\theta(\tau_1,\tau_2,\mathbf{x}) = \left(\frac{2}{1+\left(\frac{T(\tau_2,\mathbf{x})}{T(\tau_1,\mathbf{x})}\right)^\theta}\right)^{\frac{1}{\theta}}. \tag{10.11.14}$$

In terms of the notation just developed, the formula in Eq. (10.3.1) takes the explicit form,

$$\rho(\tau_1,\tau_2,\mathbf{x}) =\frac{2x_{\tau_2}e^{-|\tau_1-\tau_2|\beta}f_\theta(\tau_1,\tau_2,\mathbf{x})}{T^*(\tau_1,\mathbf{x})}, \tag{10.11.15}$$

where, by definition,

$$T^*(\tau_1,\mathbf{x}) =x_{\tau_1}+2\sum_{\tau\neq\tau_1}x_\tau e^{-|\tau_1-\tau|\beta}f_\theta(\tau_1,\tau,\mathbf{x}). \tag{10.11.16}$$

Therefore, in the structure under consideration, the probability that a susceptible individual of type $\tau_1 \in \Upsilon_S$ becomes infected during a small time interval is:

$$Q_{par}(\tau_1, \mathbf{x}) = \frac{2 \sum_{\tau_2 \in \Upsilon_I} x_{\tau_2} e^{-|\tau_1 - \tau_2|\beta} f_\theta(\tau_1, \tau_2, \mathbf{x}) q(\tau_2)}{T^*(\tau_1, \mathbf{x})}, \tag{10.11.17}$$

and the function in Eq. (10.10.7) takes the form,

$$h(\tau_1, \mathbf{x}) = x_{\tau_1} \lambda(\tau_1) \left(\frac{2 \sum_{\tau_2 \in \Upsilon_I} x_{\tau_2} e^{-|\tau_1 - \tau_2|\beta} f_\theta(\tau_1, \tau_2, \mathbf{x}) q(\tau_2)}{T^*(\tau_1, \mathbf{x})} \right). \tag{10.11.18}$$

It can be shown that the partial derivatives of this function evaluated at the vector $\mathbf{x} \in \mathfrak{P}_S$ have forms similar to the function $h(\tau_1, \mathbf{x})$ in Eq. (10.10.7). Thus, one can show that for $\tau_1 \in \Upsilon_{iS}$ the vector $\mathbf{K}_{ij}(\mathbf{x})$ in Eq. (10.9.28) at the stationary point $\widehat{\mathbf{x}} \in \mathfrak{P}_S$ has the form,

$$\mathbf{K}_{ij}(\widehat{\mathbf{x}}) = \left(0, \frac{2 \widehat{x}_{\tau_1} \lambda(\tau_1) e^{-|\tau_1 - \tau|\beta} f_\theta(\tau_1, \tau, \widehat{\mathbf{x}}) q(\tau)}{T^*(\tau_1, \widehat{\mathbf{x}})} \mid \tau \in \Upsilon_{jI} \right) \tag{10.11.19}$$

for the structure under consideration. Just as in the simpler case described in Section 10.10, it will be relatively straightforward to write software to compute the Jacobian matrix $\mathbf{J}(\widehat{\mathbf{x}})$ at a stationary point $\widehat{\mathbf{x}} \in \mathfrak{P}_S$ as a function of the parameters and determine whether it is stable.

The function $f_\theta(\tau_1, \tau_2, \mathbf{x})$ in Eq. (10.11.14) will, in some cases, have a very simple form. For example, if $\boldsymbol{\beta} = \mathbf{0}$ so that sexual partners are selected at random, then $T(\tau_1, \mathbf{x}) = T(\tau_2, \mathbf{x})$ for all $\tau_1 \neq \tau_2$ and vectors $\mathbf{x} \in \mathfrak{P}$. Thus, it follows that $f_\theta(\tau_1, \tau_2, \mathbf{x}) = 1$. Another simple form arises when there is $m = 1$ behavioral class and $n \geq 1$ stages of disease with $\tau = 0, 1, 2, \cdots, n$, types. For the case $\tau_2 = j \geq 1$ and $\tau_1 = 0$, it can be shown that:

$$f_\theta(\tau_1, \tau_2, \widehat{\mathbf{x}}) = \left(\frac{2}{1 + e^{-\theta j \beta_2}} \right)^{\frac{1}{\theta}}. \tag{10.11.20}$$

When θ is large, it is easy to see in this case that:

$$f_\theta(\tau_1, \tau_2, \widehat{\mathbf{x}}) \simeq 1 \ . \tag{10.11.21}$$

Symbolic forms of the matrices in Eqs. (10.11.12) and (10.11.13) for the structure under consideration can be written down, but this exercise will be left to the reader. Finally, the result,

$$\lim_{\beta \uparrow \infty} \mathbf{J}(\widehat{\mathbf{x}}) = \mathbf{A} \ , \tag{10.11.22}$$

also holds for the model of this section, as can be seen from the form of the vector $\mathbf{K}_{ij}(\widehat{\mathbf{x}})$ in Eq. (10.11.9). Thus, the stability of the matrix $\mathbf{A}$ will play an important role in testing the stability of the stationary vector $\widehat{\mathbf{x}}$ when the selection of sexual partners is highly assortative.

10.12 On the Probability an Epidemic Becomes Extinct

In our studies of branching process approximations to the early stages of an epidemic evolving from a few infectives being introduced into a large population of susceptibles in Chapters 6, 8, and 9, a number of examples were given in which even though the threshold parameter was greater than one, there was a positive probability that an epidemic would become extinct. Unlike the non-linear stochastic models under consideration in this chapter, models of epidemics based on branching processes are essentially linear in nature. There is, however, an analogue for these non-linear stochastic models to the extinction of an epidemic modeled as a branching process. As discussed in Section 10.9, suppose a population, composed entirely of susceptibles, has been evolving for a long period of time according to the non-linear stochastic model described in the previous sections of this chapter. Then, suppose at some time a few infectives are introduced into the population, but thereafter all recruits entering the population are susceptible. Furthermore, suppose that for the parameter settings governing the evolution of the population, it has been determined that the Jacobian matrix $\mathbf{J}(\widehat{\mathbf{x}})$ as described in Sections 10.10 and 10.11 at the stationary vector $\widehat{\mathbf{x}}$ for the embedded differential equations, is unstable, which suggests that an epidemic would develop in a population whose evolution is governed by the embedded deterministic differential equations. Yet, for the non-linear stochastic model, there may be a positive probability, depending on the number of infectives introduced into the population of susceptibles, that the epidemic becomes extinct.

To make these ideas more precise, it will be helpful to give an overview of the stochastic population process. The state space for this process is the set,

$$\mathfrak{P} = (x_\tau \mid \tau \in \Upsilon) \tag{10.12.1}$$

of all $m(n+1)$-dimensional vectors of non-negative integers, where $x_\tau = 0, 1, 2, \cdots$, for all $\tau \in \Upsilon$. For $t \in [0, \infty)$, let the vector $\mathbf{X}(t) \in \mathfrak{P}$ denote the state of the population at time t. The set in Eq. (10.12.1) is actually a subset of the set defined in Eq. (10.9.13) for the embedded differential equations, but to simplify the notation the two sets will not be distinguished except in those cases where confusion may arise. Just as in Eq. (10.9.14) and Eq. (10.9.15), the symbols $\mathfrak{P}_S$ and $\mathfrak{P}_I$ will denote, respectively, those subsets of $\mathfrak{P}$ such the population contains only susceptibles or at least one infective. It can be shown that the population stochastic process,

$$\{\mathbf{X}(t) \in \mathfrak{P} \mid t \in [0, \infty)\} \tag{10.12.2}$$

may be viewed as a multi-dimensional Markov jump process in continuous time, but from the computational point of view, it is difficult to design efficient Monte Carlo simulation algorithms to compute realizations of the process. However, it can be shown that the chain multinomial model described in Section 10.5 is a discrete time approximation to the Markov jump process in continuous time, which provides a useful and efficient approach to computing Monte Carlo realizations of the population process.

From the notational point of view, it is easier to define the probability an epidemic becomes extinct in terms of the continuous time Markov jump process in Eq. (10.12.2) rather than in terms of the chain multinomial approximation. In principle, if at some time $t \in [0, \infty)$ the population is in some state $\mathbf{X}(t) = \mathbf{x} \in \mathfrak{P}$, then one may find a latent risk function $\theta(\mathbf{x}, \mathbf{y})$, determined by the parameters of the process and the latent risk functions for individuals, such that for some state $\mathbf{y} \in \mathfrak{P}$ and $h > 0$,

$$\mathbb{P}\{\mathbf{X}(t+h) = \mathbf{y} \mid \mathbf{X}(t) = \mathbf{x}\} = \theta(\mathbf{x}, \mathbf{y})h + o(h) . \tag{10.12.3}$$

During any small time interval $(t, t+h]$, Eq. (10.12.3) may be interpreted as stating that the conditional probability is of order $o(h)$ that the vector $\mathbf{y}$ differs from $\mathbf{x}$ by more than ± 1 in some element. Given the latent risks in Eq. (10.12.3), one may view the Markov jump process as semi-Markovian and, in principle, determine a density matrix,

$$\mathbf{a}(t) = (a(\mathbf{x}, \mathbf{y}; t) \mid \mathbf{x} \in \mathfrak{P}, \mathbf{y} \in \mathfrak{P}) \tag{10.12.4}$$

for all $t \in [0, \infty)$.

For the case where only susceptible recruits enter the population, the population process is reducible and the density matrix has the partitioned form,

$$\mathbf{a}(t) = \begin{bmatrix} \mathbf{a}_{11}(t) & \mathbf{0} \\ \mathbf{a}_{21}(t) & \mathbf{a}_{22}(t) \end{bmatrix}, \tag{10.12.5}$$

where the sub-matrix $\mathbf{a}_{11}(t)$ governs transitions among states in the set $\mathfrak{P}_S$; the sub-matrix $\mathbf{a}_{21}(t)$ governs transition from states in the set $\mathfrak{P}_I$ to states in $\mathfrak{P}_S$; and the sub-matrix $\mathbf{a}_{22}(t)$ governs transitions among states in the set $\mathfrak{P}_I$. For example, the sub-matrix $\mathbf{a}_{21}(t)$ has the elements:

$$\mathbf{a}_{21}(t) = (a(\mathbf{x}, \mathbf{y}; t) \mid \mathbf{x} \in \mathfrak{P}_I, \mathbf{y} \in \mathfrak{P}_S) . \tag{10.12.6}$$

For all $t > 0$ and states $\mathbf{x}$ and $\mathbf{y}$, let

$$A(\mathbf{x}, \mathbf{y}; t) = \int_0^t a(\mathbf{x}, \mathbf{y}; s) ds , \tag{10.12.7}$$

and given that the process starts in state $\mathbf{x} \in \mathfrak{P}_I$ at time $y = 0$, let $F(\mathbf{x}, \mathbf{y}; t)$ denote the conditional probability that the population enters state $\mathbf{y} \in \mathfrak{P}_S$ sometime during the time interval $(0, t]$, $t > 0$. Then, by appealing to a renewal argument, it follows that for every $\mathbf{x} \in \mathfrak{P}_I$ and $\mathbf{y} \in \mathfrak{P}_S$ these conditional probabilities satisfy the system of renewal equations:

$$F(\mathbf{x}, \mathbf{y}; t) = A(\mathbf{x}, \mathbf{y}; t) + \sum_{\mathbf{u} \in \mathfrak{P}_I} \int_0^t a(\mathbf{x}, \mathbf{u}; s) F(\mathbf{u}, \mathbf{y}; t-s) ds . \tag{10.12.8}$$

Denote the conditional probability that the epidemic becomes extinct sometime during the time interval $(0, t]$, given that $\mathbf{x} \in \mathfrak{P}_I$ was the state of initial population, by $Q_{EXT}(\mathbf{x};t)$. Then,

$$Q_{EXT}(\mathbf{x};t) = \sum_{\mathbf{y} \in \mathfrak{P}_S} F(\mathbf{x}, \mathbf{y}; t) \, . \tag{10.12.9}$$

In most cases of interest, this extinction probability will be very difficult to calculate exactly. It may, however, be estimated with relative ease using Monte Carlo methods.

Suppose, for example, N Monte Carlo realizations of the population process are computed on the discrete time points $t = 0, 1, 2, \cdots, t_1$, given some initial vector $\mathbf{X}(0) = \mathbf{x} \in \mathfrak{P}_I$. This sample of Monte Carlo realizations may be represented by the array:

$$\left\{\mathbf{x}^{(i)}(t) \mid t = 0, 1, 2, \cdots, t_1; \; i = 1, 2, \cdots, N\right\} \, . \tag{10.12.10}$$

At time t, the ith vector in this array of N realizations has the representation,

$$\mathbf{x}^{(i)}(t) = \left(x_\tau^{(i)}(t) \mid \tau \in \Upsilon\right) \, . \tag{10.12.11}$$

For the ith realization, the total number of infectives in the population at time t is:

$$s_I^{(i)}(t) = \sum_{\tau \in \Upsilon_I} x_\tau^{(i)}(t) \, . \tag{10.12.12}$$

The next step in the Monte Carlo estimation procedure is to compute a Boolean array in terms of the following indicator functions. For $i = 1, 2, \cdots, N$, and $t = 0, 1, 2, \cdots, t_1$, let

$$\begin{aligned} \xi_i(t) &= 1 \text{ if } s_I^{(i)}(t) = 0 \\ &= 0 \text{ if } s_I^{(i)}(t) > 0 \, . \end{aligned} \tag{10.12.13}$$

Then, by the Law of Large Numbers, the Monte Carlo estimate of the extinction probability,

$$\widehat{Q}_{EXT}(\mathbf{x};t) = \frac{1}{N} \sum_{i=1}^{N} \xi_i(t) \tag{10.12.14}$$

is not only unbiased, but also has the property of consistency as $N \uparrow \infty$.

At least two caveats should be kept in mind when applying the ideas just outlined. First, the random variable in Eq. (10.12.14) is an estimate of the extinction probability for the chain multinomial population process and not for the Markov jump process discussed in this section. However, if h can be chosen sufficiently small, the chain multinomial process should be a good approximation to the Markov jump process in continuous time. A second caveat is that the properties of the random number generator used in computing the Monte Carlo realizations of the population process should have passed a sufficient number of statistical tests to convince an investigator that the sample of realizations in Eq. (10.12.10) may be regarded as independently and identically distributed.

Even though only one potential application of the non-linear stochastic epidemic process under consideration has been discussed in this section, there is at least one other application that could be investigated using ideas related to those set forth above. Suppose, for example, that a population of susceptibles has been evolving in isolation for a long period of time, but from time to time infected recruits may enter the population with small probability per unit time. In this scenario, the density matrix in Eq. (10.12.5) for the population process would no longer be reducible, because all states in $\mathfrak{P}$ may communicate with positive probability.

Nevertheless, it would be of interest to have some indicator as to whether an epidemic would become established in the population. If, for example, the Jacobian matrix $\mathbf{J}(\widehat{\mathbf{x}})$ is stable at the stationary vector $\widehat{\mathbf{x}}$ for the embedded differential equations, then this condition could be used as an indicator that an epidemic would not develop in the population whose evolution is governed by the stochastic population process. But, if the matrix $\mathbf{J}(\widehat{\mathbf{x}})$ is not stable, then this condition would be an indication that an epidemic would develop in the population with positive probability.

For those cases in which the matrix $\mathbf{J}(\widehat{\mathbf{x}})$ is not stable, given some initial vector $\mathbf{x} \in \mathfrak{P}_S$, $\widehat{Q}_{EXT}(\mathbf{x};t)$ is still the fraction of Monte Carlo realizations among N such that the population contains only susceptibles at some time $t = 1, 2, \cdots, t_1$. Therefore, $1 - \widehat{Q}_{EXT}(\mathbf{x};t)$ is the fraction of realizations such that the population contains at least one infective at time t and could be thought of as an indicator that an epidemic may be established in the population.

On the other hand, if the fraction $\widehat{Q}_{EXT}(\mathbf{x};t)$ tends to approach a limit as $t \uparrow \infty$, then for large t, the fraction $1 - \widehat{Q}_{EXT}(\mathbf{x};t)$ could be viewed as an estimate of the probability an epidemic would be established in the population. In particular, if for some t, $\widehat{Q}_{EXT}(\mathbf{x};t) = 0$, then the experimental evidence would suggest that an epidemic would become established in the population with probability one or at least with high probability.

10.13 Software for Testing Stability of the Jacobian

As suggested in the foregoing sections, the Jacobian matrix for the differential equations embedded in the stochastic process may be used to derive indicators as to whether an epidemic will occur, according to the non-linear stochastic model, when a few infectives are introduced into a population of susceptibles. From Eq. (10.9.23) it can be seen that the Jacobian matrix in question is a sum of two components; namely, the constant matrix $\mathbf{A}$ and a matrix $\mathbf{J}_V(\widehat{\mathbf{x}})$, due to non-linear terms, evaluated at the stationary vector $\widehat{\mathbf{x}}$ (see Eq. (10.9.20)), for the case where the population contains only susceptibles. When a model depends on only relatively few parameters and the Jacobian matrix is of order 2×2 or 3×3, a commonly used technique for finding conditions of stability is to derive an algebraic form for the characteristic polynomial of the matrix and then deduce conditions demarcating those regions of the parameter space where the roots of the polynomial have or do not have negative real parts.

For models with multi-dimensional state and parameter spaces, however, such techniques rarely, if ever, yield useful results, which forces an investigator to pursue alternative methods to search for threshold conditions. Fortunately, in this day of powerful desktop computers and the wide availability of programs to compute the eigenvalues of matrices, it is easy to write software to compute the eigenvalues of even relatively large matrices and test whether they have negative real parts at chosen points in the parameter space. To be sure, this approach will not yield partitions of the parameter space into regions such that the Jacobian matrix is stable or unstable, but, as will be shown by examples, it will yield threshold conditions near and around chosen points in a parameter space of particular interest to an investigator.

Some software needed to test points in the parameter space for stability of the Jacobian matrix has been written in APL for two special cases of the stochastic system under consideration. In the simplest case, the number of behavioral classes and stages of disease were chosen, respectively, as $m = 3$ and $n = 1$. With these choices, the number of types is $m(n+1) = 6$ and the Jacobian matrix is 6×6. In a more complex case, the number of behavioral classes was again chosen as $m = 3$, but the number of stages was chosen as $n = 4$, a number that is frequently used in the study of HIV/AIDS. For this case, the number of types of individuals in the population is $m(n+1) = 15$ so that the Jacobian matrix is 15×15.

For both these cases, it would be very difficult to derive usable conditions for the stability of the Jacobian matrix, using algebraic methods, but with the help of software, it is a straightforward task to test numerically at a parameter point for the stability of the matrix. The min function was used in the software implementing the stochastic model and the embedded non-linear difference equations developed in this chapter. Hence, throughout the computer experiments reported below, as well as those in subsequent sections of this chapter, the formulas set forth in Section 10.11 for computing Jacobian matrices were used. Further, by trial and error, values of the parameter θ in the differentiable function in Eq. (10.11.1) used to approximate the min function were chosen as large as possible, but small enough to stay within the accuracy of the APL software. In passing, it should be mentioned that although the software was written in APL, any programming language with a capability for manipulating matrices with ease, such as MATLAB, could have been used to obtain the results reported below.

The software used to test whether a Jacobian matrix was stable at a particular point in the parameter space was designed so that a 1 was returned if the matrix was stable and a 0 if the matrix was not stable. More precisely, suppose a particular case of the model has $\tau_{types} = m(n+1)$ types; let $\mathbf{J}(\widehat{\mathbf{x}})$ be the $\tau_{types} \times \tau_{types}$ Jacobian matrix evaluated at the stationary vector $\widehat{\mathbf{x}}$, and let λ_i, $i = 1, 2, \cdots, \tau_{types}$, be the eigenvalues of the matrix. For $i = 1, 2, \cdots, \tau_{types}$, let ϑ_i denote an indicator function such that $\vartheta_i = 1$ if $\mathrm{Re}(\lambda_i) < 0$, (the real part of λ_i), and let $\vartheta_i = 0$ otherwise. Then, the matrix $\mathbf{J}(\widehat{\mathbf{x}})$ is stable if the indicator,

$$\chi = \prod_{i=1}^{\tau_{types}} \vartheta_i \tag{10.13.1}$$

is 1 and 0 if it is unstable. The same ideas were used to test whether the matrix $\mathbf{A}$ is stable at a particular parameter point.

The illustrative examples presented below are for the case of $m = 3$ behavioral classes and $n = 1$ stage of disease. Table 10.13.1 contains three points in the parameter space for this special case of the model. The symbols q_1, q_2, and q_3 denote, respectively, the probabilities that a susceptible becomes infected per sexual contact with an infective in class $i = 1, 2, 3$.

Table 10.13.1. Points in the Parameter Space for the One-Stage Model.

Point	β_1	β_2	q_1	q_2	q_3
I	0	0	0.001	0.005	0.01
II	0	0	0.020	0.050	0.10
III	0	0	0.120	0.150	0.20

For the purposes of discussion, the three vectors of q probabilities will be referred to as low, medium, and high probabilities of infection per sexual contact. Recall that for the β-parameters in the acceptance probabilities, β_1 determines the magnitude of the probability of contact among behavioral classes, and β_2 has the same function for the stages of disease. For the particular parameter points presented in the table, the values $\beta_1 = \beta_2 = 0$ correspond to the random assortment of individuals in choices of sexual partners among the behavioral classes and stages of disease. Actually, the parameter space of this particular case of the model has a dimension greater that five, but for the sake of simplicity, attention will be focused on only five of the dimensions corresponding to the parameters known to affect whether the Jacobian matrix is stable or unstable.

Presented in Table 10.13.2 are the values of the indicator function in Eq. (10.13.1) for the **A**-matrix and the Jacobian matrix $\mathbf{J}(\widehat{\mathbf{x}})$ at the parameter points I, II, and III in Table 10.13.1. From this table, it can be seen that the matrix **A** was stable at points I, II, and II. Actually, this was anticipated, because the parameter values going into the **A**-matrix do not change at these three points. Furthermore, from the results of a number of similar numerical experiments, it is tempting to conjecture that the **A**-matrix is stable at all points in the parameter space even for cases of 15 or more types, for in no case has it been found to be unstable.

Table 10.13.2. Stability of the Matrices.

Point	A-Matrix	Jacobian Matrix
I	1	1
II	1	0
III	1	0

Nevertheless, it would be nice to have a mathematical proof as to whether the conjecture is true. As can be seen from the second column of the table, the Jacobian matrix is stable at point I but unstable at points II and III. Thus, at the low level for the probabilities of infection per sexual contact, if a few infectives were introduced into a population of susceptibles, an epidemic would not be expected to develop. However, because the Jacobian matrix is unstable at the medium and high points II and III, an epidemic would be expected to develop with a positive probability if a few infectives were introduced into a population of susceptibles.

According to Eq. (10.11.22), if the **A**-matrix is stable at a parameter point, then for sufficiently large β-values the Jacobian matrix should be stable. A question that naturally arises is how large the β-values must be in order to make the Jacobian matrix stable. To obtain answers to this question, APL software was written to test the stability of the Jacobian matrix at various combinations of values for β_1 and β_2.

Presented in Table 10.13.3 are the results of an experiment designed to explore which combinations of β-values would render the Jacobian matrix stable in regions of the parameter space near the point

II involving the medium level of probabilities of infection per sexual contact. In this experiment, nine values of each the β-parameters were chosen, ranging from 0 to 4 in increments of 0.5. The values of β_1 correspond to the rows of the table, the values of β_2 correspond to the columns, and the values of the indicator function in Eq. (10.13.1) make up the body of the table with $9 \times 9 = 81$ entries. For example, the value 1 for the indicator in the fourth row and column of the table is that for the pair of β-values $(\beta_1, \beta_2) = (1.5, 1.5)$. As can be seen from an inspection of the table, at no points such that $\beta_1 \leq 0.5$ and $\beta_2 \leq 0.5$ was the Jacobian matrix stable, but at points such that $\beta_1 \geq 1$ and $\beta_2 \geq 1$ many of the points yielded a stable matrix.

Table 10.13.3. Stability of the Jacobian Matrix for Point II as a Function of the Beta Parameters.

$\beta_1 \backslash \beta_2$	0	0.5	1.0	1.5	2.0	2.5	3.0	3.5	4.0
0	0	0	0	0	0	0	0	0	0
0.5	0	0	0	0	0	0	0	0	0
1.0	0	0	0	0	0	1	1	1	1
1.5	0	0	0	1	1	1	1	1	1
2.0	0	0	0	1	1	1	1	1	1
2.5	0	0	1	1	1	1	1	1	1
3.0	0	0	1	1	1	1	1	1	1
3.5	0	0	1	1	1	1	1	1	1
4.0	0	0	1	1	1	1	1	1	1

A similar experiment was conducted to test for regions in the parameter space such that the Jacobian matrix was stable by varying the values of the β-parameters near parameter point III, the point in Table 10.13.1 involving the high level of infection per sexual contact. In this experiment, the 81 combinations of β-values tested were the same as those in Table 10.13.3 and the results are presented in Table 10.13.4. As expected, near point III fewer combinations of β-values rendered the Jacobian matrix stable. Thus, with the exception of the point $(\beta_1, \beta_2) = (1, 4)$, at no points such that $\beta_1 \leq 1$ and $\beta_2 \leq 1$ was the Jacobian matrix stable; however, for points such that $\beta_1 \geq 1.5$ and $\beta_2 \geq 1.5$, the matrix was stable. Exploratory experiments of the kind just described are very useful in finding points in the parameter space that yield interesting projections of an epidemic, which will be described in the following sections of this chapter.

Table 10.13.4. Stability of the Jacobian Matrix for Point III as a Function of the Beta Parameters.

$\beta_1 \backslash \beta_2$	0	0.5	1.0	1.5	2.0	2.5	3.0	3.5	4.0
0	0	0	0	0	0	0	0	0	0
0.5	0	0	0	0	0	0	0	0	0
1.0	0	0	0	0	0	0	0	0	1
1.5	0	0	0	0	0	0	1	1	1
2.0	0	0	0	0	1	1	1	1	1
2.5	0	0	0	0	1	1	1	1	1
3.0	0	0	0	1	1	1	1	1	1
3.5	0	0	0	1	1	1	1	1	1
4.0	0	0	0	1	1	1	1	1	1

10.14 Invasion Thresholds: One-Stage Model, Random Assortment

Among the authors who have studied threshold concepts in stochastic and deterministic models of epidemics is Nasell,[16] who, among other things, considered invasion thresholds. The concept of an invasion threshold is of interest in a variety of circumstances, but in this section attention will be focused on computer experiments with the one-stage model in which attention was centered on a set on numerical specifications of the parameters for the following scenario. Consider a population of susceptibles that have been evolving for a long period of time so that an equilibrium has been reached according to the embedded deterministic model. Furthermore, suppose the Jacobian matrix for the embedded differential equations is stable at the stationary vector $\widehat{\mathbf{x}}$ (see Eq. (10.9.20)). Then, it seems likely that if a few infectives were introduced into the population and all recruits entering the population thereafter were also susceptibles, then the epidemic would eventually become extinct with positive probability.

Presented in Table 10.14.1 is a set of numerical assignments for some parameters of the model. By way of interpreting these parameters, observe that $m = 3$ in the first row of the table indicates that three behavioral classes, characterized by level of sexual activity per month, were considered in the experiment; while $n = 1$ in the second row indicates only one stage of disease was taken into account. The numerical assignments for λ-parameters in the third row of the table, which quantify levels of sexual activity, indicate that the expected number of sexual partners per month for individuals in behavioral classes 1, 2, and 3 were 4, 5, and 6, respectively. These levels of sexual activity are further quantified in row four of the table by assigning the η-parameters the values 0, 1, and 2. But, because a person is a sexual partner only if there is at least one sexual contact, the expected numbers of sexual contacts per partner were 1, 2, and 3, respectively, for the three behavioral classes (see Section 10.3 for details). According to the parameter assignments in the fifth row of the table, the three behavioral classes are further distinguished by cautionary procedures to avoid infection per sexual contact. Thus, the probabilities of a susceptible escaping infection per sexual contact with an infective by behavioral class were assigned the values 0.9995, 0.995 and 0.99, respectively.

Table 10.14.1. Numerical Assignments of the Parameters.

$m = 3$
$n = 1$
$(\lambda_1, \lambda_2, \lambda_3) = (4, 5, 6)$
$(\eta_1, \eta_2, \eta_3) = (0, 1, 2)$
$\mathbf{p} = (0.9995, 0.995, 0.99)$
$(\mu_0, \mu_1) = (1/720, 1/60)$
$(\beta_1, \beta_2) = (0, 0)$
$\mu_r = 10$
$\varphi = (0.7711, 0, 0.1621, 0, 0.0668, 0)$

Row six of the table contains the parameter assignments for the mortality parameters. For example, in the absence of an infection, the expectation for the life of an individual was $1/\mu_0 = 720$ months or 60 years; while for an infected person the incremental risk of death of $\mu_1 = 1/60$ corresponded to a latent expectation of 60 months or 5 years. The parameter assignments for the β-parameters in row seven of the table, $\beta_1 = \beta_2 = 0$, indicate that the selection of sexual partners according to behavioral class and state of disease was random. Finally, the parameter assignment $\mu_r = 10$ in row eight of the table indicates that the expected number of recruits per month was 10, and row nine of the table indicates that these recruits were distributed among the types of individuals according to the probability vector φ. Observe that according to this vector, all recruits entering the population were susceptibles. All that remains to complete the description of the numerical inputs used in the experiments is to specify the matrix of latent risks governing transitions among behavioral classes and the population vectors, giving the number of individuals of each type present in the initial population. The matrix of latent risks governing transitions among behavioral classes was chosen as:

$$\boldsymbol{\Psi} = (\psi_{ij}) = \begin{bmatrix} 0 & 0 & 0 \\ 0 & 0 & 1/1200 \\ 0 & 1/1200 & 0 \end{bmatrix} . \tag{10.14.1}$$

According to these parameter assignments, the latent risk governing transition from class 2 to class 3 was $\psi_{23} = 1/1,200$, corresponding to a latent expectation of 1200 months or 100 years. The latent risk ψ_{43}, governing the transition from class 4 to class 3 had the same value. Moreover, according to the matrix in Eq. (10.14.1), no transitions into or out of class 1 were possible. In summary, for populations governed by the matrix of latent risks in Eq. (10.14.1), the rates of transitions among classes 2 and 3 were low, indicating that individuals tended to remain in these behavioral classes throughout their life spans.

Presented in Table 10.14.2 are the initial population vectors used in the computer experiments. The first column contains the six types of individuals in the population, and the second column, labeled Initial 0, represents a population of susceptibles that has been evolving for a long period of time. The vector φ in Table 10.14.1 was obtained by normalizing this vector. Two invasion thresholds were studied in the computer experiments. In the first experiment with initial vector labeled Initial 10, in the third column, 10 infectives were introduced into class 3, the class with the highest level of risky behavior. In a second experiment with an initial vector labeled Initial 100, in column four of the table, this invasion threshold of infectives in class 3 was increased ten-fold to the value 100.

Table 10.14.2. Initial Population Vectors.

Type	Initial 0	Initial 10	Initial 100
(1,0)	3858	3858	3858
(1,1)	0	0	0
(2,0)	813	813	813
(2,1)	0	0	0
(3,0)	345	345	345
(3,1)	0	10	100

It should be pointed out that, given the parameter assignments in Table 10.14.1 and Eq. (10.14.1), the vector in Table 10.14.2 labeled Initial 0 is not the stationary vector for the embedded differential equations. For, with these parameter assignments, the stationary vector truncated to two decimal places is:

$$\widehat{\mathbf{x}} = \begin{bmatrix} 5551.92 \\ 0 \\ 979.98 \\ 0 \\ 668.09 \\ 0 \end{bmatrix} . \tag{10.14.2}$$

Thus, in a population with this stationary vector, the total population size is about 7200. In what follows, it will of interest to keep this number in mind with a view towards measuring the impact of an epidemic on total population size. Given the parameter assignments just described, the Jacobian matrix for the embedded differential equations was stable, suggesting that if a few infectives were introduced into the population, the epidemic would become extinct.

As explained in Section 7.9, the strategy used to condense the Monte Carlo simulation data statistically was to compute the minimum, maximum and mean of a sample of realizations of the process at each epoch $t \in S_h$ in a projection for those random functions of particular interest. The trajectories of these sample statistics were then plotted along with the trajectory computed according to the embedded non-linear difference equations in order to assess the behavior of the deterministic model in relation to a Monte Carlo sample of realizations of the process. Among the questions under consideration was in what sense is the trajectory of the embedded deterministic model a measure of central tendency for the sample functions of the stochastic process. The time unit used in all experiments reported in this section was $h = 1$ month, and the number of Monte Carlo realizations computed in each experiment was 100. However, because in preliminary experiments it was observed that the behavior of the stochastic model was very sensitive to the magnitude of the invasion threshold, the lengths of the projections differed for the two initial population vectors. For the initial vector Initial 10, the length of the projection was 1200 months or 100 years, but for the initial vector Initial 100, the length of the projection was increased to 1560 months or $1560/12 = 130$ years.

When there is reason to believe that an epidemic will eventually become extinct, then it seems natural to ask the following kinds of questions: How many people will be infected and how much variation might be expected in the number of persons infected before the epidemic becomes extinct? Presented in Table 10.14.1 are graphs of the cumulative number of individuals in behavioral class 1 who were infected following the invasion of the initial infectives, and which provide some answers to these questions. In these graphs, the minimum, mean, and maximum trajectories are labeled Min, Bar, and Max, and the trajectory for the embedded deterministic model is labeled Det. As can be seen from an inspection of the upper panel of Figure 10.14.1 for 10 initial infectives, the trajectory of the embedded deterministic model lies considerably above that for the Max trajectory; while those for the Bar (mean) and Min are relatively small. In the lower panel of the figure for the case of 100 initial infectives, the trajectory of the deterministic model again dominates the Max trajectory, but the Bar and Min trajectories occupy a more central position than in the upper panel.

As will be demonstrated subsequently, the differences in the Bar and Min trajectories in the two graphs are due to a more rapid extinction of the epidemic for the case of 10 initial infective than for the case of 100 initial infectives. With regard to variation in the total number of persons infected before an epidemic becomes extinct, it can be seen from the figures that it can be large. For example, for the case of 100 initial infectives, at 1560 months the Min trajectory is a little greater than 2250 but the Max trajectory is nearly 6000, indicating that the variability in the number of persons infected during the evolution of an epidemic can quite large. In any case, for a population governed by the parameters settings with these initial vectors, if an investigator used only a deteministic model to forecast the evolution of an epidemic, his or her forecasts would be overly pessimistic.

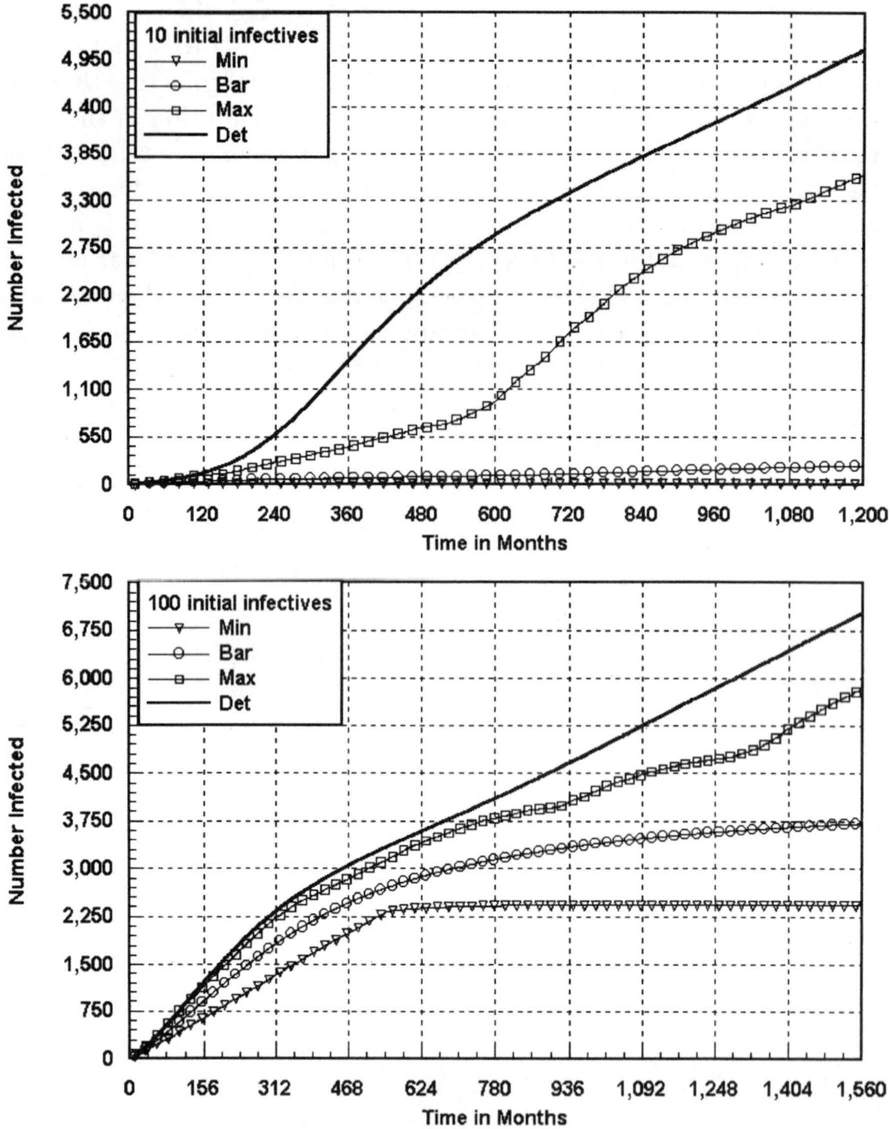

Figure 10.14.1. Cumulative Number of Individuals in Behavioral Class 1 Infected Following Invasion of Infectives.

Another perspective from which the evolution of an epidemic may be viewed is that of the number of infected individuals at each epoch $t \in S_h$ of a projection. Figure 10.14.2 contains the graphs of the Min, Bar, Max and Det trajectories for the number of infected individuals at each epoch who were members of behavioral class 1. In the upper panel of the figure, where the trajectories for the initial vector, Initial 10, are presented, it can be seen that the Det trajectory diverges significantly from the Min, Bar and Max trajectories. It can also be seen that the Max trajectory differs significantly from the small trajectories of Bar and Min, indicating that although there is an apparently high probability that the epidemic will become extinct eventually, for some realizations of the process the number of infected individuals can be quite large. When the number of initial infectives is increased tenfold, the Det and Max trajectories are quite similar throughout the projection, as can be seen from the graphs in the lower panel of Figure 10.14.2, where the initial vector was Initial 100. As can be seen from an inspection of these graphs, when there is an invasion of infectives of this size, the number of infected individuals in the population increases for about 10 years before a slow decline to eventual extinction. In this connection, it is interesting to note that if an investigator relied solely on the deterministic model to forecast the evolution an epidemic, the forecasted time to extinction would be much longer than that for the stochastic process, and, moreover, the variability in the time to extinction would be missed completely. Although the graphs for behavioral classes 2 and 3 are not shown, they are qualitatively very similar to those for class 1.

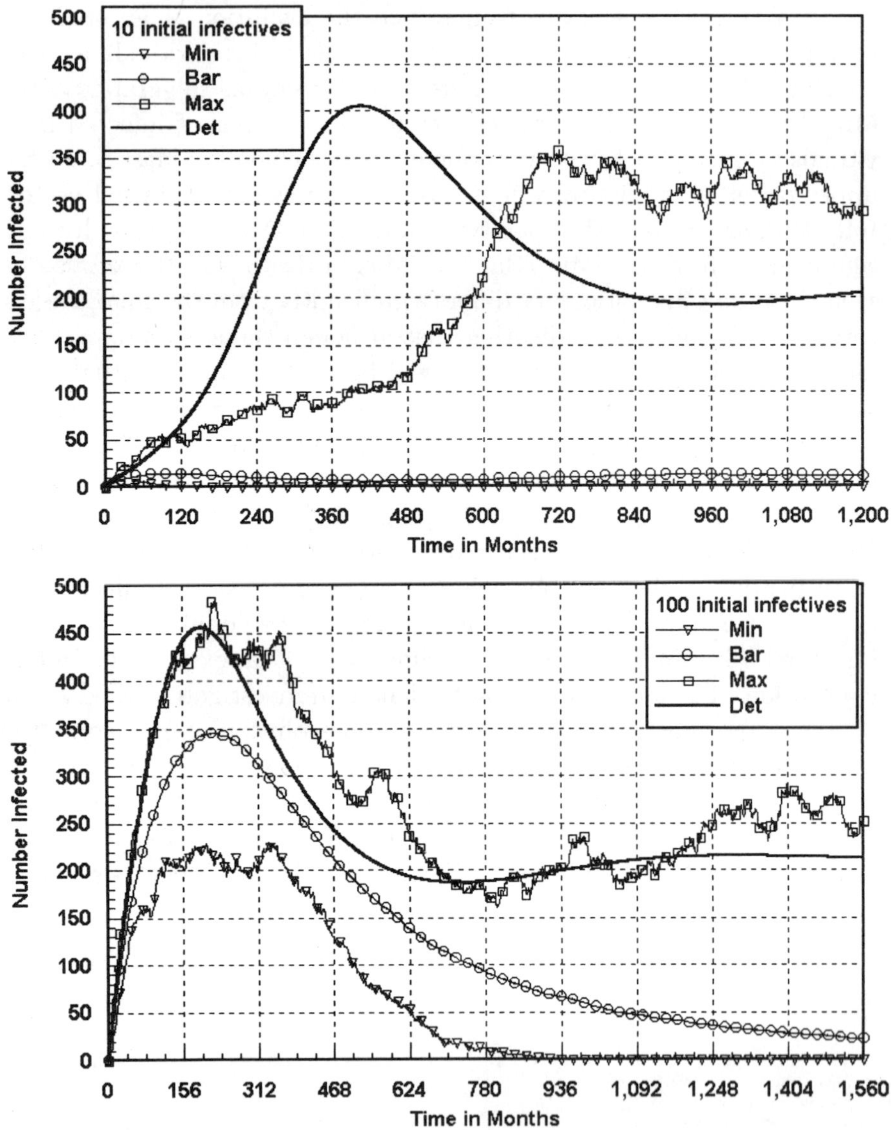

Figure 10.14.2. Number of Individuals by Epoch in Behavioral Class 1 Infected Following Invasion of Infectives.

Figure 10.14.3 contains the graphs of the estimated probability that an epidemic is extinct by each epoch $t \in S_h$ of a projection. From the graph in the upper panel of the figure, where Initial 10 was the initial vector, it is interesting to note that among the 100 Monte Carlo realizations of the process, only one realization of the epidemic had become extinct at about 14 years, 168 months, into the projections. However, after 100 years, which is a long time in terms of expected human life-spans, 95 realizations of the epidemic had become extinct. When the invasion threshold was increased to 100 infectives, the waiting times to extinction increased dramatically. For as can be seen from the lower panel of the figure, it was not until about 77 years or 924 months into the projections that only one of the Monte Carlo realizations of the epidemic had become extinct. Furthermore, by 100 years, the epidemic had become extinct in only 16 out of the 100 realizations of the process, and by 1560 months or 130 years, the epidemic was extinct in only 62 of the 100 realizations. From these examples, it can be seen that the waiting times to the extinction of an epidemic can be large, highly variable, and depend significantly on invasion thresholds.

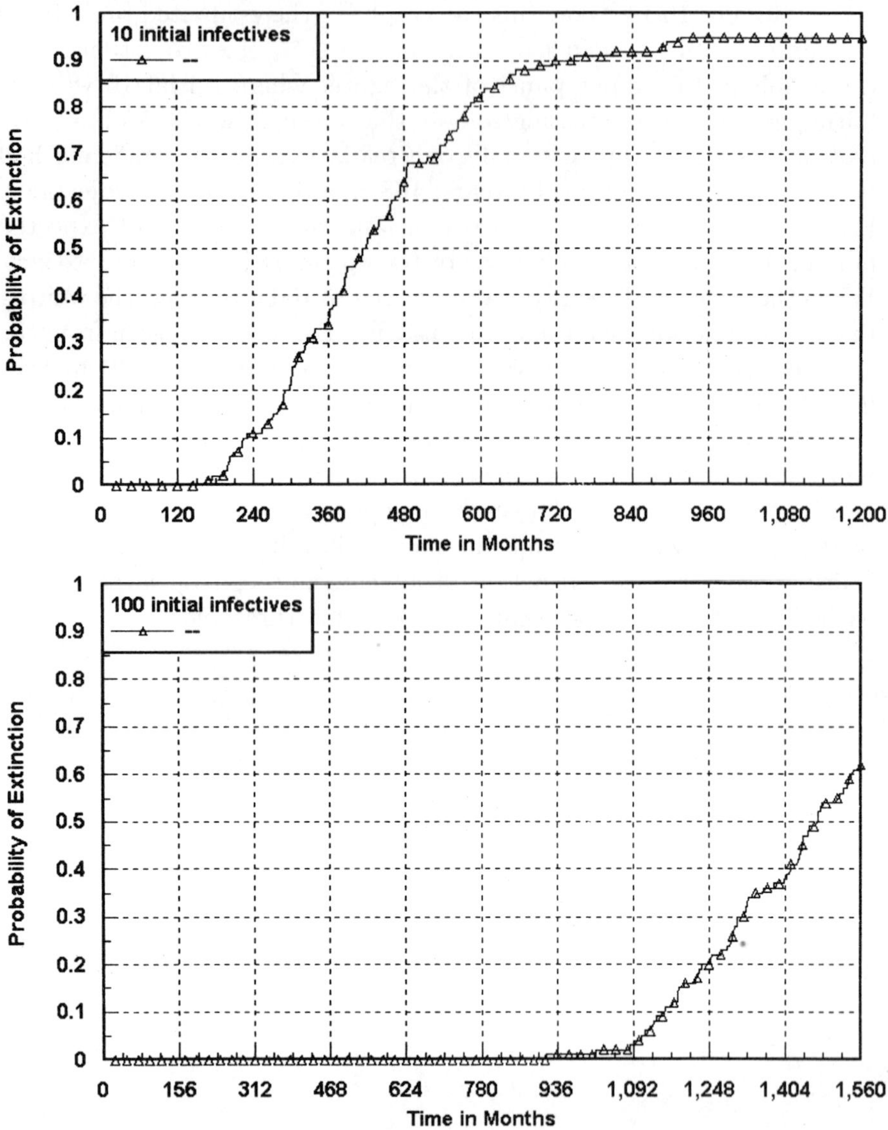

Figure 10.14.3. Probability Epidemic is Extinct by Epoch.

Although the graphs for the Min, Bar, Max and Det trajectories of the total population size in class 1 will not be presented, it is, nevertheless, of interest to present the values of these trajectories at the end of each projection and compare them to the stationary value of about 5552 in the vector in Eq. (10.14.2), which would be the total population size of class 1 if the population had evolved for a long period of time according to the deterministic model. For the projections with Initial 10 as the invasion threshold, the values of Min, Bar, Max, and Det trajectories at 1200 months or 100 years were 3255, 5133.35, 5401, and 3041.10, respectively; whereas for those projections with Initial 100 as the invasion threshold, these values at 1560 months or 130 years were 3201, 4489.18, 5058, and 3003.82, respectively. It is interesting to note that the value of the Max trajectory at the end of each set of projections was near that of the stationary value 5552, and represents the largest population size among those realizations of the process in which the epidemic had become extinct. It is also of interest to note that in both sets of projections the Min and the Det trajectories are quite close, suggesting that if an investigator confined attention to the deterministic model to forecast the evolution of an epidemic, only the worst cases of the epidemic would be included in his or her forecast.

10.15 Invasion Thresholds: One-Stage Model, Positive Assortment

As mentioned in a previous section, when both the parameters β_1 and β_2 are positive, it is more likely that persons in a given behavioral class and state of disease will prefer sexual partners in the same behavioral class and state of disease. When such conditions prevail in a population, it is sometimes said that there is positive assortment with respect to sexual partners. In all the computer experiments reported in this section, the parameter assignments described in Section 10.14 were the same except that positive values of the β-parameters were chosen. In case 1, which will be referred to as weak positive assortment, the values of the β-parameters were chosen as $\beta_1 = \beta_2 = 1$. But, in case 2 these parameter values were chosen as $\beta_1 = \beta_2 = 2$, and, in what follows, this case will be referred to as strong positive assortment. Just as in Section 10.14, the Jacobian matrix of the embedded differential equations was evaluated at the stationary vector $\widehat{\mathbf{x}}$ for the situation in which the population contained only susceptibles and checked for stability. For the case of weak assortment, the Jacobian matrix was unstable, but for the case of strong assortment, it was stable. For ease of reference, the cases of weak and strong assortment, along with the stability of the Jacobian matrix for each case, are summarized in Table 10.15.1.

Table 10.15.1. Two Cases of Positive Assortment.

Weak, Jacobian Matrix Unstable	$\beta_1 = 1$	$\beta_2 = 1$
Strong, Jacobian Matrix Stable	$\beta_1 = 2$	$\beta_2 = 2$

For case of weak assortment, the condition that the Jacobian matrix was unstable suggests that if a few infectives were introduced in a population of susceptibles, then an epidemic would develop with positive probability. However, for the case of strong assortment, the condition of a stable Jacobian matrix suggested that if a few infectives were introduced into a population of susceptibles, a small epidemic may develop but it would eventually become extinct with positive probability. As was illustrated in Section 10.14 for the case of random assortment in choosing sexual partners, whether an epidemic becomes extinct can depend significantly on the number of infectives who invade an initial population of susceptibles. To study this phenomenon for the case of positive assortment, three invasion thresholds were considered as displayed in Table 10.15.2. Observe that these initial vectors of invasion thresholds are the same as in Table 10.14.1 except for the vector Initial 1, indicating that in this situation only one infective was introduced into behavioral class 3.

Table 10.15.2. Initial Population Vectors.

Type	Initial 1	Initial 10	Initial 100
(1,0)	3858	3858	3858
(1,1)	0	0	0
(2,0)	813	813	813
(2,1)	0	0	0
(3,0)	345	345	345
(3,1)	1	10	100

For each of the initial vectors in Table 10.15.2, 100 Monte Carlo realizations of the process were computed for 1560 months or 130 years and summarized statistically as described in Section 10.14, and, to gain some insights into the behavior of the embedded deterministic model, the trajectories of various aspects of the epidemic as determined by the non-linear difference equations were also computed. Presented in Figure 10.15.1 are some selected results from these computer experiments for the initial population vector Initial 1. In the upper panel of the figure, estimates of the probability the epidemic is extinct by epoch are presented; whereas in the lower panel the Min, Bar, Max, and Det trajectories of the number infected persons in behavioral class 3 by epoch are presented. As can be seen from the upper panel of the figure, for this invasion threshold, the Monte Carlo estimates of the probability that the epidemic becomes extinct by epoch converge rather slowly to a limiting value of 0.66, a value that is quite high. Upon inspecting the lower panel of the figure, it can be seen that the Det trajectory differs significantly from those of the Min, Bar, and Max. For, according to the Det trajectory, the number of infected persons in behavioral class 3 would, eventually, converge to little over 51; yet, according to the stochastic model, 66 out of 100 realizations of the process actually became extinct. Thus, one may conclude that whenever there is a substantial probability that an epidemic will eventually become extinct, the trajectory computed according to the embedded deterministic can be quite misleading as to the actual course an epidemic may take.

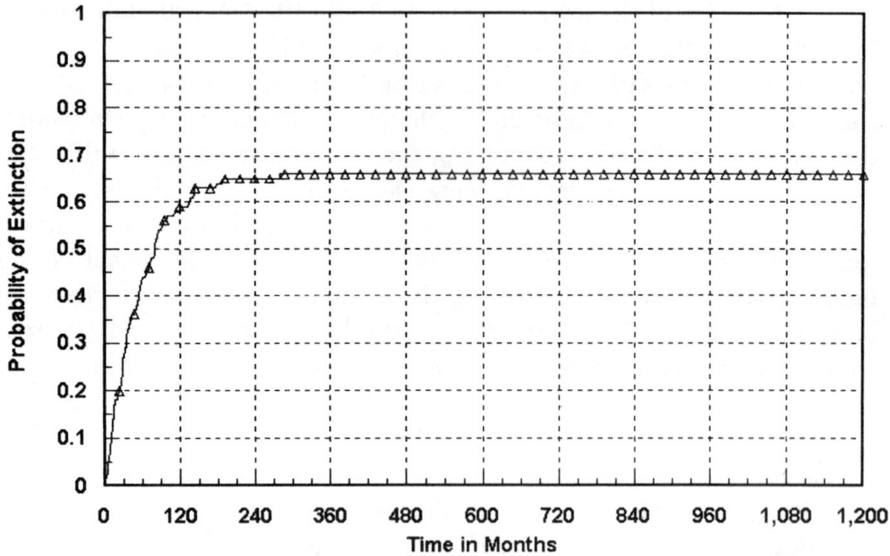

Estimated Probability Epidemic is Extinct by Epoch

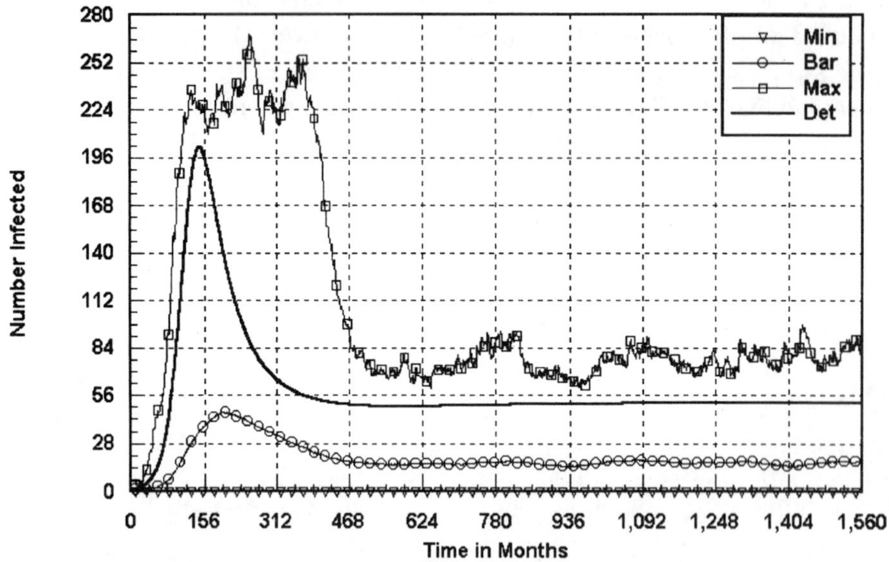

Number Infected in Behavioral Class 3 by Epoch

Figure 10.15.1. Invasion Threshold Initial 1 with Weak Assortment.

When the initial population vector was Initial 10, in only one of the 100 Monte Carlo realizations of the process did the epidemic become extinct, which suggests that, for the parameter assignments under consideration, the extinction probability decreases rather rapidly as the initial number of infectives increases. Figure 10.15.2 contains some selected graphs, summarizing the results of the computer experiments with vector Initial 10. Because information on the total number of persons infected following an invasion of infectives is of interest, the upper panel in the figure contains graphs of the Min, Bar, Max, and Det trajectories for the cumulative number of persons infected following the invasion of the initial infectives. For the sake of brevity, they are labeled as new infections. As can be seen from inspection, the Min trajectory is the constant 0, because one of the 100 Monte Carlo realizations of the process the epidemic became extinct, but throughout the projections the Det trajectory lies between the Bar and Max trajectories, indicating that with Initial 10 as the initial vector, the Det trajectory performs quite well as a measure of central tendency for the sample functions of the process.

In the lower panel of Figure 10.15.2, the graphs of the Min, Bar, Max, and Det trajectories are presented for the number of infected persons in behavioral class 3 by epoch. In these graphs, the Min trajectory converges to 0, because in one out of 100 realizations of the process the epidemic became extinct. However, from months 0 to approximately month 96, the Bar, Max, and Det trajectories increase before they commence to decline, indicating that on the set of non-extinction, infections are becoming endemic in the population. It is interesting to observe that in these projections, the Bar and Det trajectories are quite close so that again the Det trajectory performs well as a measure of central tendency for the sample functions of the process.

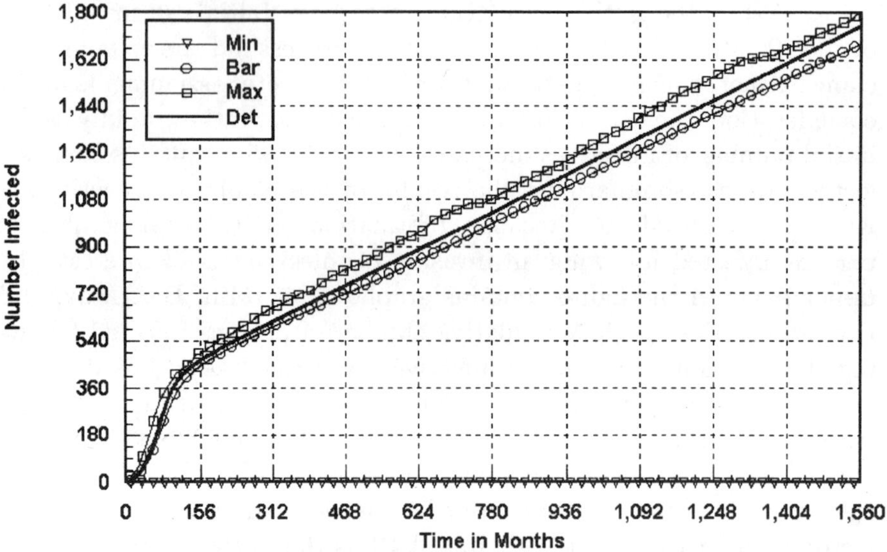

Cumulative New Infections in Behavioral Class 3

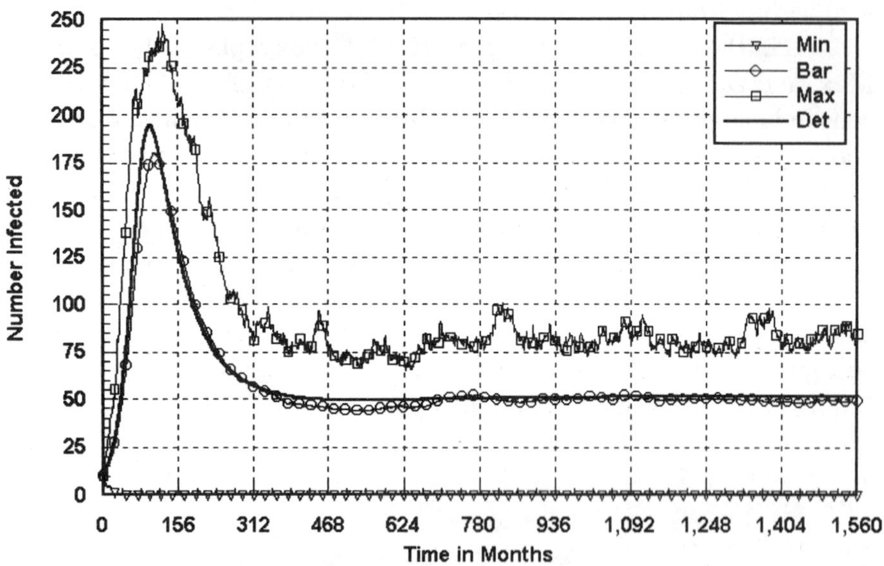

Number Infected in Behavioral Class 3 by Epoch

Figure 10.15.2. Invasion Threshold Initial 10 with Weak Assortment.

Unlike the other two initial vectors, when Initial 100 was used as the initial population vector, in none of the 100 Monte Carlo realizations of the process did the epidemic become extinct. In order to expedite comparisons between invasion thresholds Initial 10 and Initial 100, the graphs for Initial 100, corresponding to those in Figure 10.15.2 for Initial 10, are presented in Figure 10.15.3. As can be seen from the upper panel of the figure for cumulative numbers of new infections in behavioral class 3, the Min, Bar, Max, and Det trajectories are increasing throughout the projections, and the Min and Max trajectories provide a rather tight envelope within which the Bar and Det trajectories fall. Similar relationships among the Min, Bar, Max and Det trajectories are exhibited in the lower panel of Figure 10.15.3, where the trajectories are plotted for the number of infected persons in behavioral class 3 by epoch. Throughout these projections, the Bar and Det trajectories are close, suggesting that, given the present parameter assignments, if an invasion threshold of infectives is sufficiently large, then the trajectories provided by the embedded deterministic model will perform quite well as measures of central tendency for the sample functions of the process. On the other hand, as has been demonstrated by an example, if the invasion threshold of infectives is small so that there is a significant probability that the epidemic will become extinct, then the trajectories provided by the embedded deteministic model will miss much of the intrinsic variation present in the evolution of an epidemic according to the stochastic model.

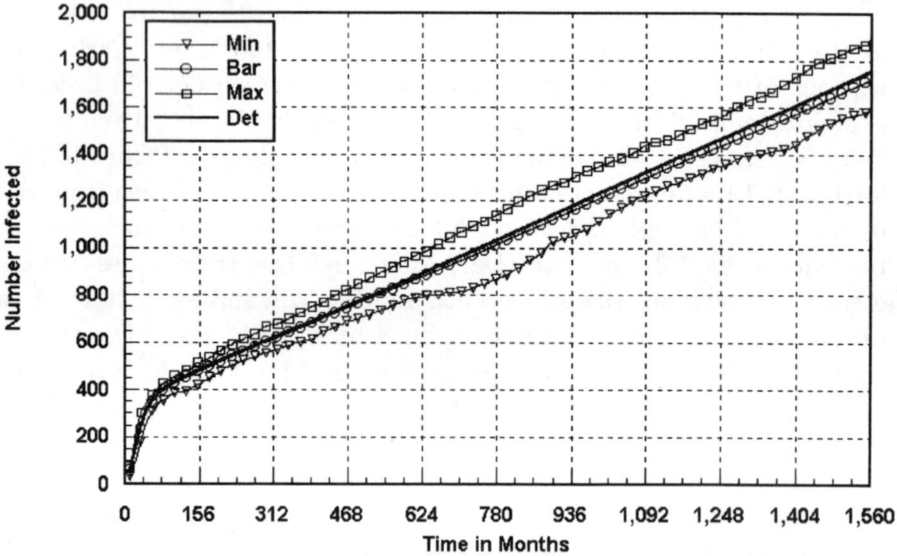

Cumulative New Infections in Behavioral Class 3

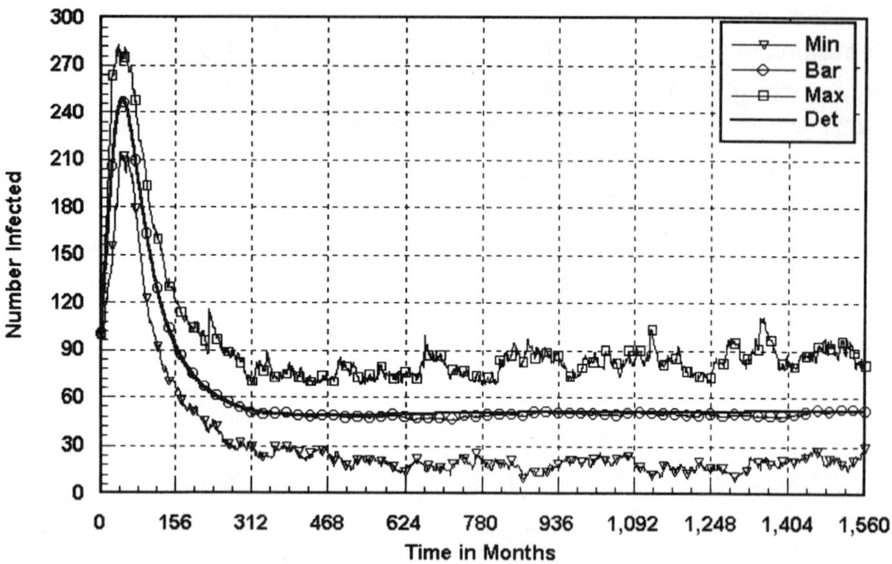

Number Infected in Behavioral Class 3 by Epoch

Figure 10.15.3. Invasion Threshold Initial 100 with Weak Assortment.

For the case of strong assortment, the only invasion threshold studied was that for the initial vector Initial 100, because it was found in preliminary experiments that an epidemic would become extinct quite rapidly for smaller invasions of infectives into a population of susceptibles. Even with 100 initial infectives in behavioral class 3, it was observed that within 60 years, or 720 months, only a few infectives would be present in the population. Consequently, it was decided to compute 100 Monte Carlo realizations of the process for a duration of 720 months. In the upper panel of Figure 10.15.4, the Min, Bar, Max, and Det trajectories are presented for the cumulative numbers of new infections in behavioral class 3, following the introduction of 100 initial infectives. It is interesting to note that at epoch 720, the values of the Min, Bar, Max, and Det trajectories were about 22, 54, 103, and 56, respectively, indicating that the initial infectives infected relatively few members of the population. That all these trajectories appear to be converging to some limit may be interpreted as an indication that the epidemic was becoming extinct. A clearer view that the epidemic is becoming extinct may be obtained from an inspection of the lower panel in Figure 10.15.4, where the Min, Bar, Max, and Det trajectories of the numbers of infected persons in behavioral class 3 by epoch are plotted. As can be seen from this figure, all these trajectories appear to be converging to 0, indicating that the epidemic was becoming extinct with high probability. It is interesting to note, however, that at epoch 720 months the population may contain at least one infective, since the Max trajectory was positive at that epoch.

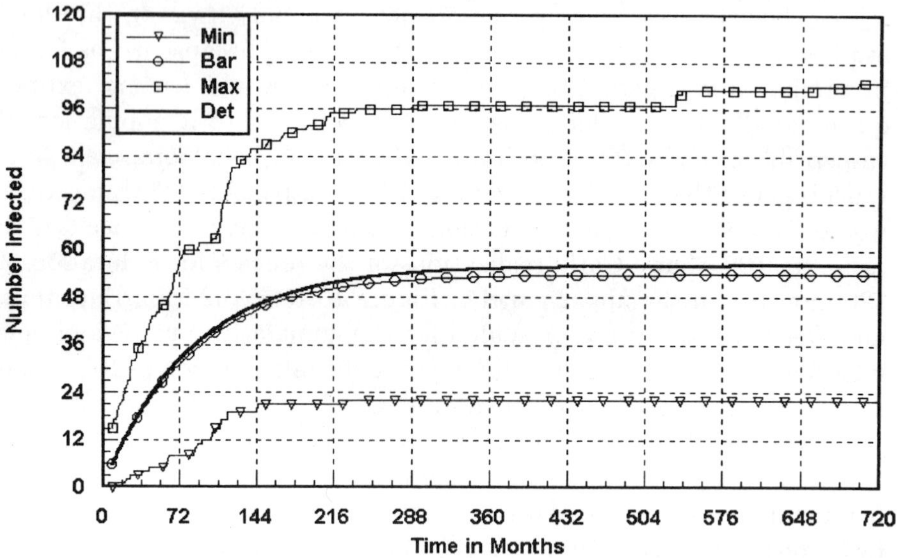

Cumulative New Infections in Behavioral Class 3

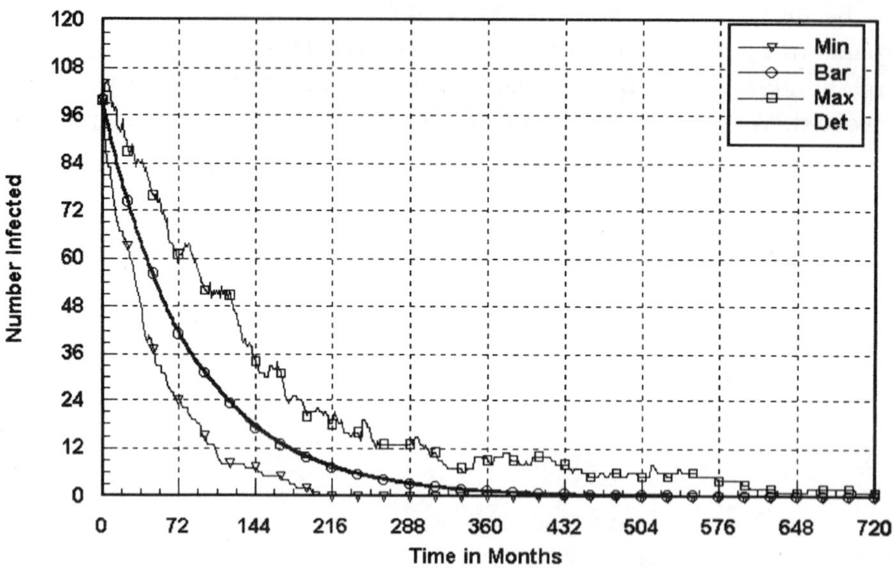

Number Infected in Behavioral Class 3 by Epoch

Figure 10.15.4. Invasion Threshold Initial 100 with Strong Assortment.

Due to space limitations, a decision was made not to display graphs depicting the number of infected persons in behavioral classes 1 and 2 as functions of time. Nevertheless, it of interest to give a brief account of the number of persons infected in these classes for the computer experiments under consideration. For the case of weak positive assortment, infections spread throughout the population in all the projections so that a substantial number of persons in classes 1 and 2 became infected. For example, when the initial population vector was Initial 100, the Min, Bar, Max and Det trajectories for the cumulative number of new infectives at epoch 1560 months for class 1 were 724, 809.73, 915, and 830.654, respectively. The corresponding numbers for behavioral class 2 were 1287, 1427.8, 1552, 1478.80. Even though the greatest number of persons belonged to class 1, a smaller proportion of them were infected than those in class 2, because, according to the assumptions of the model, persons in class 1 were less sexually active than those in class 2. For the case of strong assortment, very few individuals in classes 1 and 2 were infected and the epidemic was confined essentially to class 3, the class with the highest level of sexual activity, in all the Monte Carlo realizations of the process.

In summary, it seems appropriate to suggest some analogies between branching processes and the class of stochastic models of sexually transmitted diseases under consideration. Let $(\Omega, \mathfrak{A}, \mathbb{P})$ denote the probability space underlying the process and let $A \in \mathfrak{A}$ denote the set on which the epidemic becomes extinct. In this class of stochastic models, whether the Jacobian matrix $\mathbf{J}$ evaluated at the stationary vector $\widehat{\mathbf{x}}$ for the case where a population contains only susceptibles is stable or non-stable plays a role analogous to the threshold parameter R_0 or ρ for a branching process. If, for example, $\mathbf{J}$ is stable, analogous to $R_0 < 1$ or $\rho < 1$, then with high probability $\mathbb{P}[A]$ and the trajectories determined by the embedded deterministic model will not perform well as measures of central tendencies for the sample functions of the process. On the other hand, if $\mathbf{J}$ is not stable, analogously $R_0 > 1$ or $\rho > 1$, then there may be a positive probability $\mathbb{P}[A] > 0$ that the epidemic becomes extinct, but on the complementary set A^c of non-extinction, the trajectories determined by the embedded deterministic model may perform well as measures of central tendency for the sample functions of the process.

10.16 Recurrent Invasions by Infectious Recruits

In the two preceding sections, stochastic evolutionary scenarios of epidemics were studied following one-time invasions by various numbers of infectives into a population of susceptibles, but thereafter no infectious recruits entered the population. Such evolutionary scenarios may be applicable to those situations in which infectious recruits can be recognized and thus be denied entrance into a population. But, if no linkage has been made between disease defining symptoms and the existence of a disease causing agent, which may have a long incubation period before infected persons exhibit symptoms, then there would be no recognizable basis for denying infected recruits entrance into a population. Such a situation seems to have prevailed in the evolution of HIV/AIDS epidemics, where the causal virus, HIV, may have existed for decades or perhaps even centuries before it was recognized as a disease causing agent (see Grmek[4] for a very interesting account of the history of AIDS). It is of interest, therefore, to study computer generated stochastic evolutionary scenarios of situations in which, during each time interval, there is a small probability that one or more infective recruits enter a population consisting mainly of susceptibles.

To study scenarios of this type, as in the preceding sections, the number of behavioral classes was chosen as $m = 3$, but the number of stages of disease was chosen as $n = 4$, which gave rise to a model with $3 \times 5 = 15$ types of individuals in a population. Listed in Table 10.16.1 are the computer inputs by type used in the computer experiments reported in this section. The first column of the table contains an enumeration of the 15 types of individuals in the population, and the second column, with the heading $\mathbf{X}_0$, contains the number of individuals of each type present in the initial population. Observe that the initial population contained only susceptible individuals. The third column, with the heading $\mathbf{p}_0$, contains the probabilities that a susceptible escapes infection per sexual contact with each type of infective. Observe that for the susceptible types, $(1,0)$, $(2,0)$, and $(3,0)$, these probabilities are one, and for infective types they vary according to the stage of disease and behavioral class, with the escape probabilities being greater in behavioral class 1, the class with the lowest level of sexual activity per unit time, than in classes 2 and 3 with the higher levels of sexual activity.

Table 10.16.1. Computer Inputs by Type.

Type	$\mathbf{X}_0$	$\mathbf{p}_0$	φ
(1,0)	3461	1.000	0.48075
(1,1)	0	0.995	0
(1,2)	0	0.998	0
(1,3)	0	0.998	0
(1,4)	0	0.995	0
(2,0)	2198	1.000	0.3601363636
(2,1)	0	0.950	0
(2,2)	0	0.985	0
(2,3)	0	0.985	0
(2,4)	0	0.950	0
(3,0)	1514	1.000	0.1501136364
(3,1)	0	0.950	0.0001591136364
(3,2)	0	0.980	0
(3,3)	0	0.980	0
(3,4)	0	0.950	0

The fourth column of the table, with the heading φ, contains the probabilities governing the distribution of types of recruits entering the population during each time interval. According to this probability distribution, there was a high total probability that any recruit entering the population was susceptible, and a low probability, 0.0001591136364, that an infective of type $(3,1)$ in behavioral class 3 entered the population per unit time. The rationale for choosing this latter probability was as follows. In the probability vector that was used to determine the stationary population vector $\widehat{\mathbf{x}}$ according to the embedded deterministic differential equations, the probability a recruit belonged to behavioral class 3 was 0.1591136364. To determine a working number for the probability that a recruit of type $(3,1)$ entered the population per unit time, this number was multiplied by 10^{-3}. Thus, among recruits of behavioral class 3 with the highest level of sexual activity and greatest risk of infecting susceptibles, it was assumed that only one out of 1000 was infected, but, by assumption, no recruits in classes 1 and 2 were infected.

Whenever a model is constructed so that there is more than one stage of disease, then it is necessary to specify a matrix $\mathbf{\Gamma}$ of latent risks, governing transitions among stages of disease. For the experiments reported in this section, this matrix was chosen as

$$\mathbf{\Gamma} = \begin{bmatrix} 0 & 1/12 & 0 & 0 \\ 0 & 0 & 1/52.6316 & 0 \\ 0 & 0 & 0 & 1/62.8931 \\ 0 & 0 & 0 & 0 \end{bmatrix}, \tag{10.16.1}$$

where the time unit was a month. According to this $\mathbf{\Gamma}$-matrix, the only transitions possible among stages of HIV disease is from higher to lower $CD4^+$ counts, which seems appropriate for a population in which drugs to control the virus and diminish $CD4^+$counts had not yet been developed. All transition rates except for $\gamma_{12} = 1/12$, governing the rate of transitions from the non-seropositive state 1 to state 2, were based on estimates supplied by Longini et al.[11,9,10,12] Consequently, in the computer experiments reported in this section, the expected waiting time of 12 months in state 1 was longer than that reported by Longini and his colleagues. Among the parameters that must also be specified numerically for multiple stages of disease are those governing mortality. For the computer experiments reported in this section, these parameters were chosen as $(\mu_0, \mu_1, \mu_2, \mu_3, \mu_4) = (1/720, 1/240, 1/240, 1/23.8)$, where the time unit is again a month. All values except for $\mu_4 = 1/23.8$, which was based on results reported by Longini et al., were not based on data but were chosen purely for illustrative purposes.

Numerical values for all the other parameters of the model were chosen as in the preceding two sections. For example, the λ-vector as well as the η-vector were chosen as in Table 10.14.1, and, similarly, the expected number of recruits entering the population per month was chosen as $\mu_r = 10$. The matrix $\mathbf{\Psi}$ of latent risks, governing transitions among behavioral classes, was also chosen as in Eq. (10.14.1). Finally, the β-parameters were chosen as $\beta_1 = \beta_2 = 1$, which corresponds to the case of weak positive assortment considered in Section 10.15. At the point in the parameter space determined by the numerical values just described, it was found that the 15×15 **A**-matrix was stable as was the case for other **A**-matrices considered in this chapter. But the 15×15 Jacobian matrix **J**, evaluated at the stationary vector $\widehat{\mathbf{x}}$ for a population containing only susceptibles, was found to be unstable, which suggests that an epidemic could develop if infective recruits entered the population from time to time. In some preliminary computer experiments, it was found the number of persons who became infected could vary greatly among Monte Carlo realizations, and, in some realizations, many months may elapse before a significant number of infective were observed in the population. Consequently, to provide some further insight into the variability among realizations of the process, 100 Monte Carlo realizations of the process were computed for the period of 2400 months or 200 years and summarized statistically as described in the foregoing two sections.

Among the interesting perspectives from which to view a sample of Monte Carlo realizations of an epidemic, is to present a graph of the fraction of the realizations by epoch for which there were no infectives in the population. Fortunately, since there is a positive probability that an infective recruit may enter the population during any time period, the software used to estimate the probability that the epidemic became extinct in Sections 10.14 and 10.15, may also be used to compute this fraction by epoch. Presented in the upper panel of Figure 10.16.1 is a graph of the fraction of the Monte Carlo realizations that contained no infectives by epoch. As can be seen from this graph, at about 48 months or four years into these projections, 97 out of 100 realizations of the process contained no infectives; by 360 months this number had been reduced to 65; by 720 months this number reached 42; and by 2400 months or 200 years, this number was reduced to 3. Thus, for a population whose stochastic evolution is governed by the parameter settings under consideration, the graph of the fraction of realizations not containing any infectives suggests that, in terms of expected human life spans, the development of a noticeable epidemic would be slow for many realizations of the process, but, for some realizations an epidemic may become established in a population within a relatively short period of time. One can thus imagine that if each of these 100 realizations of the process had occurred independently among 100 isolated geographical regions and historical records were kept, then these records would show a considerable amount of variability in the severities and paces of the development of the epidemics among these regions.

An interesting perspective from which to view variability in the severities and paces with which epidemics develop in populations is that of the evolution of total population size, which reflects mortality due to disease. Presented in the lower panel of Figure 10.16.1 are the graphs of the Min, Bar, Max, and Det trajectories for total population size by epoch. During the first 60 months of the projections, these four trajectories remained in juxtaposition, but as the projections progressed they tended to diverge, indicating mortality due to disease was having an impact on the variability in total population size. At 720 months, or 60 years, into the projections the values of the Min, Bar, and Max trajectories stood at 1642, 4632.36, and 7293, respectively, and by 2400 these values were 1449, 1816.13, and 7147. To put it another way, after 200 years of evolution, the total population size in the most severe cases of the epidemic would be only $1449/7147 = 0.2027$ or about 20.27% of that for the least severe cases of the epidemic. It is interesting to note that the Det trajectory lies very close to that on the Min throughout these projections, which suggests that if an investigator relied solely on the deteministic model to forecast the evolution of an epidemic, his or her forecast would represent only the worst case and would completely miss those cases in which no epidemic developed.

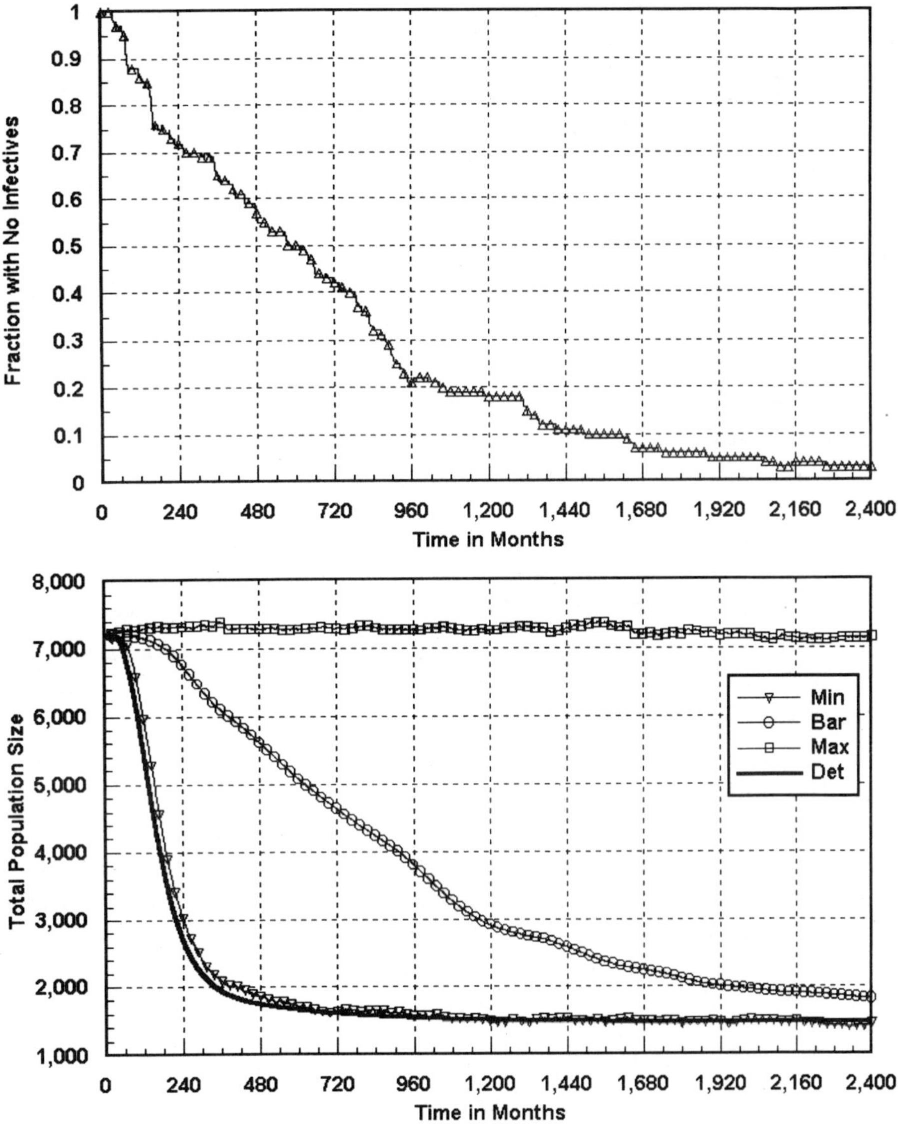

Figure 10.16.1. Fraction of Realizations with No Infectives and Total Population Size by Epoch.

Sometimes the impact of an infectious disease epidemic on a population is expressed in terms of estimates of the total number of persons infected during some time interval. Presented in Figure 10.16.2 are graphs of the Min, Bar, Max, and Det trajectories for the cumulative number of persons in behavioral class 1 infected during the projected period of 200 years. The corresponding trajectories for behavioral class 3 are presented in the lower panel of the figure. It is interesting to observe that in both these panels, the Det trajectory exceeds that of the Max at essentially all epochs, which is consistent with the observation made in connection with the total population size in that the embedded deterministic model tended to mimic those realizations of the process in which the most severe epidemics occurred. From an inspection of the trajectories in Figure 10.16.2, it is clear that, although all infectious recruits entering the population belonged to class 3, considerable numbers of persons in behavioral class 1, the class with the lowest level of sexual activity, were infected. It is of interest to compare the cumulative total number persons infected by the end of the projection period of 200 years with the size of the initial population in each class (see Table 10.16.1), by computing their ratio. For the case of the Det trajectory in behavioral class 1, this ratio was approximately $11929/3461 = 3.4$; and for the Bar trajectory this ratio was about $8690/3461 = 2.51$. The corresponding approximate ratios for the Det and Bar trajectories for behavioral class 3 were $5146/1514 = 3.40$ and $3979/1514 = 2.63$, respectively. Curiously, these ratios are nearly the same for both behavioral classes, which, perhaps, is not surprising. For, according to the embedded deterministic model, the infectious disease would eventually become endemic in the population.

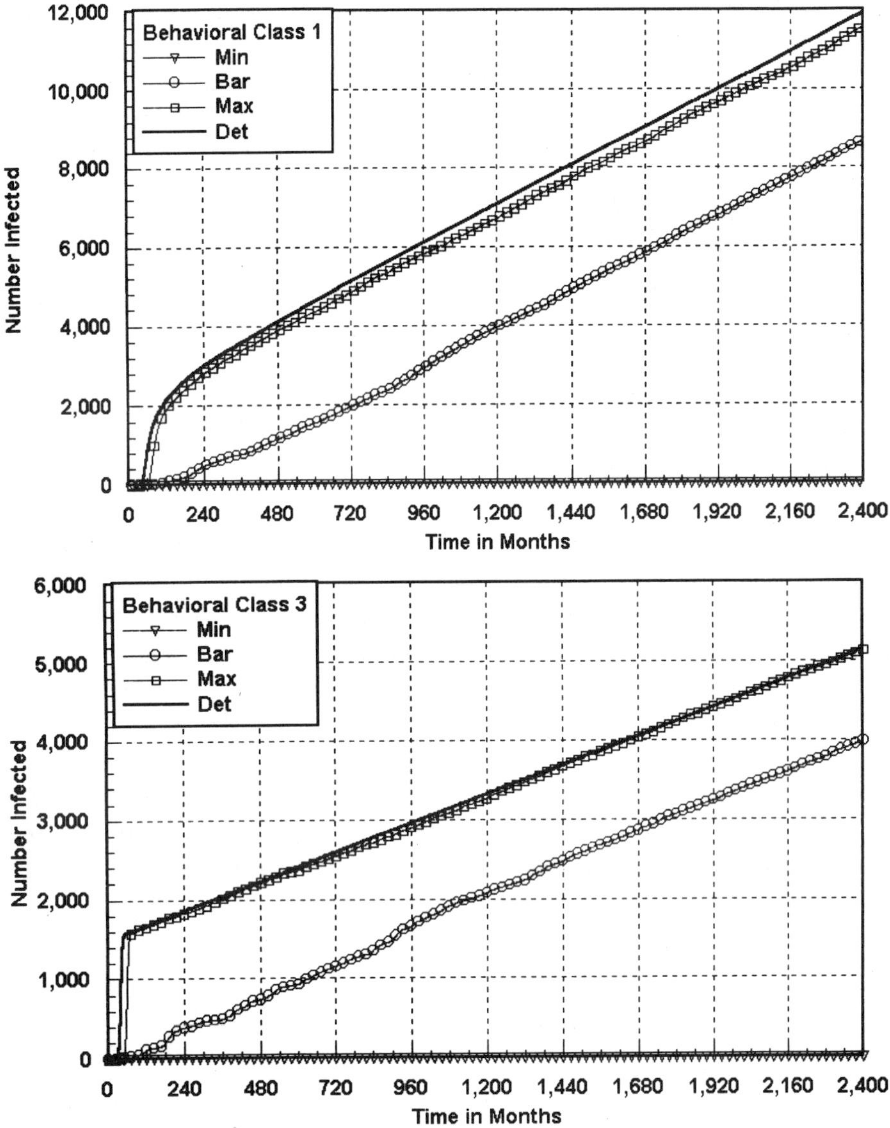

Figure 10.16.2. Cumulative Number of Individuals Infected by Epoch.

That the infectious disease did indeed become endemic in the population, according to the embedded deterministic model, may be seen by inspecting the graphs of the Min, Bar, Max, and Det trajectories for the number of persons infected by epoch in Figure 10.16.3, where those for the classes 1 and 3 appear in the upper and lower panels, respectively. Observe that, according to the Det trajectory for class 1 in the upper panel, the epidemic peaked between 84 and 120 months, or 7 to 10 years, before it started to decline to an endemic limit of about 392. But, in the lower panel of the figure for class 3, the Det trajectory peaked earlier between 36 to 60 months, or three to five years, and then declined gradually to a endemic limit of about 159. Unlike the situation in Figures 10.16.1 and 10.16.2, where the Max and Det trajectories remained fairly close throughout the projections, these trajectories diverged significantly in Figure 10.16.3, where the Det trajectory eventually came close to that for the Bar, the mean of 100 Monte Carlo realizations, but was significantly less than that of the Max in the later epochs of the projections. From the graphs presented in this and Section 10.15 for the case of weak assortment, the experimental evidence suggests that after a sufficiently long period of time, the Bar and Det trajectories tend to converge, but neither of these trajectories reflects the possibility that there may be much variation among the realizations of the process before this convergence occurs. In this connection, it is interesting to note the fluctuations that occur in the Max trajectories in the upper and lower panels of Figure 10.16.3. Although they were not shown due to space limitations, the graphs for behavioral class 2 were similar to those for classes 1 and 3.

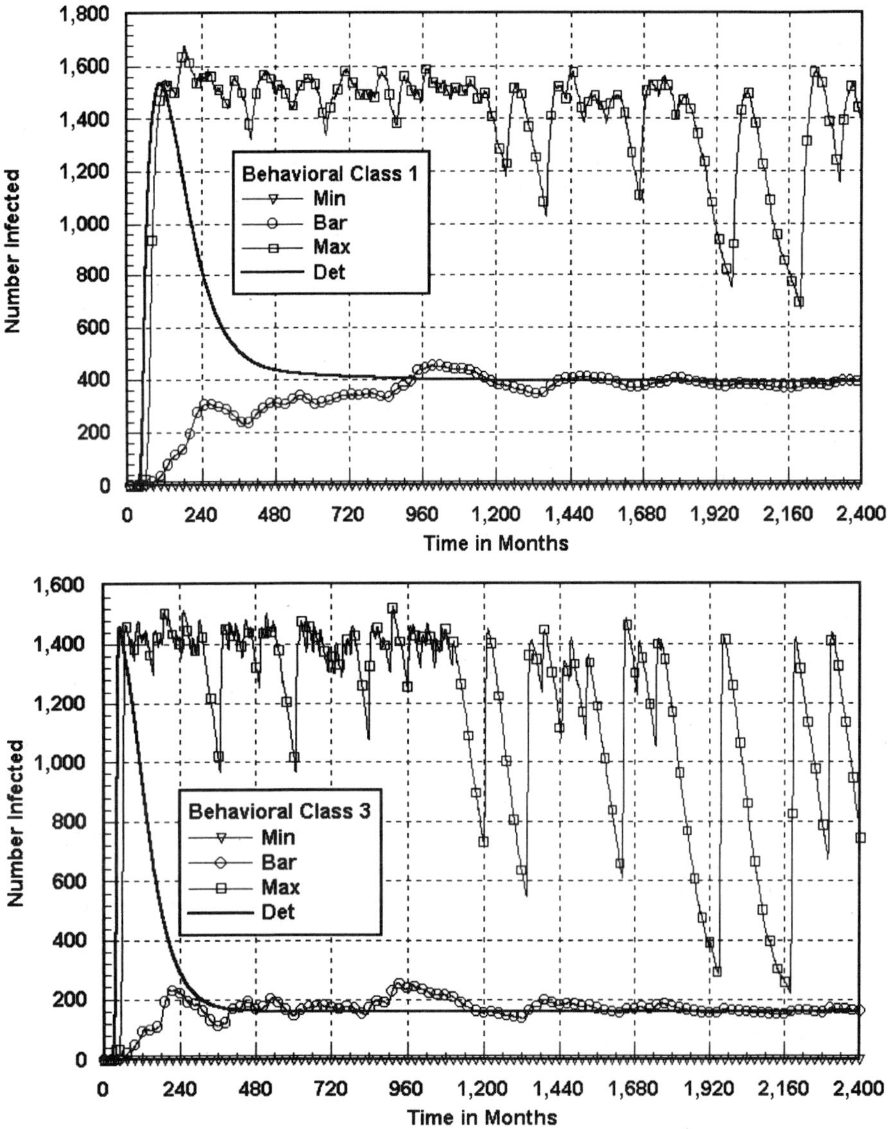

Figure 10.16.3. Number of Individuals Infected by Epoch.

In closing this chapter, it is interesting to suggest that the variability observed among Monte Carlo realizations of an epidemic of HIV/AIDS evolving according to a stochastic process, such as the one described in this section, may be helpful for interpreting data collected on the international pandemic. Among the interesting observations that a reader, who peruses the volume of papers on AIDS in the world edited by Mann and Tarantola,[13] may make is that of the rather high level of variability in the reported HIV/AIDS cases among the countries of the world and among regions within countries. As time passes, epidemiologists will probably isolate many factors underlying this variation, but among the factors to consider when analyzing such data is the intrinsic variability that occurs among realizations of a stochastic process, which may be a significant component of the observed variability among and within countries. Finally, the computer experiments reported in this section demonstrate that events, occurring with small probability during any time interval, can lead to high levels of variability among realizations of a stochastic process. Examples of events that occur with small probability in the real world are mutations in disease causing viruses, such as HIV and those causing influenza (see, for example, the recent paper by Laver et al.[8] for an interesting account of researchers' efforts to stay ahead of mutations in viruses causing this disease). Among the many challenges facing investigators who work with stochastic models of epidemics, is that of incorporating mutations in disease causing organisms into models, which would involve modeling events at the molecular level. Although this challenge is of great importance and would be of significant practical interest, no steps will be taken to meet this challenge here.

10.17 References

1. R. Bellman, *Stability Theory of Differential Equations*, McGraw-Hill, New York, Toronto, London, 1953.

2. V. Capasso, *Lecture Notes in Biomathematics* **97**, *Mathematical Structures of Epidemic Systems,* Springer-Verlag, Berlin, Heidelberg, New York, 1993.

3. F. R. Gantmacher, *The Theory of Matrices, II,* Chelsea Publishing Company, New York, New York, 1960.

4. M. D. Grmek with R. C. Maulitz and J. Duffin (translators), *History of AIDS - Emergence and Origin of a Modern Pandemic,* Princeton University Press, Princeton, New Jersey, 1990.

5. K. P. Hadeler, Pair Formation in Age-Structured Populations, *Acta Applicandae Mathematicae* **14:** 91-102, 1989.

6. J. Hale and H. Kocak, *Dynamics and Bifurcations*, Springer-Verlag, Berlin, Heidelberg, New York, 1991.

7. E. O. Laumann, J. H. Gagnon, R. T. Michael and S. Michaels, *The Social Organization of Sexuality - Sexual Practices in the United States,* The University of Chicago Press, Chicago and London, 1994.

8. W. G. Laver, N. Bischofberger and R. G. Webster, Disarming Flu Viruses, *Scientific American* **280:** 78-87, 1999.

9. I. M. Longini, Jr., B. H. Byers, N. A. Hessol and W. Y. Tan, Estimating Stage-Specific Numbers of HIV Infection Using a Markov Model and Back Calculation, *Statistics in Medicine* **11:** 831-843, 1992.

10. I. M. Longini, Jr., W. S. Clark and R. H. Byers et al., Statistical Analysis of the Stages of HIV Infection Using a Markov Model, *Statistics in Medicine* **8:** 831-843, 1989.

11. I. M. Longini, Jr., W. S. Clark, L. I. Gardner and J. F. Brundage, Modeling the Decline of CD4+ T-Lymphocyte Counts in HIV-Infected Individuals: A Markov Modeling Approach, *Journal of Acquired Immune Deficiency Syndromes* **4:** 1141-1147, 1991.

12. I. M. Longini, Jr., W. S. Clark, L. M. Haber and R. Horsburgh, Jr., The Stages of HIV Infection: Waiting Times and Infection Transmission Probabilities, *Lecture Notes in Biomathematics* **83:** 111-137, C. Castillo-Chavez (ed.), *Mathematical and Statistical Approaches in AIDS Epidemiology,* Springer-Verlag, Berlin, New York, Tokyo, 1989.

13. J. Mann and D. Tarantola, *AIDS in the World II - Global Dimensions, Social Roots, and Responses,* Oxford University Press, Oxford, New

York, 1996.

14. C. J. Mode, H. E. Gollwitzer and N. Herrmann, A Methodological Study of a Stochastic Model of an AIDS Epidemic, *Mathematical Biosciences* **92:** 201-229, 1988.
15. C. J. Mode, H. E. Gollwitzer, M. A. Salsburg and C. K. Sleeman, A Methodological Study of a Nonlinear Stochastic Model of an AIDS Epidemic with Recruitment, *IMA Journal of Mathematics Applied in Medicine and Biology* **6:** 179-203, 1989.
16. I. Nasell, The Threshold Concept in Deterministic and Stochastic Models, D. Mollison (ed.), *Epidemic Models: Their Structure and Relation to Data*, Cambridge University Press, 1995, pp. 71-83.
17. C. K. Sleeman and C. J. Mode, On Fitting a Nonlinear Stochastic Model of a HIV/AIDS Epidemic to Public Health Data for the City of Philadelphia, *Series in Mathematical Biology and Medicine* **6:** 453-476, O. Arino, D. Axelrod and M. Kimmel (eds.), *Advances in Mathematical Population Dynamics - Molecules, Cells, and Man,* World Scientific Publishing Company, Singapore, New Jersey, London, Hong Kong, 1997.
18. C. K. Sleeman and C. J. Mode, A Methodological Study on Fitting a Nonlinear Stochastic Model of the AIDS Epidemic in Philadelphia, *Mathematical and Computer Modelling* **26:** 33-51, 1997.
19. W. Y. Tan, First Passage Probability Distributions in Markov Models and the HIV Incubation Period Under Treatment, *Mathematical and Computer Modelling* **19:** 53-66, 1994.
20. W. Y. Tan, On the HIV Incubation Period Under Non-Markovian Models, *Statistics and Probability Letters* **21:** 49-57,1994.
21. W. Y. Tan and R. H. Byers, Jr. A Stochastic Model of the HIV Epidemic and HIV Infection Distribution in a Homosexual Population, *Mathematical Biosciences* **113:** 115-143, 1993.
22. W. Y. Tan and Z. Xiang, A Stochastic Model for the HIV Epidemic and Effects of Age and Race on HIV Infection in Homosexual Populations, *Series in Mathematical Biology and Medicine* **6:** 425-451, O. Arino, D. Axelrod and M. Kimmel (eds.), *Advances in Mathematical Population Dynamics - Molecules, Cells, and Man,* World Scientific Publishing Company, Singapore, New Jersey, London, Hong Kong, 1997.

Chapter 11
STOCHASTIC PARTNERSHIP MODELS IN HOMOSEXUAL POPULATIONS

11.1 Introduction

Just as in populations of heterosexuals, homosexual men form partnerships that may last over extended periods of time, or they may choose to remain single and not participate in long-standing partnerships. Yet, in the biomathematics literature on HIV/AIDS and other sexually transmitted diseases, little work has been reported on models that accommodate singles and partnerships simultaneously. Furthermore, most of the literature devoted to partnership models belongs to the deterministic paradigm and relatively little attention has been given to stochastic models that accommodate the formation and dissolution of partnerships. Accordingly, the purpose of this chapter is to extend the developments set forth in Chapter 10 and work towards the construction of classes of stochastic models that accommodate not only pairs of individuals in partnerships but also singles.

Among the earlier papers on partnership models with potential applications to the international HIV/AIDS epidemic are those Dietz and Hadeler,[4] Waldstaestatter,[9] and Blythe et al.[3] Two other papers that are also relevant to the material to be developed in this chapter are Kretzschmar et al.[6] and Kretzschmar and Dietz.[5] All models described in these papers belong to the deterministic paradigm, and, apart from some computer generated graphs to demarcate regions of the parameter space where an epidemic will spread throughout a population, die out, or exhibit other properties of the models, no computer intensive methods were used in their analysis. In short, for the most part, the working paradigms of these papers were confined essentially to what could be done using only paper and pencil. No attempt will be made to review the deterministic literature here, but an interested reader may consult the references cited in these papers for a broader view of the work that has been done on deterministic partnership models.

An early paper on stochastic partnership models is that of Mode,[8] where computer intensive methods were used to explore some of the properties of a formulation involving two sexes. Unlike the deterministic models mentioned above, which were formulated in continuous time, computer intensive methods necessarily entail discrete time formulations, which can lead to conceptual complications. Among these complications is whether, during any time interval, a transition from the single population to becoming a member of a couple or partnership while also undergoing a change of state with respect to disease is allowed. Such double transitions were allowed in the early formulation, but, subsequently, it was realized that the formulation could be greatly simplified if only one type of transition were allowed during any time interval. Accordingly, in this chapter, a stochastic partnership model will be formulated which accommodates only one type of transition during any time interval, by extending the ideas set forth in Chapter 10. From the practical point of view, it should be mentioned that when using a computer implementation of a discrete time model, an effort should be made, by trial and error, to choose the length of the time interval sufficiently small so that more than one transition occurs with negligible probability.

The class of stochastic partnership models described in this chapter differs from the earlier formulation in that attention will be confined to only one sex to accommodate HIV/AIDS epidemics in homosexual populations, where steady partnerships may occur. The formulation is also more general in that two or more behavioral classes, assortative selection of sexual partners, and extra-martial sexual contacts, i.e., sexual contacts with persons other that his steady partner, are accommodated in the formulation. When there is only one behavioral class, no extra-marital sexual contacts, and sexual partners are chosen by random assortment, the differential equations embedded in the stochastic model seem to resemble some of those considered by Kretzschmar and Dietz.[5] In passing, it should be mentioned that there are alternative approaches to considering multiple sexual partners other than those accommodated in the extra-marital component described in this chapter. Among them is the graph theoretic approach of Kretzschmar and Morris,[7] which accommodates multiple sexual partners. Another alternative formulation that may be of interest in accommodating multiple sexual partners in a model is that of attempting to extend the work of Ball[1] and Ball et al.[2] to sexually transmitted diseases. Such approaches to modelling multiple sexual partners will, however, not be undertaken in this chapter.

11.2 Types of Individuals and Partnerships

When the idea of pairs of partnerships is appended to the class of models described in Chapter 10, the notation may get rather complex. Therefore, to expedite the presentation and fix ideas, it will be expedient to set the stage for the development of stochastic models accommodating partnerships in homosexual populations by considering only $m = 1$ behavioral class and $n \geq 1$ stages of a disease. As before, the symbol 0 will stand for a susceptible person and the symbols $1, 2, \cdots, n$, will represent stages of a disease. Therefore, when there is only one behavioral class, the set of types of individuals in the population of singles will be denoted by:

$$\Upsilon_s = \{j \mid j = 0, 1, 2, \cdots, n\} \ . \qquad (11.2.1)$$

Sometimes it will be useful to refer to the elements of the set Υ_s as states, particularly when life cycle models are under consideration.

By definition, partnerships will consist of pairs of individuals or couples, and a couple type will be denoted by the ordered pair (j, k), where $j \in \Upsilon_s$ is the state of the left-hand partner and $k \in \Upsilon_s$ is the state of the right-hand partner. Thus, the set of couple types is the product set,

$$\Upsilon_c = \{\tau = (j, k) \mid (j, k) \in \Upsilon_s \times \Upsilon_s\} \ . \qquad (11.2.2)$$

Altogether, there are $n+1$ types of singles and $(n+1)^2$ types of couples, but for the case of a homosexual population, some mention should be made that it may not be possible, in an actual enumeration of the population, to identify all the elements of Υ_c, because there may not be a natural way to order the members of a couple.

For example, if $j = k$, then (j, j) is a couple type where both members are in state $j \in \Upsilon_s$, but if $j \neq k$, then the couple types (j, k) and (k, j) may not be distinguished in an enumeration so that $(j, k) = (k, j)$. If this symmetry condition holds, then the number of distinguishable types in the set Υ_c is:

$$(n+1) + \binom{n+1}{2} = \frac{1}{2}(n+2)(n+1) . \tag{11.2.3}$$

When writing software, however, particularly in such array manipulating programming languages as APL, it is easier to consider the case in which all couple types are distinguishable, because such languages have built-in structures for manipulating rectangular and hyper-rectangular arrays. In homosexual populations, there may not be straightforward ways of designating ordered pairs (j, k), but for the heterosexual populations that will be considered in the next chapter, there are natural ways to order members of a couple. For example, the left-hand partner could, by definition, be female and the right-hand partner male.

The array manipulation procedure followed in a particular case will depend on the question being asked. By way of illustration, suppose at some time $t \in S_h$ an investigator wishes to compute the total number of infective individuals in a population. At time t, let the random function $X(t; j)$ denote the number of singles of type $j \in \Upsilon_s$. Then, the number of infectives in the single population at time t is:

$$T_s(t; I) = \sum_{j=1}^{n} X(t; j) . \tag{11.2.4}$$

Similarly, let the random function $Z(t; j, k)$ denote the number of couples of type (j, k) in the population at time t. Then, the number of left-hand partners of type j at time t is:

$$Z(t; j, \cdot) = \sum_{k=0}^{n} Z(t; j, k) . \tag{11.2.5}$$

Similarly, the number of right-hand partners of type j at time t will be denoted by the random function $Z(t; \cdot, j)$. Thus, the total number of infective persons in couples at time t is:

$$T_c(t; I) = \sum_{j=1}^{n} (Z(t; j, \cdot) + Z(t; \cdot, j)) \ . \tag{11.2.6}$$

Finally, the total number of infective persons in the population at time t is, by definition,

$$T(t; I) = T_s(t; I) + T_c(t; I) \ . \tag{11.2.7}$$

Unlike models in which partnerships are not taken into account, in partnership models it is very helpful to clarify the structure of a system by introducing life cycle models for both singles and couples. Let $\mathfrak{S}_{s1}$ and $\mathfrak{S}_{s2}$ denote, respectively, the set of absorbing and transient states in a life cycle model for singles. At this juncture, these sets of states will not be enumerated, because they are essentially identical to those described in Chapter 10. But, it will be helpful to define the state space for a life cycle model for couples. It is rather more complicated than that for singles, since it must account for the evolution of both members of the couple. If the deaths of left- and right-hand partners are distinguished, then it will be useful to consider the following set of five states,

$$\mathfrak{S}_{c1} = \{E_{DIS}, E_{l1}, E_{l2}, E_{r1}, E_{r2}\} \tag{11.2.8}$$

as the set of absorbing states for the life cycle model for couples. In this case, the symbol E_{DIS} stands for couple dissolution, E_{l1} stands for the death of a left-hand partner due to a cause other than disease, and E_{l2} stands for the death of a left-hand partner from a cause due to disease. The symbols E_{r1} and E_{r2} are defined similarly for right-hand partners. If one wishes, these states could be collapsed over left- and right-hand partners, but in what follows the full set in Eq. (11.2.8) will be considered, because it paves the way for the construction of two-sex models in the next chapter. Finally, let $\mathfrak{S}_{c2}$ denote the set of transient states in the life cycle model for couples. Then, this set is $\mathfrak{S}_{c2} = \Upsilon_c$, the set of couple types defined in Eq. (11.2.2). One of the difficult problems faced by an investigator in constructing stochastic partnership models is that of defining the matrix of latent risks governing transitions among the set $\mathfrak{S}_{c2}$ of transient states, a problem that will be considered in the next section.

11.3 Life Cycle Model for Couples with One Behavioral Class

As an aid to developing more general structures, it will be helpful to consider the simplest case of $m = 1$ behavioral class and $n = 1$ stage of disease. In this case, there are four couple types

$$\Upsilon_c = \{(0,0),(0,1),(1,0),(1,1)\} \tag{11.3.1}$$

arranged in lexicographic order, and, as explained in Section 11.2, this set is also the set $\mathfrak{S}_{c2}$ of transient states of the life cycle model for couples. The first step in defining the matrices of latent risks governing the evolution of couples is to consider those governing transitions from the set $\mathfrak{S}_{c2}$ of transient states to the set $\mathfrak{S}_{c1}$ of absorbing states. Let $\mathbf{\Theta}_{c21}$ denote the 4×5 matrix of constant latent risks governing transitions from the set $\mathfrak{S}_{c2}$ to the set $\mathfrak{S}_{c1}$.

The rate of couple dissolution per unit time will be denoted by δ, and it will be assumed that this rate holds of all couple types. Just as in Chapter 10, let μ_0 denote the rate of death from causes other than disease and let μ_1 be the incremental rate of death due to disease. Then, the 4×5 matrix $\mathbf{\Theta}_{c21}$ has the form,

$$\mathbf{\Theta}_{c21} = \begin{bmatrix} \delta & \mu_0 & 0 & \mu_0 & 0 \\ \delta & \mu_0 & 0 & \mu_0 & \mu_1 \\ \delta & \mu_0 & \mu_1 & \mu_0 & 0 \\ \delta & \mu_0 & \mu_1 & \mu_0 & \mu_1 \end{bmatrix} . \tag{11.3.2}$$

By way of explanation, observe that for the first two couple types, $\tau_1 = (0,0)$ and $\tau_2 = (0,1)$, the left-hand partner is not infected. Hence, in the first two positions in the third column of the matrix, there are 0 increments of death due to disease. However, for the last two couple types, $\tau_3 = (1,0)$ and $\tau_4 = (1,1)$, the left-hand partner is infected so that there is a positive risk of death μ_1 due to disease. Similar remarks hold for the right-hand partner.

The matrix of latent risks, governing transitions among the states in the set $\mathfrak{S}_{c2}$ is 4×4 and will be denoted by $\boldsymbol{\Theta}_{c22}$. A susceptible, who is a member of couple at time t, may be infected during the time interval $(t, t+h]$ by either an infective who is his steady partner or by sexual contacts with a person or persons who are not his steady partner. Operationally, among couples any sexual contacts with persons other than their steady partners will be referred as extra-marital sexual contacts. By definition, all sexual contacts among singles will be referred to as extra-martial. For the one-behavioral class model under consideration, let λ denote the expected number of extra-martial sexual partners per unit time and let γ_{mc} denote the expected number of marital sexual contacts per unit time.

Given the state of the population at time t, a conditional probability that a susceptible person becomes infected during the time interval $(t, t+h]$ could be derived by arguments similar to those set forth in Section 10. Let $Q_{par}(t)$ denote the conditional probability that a susceptible at time t is infected during the time interval through extra-martial sexual contacts. A procedure for deriving a formula for this conditional probability will be set down in a subsequent section of this chapter. Finally, let $q(1)$ denote the probability that a susceptible is infected per sexual contact with an infective. Then, the 4×4 matrix $\boldsymbol{\Theta}_{c22}$ has the form

$$\boldsymbol{\Theta}_{c22} = \begin{bmatrix} 0 & \lambda Q_{par}(t) & \lambda Q_{par}(t) & 0 \\ 0 & 0 & 0 & \lambda Q_{par}(t) + \gamma_{mc} q(1) \\ 0 & 0 & 0 & \lambda Q_{par}(t) + \gamma_{mc} q(1) \\ 0 & 0 & 0 & 0 \end{bmatrix} . \qquad (11.3.3)$$

As an aid to interpreting the elements of this matrix, observe that the element in the first row and second column of the matrix, $\lambda Q_{par}(t)$, is that for the transition $\tau_1 = (0,0) \to \tau_2 = (0,1)$, indicating that the right-hand susceptible partner has been infected during the time interval $(t, t+h]$ through extra-marital sexual contacts with infectives. On the other hand, the element, $\lambda Q_{par}(t) + \gamma_{mc} q(1)$, in the second row and fourth column of the matrix is that for the transition $\tau_2 = (0,1) \to \tau_4 = (1,1)$, indicating that the susceptible left-hand partner has been infected during the time interval $(t, t+h]$ either through extra-marital sexual contacts with infectives or by his infective marital partner. Similar remarks hold for the other non-zero elements of the matrix in Eq. (11.3.3). A tacit assumption that has been used in constructing the matrix in Eq. (11.3.3) is that during any time interval $(t, t+h]$, only one member of a partnership can undergo a state transition.

To illustrate the types of patterns that develop in the matrices of latent risks when there are $n \geq 2$ stages of a disease, the case $n = 2$ will be considered. In this case, the set $\mathfrak{S}_{c2}$ of transient states contains 9 elements and it will be useful to partition this set into three disjoint sets according to the state of the left-hand partner. Thus, let

$$A(j) = \{(j,k) \mid k = 0,1,2\} \tag{11.3.4}$$

denote the set of couple types such that the left partner is in state $j = 0,1,2$. For example, the set $A(0)$ contains the three elements,

$$A(0) = \{(0,0),(0,1),(0,2)\} \tag{11.3.5}$$

arranged in lexicographic order. For the case of two stages of disease, the matrix $\mathbf{\Theta}_{c21}$ of latent risks governing transitions for the set of transient states $\mathfrak{S}_{c2}$ to the set $\mathfrak{S}_{c1}$ of absorbing states is 9×5, and to simplify the notation, it will be helpful to represent the matrix in a partitioned form such that the rows are grouped by elements in the sets $A(j),\ j = 0,1,2$.

In addition to those parameters defined above, let μ_2 be the incremental death rate for a person in stage 2 of disease, and let $\mathbf{1}_3$ denote a 3×1 vector of ones, and let $\mathbf{0}_3$ a 3×1 vector of zeros. It will also be convenient to let

$$\boldsymbol{\mu}_d = \begin{bmatrix} 0 \\ \mu_1 \\ \mu_2 \end{bmatrix} \tag{11.3.6}$$

be a 3×1 vector with the indicated death rates. Then, the matrix $\mathbf{\Theta}_{c21}$ may be represented in the partitioned form,

$$\mathbf{\Theta}_{c21} = \begin{bmatrix} \delta\mathbf{1}_3 & \mu_0\mathbf{1}_3 & \mathbf{0}_3 & \mu_0\mathbf{1}_3 & \boldsymbol{\mu}_d \\ \delta\mathbf{1}_3 & \mu_0\mathbf{1}_3 & \mu_1\mathbf{1}_3 & \mu_0\mathbf{1}_3 & \boldsymbol{\mu}_d \\ \delta\mathbf{1}_3 & \mu_0\mathbf{1}_3 & \mu_2\mathbf{1}_3 & \mu_0\mathbf{1}_3 & \boldsymbol{\mu}_d \end{bmatrix}. \tag{11.3.7}$$

By way of explanation of the first column, observe that, by assumption, every couple type (j, k) has the same rate of dissolution δ, and every couple type has the background death rate μ_0 as indicated in columns two and four. The first three rows of the matrix correspond to those couple types in the set $A(0)$ in which the left partner is in state 0; hence, the vector $\mathbf{0}_3$ of three zeroes represents the first three elements of the third column. Similarly, the symbols $\mu_1\mathbf{1}_3$ and $\mu_2\mathbf{1}_3$ in the third column correspond, respectively, to those sets of couple types $A(1)$ and $A(2)$, such that the left-hand partner is in states 2 and 3. Finally, the repeated use of symbol $\boldsymbol{\mu}_d$ in the fifth column of the matrix, with the indicated death rates in Eq. (11.3.6), correspond to the three sets of couple types $A(0)$, $A(1)$, and $A(2)$ such that the right-hand partner is in states $0, 1, 2$. It is clear that the pattern of the matrix in Eq. (11.3.7) may be generalized to any number of stages $n \geq 2$.

Because there are nine couples types when $m = 1$ and $n = 2$, the matrix $\boldsymbol{\Theta}_{c22}$ of latent risks, governing transitions among transient states of the life cycle model for couples, is 9×9 and may be represented in the partitioned form,

$$\boldsymbol{\Theta}_{c22} = \begin{bmatrix} \boldsymbol{\Theta}_{c22}(0,0) & \boldsymbol{\Theta}_{c22}(0,1) & \boldsymbol{\Theta}_{c22}(0,2) \\ \boldsymbol{\Theta}_{c22}(1,0) & \boldsymbol{\Theta}_{c22}(1,1) & \boldsymbol{\Theta}_{c22}(1,2) \\ \boldsymbol{\Theta}_{c22}(2,0) & \boldsymbol{\Theta}_{c22}(2,1) & \boldsymbol{\Theta}_{c22}(2,2) \end{bmatrix} \tag{11.3.8}$$

of 3×3 sub-matrices. In this case, the 3×3 sub-matrix $\boldsymbol{\Theta}_{c22}(0,0)$ contains those latent risks governing transitions from the set of states $A(0)$ into itself. Thus transitions of the form $A(0) \to A(0)$ indicate that only the right-hand partner of a couple undergoes a change of state. The 3×3 sub-matrix $\boldsymbol{\Theta}_{c22}(0,1)$, however, contains those latent risks governing transitions from the set of states $A(0)$ into the set $A(1)$ so that transitions of the form $A(0) \to A(1)$ indicate that only the left-hand partner changes state. Similar remarks hold for the other sub-matrices in Eq. (11.3.8).

In order to set down specific examples of the sub-matrices in Eq. (11.3.8), it will be necessary to define some additional parameters. Let $q(2)$ be the probability that a susceptible is infected per sexual contact when his infective partner is in stage 2 of the disease, and let

$$\mathbf{\Gamma} = \begin{bmatrix} 0 & \gamma_{12} \\ \gamma_{21} & 0 \end{bmatrix} \tag{11.3.9}$$

be the matrix of latent risks governing transitions among stages 1 and 2 of the disease. Then, because the latent risks in the sub-matrix $\mathbf{\Theta}_{c22}(0,0)$ govern transitions only for the right-hand partner, it has the form,

$$\mathbf{\Theta}_{c22}(0,0) = \begin{bmatrix} 0 & \lambda Q_{par}(t) & 0 \\ 0 & 0 & \gamma_{12} \\ 0 & \gamma_{21} & 0 \end{bmatrix} . \tag{11.3.10}$$

However, because transitions of the form $A(0) \rightarrow A(1)$ indicate that the left-hand partner has been infected, it follows that the sub-matrix $\mathbf{\Theta}_{c22}(0,1)$ has the form,

$$\mathbf{\Theta}_{c22}(0,1) = \begin{bmatrix} \lambda Q_{par}(t) & 0 & 0 \\ 0 & \lambda Q_{par}(t) + \gamma_{mc}q(1) & 0 \\ 0 & 0 & \lambda Q_{par}(t) + \gamma_{mc}q(2) \end{bmatrix} . \tag{11.3.11}$$

By assumption, transitions of the form $A(0) \rightarrow A(2)$ occur with probability zero, so that $\mathbf{\Theta}_{c22}(0,2) = \mathbf{0}_{3\times 3}$, a 3×3 zero matrix. Similarly, transitions of the forms $A(1) \rightarrow A(0)$ and $A(2) \rightarrow A(0)$ occur with probability zero so that $\mathbf{\Theta}_{c22}(1,0) = \mathbf{\Theta}_{c22}(2,0) = \mathbf{0}_{3\times 3}$.

For $j = 1, 2$, the matrices $\mathbf{\Theta}_{c22}(j,j)$ on the quasi-diagonal in Eq. (11.3.8) have the form

$$\mathbf{\Theta}_{c22}(j,j) = \begin{bmatrix} 0 & \lambda Q_{par}(t) + \gamma_{mc}q(j) & 0 \\ 0 & 0 & \gamma_{12} \\ 0 & \gamma_{21} & 0 \end{bmatrix} . \tag{11.3.12}$$

Observe that the latent risk $\lambda Q_{par}(t) + \gamma_{mc}q(j)$ for the right-hand partner to become infected during a time interval $(t, t+h]$ depends on the infective stage j of the left-hand partner. Transitions of the form $A(1) \rightarrow A(2)$ and $A(2) \rightarrow A(1)$ indicate that the left-hand partner undergoes a change in disease stage during a time interval $(t, t+h]$. Thus, the sub-matrix $\mathbf{\Theta}_{c22}(1,2)$ has the form,

$$\mathbf{\Theta}_{c22}(1,2) = \gamma_{12}\mathbf{I}_3 , \tag{11.3.13}$$

where $\mathbf{I}_3$ is a 3×3 identity matrix. Finally, the form of the sub-matrix $\mathbf{\Theta}_{c22}(2,1)$ may be obtained by substituting γ_{21} for γ_{12} in Eq. (11.3.13). From the examples just given, it is clear that a partitioned form of the matrix $\mathbf{\Theta}_{c22}$ of latent risks governing transitions among the set $\mathfrak{S}_{c2}$ of transient states of the life cycle model for couples may be written down for any number of stages $n \geq 2$.

11.4 Couple Types for Two or More Behavioral Classes

Having set the stage for the case of one behavioral class and $n \geq 1$ stages of disease, in this section the general case of $m \geq 1$ behavioral classes and $n \geq 1$ stages of disease will be considered, when couples are taken into account. Just as in Section 10.2, the set of types for the single population is the set of ordered pairs,

$$\Upsilon_s = \{\tau = (j,k) \mid j = 1,2,\cdots,m;\ k = 0,1,2,\cdots,n\}\ , \tag{11.4.1}$$

where j denotes the behavioral class and k the state with respect to disease. Therefore, the set of couple types will be chosen as the set of ordered pairs,

$$\Upsilon_c = \{\varkappa = (\tau_1,\tau_2) \mid (\tau_1,\tau_2) \in \Upsilon_s \times \Upsilon_s\} \tag{11.4.2}$$

of single types. As in Section 11.3, for ease of processing in such array manipulating languages as APL, τ_1 and τ_2 in a couple type $\varkappa = (\tau_1,\tau_2)$ will be referred to as left- and right-hand partners and all couple types will be distinguished. There are $m(n+1)$ elements in the set Υ_s of single types; therefore, the set Υ_c of couple types contains $m^2(n+1)^2$ elements.

The life cycle model for singles is the same as that set forth in Section 10.4, but the set of absorbing states will be denoted by $\mathfrak{S}_{s1}$ and the set of transient states by $\mathfrak{S}_{s2} = \Upsilon_s$. Moreover, the matrices of latent risks for singles, $\mathbf{\Theta}_{s21}$ and $\mathbf{\Theta}_{c22}$, will be chosen as in Section 10.4. With regard to the life cycle model for couples, the set of five absorbing states $\mathfrak{S}_{c1}$ will be defined as in Section 11.2, but the set of transient states will be chosen as $\mathfrak{S}_{c2} = \Upsilon_c$. The $m^2(n+1)^2 \times 5$ matrix $\mathbf{\Theta}_{c21}$ of latent risks, governing transitions from the set of transient states $\mathfrak{S}_{c2}$ to the set of absorbing states $\mathfrak{S}_{c1}$, will have the same general form as that in Eq. (11.3.7), but its explicit form will be left as an exercise for the reader. However, to describe a useful form of the $m^2(n+1)^2 \times m^2(n+1)^2$ matrix $\boldsymbol{\Theta}_{c22}$ of latent risks, governing transitions among the transient states, it will be helpful to partition the set $\mathfrak{S}_{c2}$ of couple types into sub-matrices according to the behavioral class of each member of a couple.

To this end, for a fixed pair j_1 and j_2 of behavioral classes, let $A(j_1, j_2)$ denote the set of couple types,

$$A(j_1, j_2) = \{\varkappa = ((j_1, k_1), (j_2, k_2)) \mid k_1, k_2 = 0, 1, 2, \cdots, n\} \ . \quad (11.4.3)$$

It should be noted that this set contains $(n+1)^2$ elements. Furthermore, the set $\mathfrak{S}_{c2}$ may be expressed as the disjoint union,

$$\mathfrak{S}_{c2} = \bigcup_{j_1=1}^{m} \bigcup_{j_2=1}^{m} A(j_1, j_2) \ . \quad (11.4.4)$$

For the special case of $m = 2$ behavioral classes, this disjoint union contains the four sets,

$$\{A(1,1), A(1,2), A(2,1), A(2,2)\} \ , \quad (11.4.5)$$

which will be used to partition the rows and columns of the matrix $\boldsymbol{\Theta}_{c22}$ into four sets each containing $(n+1)^2$ elements. Thus, in this case, the matrix $\boldsymbol{\Theta}_{c22}$ may be represented in the 4×4 partitioned form,

$$\begin{bmatrix} \boldsymbol{\Theta}_{c22}(1,1;1,1) & \boldsymbol{\Theta}_{c22}(1,1;1,2) & \boldsymbol{\Theta}_{c22}(1,1;2,1) & \mathbf{0} \\ \boldsymbol{\Theta}_{c22}(1,2;1,1) & \boldsymbol{\Theta}_{c22}(1,2;1,2) & \mathbf{0} & \boldsymbol{\Theta}_{c22}(1,2;2,2) \\ \boldsymbol{\Theta}_{c22}(2,1;1,1) & \mathbf{0} & \boldsymbol{\Theta}_{c22}(2,1;2,1) & \boldsymbol{\Theta}_{c22}(2,1;2,2) \\ \mathbf{0} & \boldsymbol{\Theta}_{c22}(2,2;1,2) & \boldsymbol{\Theta}_{c22}(2,2;2,1) & \boldsymbol{\Theta}_{c22}(2,2;2,2) \end{bmatrix} \quad (11.4.6)$$

where each of the 16 sub-matrices is $(n+1)^2 \times (n+1)^2$.

Partitioning the matrix $\boldsymbol{\Theta}_{c22}$ by pairs of behavioral classes is very useful in a computer implementation of the model, because the structure discussed in Section 11.3 may easily be incorporated into the sub-matrices on the quasi-principal diagonal. For example, the sub-matrix $\boldsymbol{\Theta}_{c22}(1,1;1,1)$ in the first row and column of Eq. (11.4.6) contains those latent risks such that neither the left nor right partners make a transition to behavioral class 2 (risk group 2) during a time interval $(t, t+h]$, so that the only transitions occurring would be with respect to states of disease. Therefore, the sub-matrix $\mathbf{\Theta}_{c22}(1,1;1,1)$ has a partitioned form analogous to that in Eq. (11.3.8) with sub-matrices similar to those defined in Section 11.3. Similar remarks hold for the other sub-matrices,

$$\{\mathbf{\Theta}_{c22}(1,2;1,2), \mathbf{\Theta}_{c22}(2,1;2,1), \mathbf{\Theta}_{c22}(2,2;2,2)\} \tag{11.4.7}$$

on the quasi-principal diagonal of Eq. (11.4.6), but it should be kept in mind that the λ-parameters, denoting the expected number of extra-marital partners per unit time, in the latent risks governing transitions from the susceptible state to the infected state, will depend on the behavioral class of the individual.

The sub-matrices off the quasi-principal diagonal in Eq. (11.4.6), however, correspond to those transitions in which at most one member of a couple changes to another risk group during a time interval $(t, t+h]$. For example, the sub-matrix $\mathbf{\Theta}_{c22}(1,1;1,2)$ contains those latent risks governing transitions of the right-hand partners from risk group 1 to risk group 2; whereas the sub-matrix $\mathbf{\Theta}_{c22}(1,1;2,1)$ contains those latent risk governing transitions of left-hand partners from risk group 1 to risk group 2. To illustrate the structure of these matrices, for the case $m = 2$ behavioral classes, let

$$\mathbf{\Psi} = \begin{bmatrix} 0 & \psi_{12} \\ \psi_{21} & 0 \end{bmatrix} \tag{11.4.8}$$

denote the matrix of latent risks governing transitions among risks groups 1 and 2, and let $\mathbf{I}_{(n+1)^2}$ denote a $(n+1)^2 \times (n+1)^2$ identity matrix. Then, because during any small time interval $(t, t+h]$, simultaneous changes in disease state and risk group occur with probability $o(h)$ for both members of a couple and all transitions are from risk group 1 to risk group 2, the matrices in question have the form,

$$\mathbf{\Theta}_{c22}(1,1;1,2) = \mathbf{\Theta}_{c22}(1,1;2,1) = \psi_{12}\mathbf{I}_{(n+1)^2}\,. \tag{11.4.9}$$

Finally, the sub-matrix in the first row and fourth column of Eq. (11.4.6) is $\mathbf{0}$, a $(n+1)^2 \times (n+1)^2$ zero matrix, because both members of a couple make the risk group transition $1 \to 2$ with probability $o(h)$ during any small time interval. Similar remarks hold for other sub-matrices off the quasi-principal diagonal in Eq. (11.4.6).

Matrices of the form in Eq. (11.4.6) are very useful in the computer implementation of the partnership model under consideration, because it is easy to manipulate rectangular arrays in such programming languages as APL and thus account for the number of each single and couple type in a projection of an epidemic. However, for some values of m and n, these matrices can become so large that they are beyond the capacity of a computer, but for many cases of interest these matrices will be manageable. For example, when there are $m = 3$ risk groups and $n = 1$ stage of disease, the number of rows and columns in the matrix in Eq. (11.4.6) is:

$$m^2(n+1)^2 = 9 \times 4 = 36 . \tag{11.4.10}$$

Collections of matrices of this size that arise in Monte Carlo simulations can be accommodated with ease in the random access memory of most desktop computers. But, for the case of $m = 3$ risk groups and $n = 4$ stages of disease, the number of rows and columns of the matrix $\boldsymbol{\Theta}_{c22}$ is:

$$m^2\,(n+1)^2 = 9 \times 25 = 225 , \tag{11.4.11}$$

and for some desktop computers, random access memory may not be sufficiently large to accommodate collections of matrices of this size.

Rather than accommodating every couple type in the set with 225 elements or in general with sets of $m^2\,(n+1)^2$ elements, it will suffice in many cases to account for the number of persons of some type $\tau = (j, k)$ who are members of couples at each epoch in a projection. Suppose, for example, at some time t there are $Z(t; \tau_1, \tau_2)$ couples of type $\varkappa = (\tau_1, \tau_2)$ in a computer simulation. Then, the total number of persons of type $\tau = (j, k)$ who are members of a couple at time t is given by the expression,

$$T_c(t;\tau) = \sum_{\tau' \in \Upsilon_s} \left(Z(t;\tau,\tau') + Z(t;\tau',\tau) \right) , \tag{11.4.12}$$

where Υ is the set of types of individuals (see Eq. (11.4.1)). The number of elements in the set Υ_s is $m(n+1)$, so for the case of $m = 3$ and

$n = 4$, the number of elements in an array of the form in Eq. (11.4.12) is 15. Collections of arrays of this size, which would arise in Monte Carlo simulations, can easily be accommodated in random access memory. Consequently, if it suffices to count only the number of individuals of each type $\tau \in \Upsilon$ at each epoch t in a Monte Carlo projection who are members of a couple, then it would be necessary to store only one array of size $m^2(n+1)^2 \times m^2(n+1)^2$ at each epoch in a projection, which would greatly lessen random access memory requirements in carrying out computer experiments. In passing, it should be mentioned that it is also possible to store arrays generated in each epoch of a Monte Carlo simulation on hard disk then read them back in for further processing, but such procedures can be slow in terms of processing time and should be avoided if possible, particularly in exploratory computer experiments.

11.5 Couple Formation

During any time interval $(t, t+h]$, new couples of steady sexual partners are formed from those in the singles population at time $t \in S_h$, and the definitions of the random functions involved in couple formation closely resemble those in Section 10.2. Acceptance probabilities for couple formation and extra-marital contacts will be distinguished and will be defined for $m \geq 1$ behavioral classes and $n \geq 1$ stages of disease. Accordingly, let $\alpha_c(\tau_1, \tau_2)$ denote the conditional probability that a single person of type τ_1 finds a person of type τ_2 acceptable as a steady sexual partner. For types $\tau_1 = (j_1, k_1)$ and $\tau_2 = (j_2, k_2)$, this function will be chosen as:

$$\alpha_c(\tau_1, \tau_2) = \exp\left[-\left(\beta_{c1} \mid j_1 - j_2 \mid + \beta_{c2} \mid k_1 - k_2 \mid\right)\right] , \tag{11.5.1}$$

where β_{c1} and β_{c2} are non-negative parameters. A fundamental random function involved in couple formation is the frequency of an individual of type τ in the population at time t, which is defined by:

$$U(t;\tau) = \frac{X(t;\tau)}{\sum_{\tau' \in \Upsilon} X(t;\tau')} , \tag{11.5.2}$$

provided that $X(t;\tau) > 0$ for some $\tau \in \Upsilon_s$. Given a single person of type τ_1 at time t, let $\gamma_c(t;\tau_1,\tau_2)$ be the conditional probability that a person of type τ_1 has contact with a potential sexual partner of type τ_2 during the time interval $(t, t+h]$. Then, just as in Section 10.2, by an application of Bayes' theorem it follows that:

$$\gamma_c(t; \tau_1, \tau_2) = \frac{U(t; \tau_2)\alpha_c(\tau_1, \tau_2)}{\sum_{\tau' \in \Upsilon} U(t; \tau')\alpha_c(\tau_1, \tau')} . \tag{11.5.3}$$

For each $\tau_1 \in \Upsilon$ and $t \in S_h$, let

$$\mathbf{\Gamma}_c(t; \tau_1) = (\gamma_c(t; \tau_1, \tau_2) \mid \tau_2 \in \Upsilon) \tag{11.5.4}$$

be a vector of contact probabilities for a single person of type $\tau_1 \in \Upsilon_s$. Next let the random function $Z_c(t; \tau_1, \tau_2)$ denote the number of single persons of type τ_1 at time t who seek potential partners of type τ_2 during the time interval $(t, t+h]$, and let

$$\mathbf{Z}_c(t; \tau_1) = (Z_c(t; \tau_1, \tau_2) \mid \tau_2 \in \Upsilon) \tag{11.5.5}$$

denote a vector of these random functions. Then, it will assumed that, given $X(t; \tau_1)$, the conditional distribution of this random vector is multinomial with index $X(t; \tau_1)$ and probability vector $\mathbf{\Gamma}_c(t; \tau_1)$. In symbols,

$$\mathbf{Z}_c(t; \tau_1) \sim CMultinom\left(X(t; \tau_1), \mathbf{\Gamma}_c(t; \tau_1)\right) . \tag{11.5.6}$$

According to the scheme of couple formation under consideration, members of the singles population at time t make contacts or mix, during any time interval $(t, t+h]$, according to the multinomial distribution in Eq. (11.5.6). Such mixing may, or may not, result in the formation of couples containing pairs of individuals within which sexual contacts, marital or extra-marital, may occur. It seems reasonable to suppose, however, that during any time interval there would be some maximum number of potential partnerships of type (τ_1, τ_2), with one member of type $\tau_1 \in \Upsilon_s$ and the other of type $\tau_2 \in \Upsilon_s$, that could be formed. Let the random function $N_{CF}(t; \tau_1, \tau_2)$ denote the maximum potential number of couples that may be formed during any time interval $(t, t+h]$. Because the total number of individuals of type τ_1 in partnerships of type (τ_1, τ_2) for some $\tau_2 \in \Upsilon$ cannot exceed $X(t; \tau_1)$, it follows that the inequality,

$$\sum_{\tau_2 \in \Upsilon} N_{CF}(t; \tau_1, \tau_2) \leq X(t; \tau_1) \qquad (11.5.7)$$

must be satisfied with probability one for all $\tau_1 \in \Upsilon$. Similarly, the inequality,

$$\sum_{\tau_1 \in \Upsilon} N_{CF}(t; \tau_1, \tau_2) \leq X(t; \tau_2) \qquad (11.5.8)$$

must hold with probability one for all $\tau_2 \in \Upsilon_2$.

Evidently, the random function $N_{CF}(t; \tau_1, \tau_2)$ may be chosen in a number of ways, but in the models considered in this chapter it will be chosen according to the scheme set forth in Section 10.2. If $\tau_1 \neq \tau_2$, then

$$N_{CF}(t; \tau_1, \tau_2) = \min\left(Z_{CF}(t; \tau_1, \tau_2), Z_{CF}(t; \tau_2, \tau_1)\right) . \qquad (11.5.9)$$

But, if $\tau_1 = \tau_2$, then

$$N_{CF}(t; \tau_1, \tau_1) = \left[\frac{Z_{CF}(t; \tau_1, \tau_1)}{2}\right] , \qquad (11.5.10)$$

where $[\cdot]$ stands for the greatest integer function. It can easily be checked that when the random function $N(t; \tau_1, \tau_2)$ is chosen as in Eqs. (11.5.9) and (11.5.10), then inequalities in Eqs. (11.5.7) and (11.5.8) will be satisfied with probability one.

Among the $N_{CF}(t; \tau_1, \tau_2)$ potential couples of type $\varkappa = (\tau_1, \tau_2)$ that may be formed during the time interval $(t, t+h]$, let the random function $Z_{CF}(t+h; \tau_1, \tau_2)$ denote the actual number of this type formed during the time interval. For each couple of type $\varkappa = (\tau_1, \tau_2)$, let $\rho(\varkappa)$ be a constant latent risk function governing the formation of couples of this type, and define a couple formation probability $q_{CF}(t; \varkappa)$ by:

$$q_{CF}(t; \varkappa) = 1 - \exp\left[-\rho(\varkappa)h\right] = \rho(\varkappa)h + o(h) . \qquad (11.5.11)$$

Then, by assumption,

$$Z_{CF}(t+h; \varkappa) \sim CBinom\left(N_{CF}(t; \varkappa), q_{CF}(t; \varkappa)\right) \qquad (11.5.12)$$

for all couple types $\varkappa \in \Upsilon_c$. In all computer implementations considered in this chapter, it will be assumed that there is a positive constant ρ such that $\rho(\varkappa) = \rho$ for all $\varkappa \in \Upsilon_c$. Observe that, because it is the case that $0 \leq Z_{CF}(t+h;\varkappa) \leq N_{CF}(t;\varkappa)$ for all $\varkappa \in \Upsilon_c$, the collection of random functions $\{Z_{CF}(t+h;\varkappa) \mid \varkappa \in \Upsilon_c\}$ satisfy inequalities of the type in Eqs. (11.5.7) and (11.5.8).

To ease the manipulation of computer arrays, it will be convenient to distinguish left- and right-hand partners. The total number left-hand partners of type $\tau_1 \in \Upsilon_s$, who became members of a couple during the time interval $(t, t+h]$, is:

$$Z_{CF}(t+h;\tau_1,\cdot) = \sum_{\tau_2 \in \Upsilon_s} Z_{CF}(t+h;\tau_1,\tau_2)\,. \qquad (11.5.13)$$

Similarly, the total number of right-hand partners of type τ_2, who became members of a couple during the time interval $(t, t+h]$, is:

$$Z_{CF}(t+h;\cdot,\tau_2) = \sum_{\tau_1 \in \Upsilon_s} Z_{CF}(t+h;\tau_1,\tau_2)\,. \qquad (11.5.14)$$

Therefore, the total number of singles of type τ_1 at time t, who became members of couples during time interval $(t, t+h]$, is given by the random function

$$T_{CF}(t;\tau_1) = Z_{CF}(t+h;\tau_1,\cdot) + Z_{CF}(t+h;\cdot,\tau_1) \qquad (11.5.15)$$

for all $\tau_1 \in \Upsilon_s$.

11.6 Probabilities of Being Infected by Extra-Marital Contacts

To derive a formula for the probability that a susceptible of type $\tau_1 = (j_1, 0)$ at time t is infected during the time interval $(t, t+h]$, the procedures used in Section 11.5 to construct couple formation will be extended. Although the acceptance probabilities for extra-marital contacts will have the same functional form, it will be assumed that those for couple formation and extra-marital sexual contacts may differ. To this end, let $\alpha_{em}(\tau_1, \tau_2)$ denote the conditional probability that a person of type $\tau_1 = (j_1, k_1)$ finds a person of type $\tau_2 = (j_2, k_2)$ acceptable as an extra-marital sexual partner. Just as in Section 11.5, by assumption this probability has the form,

$$\alpha_{em}(\tau_1, \tau_2) = \exp\left[-\left(\beta_{em1} \mid j_1 - j_2 \mid + \beta_{em2} \mid k_1 - k_2 \mid\right)\right] , \quad (11.6.1)$$

where β_{em1} and β_{em2} are non-negative parameters. Given a person of type τ_1 at time t who engages in extra-marital contacts, let $\gamma_{em}(t; \tau_1, \tau_2)$ be the conditional probability that a person of type τ_1 has contact with a potential extra-marital sexual partner of type τ_2 during the time interval $(t, t+h]$. This conditional probability will be defined in a manner similar to $\gamma_c(t; \tau_1, \tau_2)$ in Eq. (11.5.3), but for the case of extra-marital sexual contacts, the frequencies $U(t; \tau_1)$ must be defined differently.

At time $t \in S_h$, let the random function $X(t; \tau_1)$ denote the number of persons of type τ_1 in the population of singles, and let $Z(t; \tau_1, \tau_2)$ denote the number of couples of type (τ_1, τ_2). Just as in Eqs. (11.5.13) and (11.5.14), let the random functions $Z(t; \tau_1, \cdot)$ and $Z(t; \cdot, \tau_1)$ denote, respectively, the number of left- and right-hand partners of type τ_1 in couples at time t. Then, at time t, the total number of individuals of type τ_1 in the population is given by:

$$T(t; \tau_1) = X(t; \tau_1) + Z(t; \tau_1, \cdot) + Z(t; \cdot, \tau_1) . \quad (11.6.2)$$

Therefore, in the population as a whole, the frequency of individuals of type $\tau_1 \in \Upsilon_s$ at time t is:

$$V(t; \tau_1) = \frac{T(t; \tau_1)}{\sum_{\tau \in \Upsilon_s} T(t; \tau)} , \quad (11.6.3)$$

provided that $T(t; \tau) > 0$ for some $\tau \in \Upsilon_s$.

During any time interval $(t, t + h]$, let the random function $N_{EM}(t; \tau_1, \tau_2)$ denote the potential number of sexual contacts susceptibles of type τ_1 have with persons of type τ_2. Given the frequencies in Eq. (11.6.3), the algorithm for computing of realizations of these random functions is formally the same as that set forth in Eqs. (11.5.4) through (11.5.10). As in Section 10.3, it will assumed that this mixing and search for potential extra-martial sexual partners induces conditional probabilities $\rho_{EM}(t; \tau_1, \tau_2)$ that a susceptible of type τ_1 has an extra-marital sexual contact with a person of type τ_2 during the time interval $(t, t+h]$. According to the frequency theory of probability, these conditional probabilities have the functional form,

$$\rho_{EM}(t; \tau_1, \tau_2) = \frac{N_{EM}(t; \tau_1, \tau_2)}{\sum_{\tau' \in \Upsilon} N_{EM}(t; \tau_1, \tau')} \tag{11.6.4}$$

whenever the ratio is well-defined.

Let the random function $Q_{par}(t; \tau_1)$ denote the conditional probability that a susceptible of type τ_1 becomes infected during the time interval $(t, t+h]$ by one or more extra-martial sexual contacts. The procedure used to compute realizations of this random function runs parallel to that set forth in Section 10.3. Accordingly, let $\lambda(\tau_1)$ denote the expected number of sexual partners a person of type τ_1 has per unit time, and assume the number of partners follows a Poisson process with parameter $\lambda(\tau_1)$, so that $\lambda(\tau_1)h$ is the expected number of sexual partners during the time interval. Similarly, suppose the number of sexual contacts per partner follows a Poisson process with parameter $\eta(\tau_1)$ so that during the time interval $(t, t+h]$ the expected number of sexual contacts per partner is $1+\eta(\tau_1)h$. Observe that, by definition, a person is not a sexual partner unless at least one sexual contact occurs during any time interval.

As in Section 10.3, let $q(\tau_2)$ be the probability that a susceptible person of type τ_1 is infected per sexual contact when his partner is of type τ_2, and let $p(\tau_2) = 1 - q(\tau_2)$ be the probability of escaping infection per contact. By definition, if $\tau_2 = (j_2, 0)$ is a susceptible, then $q(\tau_2) = 0$, because a non-infected partner cannot transmit an infectious agent to his susceptible partner. Then, under the assumption that the number of sexual contacts per partner during the time interval $(t, t+h]$ occurs according to a Poisson process with support $c = 1, 2, \cdots$, the conditional probability that a susceptible person of type $\tau_1 = (j_1, 0)$ at time t escapes infection during $(t, t+h]$ when his sexual partner is of type $\tau_2 = (j_2, k_2)$ is given by:

$$\begin{aligned} p(t; \tau_1, \tau_2) &= \exp\left[-\eta(\tau_1)h\right] \sum_{c=1}^{\infty} \frac{(\eta(\tau_1)h)^{c-1}}{(c-1)!} (p(\tau_2))^c \\ &= p(\tau_2) \exp\left[-\eta(\tau_1)hq(\tau_2)\right] . \end{aligned} \tag{11.6.5}$$

By the law of total probability,

$$P_{par}(t;\tau_1) = \sum_{\tau_2 \in \Upsilon} \rho(t;\tau_1,\tau_2)p(t;\tau_1,\tau_2) \tag{11.6.6}$$

is, by definition, the conditional probability that a susceptible person of type τ_1 at time t escapes infection per extra-marital sexual partner during the time interval $(t, t+h]$. Thus,

$$Q_{par}(t;\tau_1) = 1 - P_{par}(t;\tau_1) \tag{11.6.7}$$

is the conditional probability that a susceptible person of type τ_1 becomes infected during $(t, t+h]$.

Furthermore, the number of sexual partners a person of type $\tau_1 = (j_1, 0)$ has during the time interval $(t, t+h]$, by assumption, follows a Poisson distribution with parameter $\lambda(\tau_1)$ and support $x = 0, 1, 2, \cdots$. Therefore,

$$P(t;\tau_1) = \exp\left[-\lambda(\tau_1)h\right] \sum_{x=0}^{\infty} \frac{(\lambda(\tau_1)h)^x}{x!} \left(P_{par}(t;\tau_1)\right)^x \tag{11.6.8}$$

$$= \exp\left[-\lambda(\tau_1)hQ_{par}(t;\tau_1)\right]$$

is the conditional probability that a susceptible person of type τ_1 at time t escapes infection from all extra-marital sexual partners during $(t, t+h]$. Therefore, by taking all possible extra-marital sexual partners into account,

$$Q(t;\tau_1) = 1 - P(t;\tau_1) = \lambda(i_1)Q_{par}(t;\tau_1)h + o(h) \tag{11.6.9}$$

is the conditional probability that a susceptible of type τ_1 becomes infected during $(t, t+h]$. This result justifies using the expression,

$$\lambda(i_1)Q_{par}(t;\tau_1) \tag{11.6.10}$$

as the latent risk for a susceptible of type τ_1 being infected during the time interval $(t, t+h]$, as described in semi-Markovian models for the life cycles of individuals in previous sections.

11.7 Stochastic Evolutionary Equations for the Population

Having defined matrices of latent risk for singles and couples, the purpose of this section is to set down a set of stochastic evolutionary equations for computing Monte Carlo realizations of the random functions of the population process, which are analogous to those in Section 10.5, for the case of $m \geq 1$ behavioral classes and $n \geq 1$ stages of disease. Let $\mathfrak{S}_{s1}$ and $\mathfrak{S}_{s2}$ denote, respectively, the set of absorbing and transient states of the life cycle model for individuals in the singles population. Just as in Section 10.4, the set $\mathfrak{S}_{s1}$ contains two states and the set $\mathfrak{S}_{s2}$ contains $m(n+1)$ states, and the full state space for the evolution of singles is $\mathfrak{S}_s = \mathfrak{S}_{s1} \cup \mathfrak{S}_{s2}$. Suppose that for every time interval t, a $m(n+1) \times (2 + m(n+1))$ matrix,

$$\boldsymbol{\Theta}_s(t) = (\theta_s(t; \tau_1, \tau_2) \mid \tau_1 \in \mathfrak{S}_{s1}, \tau_2 \in \mathfrak{S}_s) \tag{11.7.1}$$

of constant latent risks has been specified that is, by assumption, constant on the interval $(t, t+h]$. By definition, for every transient state $\tau_1 \in \mathfrak{S}_{s2}$, the total risk function on this interval is:

$$\theta_s(t; \tau_1) = \sum_{\tau_2 \in \mathfrak{S}_s} \theta_s(t; \tau_1, \tau_2) \,. \tag{11.7.2}$$

Whenever the risk functions are constant on the time interval $(t, t+h]$, it can be shown, by appealing to the classical theory of competing risks, that, given an individual is in state $\tau_1 \in \mathfrak{S}_{s2}$ at time t, the conditional probability $\pi(t; \tau_1, \tau_1)$ that he is still in this state at time $t + h$ is:

$$\pi_s(t; \tau_1, \tau_1) = \exp\left[-\theta_s(t; \tau_1)h\right] \,. \tag{11.7.3}$$

Therefore, the conditional probability of a jump to some other state during this time interval is $1 - \exp\left[-\theta_s(t; \tau_1)h\right]$. Consequently, another appeal to the theory of competing risks leads to the conclusion that, given a single individual in transient state τ_1 at time t,

$$\pi_s(t; \tau_1, \tau_2) = (1 - \exp\left[-\theta_s(t; \tau_1)h\right]) \frac{\theta_s(t; \tau_1, \tau_2)}{\theta_s(t; \tau_1)} \tag{11.7.4}$$

is the conditional probability of a jump to some state $\tau_2 \in \mathfrak{S}_s$ such that $\tau_2 \neq \tau_1$ during the time interval $(t, t+h]$. As they should, for every $\tau_1 \in \mathfrak{S}_{s2}$ and $t \in S_h$, these conditional probabilities satisfy the condition,

$$\sum_{\tau_2 \in \mathfrak{S}} \pi_s(t;\tau_1,\tau_2) = 1 \,. \tag{11.7.5}$$

For every $\tau_1 \in \mathfrak{S}_{s2}$ and $t \in S_h$, let

$$\mathbf{\Pi}_s(t;\tau_1) = (\pi_s(t;\tau_1,\tau_2) \mid \tau_2 \in \mathfrak{S}_s) \tag{11.7.6}$$

be a vector of these conditional probabilities.

With the exception of singles who become members of couples during any time interval $(t, t+h]$ and must be taken into account, the stochastic evolutionary equations for singles follow those in Section 10.5 quite closely. At time $t \in S_h$, let $X(t;\tau_1)$ denote the number of singles of type $\tau_1 \in \mathfrak{S}_{s2}$, and let $X_S(t;\tau_1)$ denote the number of these singles who do not become members of couples during $(t, t+h]$. Then according to Eq. (11.5.14),

$$X_S(t;\tau_1) = X(t;\tau_1) - T_{CF}(t;\tau_1) \tag{11.7.7}$$

for every $\tau_1 \in \mathfrak{S}_{s2} = \Upsilon_s$.

Given there are $X_S(t;\tau_1)$ persons of type $\tau_1 \in \mathfrak{S}_{s2}$ in the singles population at time t, let the random function $X_T(t+h;\tau_1,\tau_2)$ denote the number of persons who undergo the transition $\tau_1 \to \tau_2$ during $(t, t+h]$. Further, let

$$\mathbf{X}_T(t+h;\tau_1) = (X_T(t;\tau_1,\tau_2) \mid \tau_2 \in \mathfrak{S}) \tag{11.7.8}$$

be a vector of these random functions. It will be assumed that for every τ_1, given $X_S(t;\tau_1)$, this random vector has a conditional multinomial distribution with index $X_S(t;\tau_1)$ and probability vector $\mathbf{\Pi}_s(t;\tau_1)$. In symbols,

$$\mathbf{X}_T(t+h;\tau_1) \sim CMultinom\,(X_S(t;\tau_1), \mathbf{\Pi}_s(t;\tau_1)) \tag{11.7.9}$$

for every $\tau_1 \in \mathfrak{S}_{s2}$.

To accommodate recruits entering the population, let $\varphi_s(\tau)$ be the probability that a recruit of type $\tau \in \mathfrak{S}_{s2}$ enters the singles population during $(t, t+h]$. It will be assumed that these probabilities constitute a proper probability distribution so that the condition

$$\sum_{\tau \in \mathfrak{S}_2} \varphi_s(\tau) = 1 \tag{11.7.10}$$

is satisfied. The number of single recruits of type $\tau \in \mathfrak{S}_{s2}$ entering the population during $(t, t+h]$ will be denoted by the random function $X_R(t+h;\tau)$. If it is assumed that recruits enter the singles population according to a Poisson process at rate μ_r per unit time during this interval, then, given the state of the population at time t, it can be shown that $X_R(t+h;\tau)$ has a conditional Poisson distribution with parameter $\mu_r\varphi(\tau)h$. In symbols, for every $\tau \in \mathfrak{S}_{s2}$

$$X_R(t+h;\tau) \sim CPois\left(\mu_r\varphi_s(\tau)h\right) . \tag{11.7.11}$$

The next step in setting down the stochastic evolutionary equations for the population is to consider the matrix of latent risk functions governing the evolution of couples. Recall that, with respect to the evolution of couples, the set $\mathfrak{S}_{c1}$ of absorbing states contains 5 elements (see Eq. (11.2.8)); the set $\mathfrak{S}_{c2} = \boldsymbol{\Upsilon}_c$ of transient states contains $m^2(n+1)^2$ elements; and the state space is $\mathfrak{S}_c = \mathfrak{S}_{c1} \cup \mathfrak{S}_{c2}$. Suppose that for every time interval $(t, t+h]$, a $m^2(n+1)^2 \times (5 + m^2(n+1)^2)$ matrix of latent

$$\boldsymbol{\Theta}_c(t;\varkappa_1,\varkappa_2) = \left(\theta_c(t;\varkappa_1,\varkappa_2) \mid \varkappa_1 \in \mathfrak{S}_{c2}, \varkappa_2 \in \mathfrak{S}_c\right) \tag{11.7.12}$$

has been specified. Then, for every state $\varkappa_1 \in \mathfrak{S}_{c2}$, the total risk function is, by definition,

$$\theta_c(t;\varkappa_1) = \sum_{\varkappa_2 \in \mathfrak{S}_c} \theta_c(t;\varkappa_1,\varkappa_2) . \tag{11.7.13}$$

Given these total risk functions, the vector of π-probabilities for couples

$$\boldsymbol{\Pi}_c(t;\varkappa_1) = \left(\pi_c(t;\varkappa_1,\varkappa_2) \mid \varkappa_2 \in \mathfrak{S}_c\right) \tag{11.7.14}$$

may be defined as in Eqs. (11.7.3) through (11.7.6) for every $\varkappa_1 \in \mathfrak{S}_{c2}$.

At time t, let the random function $Z(t;\varkappa_1)$ denote the number of couples of type $\varkappa_1 = (\tau_{11}, \tau_{12}) \in \mathfrak{S}_{c2}$, and, among these couples, let the random function $Z_T(t+h;\varkappa_1,\varkappa_2)$ denote the number undergoing the state transition $\varkappa_1 \to \varkappa_2 \in \mathfrak{S}_c$ during the time interval $(t, t+h]$. Then, define a vector of the random functions as

$$\mathbf{Z}_T(t+h;\varkappa_1) = (Z_T(t+h;\varkappa_1,\varkappa_2) \mid \varkappa_2 \in \mathfrak{S}_c) \tag{11.7.15}$$

for every $\varkappa_1 = (\tau_{11}, \tau_{12}) \in \mathfrak{S}_{c2}$. Then, as in Eq. (11.7.9), by assumption

$$\mathbf{Z}_T(t+h;\varkappa_1) \sim CMultinom\,(Z(t;\varkappa_1), \mathbf{\Pi}_c(t;\varkappa_1)) \tag{11.7.16}$$

for every $\varkappa_1 \in \mathfrak{S}_{c2}$.

During any time interval $(t, t+h]$, a member of a couple at time t may return to the population of singles if the couple dissolves or there is a death of one member of the couple. As an aid to writing software that will be applicable to both one and two sex partnership models, it will be useful to distinguish left and right-hand partners of a couple. In this connection, the left member of a couple will return to the singles population during any time interval if there is a transition to any absorbing state in the subset,

$$DIS_L = \{E_{DIS}, E_{r1}, E_{r2}\}\ . \tag{11.7.17}$$

Note that states in this set include couple dissolution and the death of the right-hand partner. Similarly, the right-hand member of a couple will return to the singles population during any time interval if there is a transition in the subset,

$$DIS_R = \{E_{DIS}, E_{l1}, E_{l2}\} \tag{11.7.18}$$

of absorbing states.

Let the random function $X_{DISL}(t+h;\tau_1)$ denote the number of left-hand partners in couples at time t who return to the singles population during the time interval $(t, t+h]$. Then, for couples of type $\varkappa_1 = (\tau_1, \tau_2)$, this random function is given by

$$X_{DISL}(t+h;\tau_1) = \sum_{\tau_2 \in \Upsilon_s} \sum_{\varkappa_2 \in DIS_L} Z_T(t;\varkappa_1,\varkappa_2)\ . \tag{11.7.19}$$

Similarly, let the random function $X_{DISR}(t+h;\tau_1)$ denote the number of right partners in couple at time t who return to the singles population during the time interval $(t, t+h]$. Then, for $\varkappa_1 = (\tau_1, \tau_2)$,

$$X_{DISR}(t+h;\tau_2) = \sum_{\tau_1 \in \Upsilon_s} \sum_{\varkappa_2 \in DIS_R} Z_T(t;\varkappa_1,\varkappa_2) . \tag{11.7.20}$$

Therefore, the total number of persons who were members of couples at time t who return to the singles population during the time interval $(t, t+h]$ is given by the random function,

$$X_{DIS}(t+h;\tau_1) = X_{DISL}(t+h;\tau_1) + X_{DISR}(t+h;\tau_1) , \tag{11.7.21}$$

which is defined for every type $\tau_1 \in \mathfrak{S}_{s2} = \Upsilon_s$.

Given the above definitions, it can be seen that at time $t+h$, the number of persons in the singles population of type $\tau_1 \in \mathfrak{S}_{s2}$ is given by the random function,

$$X(t+h;\tau_1) = X_R(t+h;\tau_1) + \sum_{\tau \in \mathfrak{S}_{s2}} X_T(t+h;\tau,\tau_1) + X_{DIS}(t+h;\tau_1) , \tag{11.7.22}$$

which is the sum of the number of recruits of type τ_1 who entered the singles population during $(t, t+h]$, the number of transitions to this type among those will remained single during $(t, t+h]$, and the number of persons of this type who were members of couples at time t, but returned to the singles population during $(t, t+h]$ due to couple dissolution. By similar reasoning, if it is assumed that there are no couples among the recruits that enter the population during any time interval, then among the stochastic evolutionary equations for couples that for type $\varkappa_1$ has the form:

$$Z(t+h;\varkappa_1) = Z_{CF}(t+h;\varkappa_1) + \sum_{\varkappa \in \mathfrak{S}_{c2}} Z_T(t+h;\varkappa,\varkappa_1) \tag{11.7.23}$$

for every $\varkappa_1 \in \mathfrak{S}_{c2}$.

As described formally in Section 10.5, it is often of interest to account for the number of deaths and the number of new infections that occur during any time interval $(t, t+h]$ in the software. But, because the formal details are similar to those set forth in Section 10.5, they will be omitted here.

11.8 Embedded Non-linear Difference Equations

Just as in Section 10.6, it will be of interest to embed a system of non-linear difference equations in the stochastic process outlined in the previous section by taking conditional expectations of random functions, given the past evolution of the process, and then proceed to "estimate" the conditional expectations recursively. Given the vector,

$$\mathbf{X}_S(t) = (X_S(t;\tau) \mid \tau \in \mathfrak{S}_{s2}) \tag{11.8.1}$$

of random variables in Eq. (11.7.7), it follows that the conditional expectation of the middle term on the right in Eq. (11.7.22), the stochastic evolutionary equations for singles, is:

$$E\left[\sum_{\tau\in\mathfrak{S}_{s2}} X_T(t+h;\tau,\tau_1) \mid \mathbf{X}_S(t)\right] = \sum_{\tau\in\mathfrak{S}_{s2}} X_S(t;\tau)\pi_s(t;\tau,\tau_1)\,. \tag{11.8.2}$$

As in Section 10.6, let $\mathfrak{B}(t)$ denote a σ-sub-algebra in a probability space underlying the process induced by the sample functions of the process up to time t. To estimate the elements of the random vector in Eq. (11.8.1), the conditional expectations,

$$E\left[X_S(t;\tau) \mid \mathfrak{B}(t)\right] = X(t;\tau) - E\left[T_{CF}(t;\tau) \mid \mathfrak{B}(t)\right] \tag{11.8.3}$$

will be needed for every $\tau \in \mathfrak{S}_{s2}$. But, from Eqs. (11.5.10) through (11.5.14), it can be seen that:

$$E\left[T_{CF}(t;\tau) \mid \mathfrak{B}(t)\right] = \sum_{\tau_2\in\mathfrak{S}_{s2}} N_{CF}(t;\tau,\tau_2)q_{CF}(t;\tau,\tau_2)$$

$$+ \sum_{\tau_1\in\mathfrak{S}_{s2}} N_{CF}(t;\tau_1,\tau)q_{CF}(t;\tau_1,\tau) \tag{11.8.4}$$

for every $\tau \in \mathfrak{S}_{s2} = \Upsilon_s$.

Similarly, given $\mathfrak{B}(t)$, the conditional expectation of the third term on the right in Eq. (11.7.22) is:

$$E\left[X_{DIS}(t+h;\tau) \mid \mathfrak{B}(t)\right] = E\left[X_{DISL}(t+h;\tau) \mid \mathfrak{B}(t)\right]$$

$$+ E\left[X_{DISR}(t+h;\tau) \mid \mathfrak{B}(t)\right] . \tag{11.8.5}$$

But, for $\varkappa_1 = (\tau, \tau_2)$

$$E\left[X_{DISL}(t+h;\tau) \mid \mathfrak{B}(t)\right] = \sum_{\tau_2 \in \Upsilon_s} \sum_{\varkappa_2 \in DIS_L} Z(t;\varkappa_1)\pi_c(t;\varkappa_1,\varkappa_2) . \tag{11.8.6}$$

And, for $\varkappa_1 = (\tau_1, \tau)$

$$E\left[X_{DISR}(t+h;\tau) \mid \mathfrak{B}(t)\right] = \sum_{\tau_1 \in \Upsilon_s} \sum_{\varkappa_2 \in DIS_R} Z(t;\varkappa_1)\pi_c(t;\varkappa_1,\varkappa_2) . \tag{11.8.7}$$

It is thus clear, to estimate the random function $X_{DIS}(t+h;\tau)$ for every $\tau \in \mathfrak{S}_{s2} = \Upsilon_s$, estimates of the expressions on the right in Eqs. (11.8.6) and (11.8.7) will be needed for all types τ. Finally, with respect to Eq. (11.7.22) for the evolution of singles,

$$E\left[X_R(t+h;\tau) \mid \mathfrak{B}(t)\right] = \mu_r\varphi_s(\tau)h \tag{11.8.8}$$

for all $\tau \in \mathfrak{S}_{s2}$.

Turning to the stochastic evolutionary equations for couples in Eq. (11.7.23), it can be seen that, given $\mathfrak{B}(t)$, the conditional expectation of the second term on the right is

$$E\left[\sum_{\varkappa \in \mathfrak{S}_{c2}} Z_T(t+h;\varkappa,\varkappa_1) \mid \mathfrak{B}(t)\right] = \sum_{\varkappa \in \mathfrak{S}_{c2}} Z(t;\varkappa)\pi_c(t;\varkappa,\varkappa_1) , \tag{11.8.9}$$

and that for the first term on the right is

$$E\left[Z_{CF}(t+h;\varkappa_1) \mid \mathfrak{B}(t)\right] = N_{CF}(t;\varkappa_1)q_{CF}(t;\varkappa_1) \tag{11.8.10}$$

for all couple types $\varkappa_1 \in \mathfrak{S}_{c2}$.

By using the above formulas for conditional expectations, given the past $\mathfrak{B}(t)$, a system of non-linear difference equations may be derived, as in Section 10.6, by placing the symbol $\widehat{}$ over each random variable on the right. Thus, the embedded non-linear equation for singles may be written in the succinct form,

$$\widehat{X}(t+h;\tau_1) = \mu_r\varphi_s(\tau_1)h + \sum_{\tau \in \mathfrak{S}_{s2}} \widehat{X}_S(t;\tau)\widehat{\pi}_s(t;\tau,\tau_1) + \widehat{X}_{DIS}(t+h;\tau_1) \tag{11.8.11}$$

for all $\tau_1 \in \mathfrak{S}_{s2}$.

In order to compute the estimate $\widehat{X}_S(t;\tau)$, Eqs. (11.8.3) and (11.8.4) should be consulted; to compute the estimate $\widehat{X}_{DIS}(t+h;\tau_1)$, Eqs. (11.8.5) through (11.8.7) should be consulted. Finally, it can be seen from Eqs. (11.8.9) and (11.8.10) that the non-linear difference equation for couples takes the form,

$$\widehat{Z}(t;\varkappa_1) = \widehat{N}_{CF}(t;\varkappa_1)\widehat{q}_{CF}(t;\varkappa_1) + \sum_{\varkappa \in \mathfrak{S}_{c2}} \widehat{Z}(t;\varkappa)\widehat{\pi}_c(t;\varkappa,\varkappa_1) \ , \tag{11.8.12}$$

for every $\varkappa_1 \in \mathfrak{S}_{c2}$.

11.9 Embedded Non-linear Differential Equations

As in Section 10.7, considering the length of each time interval $(t, t+h]$ as $h \downarrow 0$, the embedded non-linear difference equations in Section 11.8 give rise to a system of differential equations. By proceeding as in Section 10.7, it can be shown that the differential equation governing the evolution of singles has the form,

$$\begin{aligned}\frac{d\widehat{X}(t;\tau_1)}{dt} &= \mu_r\varphi_s(\tau_1) - \widehat{X}(t;\tau_1)\widehat{\theta}_s(t;\tau_1) \\ &+ \sum_{\tau_1 \neq \tau \in \mathfrak{S}_{s2}} \widehat{X}(t;\tau,\tau_1)\widehat{\theta}_s(t;\tau,\tau_1) + \widehat{X}_{DIS}(t;\tau_1) - \widehat{T}_{CF}(t;\tau_1)\end{aligned} \tag{11.9.1}$$

for every $\tau_1 \in \mathfrak{S}_{s2}$. The term $\widehat{X}_{DIS}(t;\tau_1)$, which is the estimate of the number of members of couples of type τ_1 who returned to the singles population during a small time interval, is composed of two terms, corresponding to left and right members of couples. Thus,

$$\widehat{X}_{DIS}(t;\tau_1) = \widehat{X}_{DISL}(t;\tau_1) + \widehat{X}_{DISR}(t;\tau_1) \ , \tag{11.9.2}$$

where for $\varkappa_1 = (\tau_1, \tau_2)$

$$\widehat{X}_{DISL}(t;\tau_1) = \sum_{\tau_2 \in \mathfrak{S}_{s2}} \sum_{\varkappa_2 \in DISL} \widehat{Z}(t;\varkappa_1,\varkappa_2)\widehat{\theta}_c(t;\varkappa_1,\varkappa_2) \tag{11.9.3}$$

and for $\varkappa_1 = (\tau_2, \tau_1)$

$$\widehat{X}_{DISR}(t;\tau_1) = \sum_{\tau_2 \in \mathfrak{S}_{s2}} \sum_{\varkappa_2 \in DISR} \widehat{Z}(t;\varkappa_1,\varkappa_2)\widehat{\theta}_c(t;\varkappa_1,\varkappa_2) \ . \tag{11.9.4}$$

In each summation, the type $\tau_1 \in \mathfrak{S}_{s2}$ is fixed. Finally, the term $\widehat{T}_{CF}(t;\tau_1)$, representing those singles who become members of couples during a small time interval, has the form,

$$\widehat{T}_{CF}(t;\tau_1) = \sum_{\tau\in\mathfrak{S}_{s2}} \widehat{N}_{CF}(t;\tau_1,\tau)\widehat{p}(t;\tau_1,\tau) + \sum_{\tau\in\mathfrak{S}_{s2}} \widehat{N}_{CF}(t;\tau,\tau_1)\widehat{p}(t;\tau,\tau_1) \tag{11.9.5}$$

for every type $\tau_1 \in \mathfrak{S}_{s2}$.

Unlike the differential equations for the evolution of singles, those for the evolution of couples may be written in the succinct form,

$$\frac{d\widehat{Z}(t;\varkappa_1)}{dt} = -\widehat{Z}(t;\varkappa_1)\widehat{\theta}_c(t;\varkappa_1)$$

$$+ \sum_{\varkappa_1\neq\varkappa\in\mathfrak{S}_{s2}} \widehat{Z}(t;\varkappa)\widehat{\theta}_c(t;\varkappa,\varkappa_1) + \widehat{N}_{CF}(t;\varkappa_1)\widehat{p}(t;\varkappa_1) \tag{11.9.6}$$

for all couple types $\varkappa_1 \in \mathfrak{S}_{s2}$.

As an aid to the analysis of the system of differential equations just described, it will be helpful to cast them in vector-matrix form. To this end, let

$$\mathbf{R}_s = (\mu_r\varphi_s(\tau) \mid \tau \in \mathfrak{S}_{s2}) \tag{11.9.7}$$

denote a $m(n+1)\times 1$ column vector with the indicated elements, $\mathbf{0}_{m^2(n+1)^2}$ denote a $m^2(n+1)^2\times 1$ column vector of zeros, and let

$$\mathbf{R} = \begin{pmatrix} \mathbf{R}_s \\ \mathbf{0}_{m^2(n+1)^2} \end{pmatrix} \tag{11.9.8}$$

denote a $(m(n+1)+m^2(n+1)^2)\times 1$ for recruits entering the population. A $m(n+1)\times 1$ vector for singles will be denoted by:

$$\widehat{\mathbf{X}}(t) = \left(\widehat{X}(t;\tau) \mid \tau \in \mathfrak{S}_{s2}\right), \tag{11.9.9}$$

and the corresponding $m^2(n+1)^2\times 1$ vector for couples will be denoted by:

$$\widehat{\mathbf{Z}}(t) = \left(\widehat{Z}(t;\varkappa) \mid \varkappa \in \mathfrak{S}_{c2}\right). \tag{11.9.10}$$

Then, as will be shown subsequently, it will be notationally convenient to consider a partitioned $(m(n+1)+m^2(n+1)^2)\times 1$ vector defined as:

$$\widehat{\mathbf{V}}(t) = \begin{pmatrix} \widehat{\mathbf{X}}(t) \\ \widehat{\mathbf{Z}}(t) \end{pmatrix} . \tag{11.9.11}$$

Finally, let

$$\widehat{\mathbf{V}}_{CF}(t) = \begin{pmatrix} \widehat{\mathbf{V}}_{SCF}(t) \\ \widehat{\mathbf{V}}_{CCF}(t) \end{pmatrix} \tag{11.9.12}$$

denote a $(m(n+1)+m^2(n+1)^2)\times 1$ partitioned vector, whose components are defined as follows. The $m(n+1)\times 1$ component $\widehat{\mathbf{V}}_{SCF}(t)$ for singles is defined as:

$$\widehat{\mathbf{V}}_{SCF}(t) = \left(-\widehat{T}_{CF}(t;\tau) \mid \tau \in \mathfrak{S}_{s2}\right) , \tag{11.9.13}$$

and the $m^2(n+1)^2 \times 1$ component $\widehat{\mathbf{V}}_{CCR}(t)$ for couples is defined as:

$$\widehat{\mathbf{V}}_{CCF}(t) = \left(\widehat{N}_{CF}(t;\varkappa)\widehat{\rho}(t;\varkappa) \mid \varkappa \in \mathfrak{S}_{c2}\right) . \tag{11.9.14}$$

Given these definitions, just as in Section 10.7, there exists a $(m(n+1)+m^2(n+1)^2)\times(m(n+1)+m^2(n+1)^2)$ matrix $\widehat{\Xi}(t)$ such that the system of differential equations under consideration may be represented in the vector-matrix form,

$$\frac{d\widehat{\mathbf{V}}(t)}{dt} = \mathbf{R}+\widehat{\Xi}(t)\widehat{\mathbf{V}}(t)+\widehat{\mathbf{V}}_{CF}(t) . \tag{11.9.15}$$

Moreover, there is a constant matrix $\mathbf{A}$ and a matrix $\widehat{\mathbf{W}}(t)$ of non-linear terms such that:

$$\widehat{\Xi}(t) = \mathbf{A}+\widehat{\mathbf{W}}(t) . \tag{11.9.16}$$

Thus, if we define a vector,

$$\widehat{\mathbf{V}}_{EM}(t) = \widehat{\mathbf{W}}(t)\widehat{\mathbf{V}}(t) , \tag{11.9.17}$$

containing those elements arising from extra-marital sexual contacts, then the system of differential equations in Eq. (11.9.15) takes the form,

$$\frac{d\widehat{\mathbf{V}}(t)}{dt} = \mathbf{R} + \mathbf{A}\widehat{\mathbf{V}}(t) + \widehat{\mathbf{V}}_{EM}(t) + \widehat{\mathbf{V}}_{CF}(t) , \tag{11.9.18}$$

which is useful when deriving formulas for the Jacobian matrix of the system.

As an aid to a deeper analysis of the differential equation given by Eq. (11.9.18), it will be helpful to represent the transpose of matrix $\widehat{\Xi}(t)$ in the partitioned form,

$$\widehat{\Xi}'(t) = \begin{bmatrix} \widehat{\Xi}'_{ss}(t) & \mathbf{0}_{m(n+1),m^2(n+1)^2} \\ \widehat{\Xi}'_{cs}(t) & \widehat{\Xi}'_{cc}(t) \end{bmatrix} . \tag{11.9.19}$$

As the notation suggests, $\widehat{\Xi}'_{ss}(t)$ is a $m(n+1) \times m(n+1)$ matrix, containing functions of latent risks governing transitions among transient states in the life cycle models for singles; $\widehat{\Xi}'_{cs}(t)$ is a $m^2(n+1) \times m(n+1)$ matrix containing latent risks governing members of couples returning to the singles population; and $\widehat{\Xi}'_{cc}(t)$ is a $m^2(n+1) \times m^2(n+1)^2$ matrix containing functions of latent risks governing transitions among the transient states of the life cycle model for couples.

Just as in Section 10.7, the elements of the matrix $\widehat{\Xi}'_{ss}(t)$ can be identified in terms of the elements of latent risks in the life cycle model for singles. Let

$$\mathbf{\Theta}_{s2}(t) = \begin{bmatrix} \mathbf{\Theta}_{s21}(t) & \mathbf{\Theta}_{s22}(t) \end{bmatrix} \tag{11.9.20}$$

denote the $m(n+1) \times (2 + m(n+1))$ matrix of latent risks, governing transitions from transient states to absorbing states and among transient states, for the life cycle model for singles at time t. Then, for every transient state $\tau_1 \in \mathfrak{S}_{s2}$, the estimate of the total risk function for this state at time t is:

$$\widehat{\theta}_s(t;\tau_1) = \sum_{\tau \in \mathfrak{S}_s} \widehat{\theta}_s(t;\tau_1,\tau) . \tag{11.9.21}$$

Let

$$diag\left(\widehat{\theta}_s(t;\tau_1) \mid \tau_1 \in \mathfrak{S}_{s2}\right) \tag{11.9.22}$$

denote a $m(n+1) \times m(n+1)$ diagonal matrix. Then, the matrix $\widehat{\Xi}'_{ss}(t)$ is determined by:

$$\widehat{\Xi}'_{ss}(t) = \widehat{\Theta}_{s22}(t) - diag\left(\widehat{\theta}_s(t;\tau_1) \mid \tau_1 \in \mathfrak{S}_{s2}\right) \tag{11.9.23}$$

Similarly, let

$$\boldsymbol{\Theta}_{c2}(t) = \left[\ \boldsymbol{\Theta}_{c21}(t) \quad \boldsymbol{\Theta}_{c22}(t)\ \right] \tag{11.9.24}$$

denote the $m^2(n+1)^2 \times (5 + m^2(n+1)^2)$ matrix of latent risks, governing transitions from transient states to absorbing states and among transient states, for the life cycle model for couples at time t. Then, the matrix $\widehat{\Xi}'_{cc}(t)$ is determined by:

$$\widehat{\Xi}'_{cc}(t) = \widehat{\Theta}_{c22}(t) - diag\left(\widehat{\theta}_c(t;\varkappa_1) \mid \varkappa_1 \in \mathfrak{S}_{c2}\right) \tag{11.9.25}$$

at time t. Moreover, it can be shown that there are constant matrices $\mathbf{A}_{ss}$ and $\mathbf{A}_{cc}$ such that:

$$\widehat{\Xi}_{ss}(t) = \mathbf{A}_{ss} + \widehat{\mathbf{W}}_{ss}(t) \tag{11.9.26}$$

and

$$\widehat{\Xi}_{cc}(t) = \mathbf{A}_{cc} + \widehat{\mathbf{W}}_{cc}(t)\ , \tag{11.9.27}$$

where the **W**-matrices contains estimate of latent risks arising from extra-marital sexual contact. Furthermore, it can be shown that the matrix,

$$\widehat{\Xi}'_{cs}(t) = \mathbf{A}'_{cs} \tag{11.9.28}$$

is constant for all $t \in S_h$.

In summary, when displaying explicit forms of the matrices **A** and $\widehat{\mathbf{W}}(t)$ going into differential equation Eq. (11.9.18), one needs to consider the partitioned forms,

$$\mathbf{A} = \begin{bmatrix} \mathbf{A}_{ss} & \mathbf{A}_{sc} \\ \mathbf{0} & \mathbf{A}_{cc} \end{bmatrix} \tag{11.9.29}$$

and

$$\widehat{\mathbf{W}}(t) = \begin{bmatrix} \widehat{\mathbf{W}}_{ss}(t) & \mathbf{0} \\ \mathbf{0} & \widehat{\mathbf{W}}_{cc}(t) \end{bmatrix}, \tag{11.9.30}$$

where $\mathbf{A}_{sc}$ is the transpose of the matrix $\mathbf{A}'_{cs}$. Observe that, because the matrix $\mathbf{A}$ is quasi-upper triangular, its spectrum, the set of eigenvalues, is the union of those of $\mathbf{A}_{ss}$ and $\mathbf{A}_{cc}$. In symbols,

$$\sigma(\mathbf{A}) = \boldsymbol{\sigma}(\mathbf{A}_{ss}) \cup \sigma(\mathbf{A}_{cc}) \; . \tag{11.9.31}$$

Thus, to compute the spectrum of $\mathbf{A}$, it suffices to compute the spectra of the smaller matrices $\mathbf{A}_{ss}$ and $\mathbf{A}_{cc}$. In the next section, explicit forms of these matrices will be illustrated.

11.10 Examples of Coefficient Matrices for One Behavioral Class

For the class of partnership models under consideration, the simplest case is that of $m = 1$ behavioral class and $n = 1$ stage of disease. For this case, the indicator of membership class is omitted and the set of single types is:

$$\Upsilon_s = \mathfrak{S}_{s2} = \{\tau_1 = (0), \tau_2 = (1)\} \; . \tag{11.10.1}$$

Furthermore, the set of couple types for this case in lexicographic order is:

$$\Upsilon_c = \mathfrak{S}_{c2} = \{\varkappa_1 = (0,0), \varkappa_2 = (0,1), \varkappa_3 = (1,0), \varkappa_4 = (1,1)\} \; . \tag{11.10.2}$$

For the case of $m = 1$ and $n = 1$, the matrix of latent risks for the life cycle model for singles is 2×4 and will be represented in the partitioned form,

$$\boldsymbol{\Theta}_{s2}(t) = \begin{bmatrix} \boldsymbol{\Theta}_{s21} & \boldsymbol{\Theta}_{s22}(t) \end{bmatrix} , \tag{11.10.3}$$

where

$$\boldsymbol{\Theta}_{s21} = \begin{bmatrix} \mu_0 & 0 \\ \mu_0 & \mu_1 \end{bmatrix} \tag{11.10.4}$$

and

$$\boldsymbol{\Theta}_{s22}(t) = \begin{bmatrix} 0 & \lambda Q_{par}(t;\tau_1) \\ 0 & 0 \end{bmatrix} . \tag{11.10.5}$$

Given these matrices, it can be seen that the total risk functions are:

$$\theta_s(t;\tau_1) = \mu_0 + \lambda Q_{par}(t;\tau_1)$$

$$\theta_s(t;\tau_2) = \mu_0 + \mu_1 \,. \tag{11.10.6}$$

Therefore, the matrix $\widehat{\Xi}'_{ss}(t)$ has the form,

$$\begin{aligned}\widehat{\Xi}'_{ss}(t) &= \widehat{\mathbf{\Theta}}_{s22}(t) - diag\left(\widehat{\theta}_s(t;\tau_1), \widehat{\theta}_s(t;\tau_2)\right) \\ &= \mathbf{A}'_{ss} + \widehat{\mathbf{W}}'_{ss}(t)\,,\end{aligned} \tag{11.10.7}$$

where

$$\mathbf{A}'_{ss} = \begin{bmatrix} -\mu_0 & 0 \\ 0 & -(\mu_0 + \mu_1) \end{bmatrix} \tag{11.10.8}$$

and

$$\widehat{\mathbf{W}}'_{ss}(t) = \begin{bmatrix} -\lambda\widehat{Q}_{par}(t;\tau_1) & \lambda\widehat{Q}_{par}(t;\tau_1) \\ 0 & 0 \end{bmatrix} . \tag{11.10.9}$$

For the case of one behavioral class and one stage of disease, the matrix $\mathbf{\Theta}_{c2}(t)$ of latent risks for couples is 4×6 and can be represented in the partitioned form,

$$\mathbf{\Theta}_{c2}(t) = \begin{bmatrix} \mathbf{\Theta}_{c21} & \mathbf{\Theta}_{c22}(t) \end{bmatrix}, \tag{11.10.10}$$

where the 4×5 matrix $\mathbf{\Theta}_{c21}$ is displayed in Eq. (11.3.2) and the 4×4 matrix $\mathbf{\Theta}_{c22}(t)$ is displayed in Eq. (11.3.3). From inspection of Eqs. (11.3.2) and (11.3.3), it can be seen that the total risk function for couples are:

$$\begin{aligned}\theta_c(t;\varkappa_1) &= \delta + 2\mu_0 + 2\lambda Q_{par}(t;\tau_1) \\ \theta_c(t;\varkappa_2) &= \delta + 2\mu_0 + \mu_1 + \lambda Q_{par}(t;\tau_1) + \gamma_{mc}q(1) \\ \theta_c(t;\varkappa_3) &= \delta + 2\mu_0 + \mu_1 + \lambda Q_{par}(t;\tau_1) + \gamma_{mc}q(1) \\ \theta_c(t;\varkappa_4) &= \delta + 2\mu_0 + 2\mu_1 \,.\end{aligned} \tag{11.10.11}$$

The diagonal elements that enter into the diagonal of the matrix $\mathbf{A}_{cc}$ are determined by deleting all functions of t from the expression in Eq. (11.10.11). Thus,

$$\theta_c^*(\varkappa_1) = \delta + 2\mu_0$$

$$\theta_c^*(\varkappa_2) = \delta + 2\mu_0 + \mu_1 + \gamma_{mc}q(1)$$

$$\theta_c^*(\varkappa_3) = \delta + 2\mu_0 + \mu_1 + \gamma_{mc}q(1)$$

$$\theta_c^*(\varkappa_4) = \theta_c(t; \varkappa_4) = \delta + 2\mu_0 + 2\mu_1 \,. \tag{11.10.12}$$

Given these definitions, for the case under consideration the 4×4 matrix $\mathbf{A}_{cc}$ is the diagonal matrix

$$\mathbf{A}_{cc} = diag\left(-\theta_c^*(\varkappa) \mid \varkappa \in \mathfrak{S}_{c2}\right) \,, \tag{11.10.13}$$

and the transpose of the $\widehat{\mathbf{W}}_{cc}(t)$ has the form,

$$\begin{bmatrix} -2\lambda\widehat{Q}_{par}(t;\tau_1) & \lambda\widehat{Q}_{par}(t;\tau_1) & \lambda\widehat{Q}_{par}(t;\tau_1) & 0 \\ 0 & -\lambda\widehat{Q}_{par}(t;\tau_1) & 0 & \lambda\widehat{Q}_{par}(t;\tau_1) \\ 0 & 0 & -\lambda\widehat{Q}_{par}(t;\tau_1) & \lambda\widehat{Q}_{par}(t;\tau_1) \\ 0 & 0 & 0 & 0 \end{bmatrix} . \tag{11.10.14}$$

Finally, the transpose matrix $\mathbf{A}_{sc}$ of latent risk governing transitions of individuals who are members of couples to the singles population has the form

$$\mathbf{A}_{sc}^{'} = \mathbf{A}_{cs} = \begin{bmatrix} 2(\delta + \mu_0) & 0 \\ \delta + \mu_0 + \mu_1 & \delta + \mu_0 \\ \delta + \mu_0 + \mu_1 & \delta + \mu_0 \\ 0 & 2(\delta + \mu_0 + \mu_1) \end{bmatrix} . \tag{11.10.15}$$

The rows of this matrix are indexed by the set of couple types in the lexicographic order displayed in Eq. (11.10.2), and the columns of the matrix are indexed by the set of single types as displayed in Eq. (11.10.1). The element $2(\delta + \mu_0)$ in the first row and column of the matrix is the risk of either member of the couple type $\varkappa_1 = (0, 0)$, in which both members are susceptible, returning to the singles population. To justify this element, observe that either member of a couple will return to the singles population if there is a separation with risk δ or a death with risk μ_0. Thus, the total risk for either member of the couple returning to the singles population is $\delta + \mu_0$ so that the total risk for a couple returning two susceptibles to the singles population is

$2(\delta + \mu_0)$. The second row of the matrix contains those risks for a member of a couple of type $\varkappa_2 = (0,1)$ returning to the singles population. For example, the left susceptible member will return to the singles population if the couple separates with risk δ or the right infected partner dies with risk $\mu_0 + \mu_1$. Thus, $\delta + \mu_0 + \mu_1$ is the total risk the left susceptible member of a couple returns to the singles population, which is the element in the second row of first column in $\mathbf{A}_{cs}$. By following similar lines of reasoning, the other risks displayed in the matrix $\mathbf{A}_{cs}$ can be derived.

Note that the matrix $\mathbf{A}$ in this case is stable, since all the eigenvalues of $\mathbf{A}_{ss}$ and $\mathbf{A}_{cc}$ are negative (see Eq. (11.9.31)). But, when there are more than $n = 1$ stages of disease, then in most cases it will not be possible to determine whether the matrix $\mathbf{A}$ is stable by inspection. For those cases in which the number of behavioral classes $m \geq 2$ and the number of stages of disease $n \geq 2$, the matrices of latent risks described in Section 11.3 will be more complicated, but, nevertheless, some of the patterns displayed in this section will apply. However, a description of these more general matrices of latent risks will not be undertaken in this section.

11.11 Stationary Vectors and Structure of the Jacobian Matrix

In this section, some procedures for finding stationary vectors will be discussed along with an overview of the structure of the Jacobian matrix for the differential equations in Section 11.9 for the general cases for $m \geq 1$ behavioral classes and $n \geq 0$ stages of disease. As a first step in developing this overview, the differential equations in Eq. (11.9.18) are written in the notationally simpler form,

$$\frac{d\mathbf{v}}{dt} = \mathbf{R} + \mathbf{A}\mathbf{v} + \mathbf{v}_{EM}(\mathbf{v}) + \mathbf{v}_{CF}(\mathbf{v}) , \tag{11.11.1}$$

where $\mathbf{v}_{EM}(\mathbf{v})$ and $\mathbf{v}_{CF}(\mathbf{v})$ are non-linear vector-valued functions of the vector $\mathbf{v}$.

If the population consists only of susceptibles, then $\mathbf{v}_{CF}(\mathbf{v}) = \mathbf{0}$, a column vector of zeros. Therefore, if a population contains only susceptibles, then all stationary vectors $\widehat{\mathbf{v}}$ must satisfy the non-linear equation

$$\mathbf{R} + \mathbf{A}\widehat{\mathbf{v}} + \mathbf{v}_{CF}(\widehat{\mathbf{v}}) = \mathbf{0}\,. \tag{11.11.2}$$

When a population contains only susceptibles, then many elements of the vector $\widehat{\mathbf{v}}$ will be zero. Therefore, in a search for stationary vectors for the case a population contains only susceptibles, it will suffice to consider the case $n = 0$, which gives rise to the reduced form

$$\mathbf{R}_S + \mathbf{A}_S\widehat{\mathbf{v}} + \mathbf{v}_{CFS}(\widehat{\mathbf{v}}) = \mathbf{0} \tag{11.11.3}$$

of Eq. (11.11.2), where S in a subscript indicates that only a population of susceptibles is being considered. Unlike the one-sex model discussed in Chapter 10, where there was a unique stationary vector for the case in which a population contained only susceptibles (see Section 10.9), Eq. (11.11.3) may have one or more solutions due to non-linearities. However, in some special cases, the equation may be linear in $\widehat{\mathbf{v}}$.

For example, for the case of $m = 1$ behavioral class and $n = 0$ stages of disease, the differential equations for a population of susceptibles with couples takes the form,

$$\frac{dx}{dt} = \mu_r - \mu_0 x + 2(\delta + 2\mu_0)z - \rho x$$

$$\frac{dz}{dt} = -(\delta + 2\mu_0)z + \frac{\rho x}{2}\,. \tag{11.11.4}$$

Observe that in this case, the stationary equations are linear and have the symbolic solution,

$$\widehat{x} = \left(\frac{\mu_r}{\mu_0}\right)\left(\frac{\delta + 2\mu_0}{\delta + 2\mu_0 + \rho}\right)$$

$$\widehat{z} = \frac{1}{2}\left(\frac{\mu_r}{\mu_0}\right)\left(\frac{\rho}{\delta + 2\mu_0 + \rho}\right)\,. \tag{11.11.5}$$

Because it is assumed that all the parameters μ_r, μ_0, δ, and ρ are positive, it follows that $\widehat{x} > 0$ and $\widehat{z} > 0$ at all points in the parameter space. Moreover, in a stationary population, total population size is given by the formula,

$$\widehat{x} + 2\widehat{z} = \frac{\mu_r}{\mu_0}\,. \tag{11.11.6}$$

Observe that $1/\mu_0 = e_0$ is the expectation of life remaining after an individual becomes sexually active so that in this simple model total population size is $\mu_r e_0$ at equilibrium.

By way of another illustrative example, consider the case of $m = 2$ behavioral classes where $n = 0$. Then, there are two susceptible types $\tau_1 = 1$ and $\tau_2 = 2$. Furthermore, suppose there are no transition among behavioral classes so that $\psi_{12} = \psi_{21} = 0$ and that individuals choose partners only within their behavioral class. In terms of the acceptance probabilities for couple formation, this latter condition may be expressed as $\alpha_{cf}(1,1) = \alpha_{cf}(2,2) = 1$ and $\alpha_{cf}(1,2) = \alpha_{cf}(2,1) = 0$. It will also be supposed that φ_1 and φ_2 are positive and satisfy the condition $\varphi_1 + \varphi_2 = 1$. Under these assumptions, the evolution of a population of susceptibles is governed by the differential equations,

$$\frac{dx_1}{dt} = \mu_r\varphi_1 - \mu_0 x_1 + 2(\delta + 2\mu_0)z_{11} - \rho x_1$$

$$\frac{dx_2}{dt} = \mu_r\varphi_2 - \mu_0 x_2 + 2(\delta + 2\mu_0)z_{22} - \rho x_2$$

$$\frac{dz_{11}}{dt} = -(\delta + 2\mu_0)\, z_{11} + \frac{\rho x_1}{2}$$

$$\frac{dz_{22}}{dt} = -(\delta + 2\mu_0)\, z_{22} + \frac{\rho x_2}{2}\ . \tag{11.11.7}$$

Observe that in this case, Eq. (11.11.13) for the stationary vector $\widehat{\mathbf{v}}$ is linear in the unknowns and can easily be solved symbolically, just as in the first example. Thus, the elements of $\widehat{\mathbf{v}}$ for singles have the symbolic forms,

$$\widehat{x}_1 = \left(\frac{\mu_r\varphi_1}{\mu_0}\right)\left(\frac{\delta + 2\mu_0}{\delta + 2\mu_0 + \rho}\right)$$

$$\widehat{x}_2 = \left(\frac{\mu_r\varphi_2}{\mu_0}\right)\left(\frac{\delta + 2\mu_0}{\delta + 2\mu_0 + \rho}\right)\ , \tag{11.11.8}$$

and those for couples have the forms,

$$\widehat{z}_{11} = \frac{1}{2}\left(\frac{\mu_r\varphi_1}{\mu_0}\right)\left(\frac{\rho}{\delta + 2\mu_0 + \rho}\right)$$

$$\widehat{z}_{22} = \frac{1}{2}\left(\frac{\mu_r \varphi_2}{\mu_0}\right)\left(\frac{\rho}{\delta + 2\mu_0 + \rho}\right) . \tag{11.11.9}$$

As in the first example, the formula for total population size at equilibrium is:

$$\widehat{x}_1 + \widehat{x}_2 + 2\widehat{z}_{11} + 2\widehat{z}_{22} = \frac{\mu_r}{\mu_0} . \tag{11.11.10}$$

For many cases of interest, it will not be possible to derive symbolic forms for the elements of a stationary vector and one must, therefore, resort to numerical methods. The system of differential equations for a population of susceptibles has the vector-matrix form,

$$\frac{d\mathbf{v}}{dt} = \mathbf{R}_S + \mathbf{A}_S \mathbf{v} + \mathbf{v}_{CFS}(\mathbf{v}) , \tag{11.11.11}$$

and, as a first step towards finding numerical values of a stationary vector, it will be useful to convert these equations into a vector difference equation. If all time intervals are of length $h > 0$, then this difference equation has the form,

$$\mathbf{v}_{k+1} = \mathbf{v}_k + h\left(\mathbf{R}_S + \mathbf{A}_S \mathbf{v}_k + \mathbf{v}_{CFS}(\mathbf{v}_k)\right) . \tag{11.11.12}$$

Thus, if one assigns an initial vector $\mathbf{v}_0$, then, for a fixed h, the sequence of vectors $(\mathbf{v}_k \mid k = 1, 2, \cdots)$ may be computed recursively. If the limit

$$\lim_{k\uparrow\infty} \mathbf{v}_k = \widehat{\mathbf{v}} \tag{11.11.13}$$

exists, then by letting $k \uparrow \infty$ in Eq. (11.11.12), it can be seen that for every $h > 0$,

$$\mathbf{R}_S + \mathbf{A}_S \widehat{\mathbf{v}} + \mathbf{v}_{CFS}(\widehat{\mathbf{v}}) = \mathbf{0} . \tag{11.11.14}$$

At this point, however, there are no guarantees that $\widehat{\mathbf{v}}$ is a unique solution of Eq. (11.11.13), or even that the limit exists.

Fortunately, by converting differential equation into an integral equation, it can be shown that under plausible conditions its limit in Eq. (11.11.13) will indeed exist. If $\mathbf{v}_0$ is the initial vector, then an integration of Eq. (11.11.11) (see Section 10.7 for technical details) yields the integral equation,

$$\mathbf{v}(t) = e^{\mathbf{A}_S t}\mathbf{v}_0 + \int_0^t e^{\mathbf{A}_S s}\mathbf{R}_S ds + \int_0^t e^{\mathbf{A}_S s}\mathbf{v}_{CFS}(\mathbf{v}(t-s))ds \tag{11.11.15}$$

for $t > 0$. If the matrix $\mathbf{A}_S$ is stable, then

$$\lim_{t\uparrow\infty} e^{\mathbf{A}_S t}\mathbf{v}_0 = \mathbf{0} \ , \tag{11.11.16}$$

and, moreover, if the matrix $\mathbf{A}_S$ is also non-singular, then

$$\lim_{t\uparrow\infty} \int_0^t e^{\mathbf{A}_S s}\mathbf{R}_S ds = -\mathbf{A}_S^{-1}\mathbf{R}_S \ . \tag{11.11.17}$$

Thus, it suffices to find conditions such that the third term on the right in Eq. (11.11.15) approaches a limit as $t \uparrow \infty$.

To simplify the notation, for $t > 0$ let

$$\mathbf{g}(t) = \int_0^t e^{\mathbf{A}_S s}\mathbf{v}_{CFS}(\mathbf{v}(t-s))ds \ . \tag{11.11.18}$$

To establish sufficient conditions for this integral to converge as $t \uparrow \infty$, it will be help to introduce a norm for vectors and matrices. For any vector $\mathbf{x} = (x_i \mid i = 1, 2, \cdots, d)$ with $d \geq 1$ elements, real or complex, let $\|\mathbf{x}\| = \max_{\mathbf{i}} |x_i|$ be its norm.

Similarly, for any $d \times d$ matrix $\mathbf{B} = (b_{ij})$ with real or complex elements, let

$$\|\mathbf{B}\| = \max_{\mathbf{i}} \sum_{j=1}^{d} |b_{ij}| \tag{11.11.19}$$

be its norm.

It seems reasonable to assume that if the rate μ_r of recruits entering the population per unit time is sufficiently small and the death rate or rates are sufficiently large, then population size will remain bounded. Thus, it seems reasonable to suppose that there is a constant $b > 0$ such that $\|\mathbf{v}(t)\| \leq b$ for all $t > 0$. For the class of models under consideration, this assumption implies there is a constant $c > 0$ such that $\|\mathbf{v}_{CFS}(\mathbf{v}(t))\| \leq c$ for all $t > 0$. If the matrix $\mathbf{A}_S$ is stable, then it can be shown that:

$$\int_0^\infty \left\|e^{\mathbf{A}_S s}\right\| ds < \infty \ . \tag{11.11.20}$$

Furthermore, for every $\epsilon > 0$ there is a t_0 sufficiently large such that:

$$\int_{t_0}^\infty \left\|e^{\mathbf{A}_S s}\right\| ds < \frac{\epsilon}{2c} \ . \tag{11.11.21}$$

Also note that the integral in Eq. (11.11.21) is a decreasing function of t_0. Therefore, for every $k > 0$ and $t > t_0$, it follows from Eqs. (11.11.18) and (11.11.21) that

$$\|\mathbf{g}(t+k) - \mathbf{g}(t)\| \; < 2c \int_{t_0}^{\infty} \left\| e^{\mathbf{A}_S s} \right\| ds < \epsilon \, . \tag{11.11.22}$$

We can therefore conclude that the function $\mathbf{g}(t)$ has the Cauchy property and thus converges to a limit as $t \uparrow \infty$.

This result, along with Eq. (11.11.17), shows that under the conditions outlined above there will exist at least one stationary vector $\widehat{\mathbf{v}}$ determined by the formula,

$$\widehat{\mathbf{v}} = -\mathbf{A}_S^{-1}\mathbf{R}_S + \lim_{t\uparrow\infty} \int_0^t e^{\mathbf{A}_S s}\mathbf{v}_{CFS}(\mathbf{v}(t-s))ds \, . \tag{11.11.23}$$

In a number of computer experiments, it has been observed that the limit in Eq. (11.11.13) does indeed exist, although the convergence is very slow, and the number of iterations necessary to attain convergence can be large and depend significantly on the initial vector $\mathbf{v}_0$. In practice, the parameters of the system are determined according to a monthly time scale, and h is taken as a fraction of a month. Even though the number of iterations needed to attain convergence can be large, the recursive procedure is, nevertheless, a feasible method for estimating $\widehat{\mathbf{v}}$ on many desktop computers. Curiously, if the first term on the right in Eq. (11.11.23) is chosen as the initial vector $\mathbf{v}_0 = -\mathbf{A}_S^{-1}\mathbf{R}_S$, then it has been observed in many numerical experiments that convergence will occur within 2 to 10 seconds, which provides a practical way of choosing $\mathbf{v}_0$.

Having discussed procedures for estimating stationary vectors, the next item on the agenda for this section is to give an overview of the structure of Jacobian matrices associated with the differential equation. From inspection of the system of differential equations in Eq. (11.11.1), it can be seen that the Jacobian matrix of the system for a system that contains infectives has the form,

$$\mathbf{J}(\mathbf{v}) = \mathbf{A} + \mathbf{J}_{EM}(\mathbf{v}) + \mathbf{J}_{CF}(\mathbf{v}) \, , \tag{11.11.24}$$

where $\mathbf{J}_{EM}(\mathbf{v})$ and $\mathbf{J}_{CF}(\mathbf{v})$ are, respectively, the Jacobian matrices derived from the vectors $\mathbf{v}_{EM}(\mathbf{v})$ and $\mathbf{v}_{CF}(\mathbf{v})$ for extra-marital sexual contacts and couple formation. Procedures for computing the elements of the constant matrix $\mathbf{A}$ have been outlined in the examples presented Section 11.10, so that the main tasks remaining are those of describing the structure of $\mathbf{J}_{EM}(\mathbf{v})$ and $\mathbf{J}_{CF}(\mathbf{v})$. Because the differential equations in Eq. (11.11.11) for a population of susceptibles are non-linear, it will also be of interest to consider the Jacobian matrix associated with this system. From an inspection of this system, it can be seen that it Jacobian matrix has the form,

$$\mathbf{J}_S(\mathbf{v}) = \mathbf{A}_S + \mathbf{J}_{CFS}(\mathbf{v}) \,, \tag{11.11.25}$$

where $\mathbf{J}_{CFS}(\mathbf{v})$ is the Jacobian matrix that is determined by the vector $\mathbf{v}_{CFS}(\mathbf{v})$.

In deriving the structure of these Jacobian matrices, it will be helpful to represent the vector $\mathbf{v}$ in the partitioned form,

$$\mathbf{v} = \begin{pmatrix} \mathbf{v}_s \\ \mathbf{v}_c \end{pmatrix} , \tag{11.11.26}$$

where $\mathbf{v}_s$ is a $m(n+1)\times 1$ for types of singles and $\mathbf{v}_c$ is a $m^2(n+1)^2\times 1$ for types of couples. From an inspection of Eqs. (11.9.11) and (11.9.30) it can be seen that the vector for extra-marital sexual contacts in the notation of this section has the partitioned form,

$$\mathbf{v}_{EM}(\mathbf{v}) = \mathbf{W}\mathbf{v} = \begin{pmatrix} \mathbf{W}_{ss}\mathbf{v}_s \\ \mathbf{W}_{cc}\mathbf{v}_c \end{pmatrix} . \tag{11.11.27}$$

Therefore, the Jacobian matrix $\mathbf{J}_{EM}(\mathbf{v})$ has the partitioned form,

$$\mathbf{J}_{EM}(\mathbf{v}) = \frac{\partial \mathbf{W}\mathbf{v}}{\partial \mathbf{v}} = \begin{bmatrix} \dfrac{\partial \mathbf{W}_{ss}\mathbf{v}_s}{\partial \mathbf{v}} \\ \dfrac{\partial \mathbf{W}_{cc}\mathbf{v}_c}{\partial \mathbf{v}} \end{bmatrix} , \tag{11.11.28}$$

where

$$\frac{\partial \mathbf{W}_{ss}\mathbf{v}_s}{\partial \mathbf{v}} \tag{11.11.29}$$

is a $m(n+1) \times (m(n+1)+m^2(n+1)^2)$ matrix of partial derivatives and

$$\frac{\partial \mathbf{W}_{cc}\mathbf{v}_c}{\partial \mathbf{v}} \tag{11.11.30}$$

is a $m^2(n+1)^2 \times (m(n+1)+m^2(n+1)^2)$ matrix of partial derivatives. Because the matrices $\mathbf{W}_{ss}$ and $\mathbf{W}_{cc}$ are sparse, many of the elements of these matrices will be zero.

To provide an overview of the structure of the Jacobian matrix for couple formation in the notation of this section, the vector $\mathbf{v}_{CF}(\mathbf{v})$ is written in the partitioned form,

$$\mathbf{v}_{CF}(\mathbf{v}) = \begin{pmatrix} \mathbf{v}_{SCF}(\mathbf{v}) \\ \mathbf{v}_{CCF}(\mathbf{v}) \end{pmatrix}, \tag{11.11.31}$$

where $\mathbf{v}_{SCF}(\mathbf{v})$ is a $m(n+1)\times 1$ vector for types of singles and $\mathbf{v}_{CCF}(\mathbf{v})$ is a $m^2(n+1)^2 \times 1$ vector for types of couples (see Eq. (11.9.12)). Then, recall that these sub-vectors have the forms,

$$\mathbf{v}_{SCF}(\mathbf{v}) = (-T_{CF}(\tau_1, \mathbf{v}) \,|\tau_1 \in \mathfrak{S}_{s2}) \tag{11.11.32}$$

and

$$\mathbf{v}_{CCF}(\mathbf{v}) = (N_{CF}(\varkappa, \mathbf{v})\rho(\varkappa)|\varkappa \in \mathfrak{S}_{c2}) \ . \tag{11.11.33}$$

The function $T_{CF}(\mathbf{v};\tau_1)$ has the form,

$$T_{CF}(\tau_1, \mathbf{v}) = \sum_{\tau \in \mathfrak{S}_{s2}} N_{CF}(\tau_1, \tau, \mathbf{v})\rho(\tau_1, \tau) + \sum_{\tau \in \mathfrak{S}_{s2}} N_{CF}(\tau, \tau_1, \mathbf{v})\rho(\tau, \tau_1) \tag{11.11.34}$$

for every $\tau_1 \in \mathfrak{S}_{s2}$, as can be seen from Eq. (11.9.5) by writing the symbol $\varkappa$ for a couple type in vector form. Thus, as in Eq. (11.11.9), the Jacobian matrix $\mathbf{J}_{CF}(\mathbf{v})$ for couple formation may be represented in the partitioned form

$$\mathbf{J}_{CF}(\mathbf{v}) = \frac{\partial \mathbf{v}_{CF}(\mathbf{v})}{\partial \mathbf{v}} = \begin{bmatrix} \dfrac{\partial \mathbf{v}_{SCF}(\mathbf{v})}{\partial \mathbf{v}} \\ \dfrac{\partial \mathbf{v}_{CCF}(\mathbf{v})}{\partial \mathbf{v}} \end{bmatrix} = \begin{bmatrix} \mathbf{J}_{SCF}(\mathbf{v}) \\ \mathbf{J}_{CCF}(\mathbf{v}) \end{bmatrix} . \tag{11.11.35}$$

In summary, a basic step in deriving formulas for the elements of the Jacobian matrix $\mathbf{J}_{CF}(\mathbf{v})$ is that of finding partial derivatives of the function $N_{CF}(\mathbf{v};\varkappa)$ for every couple type $\varkappa \in \mathfrak{S}_{c2}$. Actually, because these functions for couple formation depend only on the elements of the vector $\mathbf{v}_s$ for singles, the problem of finding partial derivatives of these functions is very similar to that considered in Section 10.11. However, for the case of extra-marital contacts, the functions $N_{EM}(\tau_1, \tau_2, \mathbf{v})$ actually depend on all the elements of the vector $\mathbf{v}$ so that special formulas of the partial derivatives of these functions will have to derived. In the next section, the actual structure of the Jacobian matrix for extra-marital sexual contacts described in this section will be presented in a form suitable for writing software.

11.12 Overview of the Jacobian for Extra-Marital Contacts

The purpose of this section is to develop a general overview of computational formulas for the elements of the Jacobian matrix for extra-marital sexual contacts described in Section 11.11, and illustrate the concepts with a simple example. It will be helpful to have a notation to distinguish susceptibles and infectives in the population at any time with respect to extra-marital sexual contacts. As in Section 10.9, let Υ_S and Υ_I denote, respectively, the sets of susceptible and infective types of persons in the population (see Eq. (10.9.10) through (10.9.12) for definitions of these sets). At any time, either singles or members of couples can belong to these sets. Observe that $\Upsilon = \Upsilon_S \cup \Upsilon_I$ is the set of all types of individuals in the population, and, formally, the set Υ is identical to the set Υ_s of single types defined in Eq. (11.4.1).

To stress that the vector $\mathbf{v}$ defined in Eq. (11.11.7) will be emphasized in this section, the expression $T(t;\tau_1)$ in Eq. (11.6.2) for the total number of persons of type $\tau_1 \in \Upsilon$ in the population at time t will be written in the form $T(\tau_1, \mathbf{v})$. Then, the contact probabilities for potential extra-marital sexual partners may be written in the form,

$$\gamma_{EM}(\tau_1, \tau_2, \mathbf{v}) = \frac{T(\tau_2, \mathbf{v})\alpha_{em}(\tau_1, \tau_2)}{\sum_{\tau \in \Upsilon} T(\tau, \mathbf{v})\alpha_{em}(\tau_1, \tau)} \,. \tag{11.12.1}$$

From now on, to simplify the notation, let

$$W(\tau_1, \mathbf{v}) = \sum_{\tau \in \Upsilon} T(\tau, \mathbf{v})\alpha_{em}(\tau_1, \tau) \tag{11.12.2}$$

for every $\tau_1 \in \Upsilon$. Given these definitions, the derivation of formulas for the elements of the Jacobian matrix for extra-martial sexual contacts runs parallel to that in Section 10.11.

Just as in Section 10.11, the function,

$$\eta_\theta(x,y) = \frac{xy2^{\frac{1}{\theta}}}{(x^\theta + y^\theta)^{\frac{1}{\theta}}} \tag{11.12.3}$$

defined for $\theta > 0$, $x > 0$, and $y > 0$ will be used as an approximation to the function $\min(x,y)$ for θ large. For the case of extra-marital sexual contacts, the variable x in this function has the form,

$$x = \frac{T(\tau_1,\mathbf{v})T(\tau_2,\mathbf{v})\alpha_{em}(\tau_1,\tau_2)}{W(\tau_1,\mathbf{v})}\,, \tag{11.12.4}$$

and the variable y has the form,

$$y = \frac{T(\tau_2,\mathbf{v})T(\tau_1,\mathbf{v})\alpha_{em}(\tau_2,\tau_1)}{W(\tau_2,\mathbf{v})}\,. \tag{11.12.5}$$

Moreover, because the symmetry condition

$$\alpha_{em}(\tau_1,\tau_2) = \alpha_{em}(\tau_2,\tau_1) \tag{11.12.6}$$

holds for all pairs (τ_1,τ_2), the numerators in Eqs. (11.12.4) and (11.12.5) are equal.

Therefore, as in Section 10.11, it will be expedient to consider a function of the form,

$$\eta_\theta\left(\frac{x}{y_1},\frac{x}{y_2}\right) = \frac{x}{y_1}\left(\frac{2}{1+\left(\frac{y_2}{y_1}\right)^\theta}\right)^{\frac{1}{\theta}}\,, \tag{11.12.7}$$

where x is defined as the common numerator in Eqs. (11.12.4) and (11.12.5), $y_1 = W(\tau_1,\mathbf{v})$, and $y_2 = W(\tau_2,\mathbf{v})$. In order to express the results in a succinct notation, it will also be helpful to define a function

$f_\theta(\tau_1, \tau_2, \mathbf{v})$ by:

$$f_\theta(\tau_1, \tau_2, \mathbf{v}) = \left(\frac{2}{1 + \left(\frac{W(\tau_2, \mathbf{v})}{W(\tau_1, \mathbf{v})} \right)^\theta} \right)^{\frac{1}{\theta}} . \tag{11.12.8}$$

Then, in the notation of this section, if $\tau_1 \neq \tau_2$, then the formula for $N_{EM}(t; \tau_1, \tau_2)$ in Eq. (11.6.4) becomes:

$$N_{EM}(\tau_1, \tau_2, \mathbf{v}) = \frac{T(\tau_1, \mathbf{v})T(\tau_2, \mathbf{v})\alpha_{em}(\tau_1, \tau_2)}{W(\tau_1, \mathbf{v})} f_\theta(\tau_1, \tau_2, \mathbf{v}) , \tag{11.12.9}$$

but, if $\tau_1 = \tau_2$, then

$$N_{EM}(\tau_1, \tau_1, \mathbf{v}) = \frac{(T(\tau_1, \mathbf{v}))^2}{2W(\tau_1, \mathbf{v})} . \tag{11.12.10}$$

From Eqs. (11.12.9) and (11.12.10), it can be seen that the conditional probability $\rho_{EM}(t; \tau_1, \tau_2)$ that a susceptible of type τ_1 has extra-marital sexual contact with a person of type τ_2 during any time interval $(t, t+h]$ in the notation of this section has the form,

$$\rho_{EM}(t; \tau_1, \tau_2) = \frac{2T(\tau_2, \mathbf{v})\alpha_{em}(\tau_1, \tau_2) f_\theta(\tau_1, \tau_2, \mathbf{v})}{W^*(\tau_1, \mathbf{v})} , \tag{11.12.11}$$

where

$$W^*(\tau_1, \mathbf{v}) = T(\tau_1, \mathbf{v}) + 2 \sum_{\tau \neq \tau_1} T(\tau, \mathbf{v})\alpha_{em}(\tau_1, \tau) f_\theta(\tau_1, \tau, \mathbf{v}) . \tag{11.12.12}$$

Consequently, for the structure under consideration, the conditional probability $Q_{par}(t; \tau_1)$ (see Eq. (11.6.6)), that a susceptible person of type $\tau_1 \in \Upsilon_S$ becomes infected during any time interval has the form,

$$Q_{par}(\tau_1, \mathbf{v}) = \frac{2 \sum_{\tau \in \Upsilon_I} T(\tau, \mathbf{v})\alpha_{em}(\tau_1, \tau) f_\theta(\tau_1, \tau, \mathbf{v}) q_{em}(\tau)}{W^*(\tau_1, \mathbf{v})} . \tag{11.12.13}$$

By assumption, this formula holds for susceptibles who are members of the singles population as well as for susceptibles who are members of couples. Moreover, to emphasize that the probability of infection per contact for extra-marital sexual partners may differ from that of marital partners, the subscript em has been attached to $q(\tau)$ in Eq. (11.12.13).

A first step in completing the description of the Jacobian matrix $\mathbf{J}_{EM}(\mathbf{v})$ in Eq. (11.11.9) for extra-marital sexual contacts is to express the components of the vector $\mathbf{v}$ in Eq. (11.11.7) in a more explicit form, taking into account the ordering of the elements of the vector $\mathbf{v}$ used in previous sections. In the notation of this section, the vector $\mathbf{v}_s$ of dimension $m(n+1) \times 1$ for singles has the form,

$$\mathbf{v}_s = (x(\tau) \mid \tau \in \Upsilon_s = \mathfrak{S}_{s2}) \ , \tag{11.12.14}$$

where $x(\tau)$ denotes the "number" of single persons of type τ in the population at some time and the elements are arranged according to a lexicographic ordering.

As in Section 11.4 (see Eq. (11.4.3)), let the symbol $A(j_1, j_2)$ be the subset of couple types such that the left-hand partner belongs to behavioral class j_1 and the right-hand partner belongs to class j_2. For each pair (j_1, j_2), this set contains $(n+1)^2$ types of couples and the collection of these subsets as the pair (j_1, j_2) varies over all possible m^2 combinations is a partition of the set $\mathfrak{S}_{s2}$ of couple types (see Eq. (11.4.5)). For each pair (j_1, j_2), let

$$\mathbf{v}_c(j_1, j_2) = (z(\varkappa) \mid \varkappa \in A(j_1, j_2)) \tag{11.12.15}$$

denote a vector of couple numbers of the indicated types of dimension $(n+1)^2 \times 1$. Then, the $m^2(n+1)^2 \times 1$ vector $\mathbf{v}_c$ for couples may be represented the partitioned form,

$$\mathbf{v}_c = (\mathbf{v}_c(j_1, j_2) \mid j_1, j_2 = 0, 1, 2, \cdots, m) \ , \tag{11.12.16}$$

whose order conforms to that used in describing the matrix of latent risk for couples set forth in Eq. (11.4.7) for the case $m = 2$.

Given the ordering of the elements of the vector $\mathbf{v}$ just described, the Jacobian matrix for extra-marital sexual contacts may be represented in the partitioned form,

$$\mathbf{J}_{EM}(\mathbf{v}) = \begin{bmatrix} \dfrac{\partial \mathbf{W}_{ss}\mathbf{v}_s}{\partial \mathbf{v}_s} & \dfrac{\partial \mathbf{W}_{ss}\mathbf{v}_s}{\partial \mathbf{v}_c} \\ \dfrac{\partial \mathbf{W}_{cc}\mathbf{v}_c}{\partial \mathbf{v}_s} & \dfrac{\partial \mathbf{W}_{cc}\mathbf{v}_c}{\partial \mathbf{v}_c} \end{bmatrix} . \tag{11.12.17}$$

As the notation suggests,

$$\mathbf{J}_{ss}(\mathbf{v}) = \frac{\partial \mathbf{W}_{ss}\mathbf{v}_s}{\partial \mathbf{v}_s} \tag{11.12.18}$$

is a $m(n+1) \times m(n+1)$ matrix of partial derivatives, and

$$\mathbf{J}_{sc}(\mathbf{v}) = \frac{\partial \mathbf{W}_{ss}\mathbf{v}_s}{\partial \mathbf{v}_c} \tag{11.12.19}$$

is a $m(n+1) \times m^2(n+1)^2$ matrix of partial derivatives. Similarly, the sub-matrix,

$$\mathbf{J}_{cs}(\mathbf{v}) = \frac{\partial \mathbf{W}_{cc}\mathbf{v}_c}{\partial \mathbf{v}_s} \tag{11.12.20}$$

has dimensions $m^2(n+1)^2 \times m(n+1)$, and the sub-matrix,

$$\mathbf{J}_{cs}(\mathbf{v}) = \frac{\partial \mathbf{W}_{cc}\mathbf{v}_c}{\partial \mathbf{v}_c} \tag{11.12.21}$$

has dimensions $m^2(n+1)^2 \times m^2(n+1)^2$.

As a first step toward a general description of the structure of the Jacobian matrix $\mathbf{J}_{EM}(\widehat{\mathbf{v}})$ evaluated at a stationary vector $\widehat{\mathbf{v}}$ for a population of no infectives to expedite the writing of software, it will be helpful to consider the simplest case; namely, the case of $m = 1$ behavioral class and $n = 1$ stage of disease. In this case, there are two types of singles, $\tau_1 = 0$ and $\tau_2 = 1$, and four types of couples, $\varkappa_1 = (0,0)$, $\varkappa_2 = (0,1)$, $\varkappa_3 = (1,0)$ and $\varkappa_4 = (1,1)$.

Furthermore, the matrix $\mathbf{W}_{ss}$ has the simple form,

$$\mathbf{W}_{ss} = \begin{bmatrix} -\lambda Q_{par}(\tau_1, \mathbf{v}) & 0 \\ \lambda Q_{par}(\tau_1, \mathbf{v}) & 0 \end{bmatrix}. \tag{11.12.22}$$

Therefore, it follows that:

$$\mathbf{W}_{ss}\mathbf{v}_s = \begin{pmatrix} -x(0)\lambda Q_{par}(\tau_1, \mathbf{v}) \\ x(0)\lambda Q_{par}(\tau_1, \mathbf{v}) \end{pmatrix}. \tag{11.12.23}$$

It will also be helpful to observe that in this simple case,

$$Q_{par}(\tau_1, \mathbf{v}) = \frac{2T(\tau_2, \mathbf{v})\alpha_{em}(\tau_1, \tau_2) f_\theta(\tau_1, \tau_2, \mathbf{v}) q_{em}(\tau_2)}{W^*(\tau_1, \mathbf{v})}. \tag{11.12.24}$$

Let $\mathbf{J}_{ss}(\widehat{\mathbf{v}})$ denote the 2×2 Jacobian matrix in Eq. (11.12.18) evaluated at a stationary vector $\widehat{\mathbf{v}}$. To derive the formulas for this matrix from Eq. (11.12.23), it will be necessary to derive formulas for the partial derivatives of the function $x(0)\lambda Q_{par}(\tau_1, \mathbf{v})$ with respect to the elements of the vector

$$\mathbf{v}_s = \begin{pmatrix} x(0) \\ x(1) \end{pmatrix}, \tag{11.12.25}$$

and then evaluate them at a stationary vector of the form,

$$\widehat{\mathbf{v}} = \begin{pmatrix} \widehat{\mathbf{v}}_s \\ \widehat{\mathbf{v}}_c \end{pmatrix} \tag{11.12.26}$$

where

$$\widehat{\mathbf{v}}_s = \begin{pmatrix} \widehat{x}(0) \\ 0 \end{pmatrix} \tag{11.12.27}$$

and

$$\widehat{\mathbf{v}}_c = \begin{pmatrix} \widehat{z}(0,0) \\ 0 \\ 0 \\ 0 \end{pmatrix}. \tag{11.12.28}$$

Similarly, let $\mathbf{J}_{sc}(\widehat{\mathbf{v}})$ be the 2×4 Jacobian matrix defined in Eq. (11.12.19) and evaluated at a stationary vector $\widehat{\mathbf{v}}$. Then, to derive formulas for the elements of this matrix, one must take partial derivatives of the function $x(0)\lambda Q_{par}(\tau_1, \mathbf{v})$ with respect to the elements of the vector,

$$\mathbf{v}_c = \begin{pmatrix} z(0,0) \\ z(0,1) \\ z(1,0) \\ z(1,1) \end{pmatrix}. \tag{11.12.29}$$

A basic observation that will be used repeatedly in the derivation of formulas for these partial derivatives is that the function $T(\tau_2, \mathbf{v})$ in Eq. (11.12.24) has the property:

$$T(\tau_2, \widehat{\mathbf{v}}){=}0 \tag{11.12.30}$$

for every stationary vector $\widehat{\mathbf{v}}$. Another key observation is that the function $T(\tau_2, \mathbf{v})$ is linear in the elements of the vector $\mathbf{v}$ (see Eq. (11.6.2)). For example, in the notation of this section, this function has the explicit form:

$$T(\tau_2, \mathbf{v}) = x(1) + z(1,0) + z(0,1) + 2z(1,1) \,. \tag{11.12.31}$$

By using Eqs. (11.12.30) and (11.12.31), it can be seen by inspection that a constant defined by:

$$k(\tau_1, \tau_2) = \frac{\lambda 2\alpha_{em}(\tau_1, \tau_2) f_\theta(\tau_1, \tau_2, \widehat{\mathbf{v}}) q_{em}(\tau_2)}{W^*(\tau_1, \widehat{\mathbf{v}})} \tag{11.12.32}$$

arises in all partial derivatives of the function $x(0)\lambda Q_{par}(\tau_1, \mathbf{v})$ evaluated at $\widehat{\mathbf{v}}$. Thus, it can be shown that the 2×2 matrix $\mathbf{J}_{ss}(\widehat{\mathbf{v}})$ has the form,

$$\mathbf{J}_{ss}(\widehat{\mathbf{v}}) = \begin{bmatrix} 0 & -\widehat{x}(0)k(\tau_1, \tau_2) \\ 0 & \widehat{x}(0)k(\tau_1, \tau_2) \end{bmatrix} , \tag{11.12.33}$$

and the 2×4 matrix $\mathbf{J}_{sc}(\widehat{\mathbf{v}})$ has the form,

$$\mathbf{J}_{sc}(\widehat{\mathbf{v}}) = \begin{bmatrix} 0 & -\widehat{x}(0)k(\tau_1, \tau_2) & -\widehat{x}(0)k(\tau_1, \tau_2) & -2\widehat{x}(0)k(\tau_1, \tau_2) \\ 0 & \widehat{x}(0)k(\tau_1, \tau_2) & \widehat{x}(0)k(\tau_1, \tau_2) & 2\widehat{x}(0)k(\tau_1, \tau_2) \end{bmatrix} . \tag{11.12.34}$$

When the set of couple types is arranged in lexicographical order, then in the notation of this section it can be shown that the transpose of the 4×4 matrix $\mathbf{W}_{cc}$ has the form,

$$\begin{bmatrix} -2\lambda Q_{par}(\tau_1, \mathbf{v}) & \lambda Q_{par}(\tau_1, \mathbf{v}) & \lambda Q_{par}(\tau_1, \mathbf{v}) & 0 \\ 0 & -\lambda Q_{par}(\tau_1, \mathbf{v}) & 0 & \lambda Q_{par}(\tau_1, \mathbf{v}) \\ 0 & 0 & -\lambda Q_{par}(\tau_1, \mathbf{v}) & \lambda Q_{par}(\tau_1, \mathbf{v}) \\ 0 & 0 & 0 & 0 \end{bmatrix} . \tag{11.12.35}$$

Therefore, it follows that the column vector, from which formulas for the elements of the Jacobian matrices in $\mathbf{J}_{cs}(\mathbf{v})$ and $\mathbf{J}_{cc}(\mathbf{v})$ in Eqs. (11.12.20) and (11.12.21) may be derived, has the form,

$$\mathbf{W}_{cc}\mathbf{v}_c = \begin{pmatrix} -2z(0,0)\lambda Q_{par}(\tau_1, \mathbf{v}) \\ (z(0,0) - z(0,1))\lambda Q_{par}(\tau_1, \mathbf{v}) \\ (z(0,0) - z(1,0))\lambda Q_{par}(\tau_1, \mathbf{v}) \\ (z(0,1) + z(1,0))\lambda Q_{par}(\tau_1, \mathbf{v}) \end{pmatrix} . \tag{11.12.36}$$

Just as in deriving formulas for the elements of the matrices $\mathbf{J}_{ss}(\widehat{\mathbf{v}})$ and $\mathbf{J}_{sc}(\widehat{\mathbf{v}})$ for singles, Eqs. (11.12.3) and (11.12.31) play a basic role in deriving formulas for the elements of matrices $\mathbf{J}_{cs}(\widehat{\mathbf{v}})$ and $\mathbf{J}_{cc}(\widehat{\mathbf{v}})$. Thus, it can be shown that:

$$\mathbf{J}_{cs}(\widehat{\mathbf{v}}) = \begin{bmatrix} 0 & -2\widehat{z}(0,0)k(\tau_1,\tau_2) \\ 0 & \widehat{z}(0,0)k(\tau_1,\tau_2) \\ 0 & \widehat{z}(0,0)k(\tau_1,\tau_2) \\ 0 & 0 \end{bmatrix} . \tag{11.12.37}$$

To express the matrix $\mathbf{J}_{cc}(\widehat{\mathbf{v}})$ in a succinct notational form, it will be helpful to define a column vector $\mathbf{c}(\widehat{\mathbf{v}})$ by:

$$\mathbf{c}(\widehat{\mathbf{v}}) = \begin{pmatrix} -2\widehat{z}(0,0)k(\tau_1,\tau_2) \\ \widehat{z}(0,0)k(\tau_1,\tau_2) \\ \widehat{z}(0,0)k(\tau_1,\tau_2) \\ 0 \end{pmatrix} , \tag{11.12.38}$$

and let $\mathbf{0}_4$ denote a 4×1 vector of zeros. Then, the 4×4 matrix $\mathbf{J}_{cc}(\widehat{\mathbf{v}})$ may be represented in the partitioned form,

$$\mathbf{J}_{cc}(\widehat{\mathbf{v}}) = \begin{bmatrix} \mathbf{0}_4 & \mathbf{c}(\widehat{\mathbf{v}}) & \mathbf{c}(\widehat{\mathbf{v}}) & 2\mathbf{c}(\widehat{\mathbf{v}}) \end{bmatrix} . \tag{11.12.39}$$

Even though the simple case of $m = n = 1$ provides useful insights into the structure of the Jacobian matrix $\mathbf{J}_{EM}(\widehat{\mathbf{v}})$, it is not sufficient to gain insight into the structure of this matrix for more complex cases where $m \geq 2$ and $n \geq 2$. In the next section, the structure of the matrix $\mathbf{J}_{EM}(\widehat{\mathbf{v}})$ in more complex cases will be presented in a form that will be useful for writing software.

11.13 General Form of the Jacobian for Extra-Marital Contacts

As a aid to developing an overview for the general form of the Jacobian matrix for extra-marital sexual contacts, it will be helpful to illustrate the concepts for the simpler case of $m = 1$ behavioral classes and $n = 2$ stages of disease. For this case, the set of types for individuals is:

$$\Upsilon = \{\tau_1 = (0), \tau_2 = (1), \tau_3 = (2)\} \tag{11.13.1}$$

so that the set of infectious types is:

$$\Upsilon_I = \{\tau_2 = (1), \tau_3 = (2)\} \tag{11.13.2}$$

and the set Υ_S of susceptibles is $\Upsilon_S = \{\tau_1 = (0)\}$. To describe the set $\Upsilon_c = \mathfrak{S}_{c2}$ of nine types of couples, it will be helpful to partition it into three disjoint subsets according to the state of the left-hand partner. Thus, as in previous sections, for $k_1 = 0, 1, 2$, let the set

$$A(k_1) = \{(k_1, k_2) \mid k_2 = 0, 1, 2\} \tag{11.13.3}$$

denote the subset of couple types such that the left-hand partner is in state k_1. Then,

$$\Upsilon_c = \bigcup_{k_1=0}^{2} A(k_1)\,. \tag{11.13.4}$$

In this case, the matrix $\mathbf{W}_{ss}$ has the form,

$$\mathbf{W}_{ss} = \begin{bmatrix} -\lambda Q_{par}(\tau_1, \mathbf{v}) & 0 & 0 \\ \lambda Q_{par}(\tau_1, \mathbf{v}) & 0 & 0 \\ 0 & 0 & 0 \end{bmatrix}. \tag{11.13.5}$$

Therefore, the vector from which formulas for the elements of Jacobian matrices $\mathbf{J}_{ss}(\mathbf{v})$ and $\mathbf{J}_{sc}(\mathbf{v})$ may be derived has the form,

$$\mathbf{W}_{ss}\mathbf{v}_s = \begin{pmatrix} -x(0)\lambda Q_{par}(\tau_1, \mathbf{v}) \\ x(0)\lambda Q_{par}(\tau_1, \mathbf{v}) \\ 0 \end{pmatrix}. \tag{11.13.6}$$

It is easy to see that this form may be easily extended to more general cases $n > 2$.

For the case under consideration, it is helpful to represent the transpose of the 9×9 matrix $\mathbf{W}_{cc}$ for couple types in the partitioned form,

$$\mathbf{W}_{cc}' = \begin{bmatrix} \mathbf{W}_{cc}'(0,0) & \mathbf{W}_{cc}'(0,1) & \mathbf{0} \\ \mathbf{0} & \mathbf{W}_{cc}'(1,1) & \mathbf{0} \\ \mathbf{0} & \mathbf{0} & \mathbf{W}_{cc}'(2,2) \end{bmatrix}. \tag{11.13.7}$$

By way of explanation, the rows and columns of the 3×3 sub-matrix $\mathbf{W}_{cc}^{'}(0,0)$ are indexed by the elements of the set $A(0)$ of couple types; further, the rows and columns, respectively, of the 3×3 sub-matrix $\mathbf{W}_{cc}^{'}(0,1)$ are indexed by the sets of couple types $A(0)$ and $A(1)$. Similar statements hold for the other sub-matrices in Eq. (11.13.7).

The sub-matrices in the first row of the matrix in Eq. (11.13.7) have the explicit forms,

$$\mathbf{W}_{cc}^{'}(0,0) = \begin{bmatrix} -2\lambda Q_{par}(\tau_1,\mathbf{v}) & \lambda Q_{par}(\tau_1,\mathbf{v}) & 0 \\ 0 & -\lambda Q_{par}(\tau_1,\mathbf{v}) & 0 \\ 0 & 0 & -\lambda Q_{par}(\tau_1,\mathbf{v}) \end{bmatrix} \tag{11.13.8}$$

and

$$\mathbf{W}_{cc}^{'}(0,1) = \begin{bmatrix} \lambda Q_{par}(\tau_1,\mathbf{v}) & 0 & 0 \\ 0 & \lambda Q_{par}(\tau_1,\mathbf{v}) & 0 \\ 0 & 0 & \lambda Q_{par}(\tau_1,\mathbf{v}) \end{bmatrix}. \tag{11.13.9}$$

Furthermore, the other sub-matrices on the quasi-diagonal have the forms,

$$\mathbf{W}_{cc}^{'}(1,1) = \begin{bmatrix} -\lambda Q_{par}(\tau_1,\mathbf{v}) & \lambda Q_{par}(\tau_1,\mathbf{v}) & 0 \\ 0 & 0 & 0 \\ 0 & 0 & 0 \end{bmatrix} \tag{11.13.10}$$

and

$$\mathbf{W}_{cc}^{'}(2,2) = \begin{bmatrix} -\lambda Q_{par}(\tau_1,\mathbf{v}) & \lambda Q_{par}(\tau_1,\mathbf{v}) & 0 \\ 0 & 0 & 0 \\ 0 & 0 & 0 \end{bmatrix}. \tag{11.13.11}$$

To justify the elements in the matrix $\mathbf{W}_{cc}^{'}(0,0)$ in Eq. (11.13.8), observe that $\lambda Q_{par}(\tau_1,\mathbf{v})$, the element in the first row and second column, is the latent risk for the transition $(0,0) \to (0,1)$, indicating that the right-hand member of the couple type $(0,0)$ was infected during a small time interval. Similarly, the element $\lambda Q_{par}(\tau_1,\mathbf{v})$ on the principal diagonal of the matrix $\mathbf{W}_{cc}^{'}(0,1)$ in Eq. (11.13.9) is the common latent risk for transitions of the form $(0,0) \to (1,k_2)$ for $k_2 = 0,1,2$, indicating that the left-hand member of the couple type $(0,0)$ was infected during a small time interval. The negative elements on the principal diagonal of the matrix $\mathbf{W}'_{cc}(0,0)$ are the negative of the sum of the off-diagonal elements in each row. Finally, the sub-matrices $\mathbf{W}'_{cc}(1,1)$ and $\mathbf{W}'_{cc}(2,2)$ are concerned with latent risks for the transitions of the form $(k_1,0) \rightarrow (k_1,1)$ for $k_1 = 1,2$, indicating that the right-hand susceptible partner was infected during any small time interval. The 3×3 sub-matrices, denoted by $\mathbf{0}$ in Eq. (11.13.7), contain only zeros, because their elements do not contain latent risks for extra-marital contacts. From these results for the special case $n = 2$, it can be seen how the structure of the matrix $\mathbf{W}'_{cc}$ could be extended to the cases of $n > 2$ stages of disease.

As a first step in the derivation of the formulas for the vector $\mathbf{W}_{cc}\mathbf{v}_c$ from which the elements of the Jacobian matrices $\mathbf{J}_{cs}(\mathbf{v})$ and $\mathbf{J}_{cc}(\mathbf{v})$ for couples may be derived, it will be helpful to the define the 3×1 sub-vectors

$$\mathbf{v}_c(k_1) = \begin{pmatrix} z(k_1,0) \\ z(k_1,1) \\ z(k_1,2) \end{pmatrix}, \tag{11.13.12}$$

for $k_1 = 0,1,2$. Then, the 9×1 vector $\mathbf{v}_c$ may be represented in the partitioned form,

$$\mathbf{v}_c = \begin{pmatrix} \mathbf{v}_c(0) \\ \mathbf{v}_c(1) \\ \mathbf{v}_c(2) \end{pmatrix}. \tag{11.13.13}$$

Hence, the vector $\mathbf{W}_{cc}\mathbf{v}_c$ has the partitioned form

$$\mathbf{W}_{cc}\mathbf{v}_c = \begin{pmatrix} \mathbf{W}_{cc}(0,0)\mathbf{v}_c(0) \\ \mathbf{W}_{cc}(0,1)\mathbf{v}_c(0) + \mathbf{W}_{cc}(1,1)\mathbf{v}_c(1) \\ \mathbf{W}_{cc}(2,2)\mathbf{v}_c(2) \end{pmatrix}. \tag{11.13.14}$$

As a final step in the preparation for the derivation of formulas for the elements of the Jacobian matrices, it will be necessary to exhibit the elements of the sub-vectors in Eq. (11.13.14) in explicit form. Thus,

$$\mathbf{W}_{cc}(0,0)\mathbf{v}_c(0) = \begin{pmatrix} -2z(0,0)\lambda Q_{par}(\tau_1,\mathbf{v}) \\ (z(0,0) - z(0,1))\lambda Q_{par}(\tau_1,\mathbf{v}) \\ -z(0,2)\lambda Q_{par}(\tau_1,\mathbf{v}) \end{pmatrix}, \tag{11.13.15}$$

$$\mathbf{W}_{cc}(0,1)\mathbf{v}_c(0)+\mathbf{W}_{cc}(1,1)\mathbf{v}_c(1) = \begin{pmatrix} (z(0,0)-z(1,0))\lambda Q_{par}(\tau_1,\mathbf{v}) \\ (z(0,1)+z(1,0))\lambda Q_{par}(\tau_1,\mathbf{v}) \\ z(0,2)\lambda Q_{par}(\tau_1,\mathbf{v}) \end{pmatrix} \tag{11.13.16}$$

and

$$\mathbf{W}_{cc}(2,2)\mathbf{v}_c(2) = \begin{pmatrix} -z(0,2)\lambda Q_{par}(\tau_1,\mathbf{v}) \\ z(0,2)\lambda Q_{par}(\tau_1,\mathbf{v}) \\ 0 \end{pmatrix} . \tag{11.13.17}$$

Just as in Section 11.12, partial derivatives of the function $Q_{par}(\tau_1, \mathbf{v})$ will play a basic role in the derivation of formula for the elements of the Jacobian matrix $\mathbf{J}_{EM}(\widehat{\mathbf{v}})$ evaluated at a stationary vector $\widehat{\mathbf{v}}$ for the case where a population containing only susceptible types. It will, therefore, be useful to write this function in the form,

$$Q_{par}(\tau_1,\mathbf{v}) = \frac{2\sum_{\tau=1}^{2} T(\tau,\mathbf{v})\alpha_{em}(\tau_1,\tau)f_\theta(\tau_1,\tau,\mathbf{v})q_{em}(\tau)}{W^*(\tau_1,\mathbf{v})} \tag{11.13.18}$$

which is applicable to the case of $n = 2$ stages of disease with $m = 1$ behavioral class. To deduce general forms for vectors of partial derivatives evaluated at a stationary vector $\widehat{\mathbf{v}}$, it will be helpful to write the functions $T(\tau, \mathbf{v})$, $\tau = 1, 2$, in explicit forms. For the case under consideration, the explicit forms of these functions are:

$$T(1,\mathbf{v}) = x(1)+z(1,0)+z(1,1)+z(1,2)+z(0,1)+z(1,1)+z(2,1) , \tag{11.13.19}$$

and

$$T(2,\mathbf{v}) = x(2)+z(2,0)+z(2,1)+z(2,2)+z(0,2)+z(1,2)+z(2,2) . \tag{11.13.20}$$

Key observations to make at this point are that the term $z(1,1)$ occurs twice in $T(1,\mathbf{v})$, the term $z(2,2)$ occurs twice in $T(2,\mathbf{v})$, and each of the terms $z(1,2)$ and $z(2,1)$ occurs once in $T(1,\mathbf{v})$ and $T(2,\mathbf{v})$. Hence, the partial derivatives of $Q_{par}(\tau_1,\mathbf{v})$ with respect to these elements will be the sum of two terms one of which may be zero.

For $\tau = 1, 2$ let $k(\tau_1, \tau)$ denote the constant,

$$k(\tau_1,\tau) = \frac{\lambda 2\alpha_{em}(\tau_1,\tau)f_\theta(\tau_1,\tau,\widehat{\mathbf{v}})q_{em}(\tau)}{W^*(\tau_1,\widehat{\mathbf{v}})} . \tag{11.13.21}$$

Then, three 1×3 row vectors, $\mathbf{K}(0)$, $\mathbf{K}(1)$, and $\mathbf{K}(2)$, will play a basic role in enumerating the elements of the Jacobian matrices under consideration. They are defined as:

$$\mathbf{K}(0) = (0, k(\tau_1, 1), k(\tau_1, 2)) \ , \tag{11.13.22}$$

$$\mathbf{K}(1) = (k(\tau_1, 1), k(\tau_1, 1), k(\tau_1, 1)) \ , \tag{11.13.23}$$

$$\mathbf{K}(2) = (k(\tau_1, 2), k(\tau_1, 2), k(\tau_1, 2)) \ , \tag{11.13.24}$$

Using the properties discussed in connection with Eq. (11.12.13) in Section 11.12, and by taking partial derivatives in Eq. (11.13.18) with respect to the elements of the vector $\mathbf{v}_s$, it can be seen that the 3×3 Jacobian matrix $\mathbf{J}_{ss}(\widehat{\mathbf{v}})$ for this case has the partitioned form,

$$\mathbf{J}_{ss}(\widehat{\mathbf{v}}) = \begin{bmatrix} -\widehat{x}(0)\mathbf{K}(0) \\ \widehat{x}(0)\mathbf{K}(0) \\ \mathbf{0}_{1\times 3} \end{bmatrix} , \tag{11.13.25}$$

where $\mathbf{0}_{1\times 3}$ is a 1×3 vector of zeros. To describe the 3×9 Jacobian matrix $\mathbf{J}_{sc}(\widehat{\mathbf{v}})$ succinctly, it will be helpful to define a 1×9 vector $\mathbf{L}$ in the partitioned form,

$$\mathbf{L} = (\mathbf{K}(0), \mathbf{K}(1) + \mathbf{K}(0), \mathbf{K}(2) + \mathbf{K}(0)) \ . \tag{11.13.26}$$

This vector arises because every partial derivative of Eq. (11.13.18) with respect to an element of the vector $\mathbf{v}_c$ is a sum of two terms. With this in mind, it can be seen that the 3×9 Jacobian matrix $\mathbf{J}_{sc}(\widehat{\mathbf{v}})$ has the partitioned form,

$$\mathbf{J}_{sc}(\widehat{\mathbf{v}}) = \begin{bmatrix} -\widehat{x}(0)\mathbf{L} \\ \widehat{x}(0)\mathbf{L} \\ \mathbf{0}_{1\times 9} \end{bmatrix} , \tag{11.13.27}$$

where $\mathbf{0}_{1\times 9}$ is a 1×9 vector of zeros.

From an inspection of the column vectors in Eqs. (11.13.15) through (11.13.17), it can be seen that it will be useful to represent the 9×3 Jacobian sub-matrix $\mathbf{J}_{cs}(\widehat{\mathbf{v}})$ in a form partitioned according to the state of the right-hand partner. For the case in which the right-hand partner is in state k_1, let $\mathbf{J}_{cs}(k_1, \widehat{\mathbf{v}})$ denote a 3×3 sub-matrix of $\mathbf{J}_{cs}(\widehat{\mathbf{v}})$.

Note that the sub-matrix $\mathbf{J}_{cs}(0, \widehat{\mathbf{v}})$ consists of partial derivatives of the elements of the vector in Eq. (11.13.15) with respect to the elements of the vector $\mathbf{v}_s$. Thus, the matrix $\mathbf{J}_{cs}(\widehat{\mathbf{v}})$ may be represented in the partitioned form,

$$\mathbf{J}_{cs}(\widehat{\mathbf{v}}) = \begin{bmatrix} \mathbf{J}_{cs}(0, \widehat{\mathbf{v}}) \\ \mathbf{J}_{cs}(1, \widehat{\mathbf{v}}) \\ \mathbf{J}_{cs}(2, \widehat{\mathbf{v}}) \end{bmatrix} . \tag{11.13.28}$$

Next observe that when the population contains only susceptibles, the only non-zero element in the sub-vector $\widehat{\mathbf{v}}_c(0)$ is $\widehat{z}(0,0)$ and the sub-vectors $\widehat{\mathbf{v}}_c(1)$ and $\widehat{\mathbf{v}}_c(2)$ are zero vectors. Therefore, from Eq. (11.13.15) it can be seen that the matrix $\mathbf{J}_{cs}(0, \widehat{\mathbf{v}})$ has the form,

$$\mathbf{J}_{cs}(0, \widehat{\mathbf{v}}) = \begin{bmatrix} -2\widehat{z}(0,0)\mathbf{K}(0) \\ \widehat{z}(0,0)\mathbf{K}(0) \\ \mathbf{0}_{1\times 3} \end{bmatrix} , \tag{11.13.29}$$

and, from Eq. (11.13.16), it can be seen that the sub-matrix $\mathbf{J}_{cs}(1, \widehat{\mathbf{v}})$ has the form,

$$\mathbf{J}_{cs}(1, \widehat{\mathbf{v}}) = \begin{bmatrix} \widehat{z}(0,0)\mathbf{K}(0) \\ \mathbf{0}_{1\times 3} \\ \mathbf{0}_{1\times 3} \end{bmatrix} . \tag{11.13.30}$$

It can be seen from Eq. (11.13.17) that the sub-matrix $\mathbf{J}_{cs}(2, \widehat{\mathbf{v}}) = \mathbf{0}_{3\times 3}$ is a 3×3 zero matrix.

The 9×9 sub-matrix $\mathbf{J}_{cc}(\widehat{\mathbf{v}})$ has a partitioned form similar to that in Eq. (11.13.28). Let $\mathbf{J}_{cc}(k_1, \widehat{\mathbf{v}})$ denote a 3×9 of partial derivatives with respect to the elements of the vector $\mathbf{v}_c$ evaluated at $\widehat{\mathbf{v}}$, when the left-hand partner is in state k_1. Then, the matrix $\mathbf{J}_{cc}(\widehat{\mathbf{v}})$ may be represented in the partitioned form,

$$\mathbf{J}_{cc}(\widehat{\mathbf{v}}) = \begin{bmatrix} \mathbf{J}_{cc}(0, \widehat{\mathbf{v}}) \\ \mathbf{J}_{cc}(1, \widehat{\mathbf{v}}) \\ \mathbf{J}_{cc}(2, \widehat{\mathbf{v}}) \end{bmatrix} . \tag{11.13.31}$$

Moreover, by an argument similar to that just outlined, it can be shown that:

$$\mathbf{J}_{cc}(0, \widehat{\mathbf{v}}) = \begin{bmatrix} -2\widehat{z}(0,0)\mathbf{L} \\ \widehat{z}(0,0)\mathbf{L} \\ \mathbf{0}_{1\times 9} \end{bmatrix} , \tag{11.13.32}$$

$$\mathbf{J}_{cc}(1, \widehat{\mathbf{v}}) = \begin{bmatrix} \widehat{z}(0,0)\mathbf{L} \\ \mathbf{0}_{1\times 9} \\ \mathbf{0}_{1\times 9} \end{bmatrix}, \tag{11.13.33}$$

and $\mathbf{J}_{cc}(2, \widehat{\mathbf{v}}) = \mathbf{0}_{3\times 9}$, a 3×9 zero matrix. It is easy to see how the scheme just discussed for the sub-Jacobian matrices $\mathbf{J}_{cs}(\widehat{\mathbf{v}})$ and $\mathbf{J}_{cc}(\widehat{\mathbf{v}})$ can be extended to cases of $m \geq 2$ behavior classes and $n \geq 2$ stages of disease.

To illustrate the principle that the patterns just outlined can be extended in a straightforward way, it will suffice to consider cases with $m = 2$ behavioral classes and $n \geq 2$ stages of disease. Functions similar to that in Eq. (11.13.21) will play a basic role in the computational formulas, but, in the general cases to be described, the parameter λ will be a function $\lambda(\tau_1)$, depending on the behavioral class to which a susceptible of type τ_1 belongs.

For the cases of $m = 2$ and $n \geq 2$, the set Υ of types of individuals may be partitioned into two disjoint sets according to membership in a behavioral class. For example, by definition,

$$\Upsilon(1) = \{(1, k) \mid k = 0, 1, 2, \cdots, n\} \tag{11.13.34}$$

is the set of all individuals who belong to behavioral class 1, and the set $\Upsilon(2)$ is defined similarly for behavioral class 2 For $j = 1, 2$, let

$$\mathbf{v}_s(j) = (x(\tau) \mid \tau \in \Upsilon(j)) \tag{11.13.35}$$

denote a $(n+1)\times 1$ vector of variables for singles. Then, the $2(n+1)\times 1$ vector for singles variables takes the partitioned form,

$$\mathbf{v}_s = \begin{pmatrix} \mathbf{v}_s(1) \\ \mathbf{v}_s(2) \end{pmatrix}. \tag{11.13.36}$$

Given this partitioned vector, it can be seen, after inspecting the matrix of latent risks $\mathbf{\Theta}_{s2}$ in Eq. (11.10.3), that the $2(n+1)\times 2(n+1)$ matrix $\mathbf{W}_{ss}$ for singles has the quasi-diagonal form,

$$\mathbf{W}_{ss} = \begin{bmatrix} \mathbf{W}_{ss}(1) & \mathbf{0} \\ \mathbf{0} & \mathbf{W}_{ss}(2) \end{bmatrix}, \tag{11.13.37}$$

where $\mathbf{W}_{ss}(1)$ is a $(n+1) \times (n+1)$ matrix for members of class 1 and the matrix $\mathbf{W}_{ss}(2)$ is defined similarly for members of behavioral class 2. The structure of the matrices on the quasi-diagonal would be an extension of that in Eq. (11.13.5) for cases of $n > 2$ types, but each would have a different λ-parameters. From the form of the matrix in Eq. (11.13.37), it can be seen that the vector $\mathbf{W}_{ss}\mathbf{v}_s$ from which the elements of the Jacobian matrix for singles may be derived has the partitioned form,

$$\mathbf{W}_{ss}\mathbf{v}_s = \begin{pmatrix} \mathbf{W}_{ss}(1)\mathbf{v}_s(1) \\ \mathbf{W}_{ss}(2)\mathbf{v}_s(2) \end{pmatrix} . \tag{11.13.38}$$

The next step in deducing the form of the Jacobian matrix for extra-marital sexual contacts is to exhibit an extended form of the vector of variables for couples in Eq. (11.13.12) for cases of $m = 2$ behavioral classes and $n > 2$ stages of disease. Just as in Eq. (11.4.3), for every couple type $\varkappa = (\tau_1 = (j_1, k_1), \tau_2 = (j_2, k_2))$, and for a fixed pair (j_1, j_2) of behavioral classes, let

$$A(j_1, j_2) = \{\varkappa = ((\tau_1, \tau_2) \mid k_1 = 0, 1, 2, \cdots, n;\ k_1 = 0, 1, 2, \cdots, n\} \tag{11.13.39}$$

denote a subset of couples types such that the pairs (k_1, k_2) are arranged in lexicographic order. Then, for every pair (j_1, j_2) let

$$\mathbf{v}_c(j_1, j_2) = (z(\varkappa) \mid \varkappa \in A(j_1, j_2)) \tag{11.13.40}$$

denote a $(n+1)^2 \times 1$ vector of couple variables. The $4(n+1)^2 \times 1$ vector $\mathbf{v}_c$ of variables for couples then has the partitioned form,

$$\mathbf{v}_c = \begin{pmatrix} \mathbf{v}_c(1,1) \\ \mathbf{v}_c(1,2) \\ \mathbf{v}_c(2,1) \\ \mathbf{v}_c(2,2) \end{pmatrix} . \tag{11.13.41}$$

From an inspection of the matrix $\mathbf{\Theta}_{c22}$ of latent risks for couples in Eq. (11.4.7), it can be seen that for each pair (j_1, j_2) there is a $(n+1)^2 \times (n+1)^2$ matrix $\mathbf{W}_{cc}(j_1, j_2)$, whose form is an extension of that in Eq. (11.13.7), but modified to accommodate possibly different

λ-parameters for the left- and right-hand partners. Furthermore, it follows that the $4(n+1)^2 \times 4(n+1)^2$ matrix $\mathbf{W}_{cc}$ for couples has the quasi-diagonal form,

$$\mathbf{W}_{cc} = \begin{bmatrix} \mathbf{W}_{cc}(1,1) & \mathbf{0} & \mathbf{0} & \mathbf{0} \\ \mathbf{0} & \mathbf{W}_{cc}(1,2) & \mathbf{0} & \mathbf{0} \\ \mathbf{0} & \mathbf{0} & \mathbf{W}_{cc}(2,1) & \mathbf{0} \\ \mathbf{0} & \mathbf{0} & \mathbf{0} & \mathbf{W}_{cc}(2,2) \end{bmatrix}. \tag{11.13.42}$$

Consequently, the vector from which the Jacobian matrix for couples may be derived has the partitioned form,

$$\mathbf{W}_{cc}\mathbf{v}_c = \begin{pmatrix} \mathbf{W}_{cc}(1,1)\mathbf{v}_c(1,1) \\ \mathbf{W}_{cc}(1,2)\mathbf{v}_c(1,2) \\ \mathbf{W}_{cc}(2,1)\mathbf{v}_c(2,1) \\ \mathbf{W}_{cc}(2,2)\mathbf{v}_c(2,2) \end{pmatrix}. \tag{11.13.43}$$

One may thus proceed as in Eqs. (11.13.31) through (11.13.33) to derive the sub-matrices $\mathbf{J}_{ss}(j_1, j_2; \widehat{\mathbf{v}})$ and $\mathbf{J}_{sc}(j_1, j_2; \widehat{\mathbf{v}})$ for each pair of behavioral classes (j_1, j_2) in the set $\{(j_1, j_2) \mid j_1 = 1, 2;\ j_2 = 1, 2\}$ of pairs.

In summary, for cases with $m = 2$ behavioral classes and $n \geq 1$ stages of disease, the Jacobian matrix $\mathbf{J}_{EM}(\widehat{\mathbf{v}})$ may be represented in the partitioned form,

$$\mathbf{J}_{EM}(\widehat{\mathbf{v}}) = \begin{bmatrix} \mathbf{J}_s(\widehat{\mathbf{v}}) \\ \mathbf{J}_c(\widehat{\mathbf{v}}) \end{bmatrix}, \tag{11.13.44}$$

where $\mathbf{J}_s(\widehat{\mathbf{v}})$ is the $2(n+1) \times (2(n+1) + 4(n+1)^2)$ matrix for singles, and $\mathbf{J}_c(\widehat{\mathbf{v}})$ is the $4(n+1)^2 \times (2(n+1) + 4(n+1)^2)$ matrix for couples. The two behavioral classes for singles are accommodated in the partitioned matrix,

$$\mathbf{J}_s(\widehat{\mathbf{v}}) = \begin{bmatrix} \mathbf{J}_{ss}(1, \widehat{\mathbf{v}}) & \mathbf{J}_{sc}(1, \widehat{\mathbf{v}}) \\ \mathbf{J}_{ss}(2, \widehat{\mathbf{v}}) & \mathbf{J}_{sc}(2, \widehat{\mathbf{v}}) \end{bmatrix}. \tag{11.13.45}$$

For this partitioned matrix, $\mathbf{J}_{ss}(1, \widehat{\mathbf{v}})$ is a $(n+1) \times (n+1)$ sub-matrix indexed for singles in behavioral class 1, whose construction is similar to that for Eq. (11.13.25). Similarly, $\mathbf{J}_{sc}(1, \widehat{\mathbf{v}})$ is a $(n+1) \times 4(n+1)^4$

sub-matrix indexed for singles in class 1, taking into account sexual contacts with members of couples, whose construction is similar to that for Eq. (11.13.27). The sub-matrices $\mathbf{J}_{ss}(2,\widehat{\mathbf{v}})$ and $\mathbf{J}_{sc}(2,\widehat{\mathbf{v}})$ have similar interpretations for singles in behavioral class 2.

The sub-matrix $\mathbf{J}_c(\widehat{\mathbf{v}})$ in Eq. (11.13.44) has the partitioned form,

$$\mathbf{J}_c(\widehat{\mathbf{v}}) = \begin{bmatrix} \mathbf{J}_c(1,1,\widehat{\mathbf{v}}) \\ \mathbf{J}_c(1,2,\widehat{\mathbf{v}}) \\ \mathbf{J}_c(2,1,\widehat{\mathbf{v}}) \\ \mathbf{J}_c(2,2,\widehat{\mathbf{v}}) \end{bmatrix}, \tag{11.13.46}$$

corresponding to the four pairs of behavioral classes when $m = 2$. Each of these sub-matrices in turn may be partitioned into two sub-matrices. For example, for the pair $(1,1)$, the partitioned matrix has the form,

$$\mathbf{J}_c(1,1,\widehat{\mathbf{v}}) = \left[\ \mathbf{J}_{cs}(1,1,\widehat{\mathbf{v}}) \quad \mathbf{J}_{cc}(1,1,\widehat{\mathbf{v}})\ \right]. \tag{11.13.47}$$

The $4(n+1)^2 \times (n+1)$ sub-matrix $\mathbf{J}_{cs}(1,1,\widehat{\mathbf{v}})$ may be constructed by a procedure similar to that in Eqs. (11.13.28) through (11.13.30), and the $4(n+1)^2 \times 4(n+1)^2$sub-matrix $\mathbf{J}_{cc}(1,1,\widehat{\mathbf{v}})$ may be constructed by following a procedure similar to that in Eqs. (11.13.31) through (11.13.33). These two remarks also apply to the remaining three sub-matrices in Eq. (11.13.46). This completes the outline of procedures for constructing the general form of the Jacobian matrix for extra-marital sexual contacts.

11.14 Jacobian Matrix for Couple Formation

As the first step towards deriving computational formulas for the elements of the Jacobian matrix $\mathbf{J}_{CF}(\mathbf{v})$ for couple formation, it will be helpful to set down explicit forms of the couple formation functions $N_{CF}(t;\tau_1,\tau_2)$ and $N_{CF}(t;\tau_1,\tau_1)$, as defined in Eq. (11.5.8) and (11.5.9) and which occur in the embedded differential equations. Because only members of the singles population are involved in couple formation, all formulas in this section will depend only on the vector,

$$\mathbf{v}_s = (x_\tau \mid \tau \in \Upsilon_s) \tag{11.14.1}$$

of variables for singles. To simplify the writing of formulas, it will be helpful to let

$$T_c(\tau_1, \mathbf{v}_s) = \sum_{\tau \in \Upsilon_s} x_\tau \alpha_c(\tau_1, \tau) \tag{11.14.2}$$

for every $\tau_1 \in \Upsilon_s$.

Then, in the notation of this section, the contact probability $\gamma_c(\tau_1, \tau_2)$ defined in Eq. (11.5.3) takes the form,

$$\gamma_c(\tau_1, \tau_2) = \frac{x_{\tau_2} \alpha_c(\tau_1, \tau_2)}{T_c(\tau_1, \mathbf{v}_s)} \tag{11.14.3}$$

so that the multinomial expectations become,

$$x_{\tau_1} \gamma_c(\tau_1, \tau_2) = \frac{x_{\tau_1} x_{\tau_2} \alpha_c(\tau_1, \tau_2)}{T_c(\tau_1, \mathbf{v}_s)} \,. \tag{11.14.4}$$

Just as for the case of extra-marital sexual contacts, because the symmetry condition,

$$\alpha_c(\tau_1, \tau_2) = \alpha_c(\tau_2, \tau_1) \tag{11.14.5}$$

holds for all pairs (τ_1, τ_2), the numerator in Eq. (11.14.4) remains unchanged if τ_1 and τ_2 are interchanged.

With these definitions and in the notation of this section, the couple formation functions for the embedded differential equations have the following forms. If $\tau_1 = \tau_2$, then, because $\alpha_c(\tau_1, \tau_1) = 1$ for all τ_1,

$$N_{CF}(\tau_1, \tau_1, \mathbf{v}_s) = \frac{x_{\tau_1}^2}{2T_c(\tau_1, \mathbf{v}_s)} \,. \tag{11.14.6}$$

But, if $\tau_1 \neq \tau_2$, then, by using the approximation to the min function in Eq. (11.12.3) for large θ, it can be shown that:

$$N_{CF}(\tau_1, \tau_2, \mathbf{v}_s) = x_{\tau_1} x_{\tau_2} \alpha_c(\tau_1, \tau_2) \left(\frac{2}{(T_c(\tau_1, \mathbf{v}_s))^\theta + (T_c(\tau_2, \mathbf{v}_s))^\theta} \right)^{\frac{1}{\theta}} \,. \tag{11.14.7}$$

From these formulas, one may deduce that many of the elements of the Jacobian matrix $\mathbf{J}_{CF}(\widehat{\mathbf{v}})$ evaluated at a stationary vector $\widehat{\mathbf{v}}$ for the case where the population contains only susceptibles will be zero. For example, it can be shown that:

$$\frac{\partial N_{CF}(\tau_1,\tau_1,\mathbf{v}_s)}{\partial x_{\tau_1}} = \frac{1}{2}x_{\tau_1}\left(\frac{x_{\tau_1}+2\sum_{\tau\neq\tau_1}x_\tau\alpha_c(\tau_1,\tau)}{(T_c(\tau_1,\mathbf{v}_s))^2}\right), \tag{11.14.8}$$

and, if $\tau_1 \neq \tau_2$, then

$$\frac{\partial N_{CF}(\tau_1,\tau_1,\mathbf{v}_s)}{\partial x_{\tau_2}} = -\frac{1}{2}x_{\tau_1}^2\left(\frac{\alpha_c(\tau_1,\tau_2)}{(T_c(\tau_1,\mathbf{v}_s))^2}\right). \tag{11.14.9}$$

From these formulas, it can be seen that if $\tau_1 \in \Upsilon_I$, the set of infectious types, then

$$\frac{\partial N_{CF}(\tau_1,\tau_1,\mathbf{v}_s)}{\partial x_\tau} = 0 \tag{11.14.10}$$

for all types $\tau \in \Upsilon_s$ when $\mathbf{v}_s = \widehat{\mathbf{v}}_s$. Furthermore, if $\tau_1 \in \Upsilon_S$, the set susceptible types, then it can be seen from Eqs. (11.14.8) and (11.14.9) that computer code could easily be written to evaluate these functions at the vector $\widehat{\mathbf{v}}_s$.

Turning to the case $\tau_1 \neq \tau_2$, it can be seen from Eq. (11.14.7), by using the product rule for differentiation, that any partial derivative of this function will be a sum of terms, and all these terms will have x_{τ_1}, x_{τ_2} or both as factors. Consequently, if $\tau_1 \in \Upsilon_I$ and $\tau_2 \in \Upsilon_I$ and $\tau_1 \neq \tau_2$, then, it can be seen that:

$$\frac{\partial N_{CF}(\tau_1,\tau_2,\mathbf{v}_s)}{\partial x_\tau} = 0 \tag{11.14.11}$$

for all types $\tau \in \Upsilon_s$ when $\mathbf{v}_s = \widehat{\mathbf{v}}_s$. From these observations, it follows that in deriving formulas for partial derivatives of the function in Eq. (11.14.7) evaluated at $\mathbf{v}_s = \widehat{\mathbf{v}}_s$, three cases must be considered; namely, the case $\tau_1 \in \Upsilon_S$ and $\tau_2 \in \Upsilon_S$, the case $\tau_1 \in \Upsilon_S$ and $\tau_2 \in \Upsilon_I$, and the case $\tau_1 \in \Upsilon_I$ and $\tau_2 \in \Upsilon_S$. The number of formulas for partial derivatives of the function in Eq. (11.14.7), going into the Jacobian matrix for which formulas are actually required, can further be reduced by observing that the symmetry condition,

$$N_{CF}(\tau_1,\tau_2,\mathbf{v}_s) = N_{CF}(\tau_2,\tau_1,\mathbf{v}_s) \tag{11.14.12}$$

holds for all pairs (τ_1, τ_2).

As can be seen from inspecting the function in Eq. (11.14.7), the simplest formulas for the partial derivatives will arise when only one member of the pair (τ_1, τ_2) is susceptible. For example, consider the case $\tau_1 \in \Upsilon_S$ and $\tau_2 \in \Upsilon_I$. Then, because any term contain x_{τ_2} will vanish when $x_{\tau_2} = \widehat{x}_{\tau_2} = 0$, it can be seen that:

$$\frac{\partial N_{CF}(\tau_1, \tau_2, \mathbf{v}_s)}{\partial x_\tau} = 0 \tag{11.14.13}$$

for all $\tau \neq \tau_2$, but

$$\frac{\partial N_{CF}(\tau_1, \tau_2, \mathbf{v}_s)}{\partial x_{\tau_2}} = \widehat{x}_{\tau_1} \alpha_c(\tau_1, \tau_2) \left(\frac{2}{(T_c(\tau_1, \widehat{\mathbf{v}}_s))^\theta + (T_c(\tau_2, \widehat{\mathbf{v}}_s))^\theta} \right)^{\frac{1}{\theta}}, \tag{11.14.14}$$

when $\mathbf{v}_s = \widehat{\mathbf{v}}_s$. An equivalent form of this function is:

$$\frac{\partial N_{CF}(\tau_1, \tau_2, \mathbf{v}_s)}{\partial x_{\tau_2}} = \frac{\widehat{x}_{\tau_1} \alpha_c(\tau_1, \tau_2)}{T_c(\tau_1, \widehat{\mathbf{v}}_s)} \left(\frac{2}{1 + \left(\frac{T_c(\tau_2, \widehat{\mathbf{v}}_s)}{T_c(\tau_1, \widehat{\mathbf{v}}_s)} \right)^\theta} \right)^{\frac{1}{\theta}}, \tag{11.14.15}$$

which may be useful if computer overflow is encountered when computing the denominator of Eq. (11.14.14) for large θ. Formulas for partial derivatives for the case $\tau_1 \in \Upsilon_I$ and $\tau_2 \in \Upsilon_S$ may be derived from the above formulas by interchanging τ_1 and τ_2.

The most complex formulas for partial derivatives arise for the case $\tau_1 \in \Upsilon_S$ and $\tau_2 \in \Upsilon_S$ in which both types τ_1 and τ_2 are susceptibles, but with the help of MAPLE it is relatively straightforward to deduce some general formulas for these partial derivatives. From an inspection of MAPLE output, it can be seen that a function of the form,

$$f(\tau_1, \tau_2, \widehat{\mathbf{v}}_s) = \frac{1}{T_c(\tau_1, \widehat{\mathbf{v}}_s)} \left(\frac{2}{1 + \left(\frac{T_c(\tau_2, \widehat{\mathbf{v}}_s)}{T_c(\tau_1, \widehat{\mathbf{v}}_s)} \right)^\theta} \right)^{\frac{1}{\theta}} \tag{11.14.16}$$

arises as a factor in all these partial derivatives, but the other factors will depend on differentiation with respect to a particular the element in the vector $\mathbf{v}_s$.

In what follows, all formulas were derived using MAPLE, and then evaluated at the point $\mathbf{v}_s = \widehat{\mathbf{v}}_s$. For example, at the point $\mathbf{v}_s = \widehat{\mathbf{v}}_s$ it can be shown with the help of MAPLE that:

$$\frac{\partial N_{CF}(\tau_1,\tau_2,\mathbf{v}_s)}{\partial x_{\tau_1}} = -\widehat{x}_{\tau_2}\alpha_c(\tau_1,\tau_2)f_\theta(\tau_1,\tau_2,\widehat{\mathbf{v}}_s)g_{x_{\tau_1}}(\tau_1,\tau_2,\widehat{\mathbf{v}}_s)\ , \tag{11.14.17}$$

where

$$g_{x_{\tau_1}}(\tau_1,\tau_2,\widehat{\mathbf{v}}_s) = \frac{1}{T_c(\tau_1,\widehat{\mathbf{v}}_s)}\times$$

$$\left(\frac{(\widehat{x}_{\tau_1} - (T_c(\tau_1,\widehat{\mathbf{v}}_s)) + \left(\left(\frac{T_c(\tau_2,\widehat{\mathbf{v}}_s)}{T_c(\tau_1,\widehat{\mathbf{v}}_s)}\right)^{\theta-1}\right)(\widehat{x}_{\tau_1}\alpha_c(\tau_2,\tau_1) - (T_c(\tau_2,\widehat{\mathbf{v}}_s))}{1+\left(\frac{T_c(\tau_2,\widehat{\mathbf{v}}_s)}{T_c(\tau_1,\widehat{\mathbf{v}}_s)}\right)^{\theta}}\right) \tag{11.14.18}$$

by definition. Similarly, it can be shown that:

$$\frac{\partial N_{CF}(\tau_1,\tau_2,\mathbf{v}_s)}{\partial x_{\tau_2}} = -\widehat{x}_{\tau_1}\alpha_c(\tau_1,\tau_2)f_\theta(\tau_1,\tau_2,\widehat{\mathbf{v}}_s)g_{x_{\tau_2}}(\tau_1,\tau_2,\widehat{\mathbf{v}}_s)\ , \tag{11.14.19}$$

where

$$g_{x_{\tau_2}}(\tau_1,\tau_2,\widehat{\mathbf{v}}_s) = \frac{1}{T_c(\tau_1,\widehat{\mathbf{v}}_s)}\times$$

$$\left(\frac{(\widehat{x}_{\tau_2}\alpha_c(\tau_1,\tau_2) - (T_c(\tau_1,\widehat{\mathbf{v}}_s)) + \left(\left(\frac{T_c(\tau_2,\widehat{\mathbf{v}}_s)}{T_c(\tau_1,\widehat{\mathbf{v}}_s)}\right)^{\theta-1}\right)(\widehat{x}_{\tau_2} - (T_c(\tau_2,\widehat{\mathbf{v}}_s))}{1+\left(\frac{T_c(\tau_2,\widehat{\mathbf{v}}_s)}{T_c(\tau_1,\widehat{\mathbf{v}}_s)}\right)^{\theta}}\right) \tag{11.14.20}$$

by definition. Finally, if $\tau \neq \tau_1$ and $\tau \neq \tau_2$, then

$$\frac{\partial N_{CF}(\tau_1,\tau_2,\mathbf{v}_s)}{\partial x_{\tau}} = -\widehat{x}_{\tau_1}\widehat{x}_{\tau_2}\alpha_c(\tau_1,\tau_2)f_\theta(\tau_1,\tau_2,\widehat{\mathbf{v}}_s)g_{x\tau}(\tau_1,\tau_2,\widehat{\mathbf{v}}_s)\ , \tag{11.14.21}$$

where

$$g_{x\mathcal{T}}(\tau_1,\tau_2,\widehat{\mathbf{v}}_s) = \frac{1}{T_c(\tau_1,\widehat{\mathbf{v}}_s)}\left(\frac{\alpha_c(\tau_1,\mathcal{T}) + \left(\left(\frac{T_c(\tau_2,\widehat{\mathbf{v}}_s)}{T_c(\tau_1,\widehat{\mathbf{v}}_s)}\right)^{\theta-1}\right)\alpha_c(\tau_2.\mathcal{T})}{1+\left(\frac{T_c(\tau_2,\widehat{\mathbf{v}}_s)}{T_c(\tau_1,\widehat{\mathbf{v}}_s)}\right)^{\theta}}\right) \tag{11.14.22}$$

by definition

Having classified the partial derivatives that arise in deriving computational formulas for the elements of the Jacobian matrix for couple formation, the next step in developing an overview of their structure is to consider special cases with a view towards the goal of describing a general form of the matrix suitable for the writing of computer code for cases in which $m = 2$ and $n \geq 2$. The simplest case is that of $m = 1$ behavioral class and $n = 1$ stage of disease, where the set of single types is:

$$\Upsilon_s = \{\tau_1 = (0), \tau_2 = (1)\} \ , \tag{11.14.23}$$

the set of couple types is:

$$\Upsilon_c = \{(0,0),(0,1),(1,0),(1,1)\} \ , \tag{11.14.24}$$

and the vector $\widehat{\mathbf{v}}_s^{'} = (\widehat{x}_{\tau_1}, 0)$. In reference to Eq. (11.11.16), the 6×6 Jacobian matrix $\mathbf{J}_{CF}(\widehat{\mathbf{v}}_s)$ for this case evaluated at the vector $\widehat{\mathbf{v}}_s$ has the partitioned form,

$$\mathbf{J}_{CF}(\widehat{\mathbf{v}}_s) = \begin{bmatrix} \mathbf{J}_{SCF}(\widehat{\mathbf{v}}_s) \\ \mathbf{J}_{CCF}(\widehat{\mathbf{v}}_s) \end{bmatrix} \ , \tag{11.14.25}$$

where each of the sub-matrices also have partitioned forms.

For the 2×6 sub-matrix $\mathbf{J}_{SCF}(\widehat{\mathbf{v}}_s)$, this partitioned form is:

$$\mathbf{J}_{SCF}(\widehat{\mathbf{v}}_s) = \begin{bmatrix} \mathbf{J}_{SCF}(s,s,\widehat{\mathbf{v}}_s) & \mathbf{J}_{SCF}(s,c,\widehat{\mathbf{v}}_s) \end{bmatrix} \ , \tag{11.14.26}$$

where $\mathbf{J}_{SCF}(s,s,\widehat{\mathbf{v}}_s)$ is a 2×2 matrix, whose rows and columns are indexed by the set Υ_s, and $\mathbf{J}_{SCF}(s,c,\widehat{\mathbf{v}}_s)$ is a 2×4 matrix, whose rows and columns are indexed, respectively, by the sets Υ_s and Υ_c. Because the functions $N_{CF}(\tau_1,\tau_2,\mathbf{v}_s)$ do not depend on the vector $\mathbf{v}_c$ of variables for couples,

$$\mathbf{J}_{SCF}(s,c,\widehat{\mathbf{v}}_s) = \mathbf{0}_{2\times 4} \ , \tag{11.14.27}$$

where $\mathbf{0}_{2\times4}$ is a 2×4 zero matrix. Similarly, the 4×6 matrix $\mathbf{J}_{CCF}(\widehat{\mathbf{v}}_s)$ has the partitioned form,

$$\mathbf{J}_{CCF}(\widehat{\mathbf{v}}_s) = \left[\ \mathbf{J}_{CCF}(c,s,\widehat{\mathbf{v}}_s)\ \ \mathbf{J}_{CCF}(c,c,\widehat{\mathbf{v}}_s)\ \right] . \tag{11.14.28}$$

Just as in Eq. (11.14.27),

$$\mathbf{J}_{CCF}(c,c,\widehat{\mathbf{v}}_s) = \mathbf{0}_{4\times4} , \tag{11.14.29}$$

where $\mathbf{0}_{4\times4}$ is a 4×4 zero matrix, and $\mathbf{J}_{CCF}(c,s,\widehat{\mathbf{v}}_s)$ is a 4×2 matrix. Therefore, because the matrices in Eqs. (11.14.27) and (11.14.29) will be zero matrices for all $m \geq 1$ and $n \geq 1$, the problem of finding computational formulas for the elements of the Jacobian matrix for couple formation reduces to that of finding formulas for the elements of the sub-matrices $\mathbf{J}_{SCF}(s,s,\widehat{\mathbf{v}}_s)$ and $\mathbf{J}_{CCF}(c,s,\widehat{\mathbf{v}}_s)$. With reference to Eqs. (11.11.14) and (11.11.15), it will be assumed in what follows that $\rho(\tau_1,\tau_2) = \rho$, a positive constant, for all couple types (τ_1,τ_2).

With respect to the sub-matrix $\mathbf{J}_{CCF}(c,s,\widehat{\mathbf{v}}_s)$, it can be seen from Eqs. (11.14.7) and (11.14.8) that:

$$\frac{\partial N_{CF}(\tau_1,\tau_1,\widehat{\mathbf{v}}_s)}{\partial x_{\tau_1}} = \frac{1}{2} , \tag{11.14.30}$$

and

$$\frac{\partial N_{CF}(\tau_1,\tau_1,\widehat{\mathbf{v}}_s)}{\partial x_{\tau_2}} = -\frac{\alpha_c(\tau_1,\tau_2)}{2} . \tag{11.14.31}$$

For the case $\tau_1 \neq \tau_2$, the formula in Eq. (11.14.15) reduces to:

$$\frac{\partial N_{CF}(\tau_1,\tau_2,\widehat{\mathbf{v}}_s)}{\partial x_{\tau_2}} = \alpha_c(\tau_1,\tau_2) f^*(\tau_1,\tau_2,\widehat{\mathbf{v}}_s) , \tag{11.14.32}$$

where in this special case

$$f^*(\tau_1,\tau_2,\widehat{\mathbf{v}}_s) = \left(\frac{2}{1+(\alpha_c(\tau_1,\tau_2))^\theta}\right)^{\frac{1}{\theta}} . \tag{11.14.33}$$

One thus reaches the conclusion that for the case under consideration, the matrix $\mathbf{J}_{CCF}(c,s,\widehat{\mathbf{v}}_s)$ has the explicit form,

$$\mathbf{J}_{CCF}(c,s,\widehat{\mathbf{v}}_s) = \begin{bmatrix} \frac{\rho}{2} & -\frac{1}{2}\alpha_c(\tau_1,\tau_2)\rho \\ 0 & \alpha_c(\tau_1,\tau_2)\rho f^*(\tau_1,\tau_2,\widehat{\mathbf{v}}_s) \\ 0 & \alpha_c(\tau_1,\tau_2)\rho f^*(\tau_1,\tau_2,\widehat{\mathbf{v}}_s) \\ 0 & 0 \end{bmatrix} . \tag{11.14.34}$$

The elements of the 2×2 matrix $\mathbf{J}_{SCF}(s, s, \widehat{\mathbf{v}}_s)$, may be derived from those of $\mathbf{J}_{CCF}(c, s, \widehat{\mathbf{v}}_s)$ by using the formulas in Eq. (11.11.15). For the case under consideration, these formulas become:

$$T_{CF}(\tau_1, \mathbf{v}) = 2N_{CF}(\tau_1, \tau_1, \mathbf{v})\rho + N_{CF}(\tau_1, \tau_2, \mathbf{v})\rho + N_{CF}(\tau_2, \tau_1, \mathbf{v})\rho \,. \tag{11.14.35}$$

and

$$T_{CF}(\tau_2, \mathbf{v}) = N_{CF}(\tau_2, \tau_1, \mathbf{v})\rho + 2N_{CF}(\tau_2, \tau_2, \mathbf{v})\rho + N_{CF}(\tau_1, \tau_2, \mathbf{v})\rho \,. \tag{11.14.36}$$

By taking partial derivatives of these functions, evaluating them at the vector $\widehat{\mathbf{v}}_s$,and multiplying by -1 (see Eq. (11.11.13)), it can be shown that the matrix $\mathbf{J}_{SCF}(s, s, \widehat{\mathbf{v}}_s)$ has the explicit form,

$$\mathbf{J}_{SCF}(s, s, \widehat{\mathbf{v}}_s) = \begin{bmatrix} -\rho & \alpha_c(\tau_1, \tau_2)\rho(1 - 2f^*(\tau_1, \tau_2, \widehat{\mathbf{v}}_s)) \\ 0 & -\alpha_c(\tau_1, \tau_2)\rho 2f^*(\tau_1, \tau_2, \widehat{\mathbf{v}}_s) \end{bmatrix} . \tag{11.14.37}$$

This completes the derivation of the elements of the Jacobian matrix $\mathbf{J}_{CF}(\widehat{\mathbf{v}}_s)$ for the case $m = 1$ and $n = 1$.

The simple case just outlined is a helpful first step in developing an overview of the structure of the Jacobian matrix for couple formation, but it is insufficient to describe the structure of the matrix in the more general cases. The next useful step in developing a more general structure suitable for the writing of computer code is to consider the case of $m = 1$ behavioral class and $n = 2$ stages of disease. In this case, the set of single types is:

$$\Upsilon_s = \{\tau_1 = (0), \tau_2 = (1), \tau_3 = (2)\} \,, \tag{11.14.38}$$

and the set Υ_c of couple types contains nine elements arranged in lexicographical order. As in previous sections, it will be helpful to partition this set into three sets according the type of the left-hand partner. For every $\tau \in \Upsilon_s$, let

$$A(\tau) = \left\{(\tau, \tau') \mid \tau' \in \Upsilon_s\right\} \tag{11.14.39}$$

denote the subset of three couple types such that the left-hand partner is of type τ. Then, in this case, the 9×3 matrix $\mathbf{J}_{CCF}(c, s, \widehat{\mathbf{v}}_s)$ has the partitioned form,

$$\mathbf{J}_{CCF}(c, s, \widehat{\mathbf{v}}_s) = \begin{bmatrix} \mathbf{J}_{CCF}(\tau_1, c, s, \widehat{\mathbf{v}}_s) \\ \mathbf{J}_{CCF}(\tau_2, c, s, \widehat{\mathbf{v}}_s) \\ \mathbf{J}_{CCF}(\tau_3, c, s, \widehat{\mathbf{v}}_s) \end{bmatrix}, \tag{11.14.40}$$

where, for example, the 3×3 sub-matrix $\mathbf{J}_{CCF}(\tau_1, c, s, \widehat{\mathbf{v}}_s)$ rows and columns are, respectively, indexed by the sets $A(\tau_1)$ and Υ_s. A similar remark holds for each of the other sub-matrices in Eq. (11.14.40). In this case, $\widehat{\mathbf{v}}_s' = (\widehat{x}_{\tau_1}, 0, 0)$

To describe the structure of this sub-matrix in a succinct notation which may be extended, in reference to Eq. (11.4.8) it will be helpful to let

$$T^*(\tau_1, \mathbf{v}_s) = x_{\tau_1} + 2 \sum_{\tau \neq \tau_1} x\tau \alpha_c(\tau_1, \tau) \,. \tag{11.14.41}$$

Then, in view of Eqs. (11.14.8) through (11.14.16), it can be shown that $\mathbf{J}_{CCF}(\tau_1, c, s, \widehat{\mathbf{v}}_s)$ is:

$$\begin{bmatrix} \dfrac{\widehat{x}_{\tau_1} T^*(\tau_1, \widehat{\mathbf{v}}_s)}{2(T_c(\tau_1, \mathbf{v}_s))^2} & -\dfrac{\widehat{x}_{\tau_1}^2 \alpha_c(\tau_1, \tau_2)}{2(T_c(\tau_1, \mathbf{v}_s))^2} & -\dfrac{\widehat{x}_{\tau_1}^2 \alpha_c(\tau_1, \tau_3)}{2(T_c(\tau_1, \mathbf{v}_s))^2} \\ 0 & \widehat{x}_{\tau_1} \alpha_c(\tau_1, \tau_2) f(\tau_1, \tau_2, \widehat{\mathbf{v}}_s) & 0 \\ 0 & 0 & \widehat{x}_{\tau_1} \alpha_c(\tau_1, \tau_3) f(\tau_1, \tau_3, \widehat{\mathbf{v}}_s) \end{bmatrix} \tag{11.14.42}$$

Similarly, the matrix $\mathbf{J}_{CCF}(\tau_2, c, s, \widehat{\mathbf{v}}_s)$ has the form,

$$\mathbf{J}_{CCF}(\tau_2, c, s, \widehat{\mathbf{v}}_s) = \begin{bmatrix} 0 & \widehat{x}_{\tau_1} \alpha_c(\tau_1, \tau_2) f(\tau_1, \tau_2, \widehat{\mathbf{v}}_s) & 0 \\ 0 & 0 & 0 \\ 0 & 0 & 0 \end{bmatrix}, \tag{11.14.43}$$

and the matrix $\mathbf{J}_{CCF}(\tau_3, c, s, \widehat{\mathbf{v}}_s)$ has the form

$$\mathbf{J}_{CCF}(\tau_3, c, s, \widehat{\mathbf{v}}_s) = \begin{bmatrix} 0 & 0 & \widehat{x}_{\tau_1} \alpha_c(\tau_1, \tau_3) f(\tau_1, \tau_3, \widehat{\mathbf{v}}_s) \\ 0 & 0 & 0 \\ 0 & 0 & 0 \end{bmatrix}. \tag{11.14.44}$$

For the case, $m = 1$ and $n = 2$, $\mathbf{J}_{SCF}(s, s, \widehat{\mathbf{v}}_s)$ is a 3×3 matrix, whose elements are sometimes the difference of two expressions. Hence, it is difficult to represent the whole matrix in a compact form. But, if we let $\mathbf{C}_1, \mathbf{C}_2$, and $\mathbf{C}_3$ denote, respectively, the first, second and third columns of this matrix, then it may be represented in the partitioned form,

$$\mathbf{J}_{SCF}(s, s, \widehat{\mathbf{v}}_s) = \left[\begin{array}{ccc} \mathbf{C}_1 & \mathbf{C}_2 & \mathbf{C}_3 \end{array}\right] . \tag{11.14.45}$$

These column vectors have the following forms,

$$\mathbf{C}_1 = \left[\begin{array}{c} \dfrac{\widehat{x}_{\tau_1} T^*(\tau_1, \widehat{\mathbf{v}}_s)}{(T_c(\tau_1, \widehat{\mathbf{v}}_s))^2} \\ 0 \\ 0 \end{array}\right] , \tag{11.14.46}$$

$$\mathbf{C}_2 = \left[\begin{array}{c} \widehat{x}_{\tau_1} \alpha_c(\tau_1, \tau_2) \left(\dfrac{\widehat{x}_{\tau_1}}{(T_c(\tau_1, \widehat{\mathbf{v}}_s))^2} - 2f(\tau_1, \tau_2, \widehat{\mathbf{v}}_s) \right) \\ \widehat{x}_{\tau_1} 2\alpha_c(\tau_1, \tau_2) f(\tau_1, \tau_2, \widehat{\mathbf{v}}_s) \\ 0 \end{array}\right] , \tag{11.14.47}$$

$$\mathbf{C}_3 = \left[\begin{array}{c} \widehat{x}_{\tau_1} \alpha_c(\tau_1, \tau_3) \left(\dfrac{\widehat{x}_{\tau_1}}{(T_c(\tau_1, \widehat{\mathbf{v}}_s))^2} - 2f(\tau_1, \tau_3, \widehat{\mathbf{v}}_s) \right) \\ 0 \\ \widehat{x}_{\tau_1} 2\alpha_c(\tau_1, \tau_3) f(\tau_1, \tau_3, \widehat{\mathbf{v}}_s) \end{array}\right] . \tag{11.14.48}$$

These expressions may be verified by noting, for example, that if one takes the partial derivatives of the function $T_{CF}(\tau_1, \mathbf{v}_s)$ (see Eq. (11.11.15)), with respect to the elements of the vector $\mathbf{v}_s$ and evaluates them at the vector $\widehat{\mathbf{v}}_s$, then it can be shown that:

$$\frac{\partial T_{CF}(\tau_1, \widehat{\mathbf{v}}_s)}{\partial x_{\tau_1}} = \frac{\widehat{x}_{\tau_1} T^*(\tau_1, \widehat{\mathbf{v}}_s)}{(T_c(\tau_1, \mathbf{v}_s))^2} , \tag{11.14.49}$$

$$\frac{\partial T_{CF}(\tau_1, \widehat{\mathbf{v}}_s)}{\partial x_{\tau_2}} = \widehat{x}_{\tau_1} \alpha_c(\tau_1, \tau_2) \left(\frac{\widehat{x}_{\tau_1}}{(T_c(\tau_1, \mathbf{v}_s))^2} - 2f(\tau_1, \tau_2, \widehat{\mathbf{v}}_s) \right) , \tag{11.14.50}$$

$$\frac{\partial T_{CF}(\tau_1, \widehat{\mathbf{v}}_s)}{\partial x_{\tau_3}} = \widehat{x}_{\tau_1} \alpha_c(\tau_1, \tau_3) \left(\frac{\widehat{x}_{\tau_1}}{(T_c(\tau_1, \mathbf{v}_s))^2} - 2f(\tau_1, \tau_3, \widehat{\mathbf{v}}_s) \right) . \tag{11.14.51}$$

Similar arguments apply to the functions $T_{CF}(\tau_2, \mathbf{v}_s)$ and $T_{CF}(\tau_3, \mathbf{v}_s)$. The details may be checked by inspecting and differentiating expressions similar to Eqs. (11.14.35) and (11.14.36). It is clear that the derivations just outlined can be extended to cases in which $n \geq 2$.

11.15 Couple Formation for Cases m ≥ 2 and n ≥ 2

In the preceding section, explicit formulas were given for the elements of the Jacobian matrix for couple formation for cases where $m = 1$ and $n \geq 1$. However, for cases in which there are $m \geq 2$ behavioral classes, these formulas become so unwieldy that a more succinct notation must guide the numerical implementation of the Jacobian matrix. To help motivate ideas, suppose one has written software for computing numerical values of all the required partial derivatives described in Section 11.14 at some point in the parameter space of the model. Then, the problem reduces to writing code to place these numerical values in the correct positions in the Jacobian matrix for couple formation.

Suppose, for example, that one wishes to compute the numerical values of the elements in the matrix $\mathbf{J}_{SCF}(s, s, \widehat{\mathbf{v}}_s)$. To this end, observe from the symmetry conditions $N_{CF}(\tau_1, \tau_2, \mathbf{v}_s) = N_{CF}(\tau_2, \tau_1, \mathbf{v}_s)$ (see Eq. (11.14.12)), that the functions in Eq. (11.14.35) and (11.14.36) may be written in the succinct form,

$$T_{CF}(\tau_1, \mathbf{v}_s) = 2 \sum_{\tau \in \Upsilon_s} N_{CF}(\tau_1, \tau, \mathbf{v}_s) \tag{11.15.1}$$

for every $\tau_1 \in \Upsilon_s$, and let

$$\mathbf{T}_{CF}(\mathbf{v}_s) = (T_{CF}(\tau_1, \mathbf{v}_s) \mid \tau_1 \in \Upsilon_s) \tag{11.15.2}$$

be a column vector with these components. Then, symbolically, the columns of the matrix $\mathbf{J}_{SCF}(s, s, \widehat{\mathbf{v}}_s)$ are the vectors of partial derivatives,

$$\frac{\partial \mathbf{T}_{CF}(\mathbf{v}_s)}{\partial x_{\tau_1}}, \tag{11.15.3}$$

where $\tau_1 \in \Upsilon_s$. Rather than attempting to formally treat the class of general cases $m \geq 2$ and $n \geq 1$, which can lead to difficult expository problems, it will suffice to illustrate the ideas in terms of specific examples that can easily be generalized.

Consider, for example, the case $m = 2$ and $n = 1$. Then, the set of single types is:

$$\Upsilon_s = \{\tau_1 = (1,0), \tau_2 = (1,1), \tau_3 = (2,0), \tau_4 = (2,1)\} \ . \qquad (11.15.4)$$

One of the factors that complicates the structure of the Jacobian matrix $\mathbf{J}_{SCF}(s,s,\widehat{\mathbf{v}}_s)$ for cases in which $m \geq 2$ is that the set of single types contains more than one type of susceptible so that most elements of the matrix are sums of terms. For example, the set Υ_s in Eq. (11.15.4) contains susceptible types $\tau_1 = (1,0)$ and $\tau_3 = (2,0)$ in behavioral classes 1 and 2, respectively. Therefore, partial derivatives of the function $N_{CF}(\tau_1, \tau_3, \mathbf{v}_s)$ with respect to the elements of the vector $\mathbf{v}_s$ will not, in general, be zero at the stationary vector $\widehat{\mathbf{v}}_s$ (see Eq. (11.14.16) through (11.14.22)). For the case $m = 2$ and $n = 1$, the matrix $\mathbf{J}_{SCF}(s,s,\widehat{\mathbf{v}}_s)$ is 4×4, and to represent the 16 elements of this matrix in a compact notational form, it will be necessary to succinctly represent all partial derivatives. For example, the partial derivative of the function $T_{CF}(\tau_1, \mathbf{v}_s)$ with respect to x_τ evaluated at the stationary vector $\widehat{\mathbf{v}}_s$ will be denoted by $T(\tau_1)_\tau$. With reference to the function $N_{CF}(\tau_1, \tau_2, \mathbf{v}_s)$, the partial derivative $N(\tau_1, \tau_2)_\tau$ will be defined similarly. Even in this succinct notation, it will be necessary to represent the matrix $\mathbf{J}_{SCF}(s,s,\widehat{\mathbf{v}}_s)$ column by column due to the space limitations of a single printed page.

In this notation, the elements of the first column of the matrix $\mathbf{J}_{SCF}(s,s,\widehat{\mathbf{v}}_s)$ are:

$$-T(\tau_1)_{\tau_1} = -2\left(N(\tau_1,\tau_1)_{\tau_1} + N(\tau_1,\tau_3)_{\tau_1}\right) \ , \qquad (11.15.5)$$

$$-T(\tau_2)_{\tau_1} = 0 \ , \qquad (11.15.6)$$

$$-T(\tau_3)_{\tau_1} = -2\left(N(\tau_3,\tau_1)_{\tau_1} + N(\tau_3,\tau_3)_{\tau_1}\right) \ , \qquad (11.15.7)$$

$$-T(\tau_4)_{\tau_1} = 0 \ . \qquad (11.15.8)$$

By way of explanation, observe that all terms in the sum $T_{CF}(\tau_2, \mathbf{v}_s)$ contain x_{τ_2} as a factor (see Eqs. (11.14.6) and (11.14.7)), so that all partial derivative vanish when $\widehat{x}_{\tau_2} = 0$. Thus, $T(\tau_2)_{\tau_1} = 0$, which verifies Eq. (11.15.6), and a similar remark may be used in verifying Eq. (11.15.8).

By continuing in this vein, it can be shown that the second column of $\mathbf{J}_{SCF}(s,s,\widehat{\mathbf{v}}_s)$ has the following elements,

$$-T(\tau_1)_{\tau_2} = -2\left(N(\tau_1,\tau_1)_{\tau_2} + N(\tau_1,\tau_2)_{\tau_2} + N(\tau_1,\tau_3)_{\tau_2}\right) , \quad (11.15.9)$$

$$-T(\tau_2)_{\tau_2} = -2\left(N(\tau_2,\tau_1)_{\tau_2} + N(\tau_2,\tau_3)_{\tau_2}\right) , \quad (11.15.10)$$

$$-T(\tau_3)_{\tau_2} = -2\left(N(\tau_3,\tau_1)_{\tau_2} + N(\tau_3,\tau_2)_{\tau_2} + N(\tau_3,\tau_3)_{\tau_2}\right) , \quad (11.15.11)$$

$$-T(\tau_4)_{\tau_2} = 0 . \quad (11.15.12)$$

Similarly, the third column has the elements,

$$-T(\tau_1)_{\tau_3} = -2\left(N(\tau_1,\tau_1)_{\tau_3} + N(\tau_3,\tau_3)_{\tau_3}\right) , \quad (11.15.13)$$

$$-T(\tau_2)_{\tau_3} = 0 , \quad (11.15.14)$$

$$-T(\tau_3)_{\tau_3} = -2\left(N(\tau_3,\tau_1)_{\tau 3} + N(\tau_3,\tau_3)_{\tau_3}\right) , \quad (11.15.15)$$

$$-T(\tau_4)_{\tau_3} = 0 . \quad (11.15.16)$$

Finally, it can be shown that the fourth column of the matrix has the elements,

$$-T(\tau_1)_{\tau_4} = -2\left(N(\tau_1,\tau_1)_{\tau_4} + N(\tau_1,\tau_3)_{\tau_4} + N(\tau_1,\tau_4)_{\tau_4}\right) \quad (11.15.17)$$

$$-T(\tau_2)_{\tau_4} = 0 , \quad (11.15.18)$$

$$-T(\tau_3)_{\tau_4} = -2\left(N(\tau_3,\tau_1)_{\tau_4} + N(\tau_3,\tau_3)_{\tau_4} + N(\tau_3,\tau_4)_{\tau_4}\right) , \quad (11.15.19)$$

$$-T(\tau_4)_{\tau_4} = -2\left(N(\tau_4,\tau_1)_{\tau_4} + N(\tau_4,\tau_3)_{\tau_4}\right) . \quad (11.15.20)$$

Although it would be cumbersome to display formulas for the elements of the matrix $\mathbf{J}_{SCF}(s,s,\widehat{\mathbf{v}}_s)$, for cases such that $m \geq 2$ and $n \geq 2$, the ideas outlined in the above derivations could, in principle, be used to develop software to compute numerical representations of this matrix in more general cases.

The next step in developing an overview of the Jacobian matrix for couple formation is to consider the structure of the matrix $\mathbf{J}_{CCF}(c,s,\widehat{\mathbf{v}}_s)$, where the rows are indexed by the set Υ_c of couple types and the columns are indexed by the set Υ_s of single types. To elucidate the structure of this matrix, it will suffice to consider the case $m = 2$ and $n = 2$ in which the set Υ_c of couple types contains

$m^2(n+1)^2 = 36$ elements and the set Υ_s of single types contains $m(n+1) = 6$ elements. To further simplify the notation, the symbol $\widehat{\mathbf{v}}_s$ will be dropped and the matrix being considered will be denoted by $\mathbf{J}_{CCF}(c, s)$. As in Eq. (11.13.39), let $A(j_1, j_2)$ denote the subset of couple types $\varkappa = ((j_1, k_1), (j_2, k_2))$ such that the pair of behavioral classes (j_1, j_2) is fixed and the pairs of states with respect to disease (k_1, k_2) are arranged in lexicographical order. Let $\mathbf{J}_{CCF}(c, s, j_1, j_2)$ denote the sub-matrix of $\mathbf{J}_{CCF}(c, s)$ such that the rows are indexed by the elements of the set $A(j_1, j_2)$. Then, the matrix $\mathbf{J}_{CCF}(c, s)$ may be represented in the partitioned form,

$$\mathbf{J}_{CCF}(c,s) = \begin{bmatrix} \mathbf{J}_{CCF}(c,s,1,1) \\ \mathbf{J}_{CCF}(c,s,1,2) \\ \mathbf{J}_{CCF}(c,s,2,1) \\ \mathbf{J}_{CCF}(c,s,2,2) \end{bmatrix}. \tag{11.15.21}$$

Each of these sub-matrices also has a partitioned form. For every fixed state k_1 of the left-hand partner, let the set $A(j_1, j_2, k_1)$ defined by:

$$A(j_1, j_2, k_1) = \{\varkappa = ((j_1, k_1), (j_2, k_2)) \mid k_2 = 0, 1, 2\} \tag{11.15.22}$$

denote the subset of couple types such that the triple (j_1, j_2, k_1) is fixed but the index k_2 varies. Let $\mathbf{J}_{CCF}(c, s, j_1, j_2, k_1)$ denote a matrix whose rows and columns are indexed, respectively, by the sets $A(j_1, j_2, k_1)$ and Υ_s. Then, for each pair (j_1, j_2) of behavioral classes, the matrix $\mathbf{J}_{CCF}(c, s, j_1, j_2)$ has the partitioned form,

$$\mathbf{J}_{CCF}(c,s,j_1,j_2) = \begin{bmatrix} \mathbf{J}_{CCF}(c,s,j_1,j_2,0) \\ \mathbf{J}_{CCF}(c,s,j_1,j_2,1) \\ \mathbf{J}_{CCF}(c,s,j_1,j_2,2) \end{bmatrix}. \tag{11.15.23}$$

To represent the elements of these matrices in the succinct notation for the partial derivatives described above, it will be necessary to relabel the elements of the set Υ_c of single types for the case $m = 2$ and $n = 2$. The elements of the subsets of types for behavioral classes 1 and 2 will be denoted, respectively, by:

$$\Upsilon_d(1) = \{\tau_1, \tau_2, \tau_3\} \tag{11.15.24}$$

and

$$\Upsilon_s(2) = \{\tau_4, \tau_5, \tau_6\} \ . \tag{11.15.25}$$

Observe that in this case the types $\tau_1 = (1,0)$ and $\tau_4 = (2,0)$ are susceptibles, and all other types in the set $\Upsilon_s = \Upsilon_s(1) \cup \Upsilon_s(2)$ are infectives.

As a first step in describing the structure of the sub-matrices in Eq. (11.15.23), observe that for the sub-matrix $\mathbf{J}_{CCF}(c, s, 1, 1, 0)$ the left-hand partner is the susceptible type τ_1 and the types of the right-hand partners also belong to the set $\Upsilon_d(1)$ so that the rows of the matrix are indexed by the subset

$$\left\{ \begin{array}{c} (\tau_1, \tau_1) \\ (\tau_1, \tau_2) \\ (\tau_1, \tau_3) \end{array} \right\} , \tag{11.15.26}$$

of couple types. Therefore, the first 1×6 row vector of the matrix $\mathbf{J}_{CCF}(c, s, 1, 1, 0)$ has the form,

$$\mathbf{R}_1(1,1,0) = (N(\tau_1, \tau_1)_\tau \mid \tau \in \Upsilon_s) \ . \tag{11.15.27}$$

Let $\delta(\tau_1, \tau_2)$ denote the Kronecker delta, i.e., $\delta(\tau_1, \tau_2) = 0$ if $\tau_1 \neq \tau_2$ and $\delta(\tau_1, \tau_2) = 1$ if $\tau_1 = \tau_2$. Then, the second 1×6 row vector of the matrix $\mathbf{J}_{CCF}(c, s, 1, 1, 0)$ has the form

$$\mathbf{R}_2(1,1,0) = (\delta(\tau, \tau_2) N(\tau_1, \tau_2)_{\tau_2} \mid \tau \in \Upsilon_s) \ . \tag{11.15.28}$$

Similarly, the third 1×6 row vector of the matrix $\mathbf{J}_{CCF}(c, s, 1, 1, 0)$ has the form

$$\mathbf{R}_3(1,1,0) = (\delta(\tau, \tau_3) N(\tau_1, \tau_3)_{\tau_3} \mid \tau \in \Upsilon_s) \ . \tag{11.15.29}$$

For the sub-matrix $\mathbf{J}_{CCF}(c, s, 1, 1, 1)$, the rows are indexed by the subset,

$$\{(\tau_2, \tau) \mid \tau \in \Upsilon_s(1)\} \tag{11.15.30}$$

of couple types. The only type such that the right-hand partner is susceptible is (τ_2, τ_1) and in all other types both partners are infectives. Therefore, the matrix $\mathbf{J}_{CCF}(c, s, 1, 1, 1)$ has the form,

$$\mathbf{J}_{CCF}(c, s, 1, 1, 1) = \left[\begin{array}{c} \mathbf{R}_2(1,1,0) \\ \mathbf{0}_{2\times 6} \end{array} \right] , \tag{11.15.31}$$

where $\mathbf{0}_{2\times 6}$ is a 2×6 zero matrix. By a similar argument, it can be shown that the sub-matrix $\mathbf{J}_{CCF}(c, s, 1, 1, 2)$ has the partitioned form,

$$\mathbf{J}_{CCF}(c, s, 1, 1, 2) = \begin{bmatrix} \mathbf{R}_3(1, 1, 0) \\ \mathbf{0}_{2\times 6} \end{bmatrix} . \tag{11.15.32}$$

For the sub-matrix $\mathbf{J}_{CCF}(c, s, 1, 2)$, the types of the left-hand partners belong to the set $\Upsilon_d(1)$ and those of the right-hand partner to the set $\Upsilon_d(2)$. Therefore, for the case of the sub-matrix $\mathbf{J}_{CCF}(c, s, 1, 2, 0)$, the three 1×6 row vectors take the following forms,

$$\mathbf{R}_1(1, 2, 0) = (N(\tau_1, \tau_4)_\tau \mid \tau \in \Upsilon_s) \ , \tag{11.15.33}$$

$$\mathbf{R}_2(1, 2, 0) = (\delta(\tau, \tau_5) N(\tau_1, \tau_5)_{\tau_5} \mid \tau \in \Upsilon_s) \ , \tag{11.15.34}$$

$$\mathbf{R}_3(1, 2, 0) = (\delta(\tau, \tau_6) N(\tau_1, \tau_6)_{\tau_6} \mid \tau \in \Upsilon_s) \ . \tag{11.15.35}$$

Similarly, it can be shown that:

$$\mathbf{J}_{CCF}(c, s, 1, 2, 1) = \begin{bmatrix} \mathbf{R}_2(1, 2, 0) \\ \mathbf{0}_{2\times 6} \end{bmatrix} \tag{11.15.36}$$

and

$$\mathbf{J}_{CCF}(c, s, 1, 2, 2) = \begin{bmatrix} \mathbf{R}_3(1, 2, 0) \\ \mathbf{0}_{2\times 6} \end{bmatrix} . \tag{11.15.37}$$

Because the functions $N(\tau, \tau')$ are symmetric in their arguments, the matrices $\mathbf{J}_{CCF}(c, s, 1, 2)$ and $\mathbf{J}_{CCF}(c, s, 2, 1)$ have the same elements.

The last sub-matrix to be considered is $\mathbf{J}_{CCF}(c, s, 2, 2)$, where the types of both the left and right-hand partners belong to the set $\Upsilon_d(2)$. For the case of the sub-matrix $\mathbf{J}_{CCF}(c, s, 2, 2, 0)$, the three 1×6 row vectors take the following forms,

$$\mathbf{R}_1(2, 2, 0) = (N(\tau_4, \tau_4)_\tau \mid \tau \in \Upsilon_s) \ , \tag{11.15.38}$$

$$\mathbf{R}_2(2, 2, 0) = (\delta(\tau, \tau_5) N(\tau_4, \tau_5)_{\tau_5} \mid \tau \in \Upsilon_s) \ , \tag{11.15.39}$$

$$\mathbf{R}_3(2, 2, 0) = (\delta(\tau, \tau_6) N(\tau_4, \tau_6)_{\tau_6} \mid \tau \in \Upsilon_s) \ . \tag{11.15.40}$$

Just as above, it can be shown that:

$$\mathbf{J}_{CCF}(c, s, 2, 2, 1) = \begin{bmatrix} \mathbf{R}_2(2, 2, 0) \\ \mathbf{0}_{2\times 6} \end{bmatrix} \tag{11.15.41}$$

and

$$\mathbf{J}_{CCF}(c, s, 2, 2, 2) = \begin{bmatrix} \mathbf{R}_3(2, 2, 0) \\ \mathbf{0}_{2\times 6} \end{bmatrix} . \qquad (11.15.42)$$

It is clear that the above description could, in principle, be extended to cases such that $n > 2$. This completes the description of the structure of the Jacobian matrix for couple formation for cases with $m \geq 2$ behavioral classes and $n \geq 2$ stages of disease.

11.16 Invasion Thresholds for m = 2 and n = 1

As illustrated in previous sections, for the class of one sex partnership models under consideration, the number of single types $m(n+1)$ and couple types $m^2(n+1)^2$ can be quite large for moderate values of m and n. This may lead to difficulties in developing software on desktop computers to process large dimensional arrays. Therefore, to avoid potential difficulties, and as a first step toward developing more general software, a decision was made to develop code for the case of $m = 2$ behavioral classes and $n = 1$ stage of disease. For this case, there are 4 types of singles and 16 couple types, which leads to rather small arrays that may easily be processed on most desktop computers. By definition, individuals in behavioral class 1 will be the monogamous in the sense that they will consent to sexual contacts only with their marital partners; whereas those in class 2 will be assumed to be more sexually active and may have sexual contacts outside their marital partnerships. Table 11.16.1 contains the assigned values of parameters used in the numerical experiments reported in this chapter.

By way of explanation, the value $\lambda_1 = 0$ in the first row of the table is the condition that members of class 1 have no extra-marital sexual partners and are thus monogamous. On the other hand, individuals in class 2 are very active sexually in that on average, they have $\lambda_2 = 4$ extra-marital sexual partners per month. The vector $\boldsymbol{\eta} = (\eta_1, \eta_2)$ in the second row of the table contains the expected number of contacts per month per extra-marital sexual partner by behavioral class, following the first sexual contact. For example, the value $\eta_2 = 1$ indicates that on average individuals in class 2 have two sexual contacts per month with each extra-marital sexual partner. The value $\eta_1 = 0$, which was included because some value is required to make the software function properly, is not meaningful from the substantive point of view, because the monogamous members of class 1 have no extra-marital sexual partners. Within a couple, it is assumed that the expected number of sexual contacts per month is $\gamma_{mc} = 8$ (see line 3 of Table 11.16.1).

Table 11.16.1. Numerical Values of Parameters.

$(\lambda_1, \lambda_2) = (0, 4)$
$\boldsymbol{\eta} = (0, 1)$
$\gamma_{mc} = 8$
$\mathbf{p}_{mar} = (0.99, 0.97)$
$\mathbf{p}_{em} = (0.95, 0.85)$
$(\mu_0, \mu_1) = (1/720, 1/60)$
$\mu_r = 10$
$\boldsymbol{\varphi} = (0.75, 0, 0.25, 0)$
$\rho = 1/24$
$\delta = 1/120$
$\beta_{c1} = \beta_{c2} = 1$
$\beta_{em1} = \beta_{em2} = 1$

The fourth and fifth rows of the table contain the probabilities that a susceptible individual escapes infection per sexual contact with an infectious individual classified by whether a contact is with a marital or extra-marital sexual partner, and also by behavioral class. For example, the elements of the vector $\mathbf{p}_{mar} = (0.99, 0.97)$ indicate that a member of class 1 escapes infection with a probability of 0.99 per sexual contact with an infectious marital partner, but for an individual in class 2, this escape probability is 0.97. According to the second element in the vector $\mathbf{p}_{em} = (0.95, 0.85)$, extra-marital sexual contacts by members of class 2 are more risky, with a probability of 0.85 that a susceptible individual escapes infection per contact with an infectious partner. Again, the first element 0.95 in the vector $\mathbf{p}_{em}$ for monogamous individuals is not meaningful, but some value was needed for the software to function properly.

The sixth row of the table contains the assigned values for the mortality parameters $(\mu_0, \mu_1) = (1/720, 1/60)$. According to these values, a susceptible or non-infected recruit lives for an average of 720 months or 60 years after entering the sexually active population, but, when an individual is infected, the latent expectation of life remaining is 60 months or 5 years. The seventh and eighth rows of the table contain values of those parameters governing the entrance of recruits into the population. Thus, on average, $\mu_r = 10$ recruits enter the population per month, and, according to the vector $\boldsymbol{\varphi} = (0.75, 0, 0.25, 0)$, 75% are monogamous and 25% are more sexually active in that they may engage in extra-marital sexual contacts. With regard to couple formation, the value $\rho = 1/24$ in the ninth row of the table indicates that the expected latent waiting time among singles to enter into a marital partnership is 24 months or 2 years, but, after this partnership is formed the expected latent time to its dissolution is $1/\delta = 120$ months or 10 years (see line 10 of Table 11.16.1).

The values $\beta_{c1} = \beta_{c2} = 1$ and $\beta_{em1} = \beta_{em2} = 1$ in lines 11 and 12 of Table 11.16.1 indicate that is assumed that the acceptance probabilities for both couple formation and choices of extra-marital sexual partners are "weakly" assortative in the sense that there is a tendency for types to choose those types "closest" to them for both marital and extra-marital sexual partners in the sense of the distance function used in Sections 11.5 and 11.6 (see Eqs. (11.5.1) and (11.6.1)). Expressing these ideas quantitatively, the array of acceptance probabilities for couple formation used in the experiments reported in this section was determined by Eq. (11.5.1), and is as follows:

$$ALPHA_C = \begin{bmatrix} 1 & 0.3679 & 0.3679 & 0.1353 \\ 0.3679 & 1 & 0.1353 & 0.3679 \\ 0.3679 & 0.1353 & 1 & 0.3679 \\ 0.1353 & 0.3679 & 0.3679 & 1 \end{bmatrix}. \tag{11.16.1}$$

It should be mentioned that the symbols used to denote the four types of singles were $\tau_1 = (1,0)$, $\tau_2 = (1,1)$, $\tau_3 = (2,0)$ and $\tau_4 = (2,1)$. To illustrate the computation of the elements of this array, consider a potential partnership of type (τ_1, τ_4), consisting of a susceptible τ_1 in class 1, and an infective τ_4 in class 2. Then, with the parameter assignments $\beta_{c1} = \beta_{c2} = 1$, Eq. (11.5.1) yields the value

$$\alpha_c(\tau_1, \tau_4) = e^{-2} \simeq 0.1353 \tag{11.16.2}$$

for the conditional probability that an individual of type τ_1 finds an individual of type τ_4 acceptable as a marital partner, which is the element in the first row and fourth column of the array in Eq. (11.16.1). Because it was assumed that $\beta_{em1} = \beta_{em2} = 1$, the array $ALPHA_{EM}$ of extra-marital acceptance probabilities was given the same values as those in Eq. (11.16.1).

The last set of parameters needing to be assigned numerical values were those for the transition rates among the behavioral classes. In the experiments reported in this chapter, these parameters were assigned the values:

$$\mathbf{\Psi} = \begin{bmatrix} 0 & 1/1200 \\ 1/120 & 0 \end{bmatrix} . \tag{11.16.3}$$

Observe that the assumed rate $\psi_{12} = 1/1200$ of transitions of monogamous individuals to the highly sexually active class 2 implies that the latent expectation of stay in the monogamous class is $1/\psi_{12} = 1200$ months or 100 years, a value that exceeds the expected life span of a susceptible recruit entering the population. On the other hand, the assumed rate $\psi_{21} = 1/120$ of transitions from class 2 to class 1 implies that the latent expectation of the length of stay in the highly sexually active class 2 is $1/\psi_{21} = 120$ months or 10 years, the same value as that for the latent expected duration of a marital partnership.

Given the above parameter assignments, a stationary vector $\widehat{\mathbf{v}}$ with six elements for the case where a population contains only susceptibles is formed. The symbolic form of the transpose of this vector is

$$\widehat{\mathbf{v}}' = \left(\widehat{x}_1 \quad \widehat{x}_2 \quad \widehat{z}_{11} \quad \widehat{z}_{12} \quad \widehat{z}_{21} \quad \widehat{z}_{22} \right) , \tag{11.16.4}$$

where $\widehat{x}_1$ and $\widehat{x}_2$ are the number of singles in behavioral classes 1 and 2, $\widehat{z}_{11}$ is the number of couples with both members in class 1, and so on. This vector may be calculated by applying the recursive procedure outlined in Eqs. (11.11.11) through (11.11.13) with the initial value,

$$\mathbf{v}_0 = -\mathbf{A}_S^{-1}\mathbf{R}_S , \tag{11.16.5}$$

where $\mathbf{A}_S$ is the 6×6 matrix of constants, and $\mathbf{R}_S$ is the 6×1 vector for recruits in the reduced system of differential equations. In these calculations, the value of h was chosen as $h = 0.25$, which is approximately one week when the time unit is one month. The criterion used to stop the recursive procedure was to find the first k such that:

$$\|\mathbf{v}_{k+1} - \mathbf{v}_k\| < 10^{-10} , \tag{11.16.6}$$

where $\|\cdot\|$ is the vector norm used in Section 11.11.

With this initial vector and tolerance value, it was found that convergence was rapid and yielded the stationary vector,

$$\widehat{\mathbf{v}}' = \begin{pmatrix} 1278 & 188 & 2306 & 253 & 253 & 56 \end{pmatrix} , \tag{11.16.7}$$

where the elements have been rounded to the nearest integer. According to this vector, the total size of the stationary population of susceptibles is:

$$1278 + 188 + 2 \times (2306 + 253 + 253 + 56) = 7202 . \tag{11.16.8}$$

Note that this value is close to $\mu_r/\mu_0 = 7200$, the value predicted by the simpler models in Section 11.11 (see Eqs. (11.11.6) and (11.11.10)).

When considering any set of assigned parameter values, it is always of interest to test whether the reduced 6×6 matrix $\mathbf{A}_S$, as well as the full 20×20 matrix $\mathbf{A}$, are stable to determine whether the initial conditions will wear off as $t \uparrow \infty$. For the given set of parameter values, it was found that both these matrices were stable. To verify the software, it is also of interest to test whether the Jacobian matrix

$$\mathbf{J}_S(\widehat{\mathbf{v}}) = \mathbf{A}_S + \mathbf{J}_{CFS}(\widehat{\mathbf{v}}) \tag{11.16.9}$$

for the reduced system of differential equations is stable as expected when evaluated at the stationary vector $\widehat{\mathbf{v}}$. For, if this matrix is not stable for the case where a population contains only susceptibles, then one would expect there to be undetected software errors. This matrix was, however, stable as expected for the given set of parameter values, indicating that the software passed this test.

A final step in finding an indicator as to whether an epidemic may develop when a few infectives are introduced into a population of susceptibles that has been evolving for a long period of time is to test whether the full 20×20 Jacobian matrix

$$\mathbf{J}(\widehat{\mathbf{v}}) = \mathbf{A} + \mathbf{J}_{EM}(\widehat{\mathbf{v}}) + \mathbf{J}_{CF}(\widehat{\mathbf{v}}) \qquad (11.16.10)$$

is stable or not when evaluated at the stationary vector $\widehat{\mathbf{v}}$. For the given set of parameter values, this matrix was not stable, suggesting that an epidemic may develop if a few infectives were introduced into a population of susceptibles. In the remaining sections of this chapter, the results of computer experiments designed to test the extent to which an epidemic may develop in a population will be presented.

11.17 Invasion Thresholds of Highly Sexually Active Infectives

When a population is partitioned into two behavioral classes, one class monogamous and the other highly sexually active, a question that arises is what invasion threshold of highly sexually active infectives would be required to spread infections throughout the population. An attempt will be made in this section to answer this question, given the parameter assignments described in Section 11.16. As in the computer experiments presented in Chapter 10, it will be assumed that some infectives invade a population of susceptibles that have been evolving for a long period of time so that the population composition is given by the stationary vector in Eq. (11.16.4). The three invasion thresholds used in the computer experiments of this section are given in Table 11.17.1.

Table 11.17.1. Initial Numbers of Infectives.

Initial 1; $X(0;\tau_4) = 1$
Initial 2; $Z(0;\tau_4,\tau_4) = 1$
Initial 3; $Z(0;\tau_4,\tau_4) = 2$

Unlike the one-sex models considered in Chapter 10, one may assume in the one-sex model with marital partnerships studied in this chapter that the initial population contains either infective singles, or couples with one or both members infected. Thus, in projections using the first row of Table 11.17.1 as input, it was assumed that the initial population contained one single infective of type $\tau_4 = (2, 1)$ in behavioral class 2. But, in those projections using rows two and three of the table, it was assumed that the initial population contained one and two couples, respectively, in which both members were infected and belonged to type τ_4 in class 2. Another way of viewing the invasion thresholds in Table 11.17.1 is that three levels of infectives in the initial population were considered, i.e., one, two and four infectious individuals in the initial population. In all experiments reported in this section, the number of Monte Carlo replications was 100 and each projection was carried out for 1200 months or 100 years.

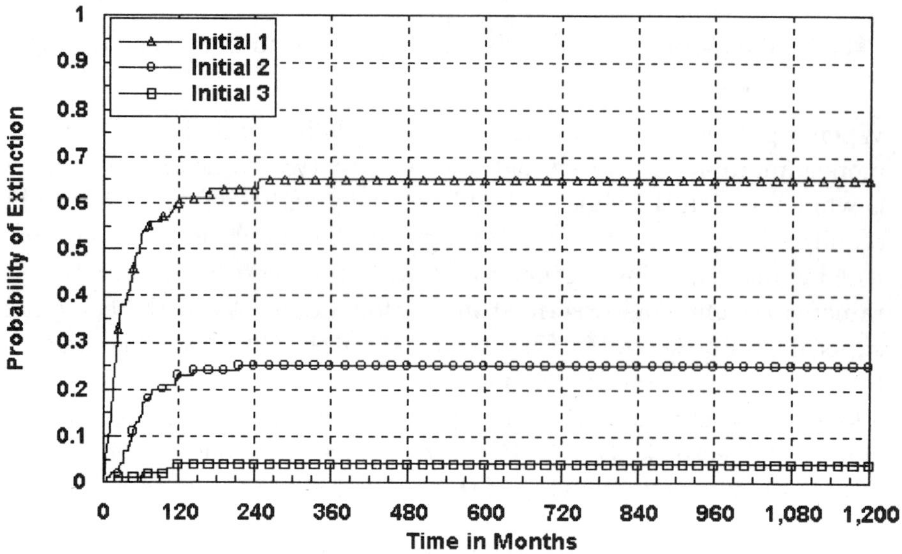

Figure 11.17.1. Probabilities of Extinction by Epoch and Invasion Threshold.

Figure 11.17.1 contains the graphs of the probabilities of extinction by epoch for the three invasion thresholds presented in Table 11.17.1. As can be seen from these graphs, the eventual probability of extinction depended significantly on the initial level of infectives. For the case of Initial 1, this graph converged to the rather high value of 0.65 at about 252 months or 21 years into the projection, indicating that in 65 of the 100 Monte Carlo realizations of the process, the epidemic eventually became extinct. However, when there were larger numbers of initial infectives in the population as in Initials 2 and 3, the eventual probability of extinction of the epidemic was much smaller. For example, for the invasion threshold Initial 2, the extinction probability converged to 0.25 at about 216 months or 18 years into the projection. But, for the case of Initial 2, the probability of eventual extinction declined to only 0.04, a limit that was reached at about 120 months or 10 years into the projection.

To gain some insight into the extent an epidemic initiated by a few infectives in highly sexually active class 2 may spread into the class of monogamous individuals, it is of interest to inspect graphs of the number of monogamous individuals in couples or singles that were infected at each epoch of the projections. When the probability that an epidemic becomes extinct is quite high, a plot of the mean trajectory of a sample of Monte Carlo realizations of the process may not be as informative as plots of other trajectories such as selected quantiles computed from the sample. A decision was made, therefore, to plot the trajectories of the 25th, 50th, and 75th quantiles of a Monte Carlo sample rather than its mean trajectory; these will be labeled Q25, Q50 and Q75, respectively. Moreover, to better understand the range of variation in a sample of Monte Carlo realizations, a decision was made to plot the Min and Max trajectories of the sample. Finally, to explore the behavior of the embedded deterministic model in relation to realizations of the stochastic process, a plot of the trajectory of the embedded deterministic model was also included and identified by the label Det.

The graphs of the Min, Q25, Q50, Q75, Max, and Det trajectories of the number of infected monogamous individuals in couples that were infected at each epoch of the projections with an invasion threshold Initial 1 are presented in Figure 11.17.2. Because the epidemic became extinct in 65 out of the 100 Monte Carlo realizations of the process, the Min, Q25 and Q50 trajectories were all zero throughout, but the Q75 and Max trajectories were positive throughout the projections. It is interesting to note that the Det trajectory remains approximately midway between the Q75 and Max trajectories throughout these projections.

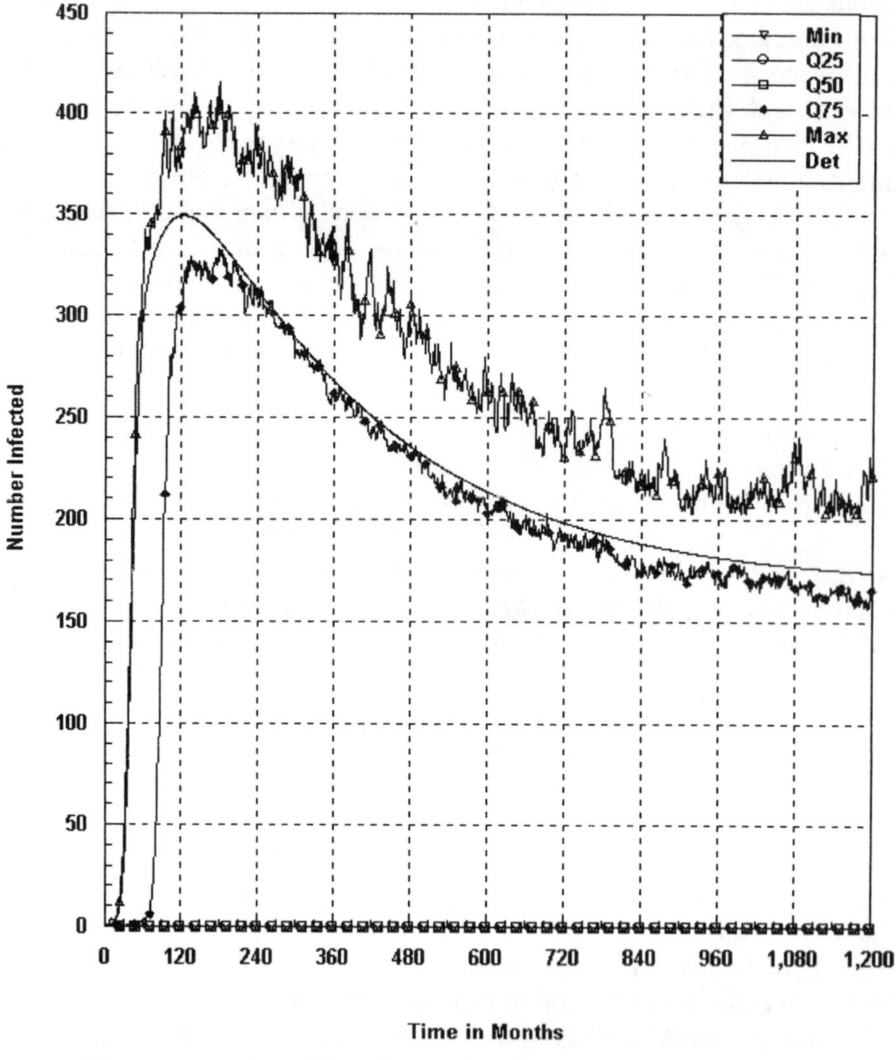

Figure 11.17.2. Number of Infected Monogamous Individuals in Couples by Epoch - Initial 1.

Figure 11.17.3 contains the graphs of the Min, Q25, Q50, Q75, Max, and Det trajectories for the number of infected monogamous individuals in couples that were infected at each epoch of the projections with the invasion threshold Initial 2. In these projections, the epidemic became extinct in 25 out of 100 of the Monte Carlo projections so that the Min trajectory was zero throughout as expected, and that of Q25 was also zero except for a few epochs during the first few years of the projection. It is interesting to note that in this projection, the Det trajectory occupies a position somewhere between the Q50 and Q75 trajectories throughout. The graphs for the Det trajectories in these figures suggest that they would eventually converge to a positive constant, indicating that infections would eventually become endemic in the population. But, just as in some of the examples presented in Chapter 10, if an investigator relied solely on the embedded deteministic model to forecast the evolution of an epidemic, such forecasts would be misleading, because, among other things, they would not take into account the possibility that an epidemic may become extinct.

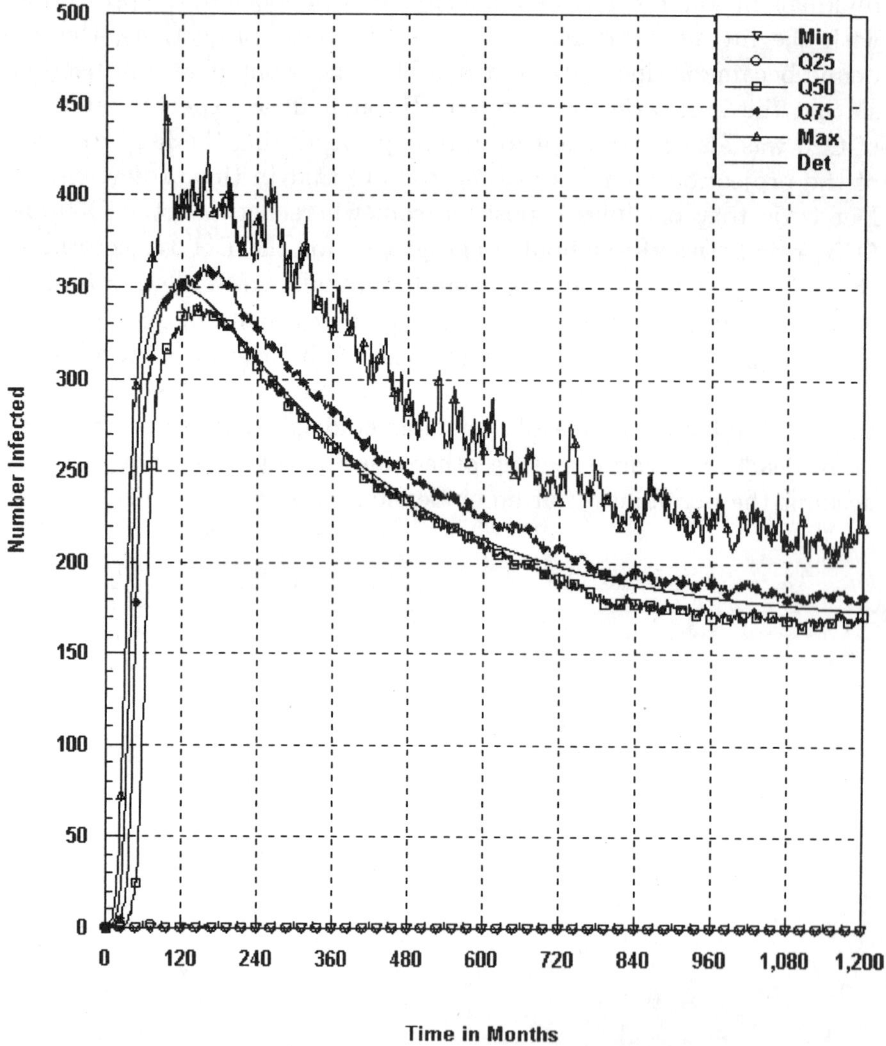

Figure 11.17.3. Number of Infected Monogamous Individuals in Couples by Epoch - Initial 2.

Another perspective from which to view the impact of an epidemic on a population is that of the evolution of total population size. Figure 11.17.4 contains the graphs of Min, Q25, Q50, Q75, Max, and Det trajectories for total population size when the invasion threshold was Initial 1. The corresponding graphs of these trajectories when Initial 2 was the invasion threshold are presented in Figure 11.17.5. The Min trajectory represents those realizations in which deaths from disease had the greatest impact. Observe that at 1200 months into the projections, the value of the Min trajectory was 2450; while that of the Q25 was somewhat higher at about 2600. Thus, with a probability of 0.25, the total population size would be less than or equal to 2600. On the other hand, the median trajectory, Q50, at 1200 months was about 7205, a value that was close to the size of the initial population. Hence, the total population size would be equal to or greater than the size of the initial population at 1200 months with probability 0.50. The pattern of trajectories displayed in Figure 11.17.4 is typical of those cases in which there is a rather high probability that an epidemic eventually becomes extinct, as was the case for Initial 1 where this probability was 0.65.

As can be seen from Figure 11.17.5, when the invasion threshold Initial 2 was used in projections of an epidemic with an eventual probability of extinction of 0.25, the graphs of the Min, Q25, Q50, Q75, Max, and Det trajectories exhibited distinctly different patterns. In these projections, at 1200 months, the quantile Q75 was about 2737; that is, it was with the probability of 0.75 that the total population size is less than or equal to 2737. The Max trajectory represents those realizations of the process in which the epidemic either became extinct or had a small impact on total population size. In these projections, the value of the Max trajectory at 1200 months was about 7420, which is greater than the initial population size of about 7200. Just as in the other figures of this section, the Det trajectories in Figures 11.17.4 and 11.17.5 tended to be closer to the worst case realizations of the epidemic. Hence, forecasts based projections of the embedded deterministic model would be unduly pessimistic.

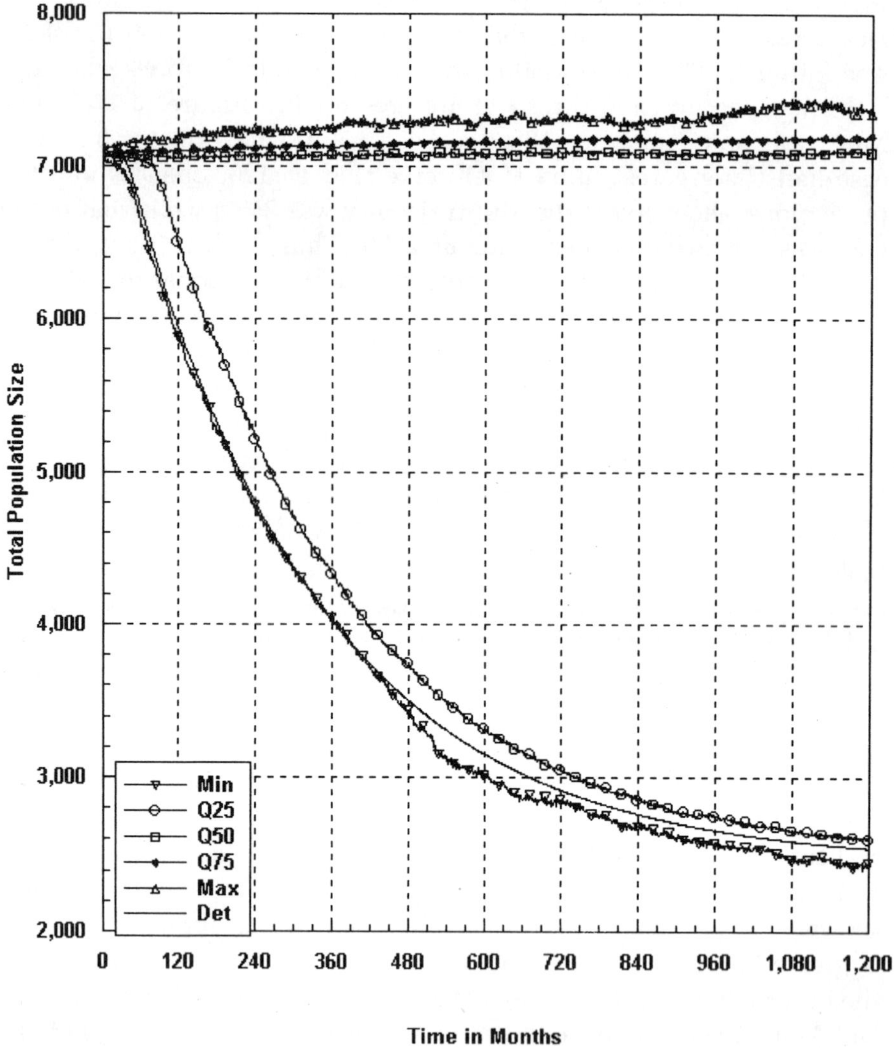

Figure 11.17.4. Total Population Size by Epoch - Initial 1.

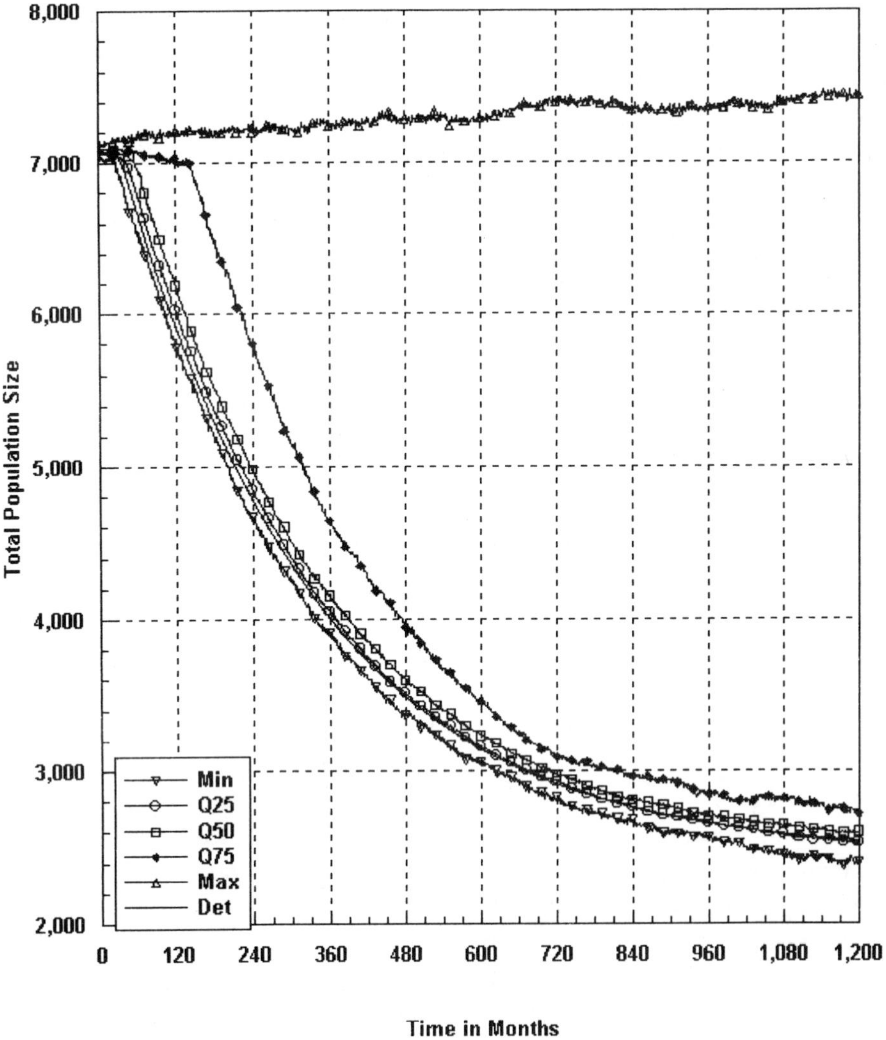

Figure 11.17.5. Total Population Size by Epoch - Initial 2.

11.18 Mutations and the Evolution of Epidemics

Strictly speaking, the models under discussion in this book do not take into account genetic mutations in the organism which is the causal agent of the disease. However, as in Section 10.16, mutational events may be simulated by supposing that among the highly sexually active recruits entering the population during any time interval, some are infected with low probability. For ease of documentation, it should be assumed throughout all computer experiments reported in this section that the inputs described in Section 11.16 were in force, except for three versions of the vector of probabilities $\boldsymbol{\varphi}$, governing the composition of recruits entering the population during each time interval.

Table 11.18.1. Distributions of Recruits.

$\boldsymbol{\varphi}_1 = (0.75, 0, 0.2499975, 0.000025)$
$\boldsymbol{\varphi}_2 = (0.75, 0, 0.24995, 0.00005)$
$\boldsymbol{\varphi}_3 = (0.75, 0, 0.24875, 0.00025)$

The three versions of this vector are displayed in Table 11.18.1. In recruit vector $\boldsymbol{\varphi}_1$, it was assumed that among the 25 out of 100 recruits that are highly sexually active, one in ten thousand was infected; hence, given that the element φ_{14} in this vector had the value $\varphi_{14} = 0.25/10000 = 0.000025$, the value of the element φ_{13} was, therefore, $\varphi_{13} = 0.25(1 - 0.000025) = 0.24999375$. Similarly, it was assumed in vector $\boldsymbol{\varphi}_2$ that one in five thousand of the highly sexually active recruits were infective so that $\varphi_{24} = 0.25/5000 = 0.00005$. Lastly, it was assumed in vector $\boldsymbol{\varphi}_3$ that one in a thousand of these recruits were infected, resulting in the value $\varphi_{34} = 0.25/1000 = 0.00025$.

It should also be emphasized that in the computer experiments reported in this section, the initial population contained no infectives so that throughout these projections the only source of infectious individuals was the highly sexually active recruits in class 2 that entered the population during any time interval according to the probabilities listed in Table 11.18.1. Because the probability that an infectious recruit entered the population during any time interval was rather small in the three cases, one would expect that rather long time spans may be required before an epidemic would develop in a population. Therefore, a decision was made to run the projections for a total of 2400 months or 200 years. As in other sections of this chapter, 100 Monte Carlo realizations of the process were computed for each of the three cases.

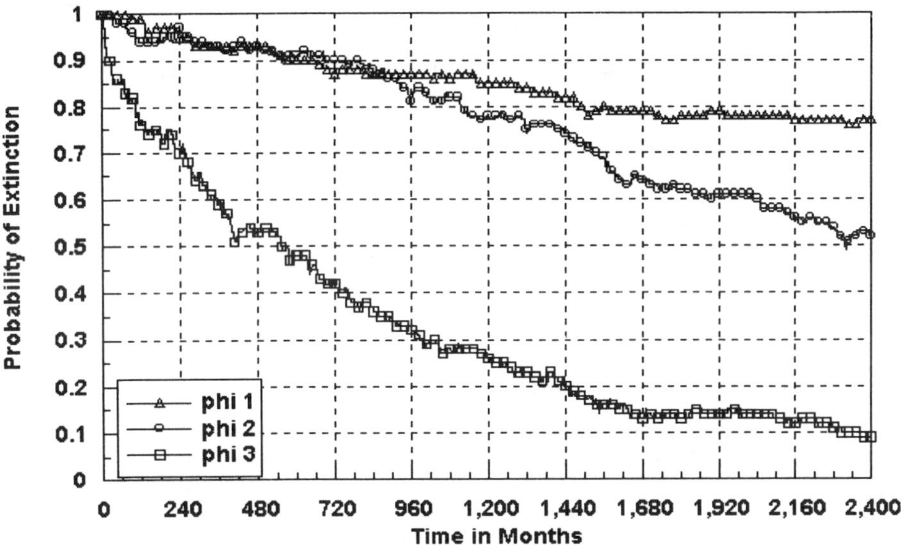

Figure 11.18.1. Fraction of Realizations that Contained No Infectives by Epoch.

The graphs of the trajectories for the fraction of the 100 Monte Carlo realizations that contained no infectives at each of the 2400 months in the projections are presented in Figure 11.18.1. For the case of recruit vector φ_1, where a highly sexually active recruit was infective with a probability of 0.0001, 77% of the realizations did not contain infectives at 2400 months into these projections, which suggests that an epidemic may become established in a population within 200 years with probability of about 0.23. However, for the case where a highly sexually active recruit was infective with a probability of 0.005 as in vector φ_2, the fraction of the realizations not containing any infectives at epoch 2400 was reduced to 0.52; and for the case of vector φ_3, where a recruit in the highly active class was infective with a probability of 0.001, none of the realizations contained infectives at 2400 months, suggesting that in this case the development of an epidemic in the population within 200 years was almost certain.

Figure 11.18.2 contains the graphs of the Max and Det trajectories of the cumulative number of infected monogamous individuals in couples for the case where one in ten thousand of the highly sexually active recruits was infective. The Min, Q25, Q50 and Q75 trajectories were not plotted, because they were zero throughout the projections, which is consistent with an estimated probability of about 0.23 that an epidemic would develop in a population within 200 years. Perhaps the most striking aspect of the graphs is that the Det trajectory often exceeds that of the Max, which is consistent with the earlier observation that the embedded deteministic model tends to mimic the worst case scenario of the epidemic. For purposes of making comparisons, note that the value of the Max trajectory at 2400 months indicates that among the worst cases, a total of about 8900 monogamous individuals in couples had been infected.

Presented in Figure 11.18.3 are the graphs of the Q25, Q50, Q75, Max and Det trajectories for the cumulative numbers of infected monogamous individuals in couples for the case of recruit vector φ_3, where a highly sexually active recruit was infective with a probability of 0.001. For this case, the Min trajectory was zero throughout the projection, indicating that among the 100 realizations of the process at each epoch, at least one realization contained no infectives. As one would expect, with this higher probability of infectious recruits entering the population during each time interval, the Q25 trajectory was positive after 100 years, suggesting that a significant epidemic would develop in a population within 200 years with probability of at least 0.75. Moreover, according to the value 7311 of the Q50 trajectory at 2400 months, the cumulative numbers of infected monogamous individuals in couples would exceed 7311 within 200 years with probability 0.50. Due to lack of space, the corresponding graphs for the case of recruit vector φ_2 will not be presented, but the graphs of quantile trajectories would occupy intermediate positions among those in Figures 11.18.2 and 11.18.3.

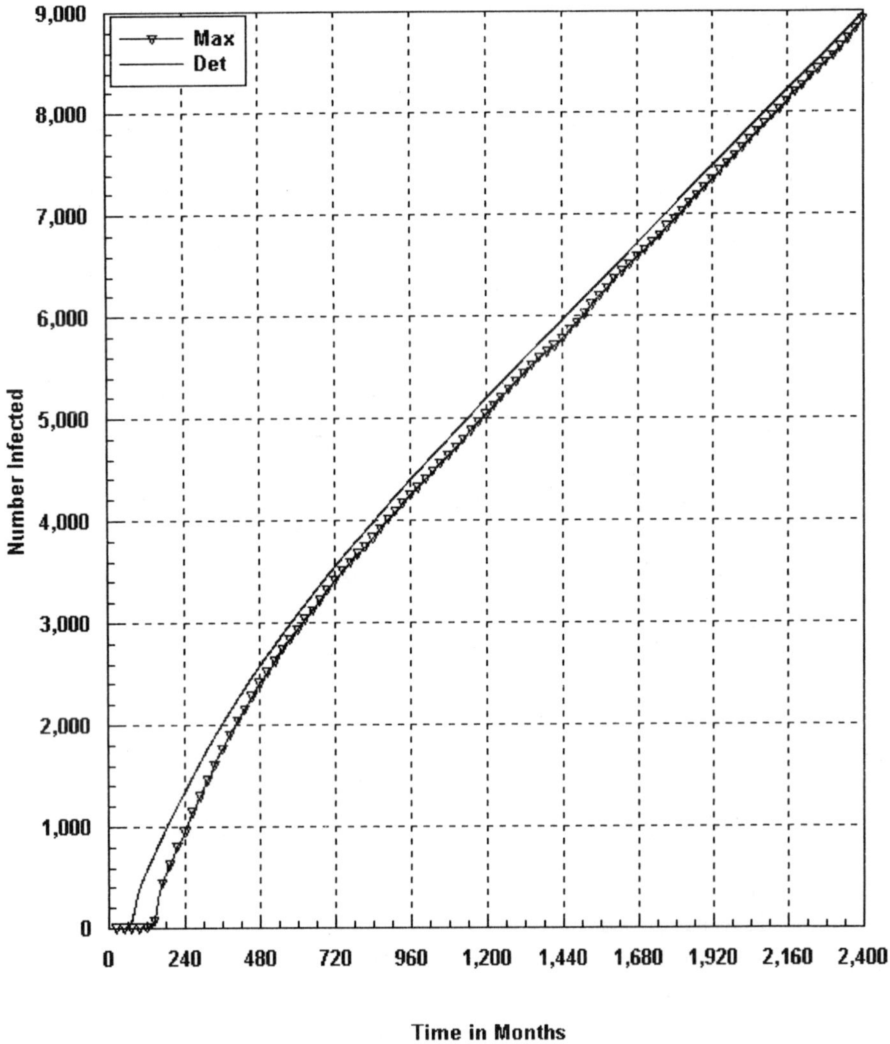

Figure 11.18.2. Cumulative Number of Infected Monogamous Individuals in Couples - 1 in 10000 Recruits Infected.

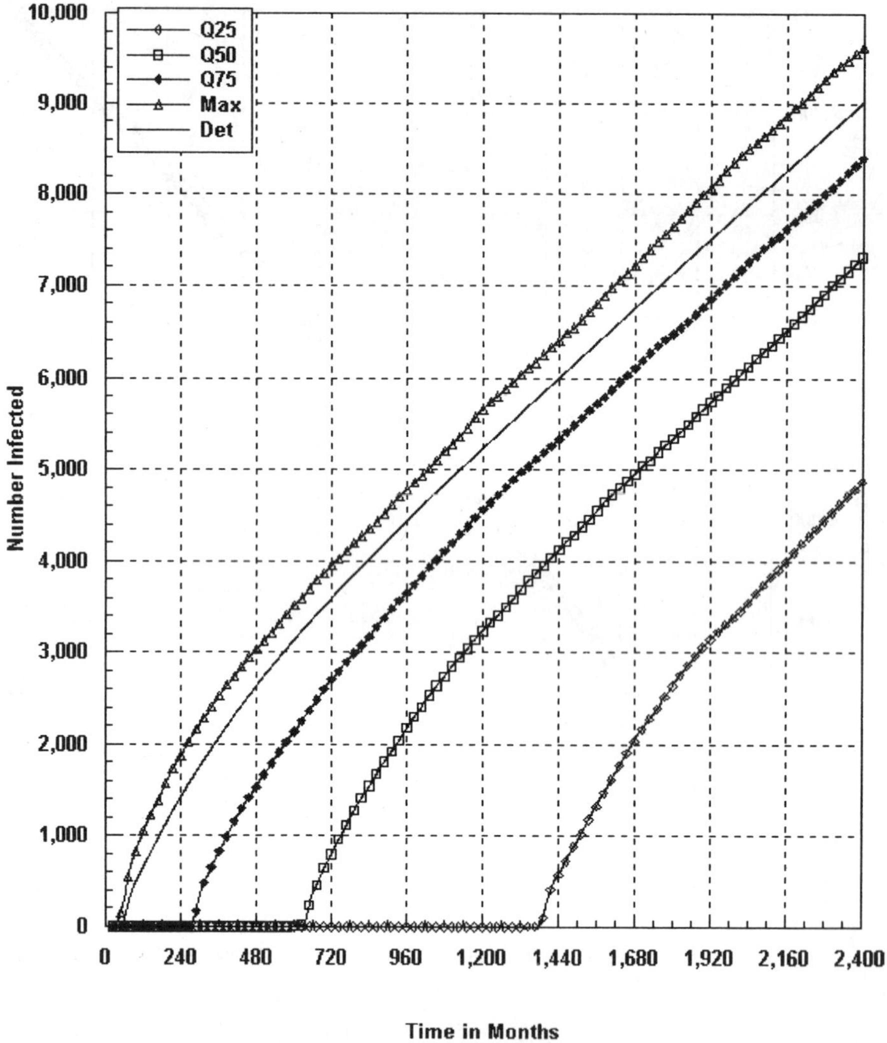

Figure 11.18.3. Cumulative Number of Infected Monogamous Individuals in Couples - 1 in 1000 Recruits Infected.

To gain some insight into how many infective individuals may need care at any epoch in the projections, the graphs of the Max and Det trajectories for the number of infected monogamous individuals in couples by epoch for recruit vector φ_1 are presented in Figure 11.18.4. The Min, Q25, Q50 and Q75 trajectories were not plotted because they were zero throughout. If an investigator relied solely on the embedded deteministic model, then the epidemic would peak somewhere between 120 and 300 months for this behavioral class, and then steadily decline to about 169 infected monogamous individuals in couples at 2400 months. Yet, according to the stochastic model, no epidemic would develop in the population with a probability of at least 0.75. Moreover, according to the Max trajectory, representing the worst case scenario of the epidemic, the number of individuals needing care at any epoch tended to lie in the range 300 to 400, indicating there was no evidence that the epidemic would peak. Relying solely on the deteministic model, the number could be underestimated by as much as 40% in those realizations in which the epidemic was most severe.

Figure 11.18.5 contains the graphs of the Q25, Q50, Q75, Max and Det trajectories for the number of infected monogamous individuals in couples by epoch for recruit vector φ_3. As might be expected, according to the trajectory of the epidemic provided by the embedded deteministic model, the epidemic would peak at about 300 to 400 individuals somewhere between 120 and 300 months. But, according to the median trajectory, Q50, the peak of the epidemic would be reached much later at about 200 individuals somewhere between 800 and 1000 months. Interestingly, the Det trajectory tended to lie at positions intermediate to those of the Q75 and Max trajectories in the early epochs, but in later epochs, the Det trajectory tended to converge to that of Q50. This suggests that, given the parameter assignments used in these projections, the Det trajectory would mimic the median trajectory of the stochastic process in the long run. Thus, with a probability of 0.50, the actual epidemic would be worse than that forecasted by the deteministic model. As in Figures 11.18.2 and 11.18.3, graphs of the quantile trajectories for recruit vector φ_2 were not presented due to lack of space, but they would occupy positions intermediate to those in Figures 11.18.4 and 11.18.5.

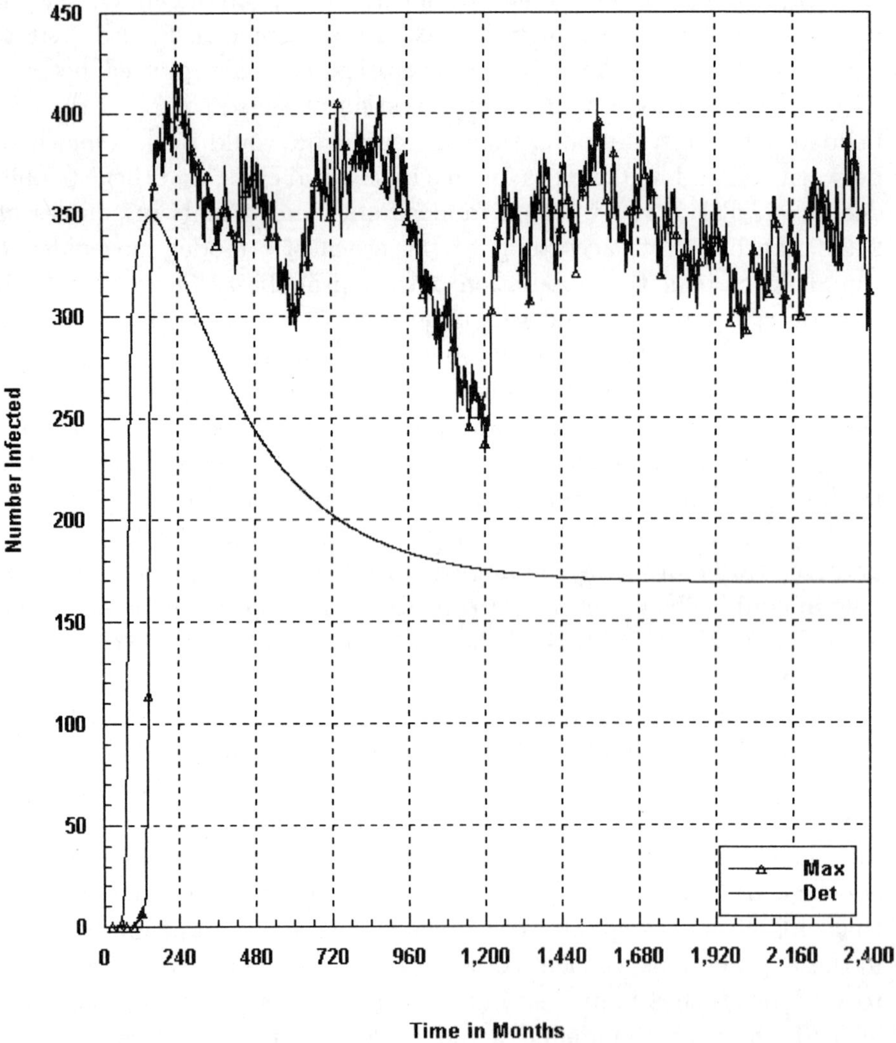

Figure 11.18.4. Number of Infected Monogamous Individuals in Couples - 1 in 10000 Recruits Infected.

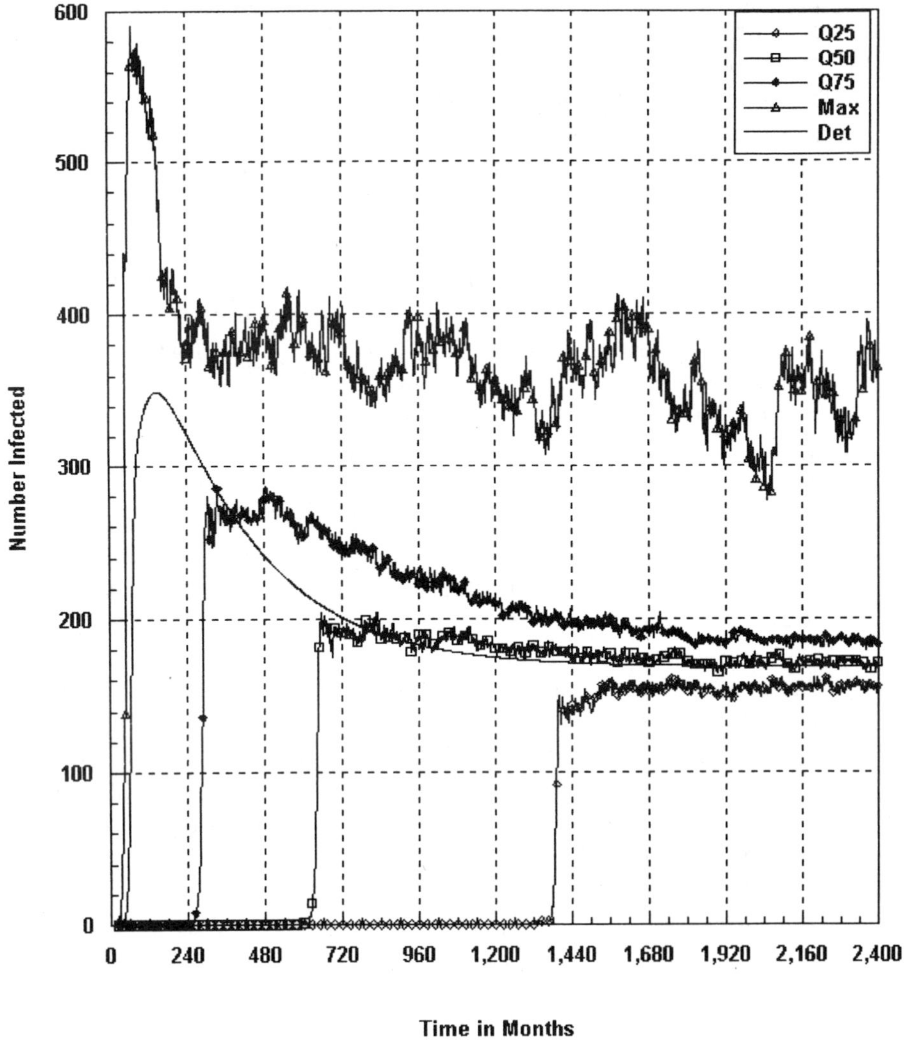

Figure 11.18.5. Number of Infected Monogamous Individuals in Couples - 1 in 1000 Recruits Infected.

11.19 References

1. F. Ball, The Threshold Behaviour of Stochastic Epidemics Among a Population Divided Into Households, *Lecture Notes in Statistics* **114**: 253-266, C. C. Heyde, Y. V. Prohorov, R. Pyke, and S. T. Rachov (eds.), *Athens Conference on Applied Probability and Time Series, I,* Springer-Verlag, Berlin, New York, Tokyo, 1995.

2. F. Ball, D. Mollison, and G. Scalia-Tomba, Epidemics with Two Levels of Mixing, *Annals of Applied Probability* **7**: 46-89, 1997.

3. S. P. Blythe et al., Towards a Unified Theory of Mixing and Pair Formation, *Mathematical Biosciences* **107**: 379-406, 1991.

4. K. Dietz and K. P. Hadeler, Epidemiological Models for Sexually Transmitted Diseases, *Journal of Mathematical Biology* **26**: 1-15, 1988.

5. M. Kretzschmar and K. Dietz, The Effect of Pair Formation and Variable Infectivity on the Spread of Infection Without Recovery, *Mathematical Biosciences* **148**: 83-113, 1998.

6. M. Kretzschmar et al., The Basic Reproduction Ratio R_0 for Sexually Transmitted Diseases in a Pair Formation Model with Two Types of Pairs, *Mathematical Biosciences* **124**: 181-205, 1994.

7. M. Kretzschmar and M. Morris, Measures of Concurrency in Networks and the Spread of Infectious Disease, *Mathematical Biosciences* **133**: 165-195, 1996.

8. C. J. Mode, A Stochastic Model for the Development of an AIDS Epidemic in a Heterosexual Population, *Mathematical Biosciences* **107**: 491-520, 1991.

9. R. Waldstaestatter, Pair Formation in Sexually Transmitted Diseases, *Lecture Notes in Biomathematics* **83**: 260-274, C. Castillo-Chavez (ed.), *Mathematical and Statistical Approaches to AIDS Epidemiology,* Springer-Verlag, 1989.

Chapter 12
HETEROSEXUAL POPULATIONS WITH PARTNERSHIPS

12.1 Introduction

In populations of heterosexuals, pairs, consisting of a female and male, often form partnerships, or couples, that may last over extended periods of time, or some females and males may choose to remain single and not participate in long-standing partnerships. Yet, in the biomathematical literature on HIV/AIDS and other sexually transmitted diseases, little work has been reported on models that accommodate single females and males as well as pairs of females and males in couples. Furthermore, most of the literature devoted to partnership models belongs to the deterministic paradigm and relatively little attention has been given to stochastic models that accommodate the formation and dissolution of partnerships in heterosexual populations. Accordingly, the purpose of this chapter is to extend the developments set forth in Chapter 11 and work toward the construction of classes of stochastic models that accommodate not only pairs of females and males in partnerships, but also single females and males.

Among those papers utilizing the stochastic paradigm, it appears that the paper by Mode[8] was among the first to attempt the formulation of a stochastic model for an epidemic of HIV/AIDS in a heterosexual population, accommodating the formation and dissolution of partnerships consisting of pairs of females and males. Because informative analyses of non-linear stochastic models are difficult to achieve using classical mathematical methods, rather than attempting to analyze the model using classical methods from applied probability in constructing it, attention was focused on developing a structure amenable to computer implementation so that computer intensive methods could be used to study some of its properties. As time passed, however, it became apparent that the formulation proposed in Mode[8] could and should be improved upon in terms of clarity of construction and ease of computer implementation. Consequently, a reformulation of the model was presented in Mode and Sleeman,[11] where some ideas from semi-Markovian processes played a basic role. In the companion paper, Sleeman and Mode,[12] a computer implementation of the model developed in Mode and Sleeman[11] was presented along with some computer experiments designed to explore threshold conditions for the model.

Among the findings of exploratory experiments was the observation that when couple formation and extra-marital sexual contacts occurred at random, the branching process approximations to the heterosexual partnership model described in Mode[10] and Mode[9] would yield useful threshold conditions as to whether an epidemic developed in a population. The reader should note that a description of these branching process approximations has been given in Chapter 9, along with the results of some computer experiments. However, if couple formation and extra-marital sexual contacts were non-random, then it was shown by numerical examples that the branching process approximations failed to provide useful threshold conditions as to whether an epidemic would develop in a population. This observation in turn suggested that the use of Jacobian matrices that arise in connection with the embedded differential equations might be more helpful in determining threshold conditions as to whether an epidemic would indeed occur in a population, whose evolution was governed by some particular point in the parameter space. The task of developing computational formulas for the elements of these Jacobian matrices, evaluated at some stationary point for the embedded differential equations, was, however, deferred to future research.

An additional limitation of the model formulated in Mode and Sleeman[11] and studied numerically in Sleeman and Mode[12] was that only $m = 1$ behavioral class with $n \geq 1$ stages of disease were included in the formulation. Nevertheless, stochastic partnership models with $m \geq 2$ behavioral classes and $n \geq 1$ stages of disease would be of more interest, because populations of heterosexuals are often heterogeneous with respect to sexual behavior. Consequently, in this chapter, a class of stochastic models will be developed with the property that $m \geq 2$ behavioral classes and $n \geq 1$ stages of disease may be accommodated in the model, and in the software necessary for its computer implementation. Furthermore, computer experiments will be reported which were designed to test the efficacy of Jacobian matrices evaluated at a stationary vector for the embedded differential equations, and to determine threshold conditions for whether an epidemic develops in a population. Like those reported in Chapter 11, most of the results reported in this chapter are new.

12.2 Types of Individuals and Partnerships

Unlike the case of one-sex populations considered in Chapter 11, when a population is viewed with respect to two sexes, partnerships consisting of a female and male may be interpreted unambiguously and there is no need to make the artificial distinction of left-hand and right-hand partners when manipulating computer arrays. However, because the population of singles consists of females and males, it will be necessary to classify both sexes by type. To this end, suppose that at any time the population of single females may be classified according to $m \geq 1$ behavioral classes and $n \geq 1$ stages of disease. As before, the symbol 0 will denote a susceptible person and the n stages of disease will be represented by $1, 2, \cdots, n$. A female will be said to be of type $\tau = (j, k)$ if she belongs to behavioral class j and is in state k with respect to disease. Then, at any time, the population of single females will consist of $m(n+1)$ types of individuals and the set of these types will be denoted by:

$$\Upsilon_f = \{\tau_f = (j, k) \mid j = 1, 2, \cdots, m;\ n = 0, 1, 2, \cdots, n\}\ . \qquad (12.2.1)$$

In reality, the number of behavioral classes for males may differ from that for females, but, to simplify the presentation, it will be assumed that the population of single males may also be classified according to $m \geq 1$ behavioral classes and $n \geq 1$ stages of disease. With this understanding, the set of $m(n+1)$ types of single males will be denoted by Υ_m with elements τ_m.

A partnership, or couple, will consist of a female and male and, by definition, is of type $\varkappa = (\tau_f, \tau_m)$ if the female is of type $\tau_f \in \Upsilon_f$ and the male is of type $\tau_m \in \Upsilon_m$. The set of couple types will be denoted by:

$$\Upsilon_c = \{\varkappa = (\tau_f, \tau_m) \mid \tau_f \in \Upsilon_f, \tau_m \in \Upsilon_m\} \ . \tag{12.2.2}$$

By definition, the left-hand partner will always be female, and the right-hand partner male, so that in the heterosexual case, each of the $m^2(n+1)^2$ types of couples can be distinguished. Let the random function $Z(t;\varkappa)$ denote the number of couples of type $\varkappa = (\tau_f, \tau_m)$ in the population at time t. Then,

$$Z(t;\tau_f,\cdot) = \sum_{\tau_m \in \Upsilon_m} Z(t;\tau_f,\tau_m) \tag{12.2.3}$$

is the number of females of type $\tau_f \in \Upsilon_f$ in the population at time t who are members of couples, and the random function $Z(t;\cdot,\tau_m)$ for males of type τ_m may be similarly and unambiguously defined.

Life cycles of all females and males end with the death of an individual, and, just as in Chapters 10 and 11, two causes of death will be recognized. But, because the latent risks governing transitions among states for females and males may differ, it will be necessary to construct life cycle models for both sexes. For the case of single females, the set of absorbing states will be denoted by:

$$\mathfrak{S}_{f1} = \{E_{f1}, E_{f2}\} \ , \tag{12.2.4}$$

where E_{f1} denotes a death from a cause other than disease and E_{f2} a death attributable to the disease under consideration. Similarly, the set $\mathfrak{S}_{m1}$ of absorbing states for single males also contains two states, E_{m1} and E_{m2}, which denote a classification of deaths by causes in the same manner as that for females. The set of transient states for the life cycle models of both females and males will correspond to sets of types of individuals defined above. Thus, if $\mathfrak{S}_{f2}$ and $\mathfrak{S}_{m2}$ denote, respectively, the sets of transient states for the life cycle models of single females and males, then $\mathfrak{S}_{f2} = \Upsilon_f$ and $\mathfrak{S}_{m2} = \Upsilon_m$. The full state spaces for single females and males will be denoted, respectively, by $\mathfrak{S}_f = \mathfrak{S}_{f1} \cup \mathfrak{S}_{f2}$

and $\mathfrak{S}_m = \mathfrak{S}_{m1} \cup \mathfrak{S}_{m2}$, and it should be noted that each of these state spaces contains $2 + m(n+1)$ elements.

The description of the state space for the life cycles for couples closely parallels that for the one-sex partnership models described in Section 11.2. For example, the set of absorbing states will be chosen as:

$$\mathfrak{S}_{c1} = \{E_{dis}, E_{f1}, E_{f2}, E_{m1}, E_{m2}\} \ , \tag{12.2.5}$$

where the state E_{dis} denotes couple dissolution and the pairs of states E_{f1}, E_{f2} and E_{m1}, E_{m2} represent the causes of death for females and males in couples. As the notation suggests, in terms of causes of death these states have the same interpretation as those in the sets of absorbing states $\mathfrak{S}_{f1}$ and $\mathfrak{S}_{m1}$ for single females and males. Just as in the one-sex model described in Chapter 11, the set of transient states of the life cycle model for couples will be chosen as $\mathfrak{S}_{c2} = \Upsilon_c$, the set of couple types defined in Eq. (12.2.2). Observe that for the two-sex model under consideration, the state space $\mathfrak{S}_c = \mathfrak{S}_{c1} \cup \mathfrak{S}_{c2}$ for couples contains $5+m^2(n+1)^2$ states. Fortunately, the description of the latent risks governing transitions among the set $\mathfrak{S}_{c2}$, which will be described in a subsequent section, closely parallels that for the one-sex model described in Chapter 11.

12.3 Matrices of Latent Risks for Life Cycle Models

The matrices of latent risks used in the construction of the semi-Markovian life cycle models for single females and males as well as for couples have many parameters in common, and, moreover, depend on the sex of an individual. Accordingly, the purpose of this section is to set forth the parameter definitions that will be used to construct the life cycle models. With respect to mortality, let the positive parameter μ_{f0} denote the death rate per unit time of females from causes other than disease, and let μ_{jk} denote the incremental death rate for females in stage $k = 1, 2, \cdots, n$, of disease. The death rates μ_{m0} and μ_{mk}, $k = 1, 2, \cdots, n$, are defined similarly for males.

As in the models described in Chapters 10 and 11, the possibilities for transitions among all stages of disease will included in the formulation, but the rates of transitions among stages may depend on the sex of an individual. With respect to females, let $\mathbf{\Gamma}_f = (\gamma_{fij})$ denote the $n \times n$ matrix of latent risks, governing transitions among stages of disease for females. For the case of $n = 2$ stages of disease, this matrix would have the simple form,

$$\mathbf{\Gamma}_f = \begin{bmatrix} 0 & \gamma_{f12} \\ \gamma_{f21} & 0 \end{bmatrix}. \tag{12.3.1}$$

Similarly, let $\mathbf{\Gamma}_m = (\gamma_{mij})$ denote the $n \times n$ matrix of latent risks, governing transitions among the stages of disease for males.

When formulating partnership models for two sexes, it seems reasonable to suppose that an individual may not remain in his or her behavioral class throughout his or her life span. Therefore, as in Chapters 10 and 11, transitions among behavioral classes will be accommodated, but the rates of transitions may depend on the sex of the individual. For the case of females, let $\mathbf{\Psi}_f = (\psi_{fij})$ denote the $m \times m$ matrix of latent risks, governing transitions among behavioral classes, and let $\mathbf{\Psi}_m = (\psi_{mij})$ denote the corresponding matrix for males. Even for the relatively simple case of $m = 3$ behavioral classes and $n = 4$ stages, the number of types of couples types can be large, for in this case $m^2(n+1)^2 = 9 \times 25 = 225$. Therefore, to avoid the necessity of processing large arrays, attention will be confined to the case of $m = 2$ behavioral classes in the software implementations of the two-sex model described in this chapter. For this case, the matrices $\mathbf{\Psi}_f$ and $\mathbf{\Psi}_m$ are 2×2, and, by way of an example, the matrix $\mathbf{\Psi}_f$ has the simple form,

$$\mathbf{\Psi}_f = \begin{bmatrix} 0 & \psi_{f12} \\ \psi_{f21} & 0 \end{bmatrix}. \tag{12.3.2}$$

With regard to the spread of infections among susceptible females and males in a population, the probabilities of infection through extra-marital sexual contacts play an important role. Given the values of the random functions of the population process up to time t, let $Q_{par}(t;\tau_f)$ denote the conditional probability that a susceptible female of type τ_f at time t becomes infected during the time interval $(t, t+h], h > 0$, through extra-marital sexual contacts, and let $Q_{par}(t;\tau_m)$ denote the corresponding conditional probability for a susceptible male of type τ_m at time t. Computational formulas for these conditional probabilities, which depend on a number of other parameters, will be derived in a subsequent section, but in this section only their definitions will be required. For a susceptible female of type τ_f, let $\lambda(\tau_f)$ denote the expected number of extra-martial male sexual partners she has per unit time and define the parameter $\lambda(\tau_m)$ similarly for males. Then, the latent risk that any susceptible female of type τ_f at time t becomes infected during the time interval $(t, t+h]$ through extra-marital sexual contacts with infectious males is $\lambda(\tau_f)Q_{par}(t;\tau_f)$. By assumption, this latent risk is the same for susceptible females who are single as well as members of couples. Similarly, whether a susceptible male of type τ_m at time t is single or a member of a couple, $\lambda(\tau_m)Q_{par}(t;\tau_m)$ is the latent risk that he is infected during the time interval $(t, t+h]$ through extra-marital sexual contacts with infectious females.

The parameters and latent risk functions just defined are sufficient to specify the matrices of latent risks in the life cycle models for single females and males. For example, let $\mathbf{\Theta}_{f21}$ denote the $m(n+1)\times 2$ matrix of latent risks for single females governing transitions from the set $\mathfrak{S}_{f2}$ of transient states to the set $\mathfrak{S}_{f1}$ of absorbing states. Then, the procedure for constructing this matrix as described in Section 10.4 (see Eq. (10.4.13) and (10.4.14)), may be used to construct this matrix for single females by using the risks of death μ_{f0} and μ_{fk}, $k = 1, 2, \cdots, n$, for females throughout. Similarly, for the life cycle model of single females, let $\mathbf{\Theta}_{f22}$ denote the $m(n+1)\times m(n+1)$ of latent risks, governing transitions among states in the set $\mathfrak{S}_{f2}$ of transient states. Then, if one uses only those latent risks pertaining to females, the procedure described in equations Eqs. (10.4.15) through (10.4.18) may be used to construct the elements of the matrix $\mathbf{\Theta}_{f22}$. In the same vein, let $\mathbf{\Theta}_{m21}$ and $\mathbf{\Theta}_{m22}$ denote the corresponding matrices of latent risks for single males. By using only those latent risks pertaining to males, the elements of these matrices may be constructed in the same manner as that described for females.

The next step in describing the structure of the model is that of focusing attention on the matrices of latent risks for the life cycle model for couples. Let $\mathbf{\Theta}_{c21}$ denote the $m^2(n+1)^2 \times 5$ matrix of latent risks, governing transitions from the set $\mathfrak{S}_{c2}$ of $m^2(n+1)^2$ transient states to the set $\mathfrak{S}_{c1}$ of five absorbing states. According to the definition of the set $\mathfrak{S}_{c1}$ of transient states in Eq. (12.2.5), the first column of the matrix $\mathbf{\Theta}_{c21}$ contains the latent risks of couple dissolution. One approach to treating these risks is to assume, as in Sections 11.3 and 11.4, that all couple types have the same risk $\delta > 0$ of dissolution per unit time. It is conceivable, however, that the risk of a couple dissolving could depend on the types of individuals in the couples. Suppose, for example, that for a couple of type $\varkappa = (\tau_f, \tau_m)$, the intrinsic positive risk for a female of type τ_f wishing to dissolve the partnership is $\delta(\tau_f)$ and that for the male is $\delta(\tau_m)$.

The larger the value of a risk δ of dissolution, the greater is the risk that a partnership actually dissolves. Therefore, for every couple type $\varkappa = (\tau_f, \tau_m) \in \Upsilon_c$, a plausible choice for the risk $\delta(\varkappa)$ couple dissolution is the function,

$$\delta(\varkappa) = \max(\delta(\tau_f), \delta(\tau_m)) \,, \tag{12.3.3}$$

indicating that the partner with the maximum wish for dissolution predominates as to whether the partnership dissolves or remains intact. If one supposes that the risk $\delta(\tau)$ for a person of type τ depends only on his or her behavioral class and not on the state with respect to disease, then for the case of $m = 2$ behavioral classes, the risk function in Eq. (12.3.3) would depend on only four parameters and could easily be implemented in the software. The remaining four columns of the matrix $\mathbf{\Theta}_{c21}$ may depend on the risks of deaths for female and males. Furthermore, the elements of these columns may be constructed by following procedures similar to those for the one-sex partnership models described in Sections 11.3 and 11.4.

To gain insight into the general case of $m \geq 2$ behavioral classes, it will be instructive to consider the case of $m = 1$ behavioral class, because the patterns that arise in the risk matrices for this case can be extended to cases in which $m \geq 2$. To illustrate the ideas, it will also be helpful to consider $n = 4$ stages of disease such as those based on CD4$^+$ counts to stage the progression of HIV/AIDS. In this case, the set,

$$\Upsilon_c = \mathfrak{S}_{c2} = \{(j, k) \mid j, k = 0, 1, 2, 3, 4\} \tag{12.3.4}$$

of couple types contains $5^2 = 25$ elements so that the matrix $\boldsymbol{\Theta}_{c21}$ of latent risks governing transitions from the set $\mathfrak{S}_{c2}$ to the set $\mathfrak{S}_{c1}$ of absorbing states is 25×5. To describe this sub-matrix succinctly, let $\mathbf{1}_5$ denote a 5×1 vector of ones, $\mathbf{0}_5$ a 5×1 vector of zeros, and define a 5×1 vector of death risks according to the state of the male by:

$$\boldsymbol{\mu}_m = \begin{bmatrix} 0 \\ \mu_{m1} \\ \mu_{m2} \\ \mu_{m3} \\ \mu_{m4} \end{bmatrix} . \tag{12.3.5}$$

Then, the 25×5 submatrix $\boldsymbol{\Theta}_{c21}$ takes the constant partitioned form,

$$\boldsymbol{\Theta}_{c21} = \begin{bmatrix} \boldsymbol{\delta} & \boldsymbol{\mu}_{f0} & \mathbf{0}_5 & \boldsymbol{\mu}_{m0} & \boldsymbol{\mu}_m \\ \boldsymbol{\delta} & \boldsymbol{\mu}_{f0} & \boldsymbol{\mu}_{f1} & \boldsymbol{\mu}_{m0} & \boldsymbol{\mu}_m \\ \boldsymbol{\delta} & \boldsymbol{\mu}_{f0} & \boldsymbol{\mu}_{f2} & \boldsymbol{\mu}_{m0} & \boldsymbol{\mu}_m \\ \boldsymbol{\delta} & \boldsymbol{\mu}_{f0} & \boldsymbol{\mu}_{f3} & \boldsymbol{\mu}_{m0} & \boldsymbol{\mu}_m \\ \boldsymbol{\delta} & \boldsymbol{\mu}_{f0} & \boldsymbol{\mu}_{f4} & \boldsymbol{\mu}_{m0} & \boldsymbol{\mu}_m \end{bmatrix} , \tag{12.3.6}$$

where $\boldsymbol{\mu}_{m0} = \mu_{m0}\mathbf{1}_5$, $\boldsymbol{\mu}_{fj} = \mu_{fj}\mathbf{1}_5$, $j = 0, 1, 2, 3, 4$, $\boldsymbol{\delta} = \delta\mathbf{1}_5$ and δ is the constant rate of dissolution for each couple type. For cases $m \geq 2$ and $n = 4$, the $m^2(n+1)^2 \times 5$ matrix $\boldsymbol{\Theta}_{c21}$ would consist of 25×5 sub-matrices whose forms would be similar to that of Eq. (12.3.6).

To describe the structure the 25×25 matrix $\boldsymbol{\Theta}_{c22}(t)$ of latent risks governing transitions among states in the set $\mathfrak{S}_{c2}$ of transient states for couples, it will be helpful to partition $\mathfrak{S}_{c2}$ according the state of the females. Thus, let

$$A(j) = \{(j, k) \mid k = 0, 1, 2, 3, 4\} \tag{12.3.7}$$

again denote the set of couple types such that the female is in state $j = 0, 1, 2, 3, 4$. Then, a lexicographic ordering of the set of 25 couple types is:

$$\mathfrak{S}_{c2} = \{A(0), A(1), A(2), A(3), A(4)\} . \tag{12.3.8}$$

As in previous discussions, this ordering of couple types will be used to order the rows and columns of the matrix $\boldsymbol{\Theta}_{c22}(t)$.

With respect to transitions among stages of disease, it will assumed that the matrix of latent risks for females has the form,

$$\mathbf{\Gamma}_f = \begin{bmatrix} 0 & \gamma_{f12} & 0 & 0 \\ \gamma_{f21} & 0 & \gamma_{f23} & 0 \\ 0 & \gamma_{f32} & 0 & \gamma_{f34} \\ 0 & 0 & \gamma_{f43} & 0 \end{bmatrix}. \tag{12.3.9}$$

Moreover, it will be assumed that the 4×4 matrix $\mathbf{\Gamma}_m$ of latent risks for males has the same form. Implicit in these assumptions is that the 25×25 matrix $\mathbf{\Theta}_{c22}(t)$ of latent risks governing transitions among states in the set of transient couple types during any small time interval, may be represented in the partitioned form,

$$\begin{bmatrix} \mathbf{\Theta}_{c22}(t;0,0) & \mathbf{\Theta}_{c22}(t;0,1) & \mathbf{0}_{5\times 5} & \mathbf{0}_{5\times 5} & \mathbf{0}_{5\times 5} \\ \mathbf{0}_{5\times 5} & \mathbf{\Theta}_{c22}(t;1,1) & \mathbf{\Theta}_{c22}(t;1,2) & \mathbf{0}_{5\times 5} & \mathbf{0}_{5\times 5} \\ \mathbf{0}_{5\times 5} & \mathbf{\Theta}_{c22}(t;2,1) & \mathbf{\Theta}_{c22}(t;2,2) & \mathbf{\Theta}_{c22}(t;2,3) & \mathbf{0}_{5\times 5} \\ \mathbf{0}_{5\times 5} & \mathbf{0}_{5\times 5} & \mathbf{\Theta}_{c22}(t;3,2) & \mathbf{\Theta}_{c22}(t;3,3) & \mathbf{\Theta}_{c22}(t;3,4) \\ \mathbf{0}_{5\times 5} & \mathbf{0}_{5\times 5} & \mathbf{0}_{5\times 5} & \mathbf{\Theta}_{c22}(t;4,3) & \mathbf{\Theta}_{c22}(t;4,4) \end{bmatrix}. \tag{12.3.10}$$

Each of the sub-matrices in Eq. (12.3.10) is 5×5, and the sub-matrix $\mathbf{\Theta}_{c22}(t;0,0)$ contains those latent risks governing transitions of the set $A(0)$ of transient states into itself, corresponding to those cases in which the male members of couples change states. On the other hand, the sub-matrix $\mathbf{\Theta}_{c22}(t;0,1)$ contains those latent risks governing transitions from the set $A(0)$ of couple types into the set $A(1)$, and represents those cases in which the female members of couples change states. Also implicit in the structure of the matrix $\mathbf{\Theta}_{c22}(t)$ is the assumption that if a female is in state 0, then, during any small time interval, the only transition possible is $0 \to 1$, indicating that she has been infected by infectious male. Similar remarks hold regarding the infection of susceptible males.

All 5×5 matrices on the quasi-principal diagonal in Eq. (12.3.10) have the same form. Let γ_{mc} denote the expected number of marital sexual contacts per unit time, and let $q_m(j)$ be the conditional probability that a susceptible male is infected per sexual contact when the female is in state $j = 0, 1, 2, 3, 4$. By definition, $q_m(0) = 0$, because a susceptible male cannot be infected by a non-infected female. The latent risk that a susceptible male of type τ_m is infected by an infectious female during any small time interval is $\lambda(\tau_m)Q_{par}(t;\tau_m) + \gamma_{mc}q_m(j)$. For $j = 0, 1, 2, 3, 4$, let

$$\mathbf{\Phi}_m(\tau_m, j) = \begin{pmatrix} \lambda(\tau_m)Q_{par}(t;\tau_m) + \gamma_{mc}q_m(j) & 0 & 0 & 0 \end{pmatrix} \quad (12.3.11)$$

denote a 1×4 vector, and let $\mathbf{0}_4$ denote a 4×1 vector of zeros. Then, for $j = 0, 1, 2, 3, 4$, the matrices on the quasi-diagonal in Eq. (12.3.10) have the partitioned form,

$$\mathbf{\Theta}_{c22}(t; j, j) = \begin{bmatrix} 0 & \mathbf{\Phi}_m(\tau_m, j) \\ \mathbf{0}_4 & \mathbf{\Gamma}_m \end{bmatrix} . \quad (12.3.12)$$

All sub-matrices off the quasi-principal diagonal in Eq. (12.3.10) have a diagonal form. Let $q_f(k)$ denote the probability that a susceptible female is infected per sexual contact with a male in state $k = 0, 1, 2, 3, 4$. By definition, $q_f(0) = 0$. A transition from the set of couple types $A(0)$ to the set $A(1)$ indicates that a susceptible female member of a couple has been infected. Hence, the matrix $\mathbf{\Theta}_{c22}(t; 0, 1)$ has the diagonal form

$$\mathbf{\Theta}_{c22}(t; 0, 1) = diag\left(\lambda(\tau_f)Q_{par}(t;\tau_f) + \gamma_{mc}q_f(k) \mid k = 0, 1, 2, 3, 4\right) . \quad (12.3.13)$$

On the other hand, a transition from the set of couple types $A(1)$ to the set $A(2)$ indicates that the female member of a couple in stage 1 of disease moved to state 2 during a small time interval. Therefore, the matrix $\mathbf{\Theta}_{c22}(t; 1, 2)$ has the diagonal form,

$$\mathbf{\Theta}_{c22}(t; 1, 2) = \gamma_{f12}\mathbf{I}_5 , \quad (12.3.14)$$

where $\mathbf{I}_5$ is a 5×5 identity matrix. The other matrices off the quasi-principal diagonal in Eq. (12.3.10) have a similar diagonal form, depending only on the transition rates for transitions among stages of disease for females.

To illustrate how the ideas just outlined may be extended to cases of $m \geq 2$ behavioral classes and $n \geq 1$ stages of disease, the structure of the matrix $\mathbf{\Theta}_{c22}(t)$ of latent risks for the case of $m = 2$

behavioral classes and $n = 4$ stages of disease will be considered. From now on, to simplify the notation, the argument t will be dropped. For a fixed pair j_1 and j_2 of behavioral classes, let $A(j_1, j_2)$ denote the set of couple types:

$$A(j_1, j_2) = \{\varkappa = ((j_1, k_1), (j_2, k_2)) \mid k_1, k_2 = 0, 1, 2, \cdots, n\} \ , \quad (12.3.15)$$

where the pairs (k_1, k_2) are arranged in lexicographical order. Then, as in Section 11.4, if the set $\mathfrak{S}_{c2}$ of couple types is ordered such that the pairs (j_1, j_2) are arranged in lexicographical order, and for each pair (j_1, j_2) of behavioral classes, the pairs (k_1, k_2) of states of disease are also arranged in lexicographical order, then the matrix $\mathbf{\Theta}_{c22}$ takes the partitioned form,

$$\begin{bmatrix} \mathbf{\Theta}_{c22}(1,1;1,1) & \mathbf{\Theta}_{c22}(1,1;1,2) & \mathbf{\Theta}_{c22}(1,1;2,1) & \mathbf{0}_{25\times 25} \\ \mathbf{\Theta}_{c22}(1,2;1,1) & \mathbf{\Theta}_{c22}(1,2;1,2) & \mathbf{0}_{25\times 25} & \mathbf{\Theta}_{c22}(1,2;2,2) \\ \mathbf{\Theta}_{c22}(2,1;1,1) & \mathbf{0}_{25\times 25} & \mathbf{\Theta}_{c22}(2,1;2,1) & \mathbf{\Theta}_{c22}(2,1;2,2) \\ \mathbf{0}_{25\times 25} & \mathbf{\Theta}_{c22}(2,2;1,2) & \mathbf{\Theta}_{c22}(2,2;2,1) & \mathbf{\Theta}_{c22}(2,2;2,2) \end{bmatrix} . \quad (12.3.16)$$

The set of couple types $\mathfrak{S}_{c2}$ contains $m^2(n+1)^2 = 4 \times 25 = 100$ elements so that $\mathbf{\Theta}_{c22}$ is a 100×100 matrix and each sub-matrix is 25×25. The sub-matrices on the quasi-principal diagonal contain those latent risks such that either the female or male member of a couple may change state with respect to disease during any small time interval. Therefore, the elements of each of the matrices in the set

$$\{\mathbf{\Theta}_{c22}(1,1;1,1), \mathbf{\Theta}_{c22}(1,2;1,2), \mathbf{\Theta}_{c22}(2,1;2,1), \mathbf{\Theta}_{c22}(2,2;2,2)\} \quad (12.3.17)$$

of 25×25 sub-matrices on the quasi-principal diagonal may be constructed by following the procedure outlined in the construction of the matrix in Eq. (12.3.10). However, care must to taken to assure that the λ-parameters, such as those appearing in Eq. (12.3.13), correspond to those for the behavioral class or classes to which the female and male member of a couple belong.

The matrices off the quasi-principal diagonal also have a simple form. For example, the matrix $\mathbf{\Theta}_{c22}(1,1;1,2)$ contains those latent risks such that, during any small time interval, a male member of a couple makes a transition from behavioral class 1 to behavioral class 2. Let $\mathbf{I}_{25}$ denote a 25×25 identity matrix. Then, it can seen that:

$$\mathbf{\Theta}_{c22}(1,1;1,2) = \psi_{m12}\mathbf{I}_{25}\ . \tag{12.3.18}$$

Similarly, the matrix $\mathbf{\Theta}_{c22}(1,1;2,1)$ contains those latent risks such that, during any time small interval, a female member of a couple undergoes a transition from behavioral class 1 to behavioral class 2. Therefore,

$$\mathbf{\Theta}_{c22}(1,1;2,1) = \psi_{f12}\mathbf{I}_{25}\ . \tag{12.3.19}$$

Analogous remarks hold for the other non-zero sub-matrices off the principal diagonal of Eq. (12.3.16).

12.4 Marital Couple Formation

A fundamental problem in formulating models for epidemics of sexually transmitted diseases is that of modelling social contacts among females and males in the singles population that may lead to the formation of couples as defined in a previous section. Many of the principles discussed in connection with couple formation in the one-sex set models forth in Section 11.6 continue to apply, but for populations with two sexes, many of the details of the couple formation process differ. Suppose, for example, that at time t there are $X(t;\tau_f)$ and $Y(t;\tau_m)$ single females and males of types $\tau_f \in \mathfrak{S}_{f2}$ and $\tau_m \in \mathfrak{S}_{m2}$, respectively, in the population. Given these numbers of singles, let the random function $N_{CF}(t;\varkappa)$ denote the potential number of couples of type $\varkappa = (\tau_f, \tau_m)$ that may be formed during any time interval $(t, t+h]$. The purpose of this section is to outline a new procedure for computing realizations of the random function $N_{CF}(t;\varkappa)$ for every pair $\varkappa \in \mathfrak{S}_{c2}$. Then, given $N_{CF}(t;\varkappa)$, the next step will be that of modelling the random function $Z_{CF}(t+h;\varkappa)$, denoting the actual number of couples of type $\varkappa$ formed during this interval from the potential number $N_{CF}(t;\varkappa)$.

Two natural constraints arise when considering the potential number of pairs of females and males; namely, the number of females (males) in contact pairs occurring during $(t, t+h]$ cannot exceed the number of single females (males) in the population at time t. Therefore, the inequalities,

$$\sum_{\tau_m \in \mathfrak{S}_{m2}} N_{CF}(t;\tau_f,\tau_m) \le X(t;\tau_f) \tag{12.4.1}$$

and

$$\sum_{\tau_f \in \mathfrak{S}_{f2}} N_{CF}(t;\tau_f,\tau_m) \le Y(t;\tau_m) \tag{12.4.2}$$

must hold with probability one for all τ_f, τ_m and t. In deterministic formulations, it is comparatively straightforward to construct contact functions such that these inequalities hold. However, in stochastic models, the construction of the random functions $N_{CF}(t;\varkappa)$, such that the above inequalities hold with probability one, involves more subtle chains of reasoning. It will be noted that by construction the inequalities $0 \le Z_{CF}(t+h;\varkappa) \le N_{CF}(t;\varkappa)$ will hold with probability one for all t and couple types $\varkappa$. Therefore, if the inequalities in Eqs. (12.4.1) and (12.4.2) hold with probability one, then so will similar inequalities for the random functions $Z_{CF}(t+h;\varkappa)$ for all $\varkappa \in \mathfrak{S}_{c2}$ and t.

A basic component of the procedure for constructing these random functions is the idea of a contact probability. Given the evolution of the process up to time t, let $\gamma_f(t;\tau_f,\tau_m)$ be the conditional probability that a single female of type τ_f contacts a single male of type τ_m. Similarly, let $\gamma_m(t;\tau_m,\tau_f)$ be the conditional probability that a single male of type τ_m contacts a single female of type τ_f. The procedure used to construct these conditional probabilities is similar to that described in Section 11.5, and further details will be given subsequently in this section. As they should, all contact probabilities for females lie in the interval $[0,1]$ and satisfy the conditions:

$$\sum_{\tau_m \in \mathfrak{S}_{m2}} \gamma_f(t;\tau_f,\tau_m) = 1 \tag{12.4.3}$$

for all t and $\tau_f \in \mathfrak{S}_{f2}$, and those for males satisfy a similar set of conditions. In what follows, the symbol,

$$\mathbf{\Gamma}_f(t;\tau_f) = (\gamma_f(t;\tau_f,\tau_m) \mid \tau_m \in \mathfrak{S}_{m2}) \tag{12.4.4}$$

will stand for the vector of contact probabilities for single females of type τ_f in the population at time t and the corresponding vector $\mathbf{\Gamma}_m(t;\tau_m)$ for single males of type τ_m is defined similarly.

For single females of type τ_f at time t, let $Z_f(t;\tau_f,\tau_m)$ denote the number of single males of type τ_m selected as potential partners, given values of the random functions for singles at time t. And, similarly, let $Z_m(t;\tau_m,\tau_f)$ be the number of females of type τ_f selected by single males of type τ_m as potential partners. It will be assumed that the vector of random variables:

$$\mathbf{Z}_f(t;\tau_f) = \{Z_f(t;\tau_f,\tau_m) \mid \tau_m \in \mathfrak{S}_{m2}\} \tag{12.4.5}$$

has a conditional multinomial distribution with index $X(t;\tau_f)$ and probability vector $\mathbf{\Gamma}_f(t;\tau_f)$. In symbols,

$$\mathbf{Z}_f(t;\tau_f) \sim CMultinom(X(t;\tau_f),\mathbf{\Gamma}_f(t;\tau_f))\ . \tag{12.4.6}$$

Similarly, the vector $\mathbf{Z}_m(t;\tau_m)$ of potential female partners for males of type τ_m will be assumed to have a conditional multinomial distribution with index $Y(t;\tau_m)$ and probability vector $\mathbf{\Gamma}_m(t;\tau_m)$. Then, because the number of pair-wise contacts of type (τ_f,τ_m) cannot exceed the number of females of type τ_f seeking males of type τ_m or the number of males of type τ_m seeking females of type τ_f, it follows that a plausible choice for the potential number of couples of $\varkappa = (\tau_f,\tau_m)$ formed during $(t,t+h]$ is:

$$N_{CF}(t;\tau_f,\tau_m) = \min\{Z_f(t;\tau_f,\tau_m), Z_m(t;\tau_m,\tau_f)\}\ . \tag{12.4.7}$$

It is important to observe that the algorithm used to compute realizations of the random function $N_{CF}(t;j,k)$ is such that the inequalities in Eqs. (12.4.1) and (12.4.2) will indeed hold with probability one. For, if the vector $\mathbf{Z}_f(t;j)$ follows a multinomial distribution, then:

$$\sum_{\tau_m\in\mathfrak{S}_{m2}} Z_f(t;\tau_f,\tau_m) = X(t;\tau_f) \tag{12.4.8}$$

with probability one for all t and $\tau_f \in \mathfrak{S}_{f2}$. But,

$$\sum_{\tau_m\in\mathfrak{S}_{m2}} N_{CF}(t;\tau_f,\tau_m) \le \sum_{\tau_m\in\mathfrak{S}_{m2}} Z_f(t;\tau_f,\tau_m) = X(t;\tau_f) \tag{12.4.9}$$

with probability one for all τ_f and t. Similarly, for the case of males of type τ_m, it can be seen that:

$$\sum_{\tau_f \in \mathfrak{S}_{f2}} N_{CF}(t; \tau_f, \tau_m) \leq \sum_{\tau_f \in \mathfrak{S}_{f2}} Z_m(t; \tau_f, \tau_m) = Y(t; \tau_m) \qquad (12.4.10)$$

holds with probability one for all τ_m and t.

The next step in developing a model for couple formation is to describe a procedure for calculating realizations of the random function $Z_{CF}(t+h; \varkappa)$, the actual number of couples formed during the time interval $(t, t+h]$ of type $\varkappa \in \mathfrak{S}_{f2} \times \mathfrak{S}_{m2}$. Given $N_{CF}(t; \varkappa)$,let $\rho(\varkappa)$ be the risk function for couple formation among contacts of type $\varkappa$. Then, $q_{CF}(\varkappa; h) = 1 - \exp[-\rho(\varkappa)h]$ is the conditional probability that a couple of type $\varkappa$ is formed during $(t, t+h]$. It will assumed that $Z_{CF}(t+h; \varkappa)$ has a conditional binomial distribution with index $N_{CF}(t; \varkappa)$ and probability $q_{CF}(\varkappa; h)$. In symbols,

$$Z_{CF}(t+h; \varkappa) \sim CBinom\left(N_{CF}(t; \varkappa), q_{CF}(\varkappa; h)\right) . \qquad (12.4.11)$$

From the above developments, it can be seen that an algorithm for computing the number $N_{CF}(t; \varkappa)$ of potential pair-wise contacts of type $\varkappa$ during the time interval $(t, t+h]$ could be developed without using any explicit functional forms for the contact probabilities $\gamma_f(t; \tau_f, \tau_m)$ and $\gamma_m(t; \tau_m, \tau_f)$. In formulating models of these probabilities, it seems reasonable to accommodate assortative schemes in the selection of potential sexual partners, because it is widely recognized that such selections in a population may not occur at random. Given a female of type τ_f, let $\alpha_f(\tau_f, \tau_m)$ be the conditional probability she finds a male of type τ_m acceptable as a sexual partner. Similarly, let $\alpha_m(\tau_m, \tau_f)$ be the conditional probability that a single male of type τ_m finds a female of type τ_f acceptable as a sexual partner. Unless these acceptance probabilities are parameterized succinctly, the number of parameters may become unwieldy. If one supposes that types of females and males may be quantified, then the acceptance probabilities can be expressed in terms of distance functions, as described in Chapter 11.

Accordingly, let $\alpha_f(\tau_1, \tau_2)$ denote the conditional probability that a single female of τ_f finds a single male of type τ_m acceptable as a marriage partner. For a single female of type $\tau_f = (j_1, k_1)$ and a single male of type $\tau_m = (j_2, k_2)$, this function will be chosen as:

$$\alpha_f(\tau_f, \tau_m) = \exp\left[-\left(\beta_{f1} \mid j_1 - j_2 \mid + \beta_{f2} \mid k_1 - k_2 \mid\right)\right] , \tag{12.4.12}$$

where β_{f1} and β_{f2} are non-negative parameters. The acceptance probability $\alpha_m(\tau_m, \tau_j)$ for single males is defined similarly in terms of two non-negative parameters β_{m1} and β_{m2}. At time t, the relative frequency of type τ_f in the single female population is:

$$U_f(t;\tau_f) = \frac{X(t;\tau_f)}{X(t;\cdot)} , \tag{12.4.13}$$

where

$$X(t;\cdot) = \sum_{\tau_f \in \mathfrak{S}_{f2}} X(t;\tau_f) > 0 \tag{12.4.14}$$

is the total size of the single female population. The relative frequency $U_m(t;\tau_m)$ of single males of type τ_m in the male population at time t is defined similarly, provided that the total size of male population is not zero.

By the law of total probability, the probability that at time t a female of type τ_f has contact with some single male is

$$\sum_{\tau_m \in \mathfrak{S}_{m2}} U_m(t;\tau_m)\alpha_f(\tau_f, \tau_m) , \tag{12.4.15}$$

and by Bayes' formula, the conditional probability that this contact is with a male of type τ_m is

$$\gamma_f(t;\tau_f,\tau_m) = \frac{U_m(t;\tau_m)\alpha_f(\tau_f,\tau_m)}{\sum_{\nu \in \mathfrak{S}_{m2}} U_m(t;\nu)\alpha_f(\tau_f,\nu)} . \tag{12.4.16}$$

Similarly, the conditional probability that a single male of type τ_m has a contact with a single female of type τ_f is given by the formula

$$\gamma_m(t;\tau_m,\tau_f) = \frac{U_f(t,\tau_f)\alpha_m(\tau_m,\tau_f)}{\sum_{\nu \in \mathfrak{S}_{f2}} U_f(t;\nu)\alpha_m(\tau_m,\nu)} . \tag{12.4.17}$$

It is easy to see that if $\beta_{f1} = \beta_{m1} = \beta_{f2} = \beta_{m2} = 0$, then it is the case that $\gamma_f(t;\tau_f,\tau_m) = U_m(t;\tau_m)$ and $\gamma_m(t;\tau_m,\tau_f) = U_f(t,\tau_f)$ so that the selection of potential sexual partners would, by definition, be random. It can also be seen that the larger the values of β-parameters, the greater the probabilities of females and males preferring potential sexual contacts with partners of their own types. As has been demonstrated in Chapters 10 and 11, the β-parameters play a significant role in determining threshold conditions such that an epidemic will or will not develop in a population of susceptibles following the introduction of a few infectives.

12.5 Probabilities of Being Infected by Extra-Marital Contacts

To derive a formula for the probability that a susceptible female of type $\tau_f = (j_1, 0)$ at time t is infected during the time interval $(t, t+h]$, the procedures used in Section 12.4 to construct the model of couple formation will be extended. Although the acceptance probabilities for female extra-marital contacts will have the same functional form, it will be assumed that those for couple formation and extra-marital sexual contacts may differ. Thus, let $\alpha_{em}(\tau_1, \tau_2)$ denote the conditional probability that a female of type $\tau_f = (j_1, k_1)$ finds a male of type $\tau_2 = (j_2, k_2)$ acceptable as an extra-marital sexual partner. As in Section 12.4, by assumption this probability has the form,

$$\alpha_{fem}(\tau_f, \tau_m) = \exp\left[-\left(\beta_{fem1} \mid j_1 - j_2 \mid + \beta_{fem2} \mid k_1 - k_2 \mid\right)\right] , \tag{12.5.1}$$

where β_{fem1} and β_{fem2} are non-negative parameters. An analogous extra-marital acceptance probability $\alpha_{mem}(\tau_m, \tau_f)$ for males is defined similarly in terms of two non-negative parameters β_{mem1} and β_{mem2}.

Given a female of type τ_f at time t who engages in extra-marital contacts, let $\gamma_{fem}(t; \tau_f, \tau_m)$ be the conditional probability that a female of type τ_f has contact with a potential extra-marital male sexual partner of type τ_m during the time interval $(t, t+h]$. This conditional probability will be defined in a manner similar to that of $\gamma_c(t; \tau_f, \tau_m)$ in Eq. (12.4.16), but for the case of extra-marital sexual contacts, the frequencies $U_m(t; \tau_1)$ for males must be defined differently. An extra-marital contact probability for males $\gamma_{mem}(t; \tau_m, \tau_f)$ will be defined similarly.

Because the risk of a susceptible being infected by extra-marital sexual contacts may differ from marital contacts, allowance will be made for the probabilities of infection per extra-marital contact to differ from those of marital contacts. Accordingly, let $p_{fem}(k)$ be the probability that a susceptible female escapes infection per sexual contact, when her male partner is in transient state k with respect to disease. Since non-infected males cannot transmit an infectious agent to their susceptible female sexual partners, $p_{fem}(0) = 1$ but $0 \leq p_{fem}(k) \leq 1$ for stage for $1 \leq k \leq n$. The probability that a susceptible female is infected per sexual contact when her male partner is in state k with respect to disease is $q_f(k) = 1 - p_f(k)$. The corresponding probabilities for males $p_{mem}(j)$ and $q_{mem}(j)$ for females in state j with respect to disease. The notation just introduced emphasizes that, by assumption, whether a susceptible female or male becomes infected depends only the disease state of his sexual partner. But, in what follows the notation will need to be extended to take into account the behavioral class of an individual. For example, if a susceptible female is of type $\tau_f = (j_1, 0)$ and the male with whom she has a sexual contact is of type $\tau_m = (j_2, k_2)$, then it will be understood that $p_{fem}(\tau_m) = p_{fem}(k_2)$, and the probability $p_{mem}(\tau_f)$ will be defined similarly.

The problem of formulating a model of extra-marital sexual contacts may be approached in several ways, but in this chapter it will be assumed that such sexual contacts may occur among singles, marital partners other than one's own, or among singles and those in partnerships. At any time t,

$$X_T(t; \tau_f) = X(t; \tau_f) + \sum_{\tau_m \in \mathfrak{S}_{m2}} Z(t; \tau_f, \tau_m) \tag{12.5.2}$$

is the total number of females of type τ_f in the population, where $Z(t; \tau_f, \tau_m)$ is the number of couples of type (τ_f, τ_m) at time t. A random function $Y_T(t, \tau_m)$ may be defined similarly for males of type τ_m at time t . With respect to extra-marital sexual contacts, the frequency of females of type τ_f in the population at time t is:

$$U_{fem}(t; \tau_f) = \frac{X_T(t; \tau_f)}{X_T(t; \cdot)}\ , \tag{12.5.3}$$

where

$$X_T(t;\cdot) = \sum_{\tau_f \in \mathfrak{S}_{f2}} X_T(t;\tau_f) > 0 \tag{12.5.4}$$

is the total number of females in the population at time $t > 0$. A similar frequency $U_{mem}(t;k)$ for males of type τ_m at time t may be defined.

Now consider a time interval $(t, t+h]$ and let the random function $N_{EMP}(t;\tau_f,\tau_m)$ denote the total number of extra-marital sexual contacts of type (τ_f,τ_m) occurring during $(t,t+h]$, involving females of type τ_f and males of type τ_m. A procedure similar to that outlined in Eqs. (12.4.12) through (12.4.17) may be used to calculate realizations of the random function $N_{EMP}(t;j,k)$. Let $\alpha_{fem}(\tau_f,\tau_m)$ be the conditional probability that a female of type τ_f finds a male of type τ_m acceptable as an extra-marital sexual partner and define a conditional probability $\alpha_{mem}(\tau_m,\tau_f)$ similarly for males of type τ_m finding females of type τ_f acceptable as sexual partners (see Eq. (12.5.1)). Then, by proceeding as in (12.4.12) – (12.4.17), extra-marital contact probabilities $\gamma_{fem}(t;\tau_f,\tau_m)$ for females and $\gamma_{mem}(t;\tau_m,\tau_f)$ for males may be computed as functions of the frequencies $\{U_{fem}(t;\tau_f) \mid \tau_f \in \mathfrak{S}_{f2}\}$ and $\{U_{mem}(t;\tau_m) \mid \tau_m \in \mathfrak{S}_{m2}\}$ and the acceptance probabilities by applications of Bayes' theorem. Finally, realizations of the random function $N_{EMP}(t;\tau_f,\tau_m)$ may be computed by utilizing a procedure similar to that used in computing realizations of $N_{CF}(t;\tau_f,\tau_m)$ (see Eq. (12.4.7)).

During any time interval $(t,t+h]$, a female or male may have several extra-marital sexual partners. For a female of type τ_f, let the random function $\rho_{fem}(t;\tau_f,\tau_m)$ denote the frequency of sexual contacts with males of type τ_m. Setting down an algorithm for calculating this frequency, pair-wise constraints for finding extra-marital sexual partners will be taken into account, which, under the frequency interpretation of probability, induce a set of conditional distributions defined as $\{\rho_{fem}(t;\tau_f,\tau_m) \mid \tau_m \in \mathfrak{S}_{m2}\}$ for every $\tau_f \in \mathfrak{S}_{f2}$. The total number of extra-marital sexual partnerships for susceptible females of type τ_f occurring during the time interval $(t,t+h]$ is:

$$\sum_{\tau \in \mathfrak{S}_{m2}} N_{EMP}(t;\tau_f,\tau)\,. \tag{12.5.5}$$

Therefore, the frequency in the population for extra-marital contacts of type (τ_f, τ_m) occurring during the time interval $(t, t+h]$, by definition, is:

$$\rho_{fem}(t; \tau_f, \tau_m) = \frac{N_{EMP}(t; \tau_f, \tau_m)}{\sum_{\tau \in \mathfrak{S}_{m2}} N_{EMP}(t; \tau_f, \tau)} \, . \tag{12.5.6}$$

A frequency $\rho_{mem}(t; \tau_m, \tau_f)$ of extra-marital contacts for susceptible males of type τ_m and females of type $\tau_f \in \mathfrak{S}_{f2}$ may be computed using a similar formula.

For any time interval $(t, t+h]$, let the random variable $N_{emf}(h)$ with range $R_{N_{emf}} = \{n \mid n = 1, 2, \cdots\}$, denote the number of sexual contacts per extra-marital male partner for any female (emf) in the population. In this case, an extra-marital partner is not counted unless there is at least one sexual contact. It will be assumed that this random variable follows a Poisson process with parameter $\eta_f > 0$ and location parameter 1 so that its expectation is $E[N_{emf}(h)] = 1 + \eta_f h$. In symbols $N_{emf}(h) \sim Pois(1, \eta_f h)$. By an argument similar to that used in deriving Eq. (11.6.5), it can be shown that:

$$p_{emf}(t; \tau_f, \tau_m; h) = p_{fem}(\tau_m) \exp[-\eta_f h q_{fem}(\tau_m)] \tag{12.5.7}$$

is the probability that a susceptible female in state type τ_f escapes infection during any time interval when her extra- marital male sexual partner is of type τ_m. A similar extra-marital escape probability $p_{emm}(t; \tau_m, \tau_f; h)$ for susceptible males of τ_m when their females sexual partners are of type τ_f is determined by substituting $p_{mem}(\tau_f)$ for $p_{fem}(\tau_m)$ in Eq. (12.5.7) and introducing the positive parameter η_m.

In the following, the symbol $\mathcal{B}(t)$ will stand for the phrase "the evolution of the process up to time t". Let $P_{femc}(t; \tau_f; h)$ be the conditional probability, given $\mathcal{B}(t)$, that a susceptible female of type τ_f participating in extra-marital sexual contacts $(femc)$ escapes infection per extra-marital sexual partner during the time interval $(t, t+h]$. By using the law of total probability, it can be seen that the random function $P_{femc}(t; \tau_f; h)$ is given by

$$P_{femc}(t; \tau_f; h) = \sum_{\tau_m \in \mathfrak{S}_{m2}} \rho_{fem}(t; \tau_f, \tau_m) p_{emf}(t; \tau_f, \tau_m; h) \, . \tag{12.5.8}$$

A formula for the corresponding conditional probability $P_{mem}(t;\tau_m;h)$ for susceptible males of type τ_m, participating in extra-marital sexual contacts may be derived by a similar argument.

Now let the random variable $N_{empf}(h)$, which has the range $R_{empf} = \{n \mid n = 0, 1, 2, \cdots\}$, be the number of extra-marital male sexual partners any female has during the time interval $(t, t+h]$. It will be assumed that this random variable follows a Poisson process with parameter $\lambda(\tau_f) \geq 0$ and location parameter 0 so that during any time interval there may be no extra-marital sexual partners. By using an argument similar to that used in the derivation of Eq. (11.6.8), it follows that the conditional probability, given $\mathcal{B}(t)$, that any susceptible female of type τ_f escapes infection during the time interval $(t, t+h]$ from all extra-marital male sexual partners ($femp$) is determined by the random function,

$$
\begin{aligned}
P_{femp}(t;\tau_f;h) &= \exp\left[\lambda(\tau_f)h(P_{femc}(t;\tau_f;h) - 1)\right] \\
&= \exp\left[-\lambda(\tau_f)hQ_{femc}(t;\tau_f;h)\right] \ , \qquad (12.5.9)
\end{aligned}
$$

where $Q_{femc}(t;\tau_f;h) = 1 - P_{femc}(t;\tau_f;h)$ is the conditional probability that a susceptible female is infected during $(t, t+h]$ per extra-marital male partner. A similar argument may be used to derive the corresponding random function $P_{memp}(t;\tau_m;h)$ for susceptible males τ_m, participating in extra-marital sexual contacts by introducing a Poisson random variable N_{empm} with expectation $E\left[N_{empm}\right] = \lambda(\tau_m) \geq 0$ and modifying Eq. (12.5.9) accordingly. In this connection, $Q_{memc}(t;\tau_m;h)$ is the conditional probability that a susceptible male of type τ_m is infected during $(t, t+h]$ per extra-marital female partner.

Finally, to connect the notation of this section with the simpler notation used for latent risks in Section 12.3, the following redefinitions,

$$
Q_{par}(t;\tau_f) = Q_{femc}(t;\tau_f;h) \qquad (12.5.10)
$$

and

$$
Q_{par}(t;\tau_m) = Q_{memc}(t;\tau_m;h) \qquad (12.5.11)
$$

will be used. Given this notation, the conditional probability (see Eq. (12.5.9)), that a susceptible female of type τ_f at time t becomes infected during the time interval $(t, t+h]$ by extra-marital sexual contacts is given by

$$1 - P_{femp}(t; \tau_f; h) = \lambda(\tau_f) Q_{par}(t; \tau_f) h + o(h) \ . \tag{12.5.12}$$

Hence, the use of the latent risk $\lambda(\tau_f)Q_{par}(t;\tau_f)$ for susceptibles females of type τ_f is justified. Similarly, the latent risk for a susceptible male of type τ_m at time t being infected by extra-marital sexual contacts during the time interval $(t, t+h]$ is given by $\lambda(\tau_m)Q_{par}(t;\tau_m)$.

12.6 Stochastic Evolutionary Equations

Having defined matrices of latent risks for the life cycle models of single females and males as well as couples, the purpose of this section is to develop a set of stochastic evolutionary equations for computing Monte Carlo realizations of the random functions of the population process, which are analogous to those in Section 10.5, for the case of $m \geq 1$ behavioral classes and $n \geq 1$ stages of disease. Let $\mathfrak{S}_{f1}$ and $\mathfrak{S}_{f2}$ denote, respectively, the set of absorbing and transient states of the life cycle model for individuals in the singles population. Just as in Section 12.3, the set $\mathfrak{S}_{f1}$ contains two states, and the set $\mathfrak{S}_{f2}$ contains $m(n+1)$ states, and the full state space for the evolution of single females is $\mathfrak{S}_f = \mathfrak{S}_{f1} \cup \mathfrak{S}_{f2}$. Suppose that for every time interval t, a $m(n+1) \times (2 + m(n+1))$ matrix,

$$\mathbf{\Theta}_{f2}(t) = (\theta_f(t; \tau_1, \tau_2) \mid \tau_1 \in \mathfrak{S}_{f1}, \tau_2 \in \mathfrak{S}_f) \tag{12.6.1}$$

of constant latent risks has been specified that is, by assumption, constant on the interval $(t, t+h]$. By definition, for every transient state $\tau_f \in \mathfrak{S}_{f2}$, the total risk function on this interval is:

$$\theta_f(t; \tau_1) = \sum_{\tau \in \mathfrak{S}_f} \theta_f(t; \tau_f, \tau) \ . \tag{12.6.2}$$

Whenever the risk functions are constant on $(t, t+h]$, it can be shown, by appealing to the classical theory of competing risks, that, given an individual female is in state $\tau_f \in \mathfrak{S}_{f2}$ at time t, the conditional probability $\pi_f(t; \tau_f, \tau_f)$ that she is still in this state at time $t+h$ is:

$$\pi_f(t; \tau_f, \tau_f) = \exp\left[-\theta_f(t; \tau_f) h\right] \ . \tag{12.6.3}$$

Therefore, the conditional probability of a jump to some other state during this time interval is $1-\exp\left[-\theta_f(t;\tau_f)h\right]$. Consequently, another appeal to the theory of competing risks leads to the conclusion that, given a single individual in transient state τ_f at time t,

$$\pi_f(t;\tau_f,\tau_2) = \left(1-\exp\left[-\theta_f(t;\tau_f)h\right]\right)\frac{\theta_f(t;\tau_f,\tau_2)}{\theta_f(t;\tau_f)} \qquad (12.6.4)$$

is the conditional probability of a jump to some state $\tau_2 \in \mathfrak{S}_f$ such that $\tau_2 \neq \tau_f$ during the time interval $(t, t+h]$. As they should, for every $\tau_f \in \mathfrak{S}_{s2}$ and $t \in S_h$, these conditional probabilities satisfy the condition,

$$\sum_{\tau_2\in\mathfrak{S}_f} \pi_f(t;\tau_f,\tau_2) = 1\,. \qquad (12.6.5)$$

For every $\tau_f \in \mathfrak{S}_{s2}$ and $t \in S_h$, let

$$\mathbf{\Pi}_f(t;\tau_f) = \left(\pi_f(t;\tau_f,\tau_2) \mid \tau_2 \in \mathfrak{S}_f\right) \qquad (12.6.6)$$

be a vector of these conditional probabilities.

With respect to single males, let $\mathfrak{S}_{m1}$ and $\mathfrak{S}_{m2}$ denote, respectively, the set of absorbing and transient states, let $\mathfrak{S}_m = \mathfrak{S}_{m1} \cup \mathfrak{S}_{m2}$ denote the full state space, and let

$$\mathbf{\Theta}_{m2}(t) = \left(\theta_m(t;\tau_1,\tau_2) \mid \tau_1 \in \mathfrak{S}_{m1}, \tau_2 \in \mathfrak{S}_m\right) \qquad (12.6.7)$$

denote a matrix of latent risks. Then, a similar vector,

$$\mathbf{\Pi}_m(t;\tau_m) = \left(\pi_m(t;\tau_m,\tau_2) \mid \tau_2 \in \mathfrak{S}_m\right) \qquad (12.6.8)$$

of conditional transition probabilities for single males may be defined for every type $\tau_m \in \mathfrak{S}_{m2}$ and $t \in S_h$ just as in Eq. (12.6.6).

The next step in setting down the stochastic evolutionary equations for the population is to consider the matrix of latent risk functions, governing the evolution of couples. Recall that, with respect to the evolution of couples, the set $\mathfrak{S}_{c1}$ of absorbing states contains 5 elements, the set $\mathfrak{S}_{c2} = \mathbf{\Upsilon}_c$ of transient states contains $m^2(n+1)^2$ elements, and the state space is $\mathfrak{S}_c = \mathfrak{S}_{c1} \cup \mathfrak{S}_{c2}$. Suppose that for every time interval $(t, t+h]$ a $m^2(n+1)^2 \times (5 + m^2(n+1)^2)$ matrix of latent risks,

$$\mathbf{\Theta}_c(t;\varkappa_1,\varkappa_2) = \left(\theta_c(t;\varkappa_1,\varkappa_2) \mid \varkappa_1 \in \mathfrak{S}_{c2}, \varkappa_2 \in \mathfrak{S}_c\right) \qquad (12.6.9)$$

has been specified that, by assumption, is constant on every interval $(t, t+h]$. Then, for every state $\varkappa_1 \in \mathfrak{S}_{c2}$, the total risk function is, by definition,

$$\theta_c(t; \varkappa_1) = \sum_{\varkappa_2 \in \mathfrak{S}_c} \theta_c(t; \varkappa_1, \varkappa_2) . \tag{12.6.10}$$

Given these total risk functions, the vector of π-probabilities for couples

$$\mathbf{\Pi}_c(t; \varkappa_1) = (\pi_c(t; \varkappa_1, \varkappa_2) \mid \varkappa_2 \in \mathfrak{S}_c) \tag{12.6.11}$$

may be defined as in Eqs. (12.6.3) through (12.6.4) for every $\varkappa_1 \in \mathfrak{S}_{c2}$.

The simplest component of these equations is that for recruits entering the population during any time interval $(t, t+h]$. Suppose single female recruits enter the population according to a Poisson process $N_f(t)$ with parameter $\mu_f > 0$. Let $\varphi_f(\tau_f)$ be the probability a female recruit is of type $\tau_f \in \mathfrak{S}_{f2}$. Let $X_R(t+h; \tau_f)$ be the number of single female recruits of type $\tau_f \in \mathfrak{S}_{f2}$ entering the population during $(t, t+h]$. Then, given the state of the population at time t, it can be shown that $X_R(t+h; \tau_f)$ has a conditional Poisson distribution with parameter $\mu_f \varphi_f(\tau_f)h$. In symbols,

$$X_R(t+h; \tau_f) \sim CPois\left(\mu_f \varphi_f(\tau_f)h\right) . \tag{12.6.12}$$

Similarly, let $Y_R(t+h; \tau_m)$ be the number of single male recruits of type $\tau_m \in \mathfrak{S}_{m2}$ entering the population during $(t, t+h]$, suppose these recruits arrive according to a Poisson process with parameter $\mu_m > 0$, and let $\varphi_m(\tau_m)$ be the probability a recruit is of type $\tau_m \in \mathfrak{S}_{m2}$. Then, just as in (12.6.12), $Y_R(t+h; k)$ has a conditional Poisson distribution with parameter $\mu_m \varphi_m(\tau_m)h$. It will be assumed it is the case that $\sum_\tau \varphi_f(\tau) = \sum_\tau \varphi_m(\tau) = 1$.

With respect to the evolution of singles, a single female of type $\tau_f \in \mathfrak{S}_{f2}$ at time t may make a transition to any state $\tau \in \mathfrak{S}_f$, become a member of a couple, or neither of these events may occur, during the time interval $(t, t+h]$. Among the $X(t; \tau_f)$ single females of type $\tau_f \in \mathfrak{S}_{f2}$ at t, the number who become members of a couple during $(t, t+h]$ is:

$$X_C(t+h; \tau_f) = \sum_{\tau_m \in \mathfrak{S}_{m2}} Z_{CF}(t+h; \tau_f, \tau_m) , \tag{12.6.13}$$

(see Eq. (12.4.11)). Therefore, the number of this type who remain single during $(t, t+h]$ is:

$$X_S(t;\tau_f) = X(t;\tau_f) - X_C(t+h;\tau_f) \ . \tag{12.6.14}$$

Among the $X_S(t;\tau_f)$ who remain single, let $X_T(t+h;\tau_f)$ be the number who make a transition to state $\tau \in \mathfrak{S}_f$, and let

$$\mathbf{X}_T(t+h;\tau_f) = (X_T(t+h;\tau_f,\tau) \mid \tau \in \mathfrak{S}_f) \tag{12.6.15}$$

be a vector with these components. Then, given $X_S(t;\tau_f)$, it is assumed the vector $\mathbf{X}_T(t+h;\tau_f)$ has a conditional multinomial distribution with index $X_S(t;\tau_f)$ and probability vector $\mathbf{\Pi}_f(t;\tau_f)$ (see Eq. (12.6.6)). In symbols,

$$\mathbf{X}_T(t+h;\tau_f) \sim CMultinom\,(X_S(t;\tau_f), \mathbf{\Pi}_f(t;\tau_f)) \tag{12.6.16}$$

for every $\tau_f \in \mathfrak{S}_{f2}$. Moreover, with respect to single males at time t, one may define in an analogous manner a random function $Y_S(t;\tau_m)$, a vector of conditional probabilities $\mathbf{\Pi}_m(t;\tau_m)$, and a vector $\mathbf{Y}_T(t;\tau_m)$ such that:

$$\mathbf{Y}_T(t+h;\tau_m) \sim CMultinom\,(Y_S(t;\tau_m), \mathbf{\Pi}_m(t;\tau_m)) \tag{12.6.17}$$

for every $\tau_m \in \mathfrak{S}_{m2}$.

Let $Z(t;\varkappa_1)$ be the number of couples of type $\varkappa_1 = (\tau_f, \tau_m)$ at time t. During the time interval $(t, t+h]$, any couple of this type may undergo a transition to a state $\varkappa_2 \in \mathfrak{S}_c$, the state space for couples. Among the $Z(t;\varkappa_1)$ couples in state $\varkappa_1 \in \mathfrak{S}_{c2}$ at time t, let the number who undergo the transition $\varkappa_1 \to \varkappa_2$ during $(t, t+h]$ be given by $Z_T(t+h;\varkappa_1,\varkappa_2)$, and let

$$\mathbf{Z}_T(t+h;\varkappa_1) = (Z_T(t+h;\varkappa_1,\varkappa_2) \mid \varkappa_2 \in \mathfrak{S}_c) \tag{12.6.18}$$

be a vector with these components. Realizations of the vector $\mathbf{Z}_T(t;\varkappa_1)$ are then computed according to:

$$\mathbf{Z}_T(t+h;\varkappa_1) \sim CMultinom\,(Z(t;\varkappa_1), \mathbf{\Pi}_c(t;\varkappa_1)) \ , \tag{12.6.19}$$

where $\mathbf{\Pi}_c(t;\varkappa_1)$ is the vector of conditional probabilities in Eq. (12.6.11).

Let $X_{DIS}(t+h;\tau_f)$ be the number of females of type τ_f at time $t+h$ who were members of couples in state $\varkappa_1 = (\tau_f, \tau_m)$ at time t who join the singles population during $(t, t+h]$ because of couple dissolution, and let

$$DIS_f = \{E_{dis}, E_{m1}, E_{m2}\} \subset \mathfrak{S}_{c1} \tag{12.6.20}$$

be the subset of states in the set $\mathfrak{S}_{c1}$ of absorbing states that signal a return of a female to the singles population. Then, because a female in partnership of type $\tau_1 = (j,k)$ joins the population of singles during $(t, t+h]$ only if the partners separate or the male dies, it follows that:

$$X_{DIS}(t+h;\tau_f) = \sum_{\tau_m \in \mathfrak{S}_{m2}} \sum_{\tau \in DIS_f} Z_T(t+h;\tau_f,\tau_m,\tau)\,. \tag{12.6.21}$$

The subset DIS_m of absorbing states $\mathfrak{S}_{c1,}$ signaling that a male has returned to the population of singles, as well as the random function $Y_{DIS}(t+h;\tau_m)$ of type τ_m, may be defined similarly. The number of single females of type τ_f who die during the time interval $(t, t+h]$ is:

$$X_D(t+h;\tau_f) = \sum_{\tau \in \mathfrak{S}_{f1}} X_T(t+h;\tau_f,\tau)\,. \tag{12.6.22}$$

The corresponding random function $Y_D(t+h;k)$ for single males of type k is defined similarly.

In the following, only those evolutionary equations counting the numbers of live single females and males at any time t along with those couples for which both members are alive will be set down. In reporting the results of computer experiments, however, it will often be of methodological interest to account for the numbers of deaths for both females and males that may occur during any time interval. At time $t+h$, the number of single females of type $\tau_f \in \mathfrak{S}_{f2}$ is a sum of three components; namely, a component due to recruitment, a component due to a possible transition to a state τ_f in $\mathfrak{S}_{f2}$, and a component due to couple dissolution. Therefore,

$$X(t+h;\tau_f) = X_R(t+h,\tau_f) + \sum_{\tau \in \mathfrak{S}_{f2}} X_T(t+h,\tau,\tau_f) + X_{DIS}(t+h;\tau_f) \tag{12.6.23}$$

for every $\tau_f \in \mathfrak{S}_{f2}$. For single males the stochastic evolutionary equations take the similar form,

$$Y(t+h;\tau_m) = Y_R(t+h,\tau_m) + \sum_{\tau \in \mathfrak{S}_{m2}} Y_T(t+h,\tau,\tau_m) + Y_{DIS}(t+h;\tau_m) \tag{12.6.24}$$

for every $\tau_m \in \mathfrak{S}_{f2}$.

Similarly, $Z(t+h,\varkappa_2)$, representing the number of couples of type $\varkappa_2 = (\tau_f, \tau_m)$ at time $t+h$, is a sum of two components. One component consists of those couples $Z_T(t+h;\varkappa_1,\varkappa_2)$, who were of some type $\varkappa_1$ at t and made a transition to type $\varkappa_2$ during $(t, t+h]$; the other component is the number $Z_{CF}(t+h;\varkappa_2)$ formed during $(t, t+h]$ from single females and males of types τ_f and τ_m, respectively, at time t. Therefore, for all $\varkappa_2 \in \mathfrak{S}_{c2}$,

$$Z(t+h,\varkappa_2) = \sum_{\varkappa_1 \in \mathfrak{S}_{c2}} Z_T(t+h;\varkappa_1,\varkappa_2) + Z_{CF}(t+h;\varkappa_2)\,. \tag{12.6.25}$$

When making projections of an epidemic, plots of the cumulative numbers of total deaths for both females and males as well as the cumulative totals of the number of susceptible females and males infected are often of interest and are frequently included in the software. Equations for these cumulative numbers may also be written down, but, for the sake of brevity, will be omitted.

12.7 Embedded Non-Linear Difference Equations

As has been demonstrated in Chapters 10 and 11, a set of non-linear difference equations embedded in a stochastic process is not only of interest for computing trajectories that are in some sense measures of central tendency for the sample functions of the process, but are also of interest because as $h \downarrow 0$, a set of non-linear differential equations arise, which are useful for deriving threshold conditions for the process. Accordingly, it is of interest to derive a system of embedded non-linear difference equations for the two-sex partnership process under consideration. A starting point in the derivation of such a system of recursive equations is that of taking conditional expectations of the random functions of the process at time $t+h$, given values of the random functions at time t.

By taking the conditional expectation given $\mathfrak{B}(t)$ for recruits in Eq. (12.6.23), it can be seen that:

$$E\left[X_R(t+h;\tau_f) \mid \mathfrak{B}(t)\right] = \mu_f \varphi_f(\tau_f)h\ , \tag{12.7.1}$$

The conditional expectation of the second term on the right hand side of Eq. (12.6.23) needs special consideration, because $X_S(t;\tau_f)$ contains an adjustment for the number of single females of type τ_f who becomes members of couples during $(t, t+h]$ (see Eq. (12.6.14)). Therefore, from Eq. (12.6.16) it follows that:

$$E\left[X_T(t+h,\tau,\tau_f) \mid X_S(t;\tau)\right] = X_S(t;\tau)\pi_f(t;\tau,\tau_f) \tag{12.7.2}$$

for all τ and τ_f. To derive a recursive system, an "estimate" of $X_S(t;\tau)$ will be required. From Eq. (12.4.11), it can be seen that:

$$E\left[X_C(t+h;\tau_f) \mid \mathfrak{B}(t)\right] = \sum_{\tau_m \in \mathfrak{S}_{m2}} N_{CF}(t;\tau_f,\tau_m) q_{CF}(\tau_f,\tau_m;h)\ . \tag{12.7.3}$$

Therefore,

$$E\left[X_S(t;\tau_f) \mid \mathfrak{B}(t)\right] = X(t;\tau_f) - \sum_{\tau_m \in \mathfrak{S}_{m2}} N_{CF}(t;\tau_f,\tau_m) q_{CF}(\tau_f,\tau_m;h)\ . \tag{12.7.4}$$

Note that the right hand sides of Eqs. (12.7.2) through (12.7.4) are functions of the sample functions at t. To express the conditional expectation of the third component on the right in Eq. (12.6.23), arising from the dissolution of couples, as a function of the sample functions at t, note that:

$$E\left[Z_T(t+h;\varkappa_1,\varkappa_2) \mid \mathfrak{B}(t)\right] = Z(t;\varkappa_1)\pi_c(t;\varkappa_1,\varkappa_2)\ . \tag{12.7.5}$$

Therefore, if $\varkappa_1 = (\tau_f, \tau_m)$, then

$$E\left[X_{DIS}(t+h;\tau_f) \mid \mathfrak{B}(t)\right] = \sum_{\tau_m \in \mathfrak{S}_{m2}} \sum_{\varkappa \in DIS_f} Z(t;\varkappa_1)\pi_c(t;\varkappa_1,\varkappa)\ . \tag{12.7.6}$$

The term for deaths among single females may be handled in a similar way and is:

$$\sum_{\tau \in \mathfrak{S}_{f1}} E\left[X_D(t+h;\tau_f,\tau) \mid X_S(t;\tau_f\right] = \sum_{\tau \in \mathfrak{S}_{f1}} X_S(t;\tau_f)\pi_f(t;\tau_f,\tau)\,. \tag{12.7.7}$$

Again the random function $X_S(t;\tau_f)$ needs to be estimated in deriving a recursive system.

Unconditional expectations may be obtained by taking expectations of the above conditional expectations. But, because the π's may be non-linear functions of the sample functions at t, equations that are linear in the unconditional expectations cannot be derived. Recall that any π-function for a transition from a susceptible to the infected state is a non-linear function of the sample functions at t. However, if the sample functions at $t = 0$ are known, then the above conditional expectations are completely determined at $h > 0$. And, in general, if estimates of these sample functions are available at t, then the above conditional expectations may be estimated at $t + h$ by substituting these estimates for the sample functions. One thus arrives at a system of recursive equations that can be implemented on a computer and will take much less time to execute than a Monte Carlo simulation.

In the following, these recursive estimates will symbolized by expressions of the form $\widehat{X}(t)$ to distinguish them from the corresponding random function $X(t)$. For example, estimates of the random functions $X_S(t;\tau_f)$ will be computed using the formula,

$$\widehat{X}_S(t;\tau_f) = \widehat{X}(t;\tau_f) - \sum_{\tau \in \mathfrak{S}_{m2}} \widehat{N}_{CF}(t;\tau_f,\tau)q_{CF}(\tau_f,\tau)\,. \tag{12.7.8}$$

With these conventions, the non-linear difference equations for single females become

$$\widehat{X}(t+h;\tau_f) = \mu_f\varphi_f(\tau_f)h \;+ \sum_{\tau \in \mathfrak{S}_{f2}} \widehat{X}_S(t;\tau)\widehat{\pi}_f(t;\tau,\tau_f)$$

$$+ \sum_{\tau \in \mathfrak{S}_{m2}} \sum_{\tau_1 \in DIS_f} \widehat{Z}(t;\tau_f,\tau)\widehat{\pi}_c(t;\tau_f,\tau;\tau_1) \tag{12.7.9}$$

for all $\tau_f \in \mathfrak{S}_{f2}$. Similarly, the non-linear difference equations for single males become

$$\widehat{Y}(t+h;\tau_m) = \mu_m \varphi_m(\tau_m) h + \sum_{\tau \in \mathfrak{S}_{m2}} \widehat{Y}_S(t;\tau)\widehat{\pi}_m(t;\tau,\tau_m)$$

$$+ \sum_{\tau \in \mathfrak{S}_{f2}} \sum_{\tau_1 \in DIS_m} \widehat{Z}(t;\tau,\tau_m)\widehat{\pi}_c(t;\tau,\tau_m;\tau_1) \tag{12.7.10}$$

for all $\tau_m \in \mathfrak{S}_{m2}$. Finally, the non-linear equations for couples take the form,

$$\widehat{Z}(t+h;\varkappa_2) = \sum_{\varkappa_1 \in \mathfrak{S}_{c2}} \widehat{Z}(t;\varkappa_1)\widehat{\pi}_c(t;\varkappa_1,\varkappa_2) + \widehat{N}_{CF}(t;\varkappa_2) q_{CF}(\varkappa_2) \tag{12.7.11}$$

for all $\varkappa_2 \in \mathfrak{S}_{c2}$. When computing these estimates recursively, h is usually chosen as $h = 1$, a time unit sufficiently small to exclude multiple transitions with high probability. Given values of all random functions at $t = 0$ and all parameters of the system, estimates of the random functions may be computed for $t = 1, 2, \cdots$. We thus arrive at a system of non-linear difference equations. A system of non-linear difference equations could also be written down for the cumulative numbers of deaths for females and males, but the details will be omitted.

12.8 Embedded Non-Linear Differential Equations

By letting the length of every time interval go to zero, i.e., $h \downarrow 0$, the system of non-linear difference equations derived in the previous section gives rise to a system of non-linear differential equations in which the latent risks appear as parameters or, more generally, as functions of t. Just as in Chapters 10 and 11, the embedded differential equations will be used to derive threshold conditions for the stochastic process, which in turn will be useful as indicators in computer simulation experiments designed to test to whether an epidemic occurs in a two-sex population following the introduction of a few infectives into a population of susceptibles. At this point in time, mathematical proofs, similar to those that arise in deriving threshold conditions for branching processes, seem to be elusive, because of the non-linearities that occur in the process.

Nevertheless, as we have seen in Chapters 10 and 11, an analysis of the system of embedded non-linear differential equations can be useful in the quest for threshold conditions for the stochastic process, which may be checked by intensive computer experimentation.

As $h \downarrow 0$, it seems plausible that the adjustment for a discrete-time approximation in Eq. (12.7.8) can be neglected so that the embedded non-linear difference equations may be expressed in an alternative form. For example, the difference equations for single females in Eq. (12.7.9) become:

$$\begin{aligned}\widehat{X}(t+h;\tau_f) &= \mu_f\varphi_f(\tau_f)h + \sum_{\nu\in\mathfrak{S}_{f2}} \widehat{X}(t;\tau)\widehat{\pi}_f(t;\tau,\tau_f;h) \\ &\quad - \sum_{\tau\in\mathfrak{S}_{m2}} \widehat{N}_{CF}(t;\tau_f,\tau)q_{CF}(\tau_f,\tau;h) \\ &\quad + \sum_{\tau\in\mathfrak{S}_{m2}}\sum_{\tau_1\in DIS_f} \widehat{Z}(t;\tau_f,\tau)\widehat{\pi}_c(t;\tau_f,\tau;\tau_1;h) \qquad (12.8.1)\end{aligned}$$

for every $\tau_f \in \mathfrak{S}_{f2}$. Similar equations may be written down for single males. But, the non-linear difference equation Eq. (12.7.11) for couples remains the same. To emphasize that the π-probabilities and other coefficients depend on h, the coefficients contain the symbol h.

To derive this system of differential equations, it suffices to observe two basic relationships that will be illustrated with single females. First, observe that for every $\tau_f \in \mathfrak{S}_{f1}$,

$$\pi_f(t;\tau_f,\tau_f;h) = 1 - \theta_f(t;\tau_f)h + o(h) \qquad (12.8.2)$$

and for $\tau_f \neq \tau$,

$$\pi_f(t;\tau_f,\tau;h) = \theta_f(t;\tau_f,\tau)h + o(h)\ , \qquad (12.8.3)$$

where $o(h)/h \to 0$ as $h \downarrow 0$. Similar equations may be written down for the π-probabilities of single males and couples as well as the function $q_{CF}(\tau_f,\tau;h)$.

Given these relationships, for every $\tau_f \in \mathfrak{S}_{f2}$ the non-linear difference equations for single females may be written in the form,

$$\widehat{X}(t+h;\tau_f) = \mu_f\varphi_f(\tau_f)h + \widehat{X}(t;\tau_f)(1-\widehat{\theta}_f(t;\tau_f)h)$$

$$+ \sum_{\tau_f \neq \tau \in \mathfrak{S}_{f2}} \widehat{X}(t;\tau)\widehat{\theta}_f(t;\tau,\tau_f)h$$

$$- \sum_{\tau \in \mathfrak{S}_{m2}} \widehat{N}_{CF}(t;\tau_f,\tau)\rho(\tau_f,\tau)h$$

$$+ \sum_{\tau \in \mathfrak{S}_{m2}} \sum_{\tau_1 \in DIS_f} \widehat{Z}(t;\tau_f,\tau)\widehat{\theta}_c(t;\tau_f,\tau;\tau_1)h \; + o(h) \, . \tag{12.8.4}$$

By forming the ratio,

$$\frac{\widehat{X}(t+h;\tau_f) - \widehat{X}(t;\tau_f)}{h} \tag{12.8.5}$$

and letting $h \downarrow 0$, it can be seen that for all $\tau_f \in \mathfrak{S}_{f2}$ the following system of differential equations for single females arises:

$$\frac{d\widehat{X}(t;\tau_f)}{dt} = \mu_f \varphi_f(\tau_f) - \widehat{X}(t;\tau_f)\widehat{\theta}_f(t;\tau_f)$$

$$+ \sum_{\tau_f \neq \tau \in \mathfrak{S}_{f2}} \widehat{X}(t;\tau)\widehat{\theta}_f(t;\tau,\tau_f)$$

$$- \sum_{\tau \in \mathfrak{S}_{m2}} \widehat{N}_{CF}(t;\tau_f,\tau)\rho(\tau_f,\tau)$$

$$+ \sum_{\tau \in \mathfrak{S}_{m2}} \sum_{\tau_2 \in DIS_f} \widehat{Z}(t;\tau_f,\tau)\widehat{\theta}_c(t;\tau_f,\tau;\tau_2) \, . \tag{12.8.6}$$

Similarly, for every $\tau_m \in \mathfrak{S}_{m2}$ the differential equation for single males takes the form,

$$\frac{d\widehat{Y}(t;\tau_m)}{dt} = \mu_m \varphi_m(\tau_m) - \widehat{Y}(t;\tau_m)\widehat{\theta}_m(t;\tau_m)$$

$$+ \sum_{\tau_m \neq \tau \in \mathfrak{S}_{m2}} \widehat{Y}(t;\tau)\widehat{\theta}_m(t;\tau,\tau_m)$$

$$- \sum_{\tau \in \mathfrak{S}_{f2}} \widehat{N}_{CF}(t;\tau,\tau_m)\rho(\tau,\tau_m)$$

$$+\sum_{\tau\in\mathfrak{S}_{f2}}\sum_{\tau_1\in DIS_m}\widehat{Z}(t;(\tau,\tau_m))\widehat{\theta}_c(t;\tau,\tau_m;\tau_1) \tag{12.8.7}$$

for all $\tau_m \in \mathfrak{S}_{m2}$.

An analogous system of differential equations for couples may be derived, and for every $\varkappa \in \mathfrak{S}_{c2}$ these equations have the form,

$$\frac{d\widehat{Z}(t;\varkappa)}{dt} = -\widehat{Z}(t;\varkappa)\widehat{\theta}_c(t;\varkappa)$$

$$+\sum_{\varkappa\neq\varkappa_1\in\mathfrak{S}_{c2}}\widehat{Z}(t;\varkappa_1)\widehat{\theta}_c(t;\varkappa_1,\varkappa)$$

$$+\widehat{N}_{CF}(t;\varkappa)\rho(\varkappa)\,. \tag{12.8.8}$$

This system of differential equations is non-linear, because some of the latent risk functions will be non-linear in the functions of the system. For the case of some sexually transmitted diseases such as HIV/AIDS, all the latent risk functions will be constant except those governing the infection of susceptibles through extra-marital sexual contacts. For example, the estimate of a latent risk function in the embedded differential equations for a susceptible female will contain non-linear terms of the form $\lambda_f(\tau_f)\widehat{Q}_{femc}(t;\tau_f)$ for a susceptible female of type τ_f (see Section 12.3 for further details). The only other source of non-linearities in these differential equations are terms of the form $\widehat{N}_{CF}(t;\varkappa)$ for new couples of type $\varkappa$. When $\varkappa = (\tau_f,\tau_m)$, it can be seen by applying expectations for the multinomial distribution that:

$$\widehat{N}_{CF}(t;\varkappa) = \min\left\{\widehat{X}(t;\tau_f)\widehat{\gamma}_f(t;\tau_f,\tau_m),\widehat{Y}(t;\tau_m)\widehat{\gamma}_m(t;\tau_m,\tau_f)\right\} \tag{12.8.9}$$

(see Section 12.4). In the deterministic differential equations, this function is clearly not only non-linear in the estimates of the sample functions at t, but also in the parameters of the system as seen in Chapter 11.

As an aid to finding threshold conditions, it will be helpful to cast the above system of differential equations in vector-matrix form. Let

$$\mathbf{R}_f = (\mu_f\varphi_f(\tau_f)\mid\tau_f\in\mathfrak{S}_{f2}) \tag{12.8.10}$$

denote a $m(n+1) \times 1$ column vector for female recruits whose elements are arranged in lexicographical order, and let $\mathbf{R}_m$ denote the corresponding column vector for male recruits. When it is assumed that no couples enter the population as recruits, then the vector for all recruits entering the population during any time interval has the partitioned form,

$$\mathbf{R} = \begin{pmatrix} \mathbf{R}_f \\ \mathbf{R}_m \\ \mathbf{0}_{m^2(n+1)^2 \times 1} \end{pmatrix}, \tag{12.8.11}$$

where $\mathbf{0}_{m^2(n+1)^2 \times 1}$ is a vector of zeros. Observe that the vector $\mathbf{R}$ has dimension $(2m(n+1) + m^2(n+1)^2) \times 1$ as will all the other column vectors to be defined in this section when females, males and couples are considered simultaneously.

At any time t, let

$$\widehat{\mathbf{X}}(t) = \left(\widehat{X}(t;\tau_f) \mid \tau_f \in \mathfrak{S}_{f2}\right), \tag{12.8.12}$$

$$\widehat{\mathbf{Y}}(t) = \left(\widehat{Y}(t;\tau_m) \mid \tau_m \in \mathfrak{S}_{m2}\right), \tag{12.8.13}$$

$$\widehat{\mathbf{Z}}(t) = \left(\widehat{Z}(t;\varkappa) \mid \varkappa \in \mathfrak{S}_{c2}\right) \tag{12.8.14}$$

denote, respectively, the column vectors of estimates for the numbers single females, single males, and couples in the population. Then, at time t the vector of estimates of these numbers for the population has the partitioned form,

$$\widehat{\mathbf{V}}(t) = \begin{pmatrix} \widehat{\mathbf{X}}(t) \\ \widehat{\mathbf{Y}}(t) \\ \widehat{\mathbf{Z}}(t) \end{pmatrix}. \tag{12.8.15}$$

With respect to couple formation, let the column vector

$$\widehat{\mathbf{V}}_{FCF}(t) = \left(-\sum_{\tau_m \in \mathfrak{S}_{m2}} \widehat{N}_{CF}(t;\tau_f,\tau_m)\widehat{\rho}(\tau_f,\tau_m) \mid \tau_f \in \mathfrak{S}_{f2}\right) \tag{12.8.16}$$

denote the estimates of the number of single females at time t who become member of couples, and let

$$\widehat{\mathbf{V}}_{MCF}(t) = \left(- \sum_{\tau_f \in \mathfrak{S}_{f2}} \widehat{N}_{CF}(t; \tau_f, \tau_m) \widehat{\rho}(\tau_f, \tau_m) \mid \tau_m \in \mathfrak{S}_{m2} \right) \tag{12.8.17}$$

denote the corresponding vector for single males. The vector

$$\widehat{\mathbf{V}}_{CCF}(t) = \left(\widehat{N}_{CF}(t; \varkappa) \widehat{\rho}(\varkappa) \mid \varkappa \in \mathfrak{S}_{c2} \right) \tag{12.8.18}$$

contains the estimates of the numbers of couples formed at time t ordered by couple types. Finally, the vector for couple formation in the population has the partitioned form,

$$\widehat{\mathbf{V}}_{CF}(t) = \begin{pmatrix} \widehat{\mathbf{V}}_{FCF}(t) \\ \widehat{\mathbf{V}}_{MCF}(t) \\ \widehat{\mathbf{V}}_{CCF}(t) \end{pmatrix} . \tag{12.8.19}$$

As in Section 11.9, it can be shown, given these definitions, that there exists a $(2m(n+1)+m^2(n+1)^2) \times (2m(n+1)+m^2(n+1)^2)$ matrix $\widehat{\Xi}(t)$ such that system of differential equations under consideration has the vector-matrix form,

$$\frac{d\widehat{\mathbf{V}}(t)}{dt} = \mathbf{R} + \widehat{\Xi}(t)\widehat{\mathbf{V}}(t) + \widehat{\mathbf{V}}_{CF}(t) . \tag{12.8.20}$$

Furthermore, there is a constant matrix $\mathbf{A}$ and a matrix $\widehat{\mathbf{W}}(t)$ of non-linear terms such that:

$$\widehat{\Xi}(t) = \mathbf{A} + \widehat{\mathbf{W}}(t) . \tag{12.8.21}$$

Therefore, if an vector containing those functions for extra-marital sexual contacts is defined by:

$$\widehat{\mathbf{V}}_{EM}(t) = \widehat{\mathbf{W}}(t)\widehat{\mathbf{V}}(t) , \tag{12.8.22}$$

then the differential equations for the system take the form,

$$\frac{d\widehat{\mathbf{V}}(t)}{dt} = \mathbf{R} + \mathbf{A}\widehat{\mathbf{V}}(t) + \widehat{\mathbf{V}}_{EM}(t) + \widehat{\mathbf{V}}_{CF}(t) , \tag{12.8.23}$$

from which formulas for the Jacobian matrix of the system may be derived.

For the two-sex model under consideration, the transpose of the matrix $\widehat{\Xi}(t)$ has the partitioned form,

$$\widehat{\Xi}'(t) = \begin{bmatrix} \widehat{\Xi}'_{ff}(t) & \mathbf{0}_{m(n+1)\times m(n+1)} & \mathbf{0}_{m(n+1)\times m^2(n+1)^2} \\ \mathbf{0}_{m(n+1)\times m(n+1)} & \widehat{\Xi}'_{mm}(t) & \mathbf{0}_{m(n+1)\times m^2(n+1)^2} \\ \widehat{\Xi}'_{cf}(t) & \widehat{\Xi}'_{cm}(t) & \widehat{\Xi}'_{cc}(t) \end{bmatrix} . \tag{12.8.24}$$

As suggested in the notation, the matrix $\widehat{\Xi}'_{ff}(t)$ is $m(n+1) \times m(n+1)$ and contains latent risks for the life cycle model for single females; a similar remark applies to the matrix $\widehat{\Xi}'_{mm}(t)$ for single males. The matrix $\widehat{\Xi}'_{cc}(t)$ is $m^2(n+1)^2 \times m^2(n+1)^2$ and contains latent risks for the life cycle model for couples, and matrices $\widehat{\Xi}'_{cf}(t)$ and $\widehat{\Xi}'_{cm}(t)$ contain those latent risks of the life cycle model for couples, governing, respectively, transitions by females and males in couples to the singles population due to couple dissolution. Observe that both these matrices are $m^2(n+1)^2 \times m(n+1)$.

As in Section 11.9, the elements of the matrix $\widehat{\Xi}'_{ff}(t)$ can be identified in terms of the elements of latent risks in the life cycle model for single females. Let

$$\mathbf{\Theta}_{f2}(t) = \begin{bmatrix} \mathbf{\Theta}_{f21}(t) & \mathbf{\Theta}_{f22}(t) \end{bmatrix} \tag{12.8.25}$$

denote the $m(n+1) \times (2 + m(n+1))$ matrix of latent risks, governing transitions from transient states to absorbing states and among transient states, for the life cycle model for single females at time t. Then, for every transient state $\tau_f \in \mathfrak{S}_{f2}$, the estimate of the total risk function for this state at time t is:

$$\widehat{\theta}_f(t;\tau_f) = \sum_{\tau\in\mathfrak{S}_f} \widehat{\theta}_f(t;\tau_f,\tau) . \tag{12.8.26}$$

Let

$$diag\left(\widehat{\theta}_f(t;\tau_f) \mid \tau_f \in \mathfrak{S}_{f2}\right) \tag{12.8.27}$$

denote a $m(n+1)\times m(n+1)$ diagonal matrix. Then, the matrix $\widehat{\Xi}'_{ff}(t)$ is determined by:

$$\widehat{\Xi}'_{ff}(t) = \widehat{\Theta}_{f22}(t) - diag\left(\widehat{\theta}_f(t;\tau_f) \mid \tau_f \in \mathfrak{S}_{f2}\right) \tag{12.8.28}$$

The elements of the matrix $\widehat{\Xi}'_{mm}(t)$ for single males are determined in a similar manner.

With regard to couples, let

$$\boldsymbol{\Theta}_{c2}(t) = \left[\begin{array}{cc} \boldsymbol{\Theta}_{c21}(t) & \boldsymbol{\Theta}_{c22}(t) \end{array} \right] \tag{12.8.29}$$

denote the $m^2(n+1)^2 \times (5 + m^2(n+1)^2)$ matrix of latent risks, governing transitions from transient states to absorbing states and among transient states, for the life cycle model for couples at time t. Then, the matrix $\widehat{\Xi}'_{cc}(t)$ is determined by:

$$\widehat{\Xi}'_{cc}(t) = \widehat{\Theta}_{c22}(t) - diag\left(\widehat{\theta}_c(t; \varkappa_1) \mid \varkappa_1 \in \mathfrak{S}_{c2}\right) \tag{12.8.30}$$

at time t. Moreover, it can be shown that there are constant matrices $\mathbf{A}_{ff}$, $\mathbf{A}_{mm}$ and $\mathbf{A}_{cc}$ such that

$$\widehat{\Xi}_{ff}(t) = \mathbf{A}_{ff} + \widehat{\mathbf{W}}_{ff}(t) \,, \tag{12.8.31}$$

$$\widehat{\Xi}_{mm}(t) = \mathbf{A}_{mm} + \widehat{\mathbf{W}}_{mm}(t) \,, \tag{12.8.32}$$

$$\widehat{\Xi}_{cc}(t) = \mathbf{A}_{cc} + \widehat{\mathbf{W}}_{cc}(t) \,, \tag{12.8.33}$$

where the $\mathbf{W}$-matrices contain estimates of the latent risks arising from extra-marital sexual contacts. Furthermore, it can be shown that there are constant matrices $\mathbf{A}'_{cf}$ and $\mathbf{A}'_{cm}$ such that:

$$\widehat{\Xi}'_{cf}(t) = \mathbf{A}'_{cf} \tag{12.8.34}$$

and

$$\widehat{\Xi}'_{cm}(t) = \mathbf{A}'_{cm} \tag{12.8.35}$$

for all $t \in S_h$.

To summarize, for the two-sex model under consideration, the constant matrix $\mathbf{A}$ has the partitioned form,

$$\mathbf{A} = \left[\begin{array}{ccc} \mathbf{A}_{ff} & \mathbf{0} & \mathbf{A}_{fc} \\ \mathbf{0} & \mathbf{A}_{mm} & \mathbf{A}_{mc} \\ \mathbf{0} & \mathbf{0} & \mathbf{A}_{cc} \end{array} \right] , \tag{12.8.36}$$

where, for example, $\mathbf{A}_{fc}$ is the transpose of the matrix $\mathbf{A}'_{cf}$. Furthermore, the matrix $\widehat{\mathbf{W}}(t)$ has the quasi-diagonal form,

$$\widehat{\mathbf{W}}(t) = \begin{bmatrix} \widehat{\mathbf{W}}_{ff}(t) & \mathbf{0} & \mathbf{0} \\ \mathbf{0} & \widehat{\mathbf{W}}_{mm}(t) & \mathbf{0} \\ \mathbf{0} & \mathbf{0} & \widehat{\mathbf{W}}_{cc}(t) \end{bmatrix} . \tag{12.8.37}$$

From the computational point of view, it is interesting to observe that because the matrix $\mathbf{A}$ is quasi-upper triangular, its spectrum $\sigma(\mathbf{A})$ is the union the spectra $\sigma(\mathbf{A}_{ff})$, $\sigma(\mathbf{A}_{mm})$ and $\sigma(\mathbf{A}_{cc})$ of smaller sub-matrices. In the next section, explicit forms of the coefficient matrices in the differential equations will be exhibited in special cases.

12.9 Coefficient Matrices for the Two-Sex Model

When stochastic two-sex partnership models are under consideration, the matrices of latent risks, particularly those for the life cycle model for couples, can become very large for cases involving $m \geq 2$ behavioral classes and $n \geq 2$ stages of disease. Consequently, it is very difficult to represent the coefficient matrices that occur in the embedded differential equations in useful and informative symbolic forms on a few pages of a book for these cases. Nevertheless, by inspecting a few simple cases, insights may be gained with respect to patterns of partitioned matrices that emerge for more general cases, which may be handled numerically with the help of software. Accordingly, the purpose of this section is to display some simple cases symbolically so as to gain insight into the patterns that arise in more complex cases.

The simplest case to consider is that of $m = 1$ behavioral class and $n = 1$ stage of disease. In this case, there are two types of females, $\tau_{f1} = (0)$, a susceptible, and $\tau_{f2} = (1)$, an infective. The two male types, τ_{m1} and τ_{m2}, are defined similarly. For this case, an inspection of the matrix of latent risks for the life cycle model for single females, shows that the sub-matrix $\mathbf{A}_{ff}$ for single females in Eq. (12.8.37) has the diagonal form,

$$\mathbf{A}_{ff} = \begin{bmatrix} -\mu_{f0} & 0 \\ 0 & -(\mu_{f0} + \mu_{f1}) \end{bmatrix} . \tag{12.9.1}$$

Similarly, the sub-matrix $\mathbf{A}_{mm}$ single males has the diagonal form,

$$\mathbf{A}_{mm} = diag\,(-\mu_{m0},\ -(\mu_{m0} + \mu_{m1}))\ . \tag{12.9.2}$$

Furthermore, from an inspection of the matrix of latent risks for single females, it can be see that the transpose of the sub-matrix $\widehat{\mathbf{W}}_{ff}(t)$ for single females in Eq. (12.8.37) has the form,

$$\widehat{\mathbf{W}}'_{ff}(t) = \begin{bmatrix} -\lambda(\tau_{f1})\widehat{Q}_{par}(t;\tau_{f1}) & \lambda(\tau_{f1})\widehat{Q}_{par}(t;\tau_{f1}) \\ 0 & 0 \end{bmatrix}\ . \tag{12.9.3}$$

It is easy to see that the corresponding matrix for single males has the form,

$$\widehat{\mathbf{W}}'_{mm}(t) = \begin{bmatrix} -\lambda(\tau_{m1})\widehat{Q}_{par}(t;\tau_{m1}) & \lambda(\tau_{m1})\widehat{Q}_{par}(t;\tau_{m1}) \\ 0 & 0 \end{bmatrix}\ . \tag{12.9.4}$$

For the simple case under consideration, there are four couple types; namely,

$$\varkappa_1 = (\tau_{f1}, \tau_{m1}),\ \varkappa_2 = (\tau_{f1}, \tau_{m2}),\ \varkappa_3 = (\tau_{f2}, \tau_{m1}),\ \varkappa_4 = (\tau_{f2}, \tau_{m2})\ . \tag{12.9.5}$$

From an inspection of the matrix of latent risks for the life cycle model for couples in Section 12.3, it can be seen that the sub-matrix $\mathbf{A}_{cc}$ for couples in Eq. (12.8.36) has a diagonal form. Let

$$\begin{aligned} \theta_1^* &= -(\mu_{f0} + \mu_{m0})\ , \\ \theta_2^* &= -(\mu_{f0} + \mu_{m0} + \mu_{m1} + \gamma_{mc} q_f(1))\ , \\ \theta_3^* &= -(\mu_{f0} + \mu_{f1} + \mu_{m0} + \gamma_{mc} q_m(1))\ , \\ \theta_4^* &= -(\mu_{f0} + \mu_{f1} + \mu_{m0} + \mu_{m1})\ . \end{aligned} \tag{12.9.6}$$

Then,

$$\mathbf{A}_{cc} = diag\,(\theta_1^*, \theta_2^*, \theta_3^*, \theta_4^*)\ . \tag{12.9.7}$$

To simplify the notation for the elements of the sub-matrix $\widehat{\mathbf{W}}_{cc}(t)$ for couples in Eq. (12.8.37), let

$$\widehat{S}_{par}(t) = \lambda(\tau_{m1})\widehat{Q}_{par}(t;\tau_{m1}) + \lambda(\tau_{f1})\widehat{Q}_{par}(t;\tau_{f1})\ . \tag{12.9.8}$$

Then, another inspection of the matrix of latent risks for the life cycle model for couples in Section 12.3 yields the result,

$$\widehat{\mathbf{W}}'_{cc}(t) = \begin{bmatrix} -\widehat{S}_{par}(t) & M & F & 0 \\ 0 & -F & 0 & F \\ 0 & 0 & -M & M \\ 0 & 0 & 0 & 0 \end{bmatrix}, \tag{12.9.9}$$

where $M = \lambda(\tau_{m1})\widehat{Q}_{par}(t;\tau_{m1})$ and $F = \lambda(\tau_{f1})\widehat{Q}_{par}(t;\tau_{f1})$.

The last step in describing the coefficient matrices for the embedded differential equations for the simple case under consideration is to set down those sub-matrices of latent risks governing transitions, during any time interval, of females and males in couples to the singles population. For the case of females, this matrix has the form,

$$\mathbf{A}_{cf} = \begin{bmatrix} \delta + \mu_{m0} & 0 \\ \delta + \mu_{m0} + \mu_{m1} & 0 \\ 0 & \delta + \mu_{m0} \\ 0 & \delta + \mu_{m0} + \mu_{m1} \end{bmatrix}. \tag{12.9.10}$$

Similarly, for the case of males, this matrix has the form,

$$\mathbf{A}_{cm} = \begin{bmatrix} \delta + \mu_{f0} & 0 \\ 0 & \delta + \mu_{f0} \\ \delta + \mu_{f0} + \mu_{f1} & 0 \\ 0 & \delta + \mu_{f0} + \mu_{f1} \end{bmatrix}. \tag{12.9.11}$$

Finally, the sub-matrices $\mathbf{A}_{fc}$ and $\mathbf{A}_{mc}$ in Eq. (12.8.36) are the transposes $\mathbf{A}_{fc} = \mathbf{A}'_{cf}$ and $\mathbf{A}_{mc} = \mathbf{A}'_{cm}$.

As can be seen from an inspection of the above matrices, for the case of $m = 1$ behavioral class and $n = 1$ stage of disease, the 8×8 matrix $\mathbf{A}$ in Eq. (12.8.36) is upper-triangular. Therefore, the matrix is stable at all points in the parameter space, because its eigenvalues are merely the negative elements on the principal diagonal. For more general cases of $m \geq 2$ behavioral classes and $n \geq 2$ stages of disease, however, the stability of the matrix $\mathbf{A}$ cannot be determined by inspection of its symbolical form, but, fortunately, it is easy to write computer programs to check numerically whether the matrix is stable at any point in the parameter space. Just as for the one-sex partnership models considered in Chapter 11, the matrix **A** will be a component of the Jacobian matrix of the embedded differential equations with functions of the $\widehat{W}$-matrices. But, rather than exhibiting more general symbolic forms of the $\widehat{W}$-matrices for more general cases of $m \geq 2$ behavioral classes and $n \geq 2$ stages of disease, only functions derived from them through partial differentiation will be described in the next section and exhibited in subsequent sections of this chapter.

As illustrated in Chapters 10 and 11, all Jacobian matrices are evaluated at a stationary vector for the case where a population contains only susceptibles. In the next section, an A-matrix will be considered for the case of $m = 2$ behavioral classes and $n = 0$ stages of disease, so, by way of another illustrative example, the 8×8 matrix **A** for this case will be exhibited. Because there are no infectives in the population, all types may be identified by their behavioral class. For this case, there are two types of single females, $\tau_{f1} = 1$ and $\tau_{f2} = 2$, representing behavioral class 1 and behavioral class 2, respectively. Similarly, the types of single males are $\tau_{m1} = 1$ and $\tau_{m2} = 2$. In this version of the model, the matrix of latent risks for single females has the form,

$$\begin{bmatrix} \mu_{f0} & 0 & \psi_{f12} \\ \mu_{f0} & \psi_{f21} & 0 \end{bmatrix} . \tag{12.9.12}$$

Therefore, the sub-matrix $\mathbf{A}'_{ff}$ for single females has the form,

$$\mathbf{A}'_{ff} = \begin{bmatrix} -(\mu_{f0} + \psi_{f12}) & \psi_{f12} \\ \psi_{f21} & -(\mu_{f0} + \psi_{f21}) \end{bmatrix} . \tag{12.9.13}$$

From the structure of the matrix in Eq. (12.9.13), it is easy to see that the sub-matrix $\mathbf{A}'_{mm}$ for single males has the form,

$$\mathbf{A}'_{mm} = \begin{bmatrix} -(\mu_{mf0} + \psi_{m12}) & \psi_{m12} \\ \psi_{m21} & -(\mu_{m0} + \psi_{m21}) \end{bmatrix} . \tag{12.9.14}$$

For the case of $m = 2$ and $n = 0$, the set of four couples types may be represented by:

$$\{\varkappa_1 = (1,1),\ \varkappa_2 = (1,2),\ \varkappa_3 = (2,1),\ \varkappa_4 = (2,2)\} , \tag{12.9.15}$$

and the 4×5 matrix $\boldsymbol{\Theta}_{c1}$ of latent risks, governing transitions of females and males in couples from the transient states to the absorbing states, has the form,

$$\boldsymbol{\Theta}_{c1} = \begin{bmatrix} \delta & \mu_{f0} & 0 & \mu_{m0} & 0 \\ \delta & \mu_{f0} & 0 & 0 & \mu_{m0} \\ \delta & 0 & \mu_{f0} & \mu_{m0} & 0 \\ \delta & 0 & \mu_{f0} & 0 & \mu_{m0} \end{bmatrix} . \tag{12.9.16}$$

The 4×4 matrix $\boldsymbol{\Theta}_{c2}$ of latent risks, governing transitions among couple types, i.e., the set of transient states for couples, has the form,

$$\boldsymbol{\Theta}_{c2} = \begin{bmatrix} 0 & \psi_{m12} & \psi_{f12} & 0 \\ \psi_{m21} & 0 & 0 & \psi_{f12} \\ \psi_{f21} & 0 & 0 & \psi_{m12} \\ 0 & \psi_{f21} & \psi_{m21} & 0 \end{bmatrix} . \tag{12.9.17}$$

Thus, the total risks determined by the matrices in Eqs. (12.9.16) and (12.9.17) are:

$$\theta_c(1,1) = \delta + \mu_{f0} + \mu_{m0} + \psi_{m12} + \psi_{f12}$$

$$\theta_c(1,2) = \delta + \mu_{f0} + \mu_{m0} + \psi_{m21} + \psi_{f12}$$

$$\theta_c(2,1) = \delta + \mu_{f0} + \mu_{m0} + \psi_{f21} + \psi_{m12}$$

$$\theta_c(2,2) = \delta + \mu_{f0} + \mu_{m0} + \psi_{f21} + \psi_{m21} \, . \tag{12.9.18}$$

From these equations, it follows that the 4×4 matrix $\mathbf{A}'_{cc}$ for couples has the form,

$$\mathbf{A}'_{cc} = \begin{bmatrix} -\theta_c(1,1) & \psi_{m12} & \psi_{f12} & 0 \\ \psi_{m21} & -\theta_c(1,2) & 0 & \psi_{f12} \\ \psi_{f21} & 0 & -\theta_c(2,1) & \psi_{m12} \\ 0 & \psi_{f21} & \psi_{m21} & -\theta_c(2,2) \end{bmatrix} . \tag{12.9.19}$$

The last task is to specify those matrices of latent risks governing transitions of females and males in couples to the singles population.

The 4×2 matrix $\mathbf{A}_{cf}$, governing transitions of females in couples to the singles population has the form,

$$\mathbf{A}'_{fc} = \mathbf{A}_{cf} = \begin{bmatrix} \delta + \mu_{m0} & 0 \\ \delta + \mu_{m0} & 0 \\ 0 & \delta + \mu_{m0} \\ 0 & \delta + \mu_{m0} \end{bmatrix} . \tag{12.9.20}$$

Similarly, the 4×2 matrix $\mathbf{A}_{cm}$, governing transitions of males in couples to the singles population has the form,

$$\mathbf{A}'_{mc} = \mathbf{A}_{cm} = \begin{bmatrix} \delta + \mu_{f0} & 0 \\ 0 & \delta + \mu_{f0} \\ \delta + \mu_{f0} & 0 \\ 0 & \delta + \mu_{f0} \end{bmatrix} . \tag{12.9.21}$$

Finally, given the above sub-matrices, the transpose of the 8×8 matrix $\mathbf{A}$ has the partitioned form,

$$\mathbf{A}' = \begin{bmatrix} \mathbf{A}'_{ff} & \mathbf{0} & \mathbf{0} \\ \mathbf{0} & \mathbf{A}'_{mm} & \mathbf{0} \\ \mathbf{A}'_{fc} & \mathbf{A}'_{mc} & \mathbf{A}'_{cc} \end{bmatrix} . \tag{12.9.22}$$

In the next section, the matrix $\mathbf{A}$, the transpose of which is defined in Eq. (12.9.22), will denoted by $\mathbf{A}_S$ in a system of differential equations governing the evolution of a population containing only susceptibles with $m = 2$ behavioral classes.

12.10 The Jacobian Matrix and Stationary Points

In many ways, providing an overview of the structure of the Jacobian matrix for the embedded differential equations for the two-sex partnership model considered in this chapter runs parallel to that for the one-sex partnership model presented in Section 11.11. Nevertheless, because many of the details for the two-sex case differ from those for the one-sex, it seems worthwhile to present an overview of the Jacobian matrix for the two-sex case. As a starting point, write the system of differential equations in Eq. (12.8.23) in the compact form,

$$\frac{d\mathbf{v}}{dt} = \mathbf{R} + \mathbf{A}\mathbf{v} + \mathbf{v}_{EM}(\mathbf{v}) + \mathbf{v}_{CF}(\mathbf{v}) , \tag{12.10.1}$$

where $\mathbf{v}_{EM}(\mathbf{v})$ and $\mathbf{v}_{CF}(\mathbf{v})$ are non-linear functions of the vector $\mathbf{v}$ attributable, respectively, to extra-marital sexual contacts and couple formation and are of dimension $(2m(n+1)+m^2(n+1)^2)\times 1$. From Eq. (12.10.1), it is clear that the Jacobian matrix of the system has the form,

$$\mathbf{J}(\mathbf{v}) = \mathbf{A} + \mathbf{J}_{EM}(\mathbf{v}) + \mathbf{J}_{CF}(\mathbf{v}) , \tag{12.10.2}$$

where the Jacobian matrices $\mathbf{J}_{EM}(\mathbf{v})$ and $\mathbf{J}_{CF}(\mathbf{v})$ are derived from the vectors $\mathbf{v}_{EM}(\mathbf{v})$ and $\mathbf{v}_{CF}(\mathbf{v})$. The dimensions of all matrices in Eq. (12.10.2) are $(2m(n+1)+m^2(n+1)^2)\times(2m(n+1)+m^2(n+1)^2)$.

For the case where the population contains only susceptibles, the term in Eq. (12.10.1) for extra-marital sexual contacts vanishes, i.e., $\mathbf{v}_{EM}(\mathbf{v}) = \mathbf{0}$, a zero vector. Moreover, rather than considering the full system in Eq. (12.10.1), it is sufficient to consider the case $n = 0$, indicating the population contains only susceptibles. For this case, the differential equations in Eq. (12.10.1) have the reduced form,

$$\frac{d\mathbf{v}}{dt} = \mathbf{R}_S + \mathbf{A}_S\mathbf{v} + \mathbf{v}_{CFS}(\mathbf{v}) , \tag{12.10.3}$$

where $\mathbf{R}_S$ and $\mathbf{v}_{CFS}(\mathbf{v})$ are $(2m+m^2)\times 1$ vectors and the matrix $\mathbf{A}_S$ is a $(2m+m^2)\times(2m+m^2)$ matrix of constants. Observe that for the case $m = 2$, Eq. (12.10.3) is a system of 8 differential equations, which are cumbersome to represent symbolically on one printed page (see Eq. (12.9.22) for a symbolic representation of the matrix $\mathbf{A}_S'$ when $m = 2$).

However, for the case $m = 1$, the system reduces to three differential equations of the form,

$$\begin{aligned}
\frac{dx}{dt} &= \mu_{rf} - \mu_{f0}x + (\delta + \mu_{m0})z - \rho N_{CF}(x,y) \\
\frac{dy}{dt} &= \mu_{rm} - \mu_{m0}y + (\delta + \mu_{f0})z - \rho N_{CF}(x,y) \\
\frac{dz}{dt} &= -(\delta + \mu_{f0} + \mu_{m0})z + \rho N_{CF}(x,y) ,
\end{aligned} \tag{12.10.4}$$

which are useful for illustrating concepts, where $N_{CF}(x,y) = \min(x,y)$ by definition. For points in the parameter space such that $y < x$, these differential equations have the simple form,

$$\frac{dx}{dt} = \mu_{rf} - \mu_{f0}x + (\delta + \mu_{m0})z - \rho y$$

$$\frac{dy}{dt} = \mu_{rm} - \mu_{m0}y + (\delta + \mu_{f0})z - \rho y$$

$$\frac{dz}{dt} = -(\delta + \mu_{f0} + \mu_{m0})z + \rho y \ , \tag{12.10.5}$$

such that all terms on the right hand side are linear in x, y, and z.

For this case, it is possible to find symbolic forms for the elements of a stationary vector $\widehat{\mathbf{v}}$ for this system, and, with the help of MAPLE, it can be shown that:

$$\widehat{x} = \frac{\mu_{rf}\mu_{m0}\delta + \mu_{rf}\mu_{m0}\mu_{f0} + \mu_{rf}\mu_{m0}^2 + \mu_{rf}\mu_{m0}\rho - \rho\mu_{rm}\mu_{f0}}{\mu_{f0}\mu_{m0}\left(\delta + \mu_{f0} + \mu_{m0} + \rho\right)}$$

$$\widehat{y} = \frac{\delta + \mu_{f0} + \mu_{m0}}{\mu_{m0}\left(\delta + \mu_{f0} + \mu_{m0} + \rho\right)}\mu_{rm}$$

$$\widehat{z} = \frac{\rho}{\mu_{m0}\left(\delta + \mu_{f0} + \mu_{m0} + \rho\right)}\mu_{rm} \ . \tag{12.10.6}$$

From an inspection of these expressions for the stationary values, it can be seen that because all parameters are positive, the values of $\widehat{y}$ and $\widehat{z}$ will be positive at all points in the parameter space. But, because the numerator of the expression for $\widehat{x}$ contains the negative term $-\rho\mu_{rm}\mu_{f0}$, $\widehat{x}$ may not be positive at all points in the parameter space.

However, if the rate of female recruits entering the population is greater than that for males, $\mu_{rf} > \mu_{rm}$, and the death rate of males is greater than that of females, $\mu_{m0} > \mu_{f0}$, then:

$$\mu_{rf}\mu_{m0}\rho - \rho\mu_{rm}\mu_{f0} > \rho(\mu_{rm}\mu_{f0} - \mu_{rm}\mu_{f0}) = 0 \ . \tag{12.10.7}$$

Therefore, at points in the parameter space such that $\mu_{rf} > \mu_{rm}$ and $\mu_{m0} > \mu_{f0}$, $\widehat{x} > 0$. From the biological point of view, these conditions seem reasonable, because death rates among sexually active males are greater than those for females in most populations. A greater death rate for males is also consistent with the condition that more female recruits enter the population per unit time than male recruits. As in the one-sex models with partnerships studied in Section 11.11, it can be shown, with the help of MAPLE, that at equilibrium, the total population size is:

$$\widehat{x}+\widehat{y}+2\widehat{z}=\frac{\mu_{rf}}{\mu_{f0}}+\frac{\mu_{rm}}{\mu_{m0}}=\mu_{rf}E[T_f]+\mu_{rm}E\left[T_m\right] , \tag{12.10.8}$$

where $E[T_f]$ and $E\left[T_m\right]$ are, respectively, the expectations for remaining life spans for females and males after becoming sexually active.

For more complicated models of cases such that $m > 1$ and $n = 0$, it will, in general, not be possible to derive useful symbolic forms of a stationary vector that can be printed on one or two pages. Useful results may, however, be obtained by resorting to numerical methods for finding stationary vectors. The vector-valued non-linear difference equation version of the system of differential equations in Eq. (12.10.3) is:

$$\mathbf{v}_{n+1}=\mathbf{v}_n+h\left(\mathbf{R}_S+\mathbf{A}_S\mathbf{v}_n+\mathbf{v}_{CFS}(\mathbf{v}_n)\right) . \tag{12.10.9}$$

Hence, if the limit

$$\lim_{n\uparrow\infty}\mathbf{v}_n=\widehat{\mathbf{v}} \tag{12.10.10}$$

exits, then for every $h > 0$,

$$\mathbf{R}_S+\mathbf{A}_S\widehat{\mathbf{v}}+\mathbf{v}_{CFS}(\widehat{\mathbf{v}})=\mathbf{0} \tag{12.10.11}$$

so that $\widehat{\mathbf{v}}$ is a stationary vector. By using arguments similar to those outlined in Section 11.11, it would be possible to find plausible conditions for the limit in Eq. (12.10.10) to exist. Furthermore, given an initial vector $\mathbf{v}_0$, it is a straightforward exercise to write software to implement the non-linear vector-valued difference equation in Eq. (12.10.9) to find a stationary vector $\widehat{\mathbf{v}}$ at any point in the parameter space.

Having found a stationary vector $\widehat{\mathbf{v}}$, the next step would be that of evaluating the Jacobian matrix in Eq. (12.10.2) at this vector. For the two-sex partnership model under consideration, the population vector $\mathbf{v}$ has the partitioned form,

$$\mathbf{v}=\begin{pmatrix}\mathbf{v}_f\\ \mathbf{v}_m\\ \mathbf{v}_m\end{pmatrix} , \tag{12.10.12}$$

where $\mathbf{v}_f$ is a $m(n+1) \times 1$ vector for single females, $\mathbf{v}_m$ is a similar vector for single males, and $\mathbf{v}_c$ is a $m^2(n+1)^2 \times 1$ for couples. From the quasi-diagonal matrix in Eq. (12.8.36), it can be seen that:

$$\mathbf{v}_{EM}(\mathbf{v}) = \mathbf{W}\mathbf{v} = \begin{pmatrix} \mathbf{W}_{ff}\mathbf{v}_f \\ \mathbf{W}_{mm}\mathbf{v}_m \\ \mathbf{W}_{cc}\mathbf{v}_c \end{pmatrix} . \tag{12.10.13}$$

Consequently, the Jacobian matrix $\mathbf{J}_{EM}(\mathbf{v})$ for extra-marital contacts has the partitioned form,

$$\mathbf{J}_{EM}(\mathbf{v}) = \begin{bmatrix} \dfrac{\partial \mathbf{W}_{ff}\mathbf{v}_f}{\partial \mathbf{v}} \\ \dfrac{\partial \mathbf{W}_{mm}\mathbf{v}_m}{\partial \mathbf{v}} \\ \dfrac{\partial \mathbf{W}_{cc}\mathbf{v}_c}{\partial \mathbf{v}} \end{bmatrix} . \tag{12.10.14}$$

By way of explanation,

$$\frac{\partial \mathbf{W}_{ff}\mathbf{v}_f}{\partial \mathbf{v}} \tag{12.10.15}$$

is a $m(n+1) \times (2m(n+1) + m^2(n+1)^2)$ matrix of partial derivatives for single females; the matrix for single males,

$$\frac{\partial \mathbf{W}_{mm}\mathbf{v}_m}{\partial \mathbf{v}} \tag{12.10.16}$$

has the same dimensions; and the matrix of partial derivatives for couples,

$$\frac{\partial \mathbf{W}_{cc}\mathbf{v}_c}{\partial \mathbf{v}} \tag{12.10.17}$$

has dimensions $m^2(n+1)^2 \times (2m(n+1)+m^2(n+1)^2)$. Just as in the one-sex partnership model, these matrices will be sparse, when evaluated at a stationary vector $\widehat{\mathbf{v}}$.

In the simplified notation of this section, the vector $\mathbf{v}_{CF}(\mathbf{v})$ for couple formation has the partitioned form,

$$\mathbf{v}_{CF}(\mathbf{v}) = \begin{pmatrix} \mathbf{v}_{FCF}(\mathbf{v}) \\ \mathbf{v}_{MCF}(\mathbf{v}) \\ \mathbf{v}_{CCF}(\mathbf{v}) \end{pmatrix} , \tag{12.10.18}$$

(see Eqs. (12.8.15) through (12.8.17) for the definitions of the elements of the sub-vectors in Eq. (12.10.18)). Therefore, the Jacobian matrix corresponding to this vector has the partitioned form,

$$\mathbf{J}_{CF}(\mathbf{v}) = \frac{\partial \mathbf{v}_{CF}(\mathbf{v})}{\partial \mathbf{v}} = \begin{bmatrix} \dfrac{\partial \mathbf{v}_{FCF}(\mathbf{v})}{\partial \mathbf{v}} \\ \dfrac{\partial \mathbf{v}_{MCF}(\mathbf{v})}{\partial \mathbf{v}} \\ \dfrac{\partial \mathbf{v}_{CCF}(\mathbf{v})}{\partial \mathbf{v}} \end{bmatrix} = \begin{bmatrix} \mathbf{J}_{FCF}(\mathbf{v}) \\ \mathbf{J}_{MCF}(\mathbf{v}) \\ \mathbf{J}_{CCF}(\mathbf{v}) \end{bmatrix}. \tag{12.10.19}$$

The dimensions of these matrices are the same as the corresponding ones in Eqs. (12.10.15) through (12.10.17). Because the elements of the sub-vectors in Eq. (12.10.19) depend only on the sub-vectors $\mathbf{v}_f$ and $\mathbf{v}_m$ for single females and males, all partial derivatives with respect to the elements of the vector $\mathbf{v}_c$ for couples will be zero. Thus, all $m^2(n+1)^2$ column vectors of the Jacobian matrix in Eq. (12.10.19), which arise from differentiation with respect to the vector $\mathbf{v}_c$, will be zero vectors.

12.11 Overview of the Jacobian for Extra-Marital Contacts

The structure of the Jacobian matrix for extra-marital sexual contacts for the two-sex partnership model under consideration is similar to that for the one-sex partnership models discussed in Section 11.12. But, because many of the details are significantly different from those for the one-sex model, a detailed exposition of the structure of the Jacobian matrix for the two-sex model is justified. To this end, let the symbols Υ_{SF} and Υ_{IF} denote, respectively, the sets of susceptible and infectious females types. Then, then $\Upsilon_{SF} \cup \Upsilon_{IF} = \Upsilon_f = \mathfrak{S}_{f2}$, the set of females types (see Eq. (12.2.1)). The sets Υ_{SM} and Υ_{IM} are defined similarly for males with $\Upsilon_{SM} \cup \Upsilon_{IM} = \Upsilon_m = \mathfrak{S}_{m2}$. The objective of this section is to derive some general formulas for non-zero elements of the Jacobian matrix for extra-marital sexual contacts and then illustrate their use in the simple case of $m = 1$ behavioral class and $n = 1$ stage of disease.

In the succinct notation of this section (see Eq. (12.5.2)), the total number of females of type $\tau_f \in \Upsilon_f$ in the population at any time is:

$$x_T(\tau_f) = x(\tau_f) + \sum_{\tau_m \in \Upsilon_m} z(\tau_f, \tau_m) . \tag{12.11.1}$$

Similarly, the total number of males of type $\tau_m \in \Upsilon_m$ in the population at any time is:

$$y_T(\tau_m) = y(\tau_m) + \sum_{\tau_f \in \Upsilon_f} z(\tau_f, \tau_m) . \tag{12.11.2}$$

For every female type $\tau_f \in \Upsilon_f$, let

$$T_f(\tau_f, \mathbf{v}) = \sum_{\tau_m \in \Upsilon_m} y_T(\tau_m)\alpha_{fem}(\tau_f, \tau_m) , \tag{12.11.3}$$

where $\mathbf{v}$ is the population vector defined in Eq. (12.10.5). Similarly, to avoid ambiguity, for every male type $\tau_m \in \Upsilon_m$ and population vector $\mathbf{v}$, let

$$T_m(\tau_m, \mathbf{v}) = \sum_{\tau_f \in \Upsilon_f} x_T(\tau_f)\alpha_{mem}(\tau_m, \tau_f) . \tag{12.11.4}$$

From Eq. (12.11.1), it can be seen that the function $T_f(\tau_f, \mathbf{v})$ depends only on the sub-vector $\mathbf{v}_m$ for single males and on the sub-vector $\mathbf{v}_c$ for couples. Similarly, the function $T_m(\tau_m, \mathbf{v})$ depends only on the sub-vector $\mathbf{v}_f$ for single females and on the sub-vector $\mathbf{v}_c$ for couples.

Given the above definitions, the conditional probability that a female of type τ_f has contact with a male of type τ_m as a potential extra-marital sexual partner is:

$$\gamma_{fem}(\tau_f, \tau_m) = \frac{y_T(\tau_m)\alpha_{fem}(\tau_f, \tau_m)}{T_f(\tau_f, \mathbf{v})} . \tag{12.11.5}$$

Analogously, the conditional probability that a male of type τ_m has contact with a female of type τ_f as a potential extra-marital sexual partner is:

$$\gamma_{mem}(\tau_m, \tau_f) = \frac{x_T(\tau_f)\alpha_{mem}(\tau_m, \tau_f)}{T_m(\tau_m, \mathbf{v})} . \tag{12.11.6}$$

For the embedded differential equations, the multinomial expectations,

$$x_T(\tau_f)\gamma_{fem}(\tau_f,\tau_m) = \frac{x_T(\tau_f)y_T(\tau_m)\alpha_{fem}(\tau_f,\tau_m)}{T_f(\tau_f,\mathbf{v})} \tag{12.11.7}$$

and

$$y_T(\tau_m)\gamma_{mem}(\tau_m,\tau_f) = \frac{y_T(\tau_m)x_T(\tau_f)\alpha_{mem}(\tau_m,\tau_f)}{T_m(\tau_m,\mathbf{v})} \tag{12.11.8}$$

are the arguments used in the approximation,

$$\eta_\theta(x,y) = \frac{xy2^{\frac{1}{\theta}}}{(x^\theta + y^\theta)^{\frac{1}{\theta}}} \tag{12.11.9}$$

to the min function, $\min(x,y)$, for $x > 0$ and $y > 0$. Moreover, just as in Section 11.12, if one can define variables x, y_1 and y_2 such that the approximation to the min function has the form,

$$\eta_\theta(\frac{x}{y_1},\frac{x}{y_2}) = \frac{x}{y_1}\left(\frac{2}{1+\left(\frac{y_2}{y_1}\right)^\theta}\right)^{\frac{1}{\theta}}, \tag{12.11.10}$$

then computationally useful formulas for the elements of the Jacobian matrix for extra-marital sexual contacts may be derived. It is easy to see that the symbols y_1 and y_2 may be interchanged.

To apply this formula let

$$x = x_T(\tau_f)y_T(\tau_m)\ , \tag{12.11.11}$$

$$y_1 = \frac{T_f(\tau_f,\mathbf{v})}{\alpha_{fem}(\tau_f,\tau_m)} \tag{12.11.12}$$

and

$$y_2 = \frac{T_m(\tau_m,\mathbf{v})}{\alpha_{mem}(\tau_m,\tau_f)}\ . \tag{12.11.13}$$

Then, to simplify the notation, let

$$R_f(\tau_f,\tau_m,\mathbf{v}) = \frac{y_2}{y_1} = \frac{\alpha_{fem}(\tau_f,\tau_m)T_m(\tau_m,\mathbf{v})}{\alpha_{mem}(\tau_m,\tau_f)T_f(\tau_f,\mathbf{v})} \tag{12.11.14}$$

and

$$g_{f\theta}(\tau_f, \tau_m, \mathbf{v}) = \left(\frac{2}{1 + (R_f(\tau_f, \tau_m, \mathbf{v}))^{\theta}} \right)^{\frac{1}{\theta}} \tag{12.11.15}$$

If $\tau_f \in \Upsilon_{SF}$ is a susceptible female, then in the notation of this section the number of extra-marital sexual contacts of type (τ_f, τ_m) occurring during a small time interval (see Eq. (12.5.5)), is:

$$N_{EMP}(\tau_f, \tau_m, \mathbf{v}) = \frac{x_T(\tau_f) y_T(\tau_m) \alpha_{fem}(\tau_f, \tau_m)}{T_f(\tau_f, \mathbf{v})} g_{f\theta}(\tau_f, \tau_m, \mathbf{v}) \tag{12.11.16}$$

for every $\tau_m \in \mathfrak{S}_{m2}$. Therefore, from Eq. (12.5.6) the conditional probability $\rho_{fem}(\tau_f, \tau_m, \mathbf{v})$ that a susceptible female of type has τ_f has an extra-marital sexual contact with a male of type τ_m is:

$$\rho_{fem}(\tau_f, \tau_m, \mathbf{v}) = \frac{y_T(\tau_m) \alpha_{fem}(\tau_f, \tau_m) g_{f\theta}(\tau_f, \tau_m, \mathbf{v})}{W_f(\tau_f, \mathbf{v})}, \tag{12.11.17}$$

where

$$W_f(\tau_f, \mathbf{v}) = \sum_{\tau_m \in \mathfrak{S}_{m2}} y_T(\tau_m) \alpha_{fem}(\tau_f, \tau_m) g_{f\theta}(\tau_f, \tau_m, \mathbf{v}) . \tag{12.11.18}$$

From these formulas it follows that, during any small time interval, the conditional probability that a susceptible female of type $\tau_f \in \Upsilon_{SF}$ is infected through extra-marital sexual contacts with an infectious male is:

$$Q_{par}(\tau_f, \mathbf{v}) = \frac{1}{W_f(\tau_f, \mathbf{v})} \times$$

$$\sum_{\tau_m \in \Upsilon_{IM}} y_T(\tau_m) \alpha_{fem}(\tau_f, \tau_m) g_{f\theta}(\tau_f, \tau_m, \mathbf{v}) q_{fem}(\tau_m) . \tag{12.11.19}$$

The corresponding conditional probability $Q_{par}(\tau_m, \mathbf{v})$ for susceptible male of type $\tau_m \in \Upsilon_{SM}$ to be infected during any small time interval may derived by an analogous argument. To this end, let

$$R_m(\tau_m, \tau_f, \mathbf{v}) = \frac{1}{R_f(\tau_f, \tau_m, \mathbf{v})}, \tag{12.11.20}$$

and let

$$g_{m\theta}(\tau_m,\tau_f,\mathbf{v})=\left(\frac{2}{1+(R_m(\tau_m,\tau_f,\mathbf{v}))^{\theta}}\right)^{\frac{1}{\theta}} . \qquad (12.11.21)$$

Then, it can be shown that:

$$Q_{par}(\tau_m,\mathbf{v})=\frac{1}{W_m(\tau_m,\mathbf{v})}\times$$

$$\sum_{\tau_f\in\Upsilon_{IF}} x_T(\tau_f)\alpha_{mem}(\tau_m,\tau_f)g_{mf\theta}(\tau_m,\tau_f,\mathbf{v})q_{mem}(\tau_f)\,, \qquad (12.11.22)$$

where

$$W_m(\tau_m,\mathbf{v})=\sum_{\tau_f\in\mathfrak{S}_{f2}} x_T(\tau_m)\alpha_{mem}(\tau_m,\tau_f)g_{m\theta}(\tau_m,\tau_f,\mathbf{v})\,. \qquad (12.11.23)$$

As in Section 12.10, let $\widehat{\mathbf{v}}$ denote a stationary vector of the differential equations in Eq. (12.10.1) such that the population contains only susceptible females and males. Because the numerators in the functions $Q_{par}(\tau_f,\widehat{\mathbf{v}})$ and $Q_{par}(\tau_m,\widehat{\mathbf{v}})$ vanish at $\widehat{\mathbf{v}}$ for all susceptible female and male types τ_f and τ_m, formulas for their partial derivatives evaluated at the vector $\widehat{\mathbf{v}}$ are either zero or relatively simple. Many elements of the Jacobian matrix are also zero, because $Q_{par}(\tau_f,\mathbf{v})$ depends only the sub-vectors $\mathbf{v}_m$, and $\mathbf{v}_c$ and $Q_{par}(\tau_m,\mathbf{v})$ depends only on the sub-vectors $\mathbf{v}_f$ and $\mathbf{v}_c$. In the following, the notation is to be interpreted such that a formula for a partial derivative with respect to any element of $\mathbf{v}$ is derived and then evaluated at a stationary vector $\widehat{\mathbf{v}}$. Thus, for every susceptible female type $\tau_f\in\Upsilon_{SF}$ and infectious male type $\tau_m\in\Upsilon_{IM}$, it follows from Eq. (12.11.2) that:

$$\frac{\partial Q_{par}(\tau_f,\widehat{\mathbf{v}})}{\partial y(\tau_m)}=\frac{1}{W_f(\tau_f,\widehat{\mathbf{v}})}\alpha_{fem}(\tau_f,\tau_m)g_{f\theta}(\tau_f,\tau_m,\widehat{\mathbf{v}})q_{fem}(\tau_m)\,. \qquad (12.11.24)$$

Similarly, for every susceptible female type $\tau_f\in\Upsilon_{SF}$, infectious male type $\tau_m\in\Upsilon_{IM}$ and couple type (τ,τ_m), it also follows from Eq. (12.11.2) that:

$$\frac{\partial Q_{par}(\tau_f,\widehat{\mathbf{v}})}{\partial z(\tau,\tau_m)}=\frac{1}{W_f(\tau_t,\widehat{\mathbf{v}})}\alpha_{fem}(\tau_f,\tau_m)g_{f\theta}(\tau,\tau_m,\widehat{\mathbf{v}})q_{fem}(\tau_m) \qquad (12.11.25)$$

for all female types $\tau \in \Upsilon_f$.

As an aid to writing software, the corresponding formulas of susceptible male types will also be exhibited. For every susceptible male type $\tau_m \in \Upsilon_{SM}$ and infectious female type $\tau_f \in \Upsilon_{IF}$, it follows from Eq. (12.11.1) that

$$\frac{\partial Q_{par}(\tau_m, \widehat{\mathbf{v}})}{\partial x(\tau_f)} = \frac{1}{W_m(\tau_m, \widehat{\mathbf{v}})} \alpha_{mem}(\tau_m, \tau_f) g_{m\theta}(\tau_m, \tau_f, \widehat{\mathbf{v}}) q_{mem}(\tau_f) \,. \tag{12.11.26}$$

And, for every susceptible male type $\tau_m \in \Upsilon_{SM}$, infectious female type $\tau_f \in \Upsilon_{IF}$ and couple type (τ_f, τ), it also follows from Eq. (12.11.2) that:

$$\frac{\partial Q_{par}(\tau_m, \widehat{\mathbf{v}})}{\partial z(\tau_f, \tau)} = \frac{1}{W_m(\tau_m, \widehat{\mathbf{v}})} \alpha_{mem}(\tau_m, \tau_f) g_{m\theta}(\tau, \tau_f, \widehat{\mathbf{v}}) q_{mem}(\tau_f) \tag{12.11.27}$$

for all $\tau \in \Upsilon_m$.

From the formulas just derived, it can be seen that the Jacobian matrix for extra-marital sexual contacts exhibited in Eq. (12.10.14) has the partitioned form,

$$\mathbf{J}_{EM}(\mathbf{v}) = \begin{bmatrix} \mathbf{J}_{ff}(\mathbf{v}) & \mathbf{J}_{fm}(\mathbf{v}) & \mathbf{J}_{fc}(\mathbf{v}) \\ \mathbf{J}_{mf}(\mathbf{v}) & \mathbf{J}_{mm}(\mathbf{v}) & \mathbf{J}_{mc}(\mathbf{v}) \\ \mathbf{J}_{cf}(\mathbf{v}) & \mathbf{J}_{cm}(\mathbf{v}) & \mathbf{J}_{cc}(\mathbf{v}) \end{bmatrix} \,. \tag{12.11.28}$$

By way of explanation, observe that the sub-matrix,

$$\mathbf{J}_{fm}(\mathbf{v}) = \frac{\partial \mathbf{W}_{ff}\mathbf{v}_f}{\partial \mathbf{v}_m} \tag{12.11.29}$$

is $m(n+1) \times m(n+1)$ and the sub-matrix,

$$\mathbf{J}_{fc}(\mathbf{v}) = \frac{\partial \mathbf{W}_{ff}\mathbf{v}_f}{\partial \mathbf{v}_c} \tag{12.11.30}$$

is $m(n+1) \times m^2(n+1)^2$. The sub-matrices $\mathbf{J}_{mf}(\mathbf{v})$ and $\mathbf{J}_{mc}(\mathbf{v})$ as well as $\mathbf{J}_{ff}(\mathbf{v})$ and $\mathbf{J}_{mm}(\mathbf{v})$ are defined similarly. However, the sub-matrix,

$$\mathbf{J}_{cf}(\mathbf{v}) = \frac{\partial \mathbf{W}_{cc}\mathbf{v}_c}{\partial \mathbf{v}_f} \tag{12.11.31}$$

is $m^2(n+1)^2 \times m(n+1)$ and the sub-matrix,

$$\mathbf{J}_{cc}(\mathbf{v}) = \frac{\partial \mathbf{W}_{cc}\mathbf{v}_c}{\partial \mathbf{v}_c} \tag{12.11.32}$$

is $m^2(n+1)^2 \times m^2(n+1)^2$. Finally, the sub-matrix $\mathbf{J}_{cm}(\mathbf{v})$ is defined in a manner similar to that in Eq. (12.11.31).

In the remainder of this section, examples of these sub-matrices evaluated at a stationary vector $\widehat{\mathbf{v}}$ will be given for the simple case of $m = 1$ behavioral class and $n = 1$ stage of disease. For this case, the susceptible female and male types are $\tau_{f1} = (0)$ and $\tau_{m1} = (0)$ and the infectious female and male types are $\tau_{f2} = (1)$ and $\tau_{m2} = (1)$. The set of four couple types in lexicographical order has the elements $\varkappa_1 = (\tau_{f1}, \tau_{m1})$, $\varkappa_2 = (\tau_{f1}, \tau_{m2})$, $\varkappa_3 = (\tau_{f_2}, \tau_{m1})$ and $\varkappa_3 = (\tau_{f_2}, \tau_{m1})$.

Therefore, from Eqs. (12.9.3) and (12.9.4), it can be seen that:

$$\mathbf{W}_{ff}\mathbf{v}_f = \begin{pmatrix} -x(\tau_{f1})\lambda(\tau_{f1})Q_{par}(\tau_f, \mathbf{v}) \\ x(\tau_{f1})\lambda(\tau_{f1})Q_{par}(\tau_f, \mathbf{v}) \end{pmatrix} \tag{12.11.33}$$

and

$$\mathbf{W}_{mm}\mathbf{v}_m = \begin{pmatrix} -y(\tau_{m1})\lambda(\tau_{m1})Q_{par}(\tau_m, \mathbf{v}) \\ y(\tau_{m1})\lambda(\tau_{m1})Q_{par}(\tau_m, \mathbf{v}) \end{pmatrix} . \tag{12.11.34}$$

To compact and augment the notation in Eq. (12.11.24), let

$$k_f(\tau_{f1}, \tau_{m2}, \widehat{\mathbf{v}}) = \frac{\lambda(\tau_{f1})}{W_f(\tau_{f1}, \widehat{\mathbf{v}})} \alpha_{fem}(\tau_{f1}, \tau_{m2}) g_{f\theta}(\tau_{f1}, \tau_{m2}, \widehat{\mathbf{v}}) q_{fem}(\tau_{m2}) . \tag{12.11.35}$$

Then, it can be shown that:

$$\mathbf{J}_{fm}(\widehat{\mathbf{v}}) = \begin{bmatrix} 0 & -\widehat{x}(\tau_{f1})k_f(\tau_{f1}, \tau_{m2}, \widehat{\mathbf{v}}) \\ 0 & \widehat{x}(\tau_{f1})k_f(\tau_{f1}, \tau_{m2}, \widehat{\mathbf{v}}) \end{bmatrix} . \tag{12.11.36}$$

Furthermore, it can be shown that:

$$\mathbf{J}_{fc}(\widehat{\mathbf{v}}) = \begin{bmatrix} 0 & -\widehat{x}(\tau_{f1})k_f(\tau_{f1}, \tau_{m2}, \widehat{\mathbf{v}}) & 0 & -\widehat{x}(\tau_{f1})k_f(\tau_{f1}, \tau_{m2}, \widehat{\mathbf{v}}) \\ 0 & \widehat{x}(\tau_{f1})k_f(\tau_{f1}, \tau_{m2}, \widehat{\mathbf{v}}) & 0 & \widehat{x}(\tau_{f1})k_f(\tau_{f1}, \tau_{m2}, \widehat{\mathbf{v}}) \end{bmatrix} . \tag{12.11.37}$$

It can also be seen from Eq. (12.11.33) that $\mathbf{J}_{ff}(\mathbf{v}) = \mathbf{0}_{2\times 2}$, a 2×2 zero matrix.

In a similar vein for males, let

$$k_m(\tau_{m1}, \tau_{f2}, \widehat{\mathbf{v}}) = \frac{\lambda(\tau_{m1})}{W_m(\tau_{m1}, \widehat{\mathbf{v}})} \alpha_{mem}(\tau_{m1}, \tau_{f2}) g_{m\theta}(\tau_{m1}, \tau_{f2}, \widehat{\mathbf{v}}) q_{mem}(\tau_{f2}) . \tag{12.11.38}$$

Then, it can be shown that:

$$\mathbf{J}_{mf}(\widehat{\mathbf{v}}) = \begin{bmatrix} 0 & -\widehat{y}(\tau_{m1}) k_m(\tau_{m1}, \tau_{f2}, \widehat{\mathbf{v}}) \\ 0 & \widehat{y}(\tau_{m1}) k_m(\tau_{m1}, \tau_{f2}, \widehat{\mathbf{v}}) \end{bmatrix} \tag{12.11.39}$$

and

$$\mathbf{J}_{mc}(\widehat{\mathbf{v}}) = \begin{bmatrix} 0 & 0 & -\widehat{y}(\tau_{m1}) k_m(\tau_{m1}, \tau_{f2}, \widehat{\mathbf{v}}) & -\widehat{y}(\tau_{m1}) k_m(\tau_{m1}, \tau_{f2}, \widehat{\mathbf{v}}) \\ 0 & 0 & \widehat{y}(\tau_{m1}) k_m(\tau_{m1}, \tau_{f2}, \widehat{\mathbf{v}}) & \widehat{y}(\tau_{m1}) k_m(\tau_{m1}, \tau_{f2}, \widehat{\mathbf{v}}) \end{bmatrix} . \tag{12.11.40}$$

Similarly, it can be seen that $\mathbf{J}_{mm}(\mathbf{v}) = \mathbf{0}_{2\times 2}$, a 2×2 zero matrix.

The last step in displaying the Jacobian matrix in Eq. (12.11.28) is to consider the elements of the sub-matrices $\mathbf{J}_{cf}(\mathbf{v})$, $\mathbf{J}_{cm}(\mathbf{v})$ and $\mathbf{J}_{cc}(\mathbf{v})$ at $\mathbf{v} = \widehat{\mathbf{v}}$. In terms of the notation of this section, let $S_{par}(\mathbf{v})$ denote the sum,

$$S_{par}(\mathbf{v}) = \lambda(\tau_{m1}) Q_{par}(\tau_m, \mathbf{v}) + \lambda(\tau_{f1}) Q_{par}(\tau_f, \mathbf{v}) \tag{12.11.41}$$

as defined in Eq. (12.9.8). Moreover, in the notation of this section, the column vector for couples is:

$$\mathbf{v}_c = \begin{pmatrix} z(\varkappa_1) \\ z(\varkappa_2) \\ z(\varkappa_3) \\ z(\varkappa_4) \end{pmatrix} . \tag{12.11.42}$$

Then, from Eq. (12.9.9), it can be seen that:

$$\mathbf{W}_{cc}\mathbf{v}_c = \begin{pmatrix} -z(\varkappa_1) S_{par}(\mathbf{v}) \\ z(\varkappa_1)\lambda(\tau_{m1}) Q_{par}(\tau_m, \mathbf{v}) - z(\varkappa_2)\lambda(\tau_{f1}) Q_{par}(\tau_f, \mathbf{v}) \\ z(\varkappa_1)\lambda(\tau_{f1}) Q_{par}(\tau_f, \mathbf{v}) - z(\varkappa_3)\lambda(\tau_{m1}) Q_{par}(\tau_m, \mathbf{v}) \\ z(\varkappa_2)\lambda(\tau_{f1}) Q_{par}(\tau_f, \mathbf{v}) + z(\varkappa_3)\lambda(\tau_{m1}) Q_{par}(\tau_m, \mathbf{v}) \end{pmatrix} . \tag{12.11.43}$$

A key observation in deriving formulas for the elements of the sub-Jacobian matrices under consideration is that the stationary vector $\widehat{\mathbf{v}}_c$ for couples has the form,

$$\widehat{\mathbf{v}}_c = \begin{pmatrix} \widehat{z}(\varkappa_1) \\ 0 \\ 0 \\ 0 \end{pmatrix}, \tag{12.11.44}$$

where $\widehat{z}(\varkappa_1) > 0$.

Then, because $Q_{par}(\tau_m, \mathbf{v})$ is a function of the vector $\mathbf{v}_f$ for single females, it follows from Eq. (12.11.43) that:

$$\mathbf{J}_{cf}(\widehat{\mathbf{v}}) = \begin{bmatrix} 0 & -\widehat{z}(\varkappa_1)k_m(\tau_{m1}, \tau_{f2}, \widehat{\mathbf{v}}) \\ 0 & \widehat{z}(\varkappa_1)k_m(\tau_{m1}, \tau_{f2}, \widehat{\mathbf{v}}) \\ 0 & 0 \\ 0 & 0 \end{bmatrix}. \tag{12.11.45}$$

Similarly, because $Q_{par}(\tau_f, \mathbf{v})$ is a function of the vector $\mathbf{v}_m$ for single males, it can be shown that:

$$\mathbf{J}_{cm}(\widehat{\mathbf{v}}) = \begin{bmatrix} 0 & -\widehat{z}(\varkappa_1)k_f(\tau_{f1}, \tau_{m2}, \widehat{\mathbf{v}}) \\ 0 & 0 \\ 0 & \widehat{z}(\varkappa_1)k_f(\tau_{f1}, \tau_{m2}, \widehat{\mathbf{v}}) \\ 0 & 0 \end{bmatrix}. \tag{12.11.46}$$

The last sub-Jacobian matrix to be considered it that for couples in Eq. (12.11.32). To represent this matrix in a succinct form, it will be helpful to display its column vectors separately. Let $\mathbf{0}_4$ denote a 4×1 column vector of zeros, let

$$\mathbf{c}_2(\widehat{\mathbf{v}}) = \begin{pmatrix} -\widehat{z}(\varkappa_1)k_f(\tau_{f1}, \tau_{m2}, \widehat{\mathbf{v}}) \\ 0 \\ \widehat{z}(\varkappa_1)k_f(\tau_{f1}, \tau_{m2}, \widehat{\mathbf{v}}) \\ 0 \end{pmatrix}, \tag{12.11.47}$$

let

$$\mathbf{c}_3(\widehat{\mathbf{v}}) = \begin{pmatrix} -\widehat{z}(\varkappa_1)k_m(\tau_{m1}, \tau_{f2}, \widehat{\mathbf{v}}) \\ \widehat{z}(\varkappa_1)k_m(\tau_{m1}, \tau_{f2}, \widehat{\mathbf{v}}) \\ 0 \\ 0 \end{pmatrix}, \tag{12.11.48}$$

and let

$$\mathbf{c}_4(\widehat{\mathbf{v}}) = \begin{pmatrix} -\widehat{z}(\varkappa_1)(k_f(\tau_{f1}, \tau_{m2}, \widehat{\mathbf{v}}) + k_m(\tau_{m1}, \tau_{f2}, \widehat{\mathbf{v}})) \\ \widehat{z}(\varkappa_1) k_m(\tau_{m1}, \tau_{f2}, \widehat{\mathbf{v}}) \\ \widehat{z}(\varkappa_1) k_f(\tau_{f1}, \tau_{m2}, \widehat{\mathbf{v}}) \\ 0 \end{pmatrix} \tag{12.11.49}$$

By using equations Eqs. (12.11.1) and (12.11.2) and the foregoing results on formulas for partial derivatives, it can be shown that:

$$\mathbf{J}_{cc}(\widehat{\mathbf{v}}) = \left[\ \mathbf{0}_4 \quad \mathbf{c}_2(\widehat{\mathbf{v}}) \quad \mathbf{c}_3(\widehat{\mathbf{v}}) \quad \mathbf{c}_4(\widehat{\mathbf{v}})\ \right] . \tag{12.11.50}$$

12.12 General Form of the Jacobian for Extra-Marital Contacts

Before proceeding to the general form of the Jacobian matrix for extra-marital sexual contacts, it will be helpful in illustrating the concepts to consider the case of $m = 1$ behavioral class and $n = 2$ stages of disease. In this case, the set Υ_f of female types contains the elements $\tau_{f1} = (0)$, a susceptible, and two infectious types $\tau_{f2} = (1)$ and $\tau_{f2} = (2)$. Similarly, the set Υ_m of male types contains the elements $\tau_{m1} = (0)$, $\tau_{m2} = (1)$ and $\tau_{m3} = (2)$. Hence, the product set,

$$\Upsilon_c = \mathfrak{S}_{c2} = \Upsilon_f \times \Upsilon_c \tag{12.12.1}$$

of couple types contains 9 elements. There are notational advantages to representing this set in the form,

$$\Upsilon_c = \{\varkappa = (k_1, k_2) \mid k_1 = 0, 1, 2;\ k_2 = 0, 1, 2\} \ , \tag{12.12.2}$$

which is particularly useful in representing the 9×9 matrix W_{cc} in the partitioned form of 3×3 sub-matrices. In this connection, let

$$A(k_1) = \{\varkappa = (k_1, k_2) \mid k_2 = 0, 1, 2\} \tag{12.12.3}$$

be the set of couple types such that the female is in state k_1 with respect to disease. Then, Υ_c is the disjoint union

$$\Upsilon_c = \bigcup_{k_k=0}^{2} A(k_1) \ . \tag{12.12.4}$$

In this case the 3×3 matrix $\mathbf{W}_{ff}$ for single females has the form,

$$\mathbf{W}_{ff} = \begin{bmatrix} -\lambda(\tau_{f1})Q_{par}(\tau_{f1}, \mathbf{v}) & 0 & 0 \\ \lambda(\tau_{f1})Q_{par}(\tau_{f1}, \mathbf{v}) & 0 & 0 \\ 0 & 0 & 0 \end{bmatrix} . \tag{12.12.5}$$

Thus, the vector from which the elements of the sub-Jacobian matrices $\mathbf{J}_{ff}(\mathbf{v})$ and $\mathbf{J}_{fc}(\mathbf{v})$ are derived has the form,

$$\mathbf{W}_{ff}\mathbf{v}_f = \begin{pmatrix} -x(\tau_{f1})\lambda(\tau_{f1})Q_{par}(\tau_{f1}, \mathbf{v}) \\ x(\tau_{f1})\lambda(\tau_{f1})Q_{par}(\tau_1, \mathbf{v}) \\ 0 \end{pmatrix} . \tag{12.12.6}$$

Similarly, the corresponding vector for single males from which the elements of the sub-Jacobian matrices $\mathbf{J}_{mm}(\mathbf{v})$ and $\mathbf{J}_{mc}(\mathbf{v})$ are derived has the form,

$$\mathbf{W}_{mm}\mathbf{v}_m = \begin{pmatrix} -y(\tau_{m1})\lambda(\tau_{m1})Q_{par}(\tau_{m1}, \mathbf{v}) \\ y(\tau_{m1})\lambda(\tau_{m1})Q_{par}(\tau_{m1}, \mathbf{v}) \\ 0 \end{pmatrix} . \tag{12.12.7}$$

As in Section 11.13, for the one-sex partnership model, the transpose of the 9×9 matrix $\mathbf{W}_{cc}$ for couples has the partitioned form,

$$\mathbf{W}'_{cc} = \begin{bmatrix} \mathbf{W}'_{cc}(0,0) & \mathbf{W}'_{cc}(0,1) & \mathbf{0} \\ \mathbf{0} & \mathbf{W}'_{cc}(1,1) & \mathbf{0} \\ \mathbf{0} & \mathbf{0} & \mathbf{W}'_{cc}(2,2) \end{bmatrix} \tag{12.12.8}$$

of 3×3 sub-matrices. In the sub-matrix $\mathbf{W}'_{cc}(0,0)$ in Eq. (12.12.10), the rows and columns are indexed by the elements of the set $A(0)$; whereas in the sub-matrix $\mathbf{W}'_{cc}(0,1)$, the rows are indexed by the set $A(0)$ and the columns by the set $A(1)$. Similar remarks apply to the sub-matrices $\mathbf{W}'_{cc}(0,1)$ and $\mathbf{W}'_{cc}(2,2)$. The structures of the sub-matrices in Eq. (12.12.8) are very similar to those in Eqs. (11.13.8) through (11.13.11) for a one-sex partnership model, but, because the details differ significantly, the case of two sexes needs more careful consideration.

As in Section 12.11 (see Eq. (12.11.41)), let $S_{par}(\mathbf{v})$ denote the sum:

$$S_{par}(\mathbf{v}) = \lambda(\tau_{m1})Q_{par}(\tau_m, \mathbf{v}) + \lambda(\tau_{f1})Q_{par}(\tau_f, \mathbf{v}) . \qquad (12.12.9)$$

Then,

$$\mathbf{W}'_{cc}(0,0) = \begin{bmatrix} -S_{par}(\mathbf{v}) & M & 0 \\ 0 & -F & 0 \\ 0 & 0 & -F \end{bmatrix} \qquad (12.12.10)$$

and

$$\mathbf{W}'_{cc}(0,1) = \begin{bmatrix} F & 0 & 0 \\ 0 & F & 0 \\ 0 & 0 & F \end{bmatrix} . \qquad (12.12.11)$$

where $M = \lambda(\tau_{m1})Q_{par}(\tau_{m1}, \mathbf{v})$ and $F = \lambda(\tau_{f1})Q_{par}(\tau_{f1}, \mathbf{v})$. Moreover, the other sub-matrices in Eq. (12.12.8) have the forms,

$$\mathbf{W}'_{cc}(1,1) = \begin{bmatrix} -M & M & 0 \\ 0 & 0 & 0 \\ 0 & 0 & 0 \end{bmatrix} \qquad (12.12.12)$$

and

$$\mathbf{W}'_{cc}(2,2) = \begin{bmatrix} -M & M & 0 \\ 0 & 0 & 0 \\ 0 & 0 & 0 \end{bmatrix} . \qquad (12.12.13)$$

Justifying the elements in the matrix $\mathbf{W}'_{cc}(0,0)$ in Eq. (12.12.10), observe that $\lambda(\tau_{m1})Q_{par}(\tau_{m1}, \mathbf{v})$, the element in the first row and second column, is the latent risk for the transition, $(0,0) \to (0,1)$, indicating that the male member of the couple type $(0,0)$ was infected during a small time interval. Similarly, the common element $\lambda(\tau_{f1})Q_{par}(\tau_{f1}, \mathbf{v})$ on the principal diagonal of the matrix $\mathbf{W}'_{cc}(0,1)$ in Eq. (12.12.11) is the latent risk for transitions of the form $(0,0) \to (1, k_2)$ for $k_2 = 0, 1, 2$, indicating that the female member of the couple type $(0,0)$ was infected during a small time interval. Further, the negative elements on the principal diagonal of the matrix $\mathbf{W}'_{cc}(0,0)$ are the negatives of the sums of the off-diagonal elements for each row. Finally, the sub-matrices $\mathbf{W}'_{cc}(1,1)$ and $\mathbf{W}'_{cc}(2,2)$ are concerned with latent risks for the transitions of the form $(k_1, 0) \rightarrow (k_1, 1)$ for $k_1 = 1, 2$, indicating that the male susceptible partner was infected during any small time interval. The 3×3 sub-matrices, denoted by $\mathbf{0}$ in Eq. (12.12.10), contain only zeros because their elements do not contain latent risks for extra-marital contacts. From these results for the special case $n = 2$, it can be seen how the structure of the matrix $\mathbf{W}_{cc}^{'}$ could be extended to the cases of $n > 2$ stages of disease.

As a first step in the derivation of the formulas of the vector $\mathbf{W}_{cc}\mathbf{v}_c$ from which the elements of the Jacobian matrices $\mathbf{J}_{cf}(\mathbf{v})$, $\mathbf{J}_{cf}(\mathbf{v})$ and $\mathbf{J}_{cc}(\mathbf{v})$ for couples may be derived, it will be helpful to the define the 3×1 sub-vectors,

$$\mathbf{v}_c(k_1) = \begin{pmatrix} z(k_1, 0) \\ z(k_1, 1) \\ z(k_1, 2) \end{pmatrix}, \tag{12.12.14}$$

for $k_1 = 0, 1, 2$. Then, the 9×1 vector $\mathbf{v}_c$ may be represented in the partitioned form,

$$\mathbf{v}_c = \begin{pmatrix} \mathbf{v}_c(0) \\ \mathbf{v}_c(1) \\ \mathbf{v}_c(2) \end{pmatrix}. \tag{12.12.15}$$

Hence, it follows from Eq. (12.12.8) that the vector $\mathbf{W}_{cc}\mathbf{v}_c$ has the partitioned form,

$$\mathbf{W}_{cc}\mathbf{v}_c = \begin{pmatrix} \mathbf{W}_{cc}(0,0)\mathbf{v}_c(0) \\ \mathbf{W}_{cc}(0,1)\mathbf{v}_c(0) + \mathbf{W}_{cc}(1,1)\mathbf{v}_c(1) \\ \mathbf{W}_{cc}(2,2)\mathbf{v}_c(2) \end{pmatrix}. \tag{12.12.16}$$

As a final step in the preparation for the derivation of formulas for the elements of the Jacobian matrices, it will be necessary to exhibit the elements of the sub-vectors in Eq. (12.12.16) in their explicit forms. Thus,

$$\mathbf{W}_{cc}(0,0)\mathbf{v}_c(0) = \begin{pmatrix} -z(0,0)S_{par}(\mathbf{v}) \\ z(0,0)M - z(0,1)F \\ -z(0,2)F \end{pmatrix}, \tag{12.12.17}$$

$$\mathbf{W}_{cc}(0,1)\mathbf{v}_c(0) + \mathbf{W}_{cc}(1,1)\mathbf{v}_c(1) = \begin{pmatrix} z(0,0)F - z(1,0)M \\ z(0,1)F + z(1,0)M \\ z(0,2)F \end{pmatrix}, \tag{12.12.18}$$

and

$$\mathbf{W}_{cc}(2,2)\mathbf{v}_c(2) = \begin{pmatrix} -z(0,2)M \\ z(0,2)M \\ 0 \end{pmatrix}. \tag{12.12.19}$$

Just as in the simple case of $m = 1$ behavioral class and $n = 1$ stage of disease, the following functions for females and males will be helpful in presenting the elements of the sub-Jacobian matrices in a succinct form. Thus, for susceptible females of type τ_{f1}, let

$$k_f(\tau_{f1}, \tau_{m\nu}, \widehat{\mathbf{v}}) = \frac{\lambda(\tau_{f1})}{W_f(\tau_{f1}, \widehat{\mathbf{v}})} \alpha_{fem}(\tau_{f1}, \tau_{m\nu}) g_{f\theta}(\tau_{f1}, \tau_{m\nu}, \widehat{\mathbf{v}}) q_{fem}(\tau_{m\nu}) \tag{12.12.20}$$

for $\nu = 1, 2$. And, similarly for susceptible males of type τ_{m1}, let

$$k_m(\tau_{m1}, \tau_{f\nu}, \widehat{\mathbf{v}}) = \frac{\lambda(\tau_{m1})}{W_m(\tau_{m1}, \widehat{\mathbf{v}})} \alpha_{mem}(\tau_{m1}, \tau_{f\nu}) g_{m\theta}(\tau_{m1}, \tau_{f\nu}, \widehat{\mathbf{v}}) q_{mem}(\tau_{f\nu}) \tag{12.12.21}$$

for $\nu = 1, 2$. The following row vectors will also be useful in representing the sub-Jacobian matrices in a succinct form. Let

$$\mathbf{K}_f(\tau_{f1}, \widehat{\mathbf{v}}) = \begin{pmatrix} 0 & k_f(\tau_{f1}, \tau_{m1}, \widehat{\mathbf{v}}) & k_f(\tau_{f1}, \tau_{m2}, \widehat{\mathbf{v}}) \end{pmatrix} \tag{12.12.22}$$

and

$$\mathbf{K}_m(\tau_{m1}, \widehat{\mathbf{v}}) = \begin{pmatrix} 0 & k_m(\tau_{m1}, \tau_{f1}, \widehat{\mathbf{v}}) & k_m(\tau_{m1}, \tau_{f2}, \widehat{\mathbf{v}}) \end{pmatrix}. \tag{12.12.23}$$

Given these definitions, it can be shown from an inspection of Eq. (12.12.6) that the 3×3 sub-Jacobian matrix for $\mathbf{J}_{fm}(\widehat{\mathbf{v}})$ single females (see Eq. (12.11.29)), has the form,

$$\mathbf{J}_{fm}(\widehat{\mathbf{v}}) = \begin{bmatrix} -\widehat{x}(\tau_{f1})\mathbf{K}_f(\tau_{f1}, \widehat{\mathbf{v}}) \\ \widehat{x}(\tau_{f1})\mathbf{K}_f(\tau_{f1}, \widehat{\mathbf{v}}) \\ \mathbf{0}_{1\times 3} \end{bmatrix}. \tag{12.12.24}$$

It is easy to see that the corresponding sub-Jacobian matrix for single males has the form,

$$\mathbf{J}_{mf}(\widehat{\mathbf{v}}) = \begin{bmatrix} -\widehat{y}(\tau_{m1})\mathbf{K}_m(\tau_{m1}, \widehat{\mathbf{v}}) \\ \widehat{y}(\tau_{m1})\mathbf{K}_m(\tau_{m1}, \widehat{\mathbf{v}}) \\ \mathbf{0}_{1\times 3} \end{bmatrix}, \tag{12.12.25}$$

as can be seen by inspecting Eq. (12.12.7).

In this case, the sub-Jacobian matrix $\mathbf{J}_{fc}(\widehat{\mathbf{v}})$ (see Eq. (12.11.30)) for single females is 3×9. To describe this matrix succinctly, for a susceptible female of type τ_{f1} it will be helpful to define a 1×9 row vector by:

$$\mathbf{L}_f(\tau_{f1}, \widehat{\mathbf{v}}) = \begin{pmatrix} \mathbf{K}_f(\tau_{f1}, \widehat{\mathbf{v}}) & \mathbf{K}_f(\tau_{f1}, \widehat{\mathbf{v}}) & \mathbf{K}_f(\tau_{f1}, \widehat{\mathbf{v}}) \end{pmatrix}. \tag{12.12.26}$$

Then, from Eq. (12.12.6) it can be shown that:

$$\mathbf{J}_{fc}(\widehat{\mathbf{v}}) = \begin{bmatrix} -\widehat{x}(\tau_{f1})\mathbf{L}_f(\tau_{f1}, \widehat{\mathbf{v}}) \\ \widehat{x}(\tau_{f1})\mathbf{L}_f(\tau_{f1}, \widehat{\mathbf{v}}) \\ \mathbf{0}_{1\times 9} \end{bmatrix}, \tag{12.12.27}$$

where $\mathbf{0}_{1\times 9}$ is 1×9 row vector of zeros. By way of justifying these formulas, observe that the columns in the sub-vectors in Eq. (12.12.16) are indexed, respectively, by the sets of couple types $A(0)$, $A(1)$, and $A(2)$. And, for each of these sets, the state of the male in the couple types runs over the indices $k_2 = 0, 1, 2$. Hence, the vector $\mathbf{K}_f(\tau_{f1}, \widehat{\mathbf{v}})$ is repeated three times in Eq. (12.12.26).

On the other hand, in each of the sets of couple types $A(0)$, $A(1)$, and $A(2)$, the state of the female is held constant with respect to disease. Therefore, for the case of the matrix $\mathbf{J}_{mc}(\widehat{\mathbf{v}})$ for single males, the analogue of the row vector in Eq. (12.12.26) has the following form. Let $\mathbf{1}_{1\times 3}$ denote a 1×3 row vector of ones and then define the following row vectors by:

$$\mathbf{L}_{m1}(\tau_{m1}, \widehat{\mathbf{v}}) = k_m(\tau_{m1}, \tau_{f1}, \widehat{\mathbf{v}})\mathbf{1}_{1\times 3} \tag{12.12.28}$$

and

$$\mathbf{L}_{m2}(\tau_{m1}, \widehat{\mathbf{v}}) = k_m(\tau_{m1}, \tau_{f2}, \widehat{\mathbf{v}})\mathbf{1}_{1\times 3} \tag{12.12.29}$$

Then, the analogue of the vector in Eq. (12.12.26) for single males has the partitioned form,

$$\mathbf{L}_m(\tau_{m1},\widehat{\mathbf{v}}) = \left[\begin{array}{ccc} \mathbf{0}_{1\times 3} & \mathbf{L}_{m1}(\tau_{m1},\widehat{\mathbf{v}}) & \mathbf{L}_{m2}(\tau_{m1},\widehat{\mathbf{v}}) \end{array}\right] . \tag{12.12.30}$$

From these definitions, it can be seen from Eq. (12.12.7) that:

$$\mathbf{J}_{mc}(\widehat{\mathbf{v}}) = \left[\begin{array}{c} -\widehat{y}(\tau_{m1})\mathbf{L}_m(\tau_{m1},\widehat{\mathbf{v}}) \\ \widehat{y}(\tau_{m1})\mathbf{L}_m(\tau_{m1},\widehat{\mathbf{v}}) \\ \mathbf{0}_{1\times 9} \end{array}\right] . \tag{12.12.31}$$

With respect to those sub-Jacobian matrices whose rows are indexed by the set Υ_c of couple types, it can be seen from Eqs. (12.12.17) through (12.12.19) that it will be helpful to partitions these matrices according to the state of the female in the set of couple types. For example, for the 9×3 matrix $\mathbf{J}_{cf}(\widehat{\mathbf{v}})$, consider the partitioned form,

$$\mathbf{J}_{cf}(\widehat{\mathbf{v}}) = \left[\begin{array}{c} \mathbf{J}_{cf}(0,\widehat{\mathbf{v}}) \\ \mathbf{J}_{cf}(1,\widehat{\mathbf{v}}) \\ \mathbf{J}_{cf}(2,\widehat{\mathbf{v}}) \end{array}\right] , \tag{12.12.32}$$

where each of the sub-matrices are 3×3. At this juncture, it should be noted that all the elements in the stationary sub-vector $\widehat{\mathbf{v}}_c$ for couples are zero except for $\widehat{z}(0,0)$. From an inspection of Eq. (12.12.17), it can be seen that the matrix $\mathbf{J}_{cf}(0,\widehat{\mathbf{v}})$ has the partitioned form,

$$\mathbf{J}_{cf}(0,\widehat{\mathbf{v}}) = \left[\begin{array}{c} -\widehat{z}(0,0)\mathbf{K}_m(\tau_{m1},\widehat{\mathbf{v}}) \\ \widehat{z}(0,0)\mathbf{K}_m(\tau_{m1},\widehat{\mathbf{v}}) \\ \mathbf{0}_{1\times 3} \end{array}\right] , \tag{12.12.33}$$

and, from an inspection of Eqs. (12.12.18) and (12.12.19), it can be seen that $\mathbf{J}_{cf}(1,\widehat{\mathbf{v}}) = \mathbf{J}_{cf}(2,\widehat{\mathbf{v}}) = \mathbf{0}_{3\times 3}$, a 3×3 zero matrix.

Similarly, the 9×3 matrix $\mathbf{J}_{cm}(\widehat{\mathbf{v}})$ has the partitioned form,

$$\mathbf{J}_{cm}(\widehat{\mathbf{v}}) = \left[\begin{array}{c} \mathbf{J}_{cm}(0,\widehat{\mathbf{v}}) \\ \mathbf{J}_{cm}(1,\widehat{\mathbf{v}}) \\ \mathbf{J}_{cm}(2,\widehat{\mathbf{v}}) \end{array}\right] \tag{12.12.34}$$

of 3×3 sub-matrices. From an inspection of Eq. (12.12.17), it can be seen that:

$$\mathbf{J}_{cm}(0, \widehat{\mathbf{v}}) = \begin{bmatrix} -\widehat{z}(0,0)\mathbf{K}_f(\tau_{f1}, \widehat{\mathbf{v}}) \\ \mathbf{0}_{1\times 3} \\ \mathbf{0}_{1\times 3} \end{bmatrix}, \tag{12.12.35}$$

from Eq. (12.12.18) it can be seen that:

$$\mathbf{J}_{cm}(1, \widehat{\mathbf{v}}) = \begin{bmatrix} \widehat{z}(0,0)\mathbf{K}_f(\tau_{f1}, \widehat{\mathbf{v}}) \\ \mathbf{0}_{1\times 3} \\ \mathbf{0}_{1\times 3} \end{bmatrix}, \tag{12.12.36}$$

and from Eq. (12.12.19) it can be seen that $\mathbf{J}_{cm}(2, \widehat{\mathbf{v}}) = \mathbf{0}_{3\times 3}$.

The 9×9 sub-matrix $\mathbf{J}_{cc}(\widehat{\mathbf{v}})$ for couples has a partitioned form similar to that just discussed. For, let $\mathbf{J}_{cc}(k_1, \widehat{\mathbf{v}})$ denote a 3×9 matrix of partial derivatives with respect to the elements of the vector $\mathbf{v}_c$ evaluated at $\widehat{\mathbf{v}}$, when the female member of the couple is in state k_1. Then, the matrix $\mathbf{J}_{cc}(\widehat{\mathbf{v}})$ may be represented in the partitioned form,

$$\mathbf{J}_{cc}(\widehat{\mathbf{v}}) = \begin{bmatrix} \mathbf{J}_{cc}(0, \widehat{\mathbf{v}}) \\ \mathbf{J}_{cc}(1, \widehat{\mathbf{v}}) \\ \mathbf{J}_{cc}(2, \widehat{\mathbf{v}}) \end{bmatrix}. \tag{12.12.37}$$

Then, from Eqs. (12.12.17), (12.12.26) and (12.12.30), it can be seen that:

$$\mathbf{J}_{cc}(0, \widehat{\mathbf{v}}) = \begin{bmatrix} -\widehat{z}(0,0)(\mathbf{L}_f(\tau_{f1}, \widehat{\mathbf{v}}) + \mathbf{L}_m(\tau_{m1}, \widehat{\mathbf{v}})) \\ \widehat{z}(0,0)\mathbf{L}_m(\tau_{m1}, \widehat{\mathbf{v}}) \\ \mathbf{0}_{1\times 9} \end{bmatrix}. \tag{12.12.38}$$

Similarly, an inspection of Eqs. (12.12.18) and (12.12.26) yields the result,

$$\mathbf{J}_{cc}(1, \widehat{\mathbf{v}}) = \begin{bmatrix} \widehat{z}(0,0)\mathbf{L}_f(\tau_{f1}, \widehat{\mathbf{v}}) \\ \mathbf{0}_{1\times 9} \\ \mathbf{0}_{1\times 9} \end{bmatrix}. \tag{12.12.39}$$

Finally, from Eq. (12.12.19), it can be seen that $\mathbf{J}_{cc}(2, \widehat{\mathbf{v}}) = \mathbf{0}_{3\times 9}$. At this juncture it can be seen that the pattern of the Jacobian matrix for extra-marital sexual contacts for the case $m = 1$ and $n = 2$ can easily be extended to cases such that $m = 1$ and $n > 2$.

As in Section 11.13, the patterns in the Jacobian matrices just described can be extended to cases of $m \geq 2$ behavior classes and $n \geq 2$ stages of disease in a straightforward way, and, to illustrate the principles, it will suffice to consider cases with $m = 2$ behavioral classes and $n \geq 2$ stages of disease. The functions $k_f(\tau_f, \tau_{m\nu}, \widehat{\mathbf{v}})$ and $k_m(\tau_m, \tau_{f\nu}, \widehat{\mathbf{v}})$, defined for every behavioral class and stage ν of disease for susceptible females and males as in Eqs. (12.12.20) and (12.12.21), will play a basic role in the computational formulas, but, in the general cases to be described, the λ-parameters, denoted by $\lambda(\tau_f)$ or $\lambda(\tau_m)$, will depend on the behavioral class to which a susceptible female or male belongs.

For the cases of $m = 2$ and $n \geq 2$, the set Υ_f of types of females may be partitioned into two disjoint sets according to membership in a behavioral class. For example, by definition,

$$\Upsilon_f(1) = \{(1, k) \mid k = 0, 1, 2, \cdots, n\} \tag{12.12.40}$$

is the set of all female types belonging to behavioral class 1, and the set $\Upsilon_f(2)$ is defined similarly for females belonging to behavioral class 2. For $j = 1, 2$, let

$$\mathbf{v}_f(j) = (x(\tau) \mid \tau \in \Upsilon_f(j)) \tag{12.12.41}$$

denote a $(n+1) \times 1$ vector of variables for singles. Then, the $2(n+1) \times 1$ vector of variables for single females takes the partitioned form,

$$\mathbf{v}_f = \begin{pmatrix} \mathbf{v}_f(1) \\ \mathbf{v}_f(2) \end{pmatrix} . \tag{12.12.42}$$

Similarly, the $2(n + 1) \times 1$ vector of variables for single males has the partitioned form,

$$\mathbf{v}_m = \begin{pmatrix} \mathbf{v}_m(1) \\ \mathbf{v}_m(2) \end{pmatrix} . \tag{12.12.43}$$

Given the partitioned form of the vector for single females in Eq. (12.12.42), it can be seen, after inspecting the explicit forms of the matrix of latent risks $\mathbf{\Theta}_{f2}$ for single females in Eq. (12.6.1), that the

$2(n+1) \times 2(n+1)$ matrix $\mathbf{W}_{ff}$ for single females has the quasi-diagonal form,

$$\mathbf{W}_{ff} = \begin{bmatrix} \mathbf{W}_{ff}(1) & \mathbf{0} \\ \mathbf{0} & \mathbf{W}_{ff}(2) \end{bmatrix}, \tag{12.12.44}$$

where $\mathbf{W}_{ff}(1)$ is a $(n+1) \times (n+1)$ matrix for members of class 1 and the matrix $\mathbf{W}_{ff}(2)$ is defined similarly for members of behavioral class 2. The structure of the matrices on the quasi-diagonal would be an extension of that in Eq. (12.12.5) for cases of $n > 2$ types, but each would have different λ-parameters. From the form of the matrix in Eq. (12.12.44), it can be seen that the vector $\mathbf{W}_{ff}\mathbf{v}_f$ from which the elements of the Jacobian matrix for single females may be derived has the partitioned form,

$$\mathbf{W}_{ff}\mathbf{v}_f = \begin{pmatrix} \mathbf{W}_{ff}(1)\mathbf{v}_f(1) \\ \mathbf{W}_{ff}(2)\mathbf{v}_f(2) \end{pmatrix}. \tag{12.12.45}$$

The corresponding vector $\mathbf{W}_{mm}\mathbf{v}_m$ for single males would have a similar partitioned form.

The next step in deducing the form of the Jacobian matrix for extra-marital sexual contacts is to exhibit an extended form of the vector of variables for couples in Eqs. (12.12.14) and (12.12.15) for cases of $m = 2$ behavioral classes and $n > 2$ stages of disease. As in Section 11.13, for every couple type $\varkappa = (\tau_f = (j_1, k_1), \tau_m = (j_2, k_2))$ and for a fixed pair (j_1, j_2) of behavioral classes for females and males, let

$$A(j_1, j_2) = \{\varkappa = ((\tau_f, \tau_m) \mid k_1 = 0, 1, 2, \cdots, n;\ k_1 = 0, 1, 2, \cdots, n\} \tag{12.12.46}$$

denote a subset of couples types such that the pairs (k_1, k_2) are arranged in lexicographic order. Then, for every pair (j_1, j_2) let

$$\mathbf{v}_c(j_1, j_2) = (z(\varkappa) \mid \varkappa \in A(j_1, j_2)) \tag{12.12.47}$$

denote a $(n+1)^2 \times 1$ vector of couple variables. The $4(n+1)^2 \times 1$ vector $\mathbf{v}_c$ of variables for couples then has the partitioned form,

$$\mathbf{v}_c = \begin{pmatrix} \mathbf{v}_c(1,1) \\ \mathbf{v}_c(1,2) \\ \mathbf{v}_c(2,1) \\ \mathbf{v}_c(2,2) \end{pmatrix}. \tag{12.12.48}$$

Moreover, each of the sub-vectors in Eq. (12.12.48) may be partitioned as in Eqs. (12.12.14) and (12.12.15).

From an inspection of the matrix $\mathbf{\Theta}_{c22}$ of latent risks for couples in Eq. (12.12.9), it can be seen that for each pair (j_1, j_2) there is a $(n+1)^2 \times (n+1)^2$ matrix $\mathbf{W}_{cc}(j_1, j_2)$, whose form is an extension of that in Eq. (12.12.8) but modified to accommodate possible different λ-parameters for the female and male partners. Furthermore, it follows that the $4(n+1)^2 \times 4(n+1)^2$ matrix $\mathbf{W}_{cc}$ for couples has the quasi-diagonal form,

$$\mathbf{W}_{cc} = \begin{bmatrix} \mathbf{W}_{cc}(1,1) & \mathbf{0} & \mathbf{0} & \mathbf{0} \\ \mathbf{0} & \mathbf{W}_{cc}(1,2) & \mathbf{0} & \mathbf{0} \\ \mathbf{0} & \mathbf{0} & \mathbf{W}_{cc}(2,1) & \mathbf{0} \\ \mathbf{0} & \mathbf{0} & \mathbf{0} & \mathbf{W}_{cc}(2,2) \end{bmatrix} . \tag{12.12.49}$$

Consequently, the vector from which the Jacobian matrix for couples may be derived has the partitioned form,

$$\mathbf{W}_{cc}\mathbf{v}_c = \begin{pmatrix} \mathbf{W}_{cc}(1,1)\mathbf{v}_c(1,1) \\ \mathbf{W}_{cc}(1,2)\mathbf{v}_c(1,2) \\ \mathbf{W}_{cc}(2,1)\mathbf{v}_c(2,1) \\ \mathbf{W}_{cc}(2,2)\mathbf{v}_c(2,2) \end{pmatrix} . \tag{12.12.50}$$

One may thus proceed as in Eqs. (12.12.10) through (12.12.13) to derive sub-matrices $\mathbf{J}_{fc}(j_1, j_2; \widehat{\mathbf{v}})$, $\mathbf{J}_{mc}(j_1, j_2; \widehat{\mathbf{v}})$, and $\mathbf{J}_{cc}(j_1, j_2; \widehat{\mathbf{v}})$ for each pair of behavioral classes (j_1, j_2) in the set $\{(j_1, j_2) \mid j_1 = 1, 2;\ j_2 = 1, 2\}$ of pairs.

In summary, for cases with $m = 2$ behavioral classes and $n \geq 1$ stages of disease, the Jacobian matrix $\mathbf{J}_{EM}(\widehat{\mathbf{v}})$ may be represented in the partitioned form,

$$\mathbf{J}_{EM}(\widehat{\mathbf{v}}) = \begin{bmatrix} \mathbf{J}_f(\widehat{\mathbf{v}}) \\ \mathbf{J}_m(\widehat{\mathbf{v}}) \\ \mathbf{J}_c(\widehat{\mathbf{v}}) \end{bmatrix} , \tag{12.12.51}$$

where $\mathbf{J}_f(\widehat{\mathbf{v}})$ is the $2(n+1) \times (2(n+1) + 4(n+1)^2)$ matrix for single females, $\mathbf{J}_m(\widehat{\mathbf{v}})$ is a matrix with the same dimensions for single males, and $\mathbf{J}_c(\widehat{\mathbf{v}})$ is a $4(n+1)^2 \times (2(n+1) + 4(n+1)^2)$ matrix for couples.

For the case of single females, the two behavioral classes are accommodated in the partitioned matrix,

$$\mathbf{J}_f(\widehat{\mathbf{v}}) = \begin{bmatrix} \mathbf{0}_{(n+1)\times(n+1)} & \mathbf{J}_{fm}(1,\widehat{\mathbf{v}}) & \mathbf{J}_{fc}(1,\widehat{\mathbf{v}}) \\ \mathbf{0}_{(n+1)\times(n+1)} & \mathbf{J}_{fm}(2,\widehat{\mathbf{v}}) & \mathbf{J}_{fc}(2,\widehat{\mathbf{v}}) \end{bmatrix}. \tag{12.12.52}$$

In this partitioned matrix, $\mathbf{J}_{fm}(1,\widehat{\mathbf{v}})$ is a $(n+1)\times(n+1)$ sub-matrix indexed for singles in behavioral class 1, whose construction is similar to that in Eq. (12.12.24). Similarly, $\mathbf{J}_{fc}(1,\widehat{\mathbf{v}})$ is a $(n+1)\times 4(n+1)^2$ sub-matrix indexed for singles in class 1, taking into account sexual contacts with members of couples, whose construction is similar to that in Eq. (12.12.27). The sub-matrices $\mathbf{J}_{fm}(2,\widehat{\mathbf{v}})$ and $\mathbf{J}_{fc}(2,\widehat{\mathbf{v}})$ have similar interpretations for single females in behavioral class 2. For the case of single males, the matrix $\mathbf{J}_m(\widehat{\mathbf{v}})$ has the partitioned form,

$$\mathbf{J}_m(\widehat{\mathbf{v}}) = \begin{bmatrix} \mathbf{J}_{mf}(1,\widehat{\mathbf{v}}) & \mathbf{0}_{(n+1)\times(n+1)} & \mathbf{J}_{mc}(1,\widehat{\mathbf{v}}) \\ \mathbf{J}_{mf}(2,\widehat{\mathbf{v}}) & \mathbf{0}_{(n+1)\times(n+1)} & \mathbf{J}_{mc}(2,\widehat{\mathbf{v}}) \end{bmatrix}, \tag{12.12.53}$$

whose sub-matrices are analogous to those in Eq. (12.12.52).

The sub-matrix $\mathbf{J}_c(\widehat{\mathbf{v}})$ in Eq. (12.12.51) has the partitioned form,

$$\mathbf{J}_c(\widehat{\mathbf{v}}) = \begin{bmatrix} \mathbf{J}_c(1,1,\widehat{\mathbf{v}}) \\ \mathbf{J}_c(1,2,\widehat{\mathbf{v}}) \\ \mathbf{J}_c(2,1,\widehat{\mathbf{v}}) \\ \mathbf{J}_c(2,2,\widehat{\mathbf{v}}) \end{bmatrix}, \tag{12.12.54}$$

corresponding to the four pairs of behavioral classes when $m = 2$. Each of these sub-matrices in turn may be partitioned into three sub-matrices. For example, for the pair $(1,1)$, the partitioned matrix has the form,

$$\mathbf{J}_c(1,1,\widehat{\mathbf{v}}) = \begin{bmatrix} \mathbf{J}_{cf}(1,1,\widehat{\mathbf{v}}) & \mathbf{J}_{cm}(1,1,\widehat{\mathbf{v}}) & \mathbf{J}_{cc}(1,1,\widehat{\mathbf{v}}) \end{bmatrix}. \tag{12.12.55}$$

The sub-matrix $\mathbf{J}_{cf}(1,1,\widehat{\mathbf{v}})$ has dimensions $4(n+1)^2 \times (n+1)$ and can be constructed by a procedure similar to that in Eqs. (12.12.32) and (12.12.33), the sub-matrix $\mathbf{J}_{cm}(1,1,\widehat{\mathbf{v}})$ has the same dimensions and can be constructed along lines similar to those in Eqs. (12.12.35) and (12.12.36), and the $4(n+1)^2 \times 4(n+1)^2$ sub-matrix $\mathbf{J}_{cc}(1,1,\widehat{\mathbf{v}})$ may be constructed by following a procedure similar to that in Eqs. (12.12.38) and (12.12.39). These remarks also apply to the remaining three submatrices in Eq. (12.12.54), and this completes the outline of procedures for constructing the general form of the Jacobian matrix for extramarital sexual contacts.

12.13 Jacobian Matrix for Couple Formation

Just as in Section 11.14, as a first step in deriving computational formulas for the elements of the Jacobian matrix for marital couple formation $\mathbf{J}_{CF}(\widehat{\mathbf{v}})$ evaluated at a stationary vector $\widehat{\mathbf{v}}$ such that the population contains only susceptibles, a formula for the function $N_{CF}(t;\tau_f,\tau_m)$ defined in Eq. (12.4.7) will be derived in the notation for the embedded differential equations. In this section, this function will be denoted by $N_{CF}(\tau_f,\tau_m,\mathbf{v})$. Because only single females and males are involved in marital couple formation, $N_{CF}(\tau_f,\tau_m,\mathbf{v})$ will depend only on the vector,

$$\mathbf{v}_f = (x(\tau_f) \mid \tau_f \in \Upsilon_f) \tag{12.13.1}$$

for single females, and on the vector,

$$\mathbf{v}_m = (y(\tau_m) \mid \tau_m \in \Upsilon_m) \tag{12.13.2}$$

for single males.

Let

$$T_{fc}(\tau_f,\mathbf{v}) = \sum_{\tau_m \in \Upsilon_m} y(\tau_m)\alpha_f(\tau_f,\tau_m)\,. \tag{12.13.3}$$

Then, in the notation of this section, the contact probability for single females in Eq. (12.4.16) takes the form,

$$\gamma_f(\tau_f,\tau_m) = \frac{y(\tau_m)\alpha_f(\tau_f,\tau_m)}{T_{fc}(\tau_f,\mathbf{v})} \tag{12.13.4}$$

for every single female of type $\tau_f \in \Upsilon_f$. Similarly, with respect to single males, let

$$T_{mc}(\tau_m,\mathbf{v}) = \sum_{\tau_f \in \Upsilon_f} x(\tau_f)\alpha_m(\tau_m,\tau_f)\,. \tag{12.13.5}$$

Then, the contact probability in Eq. (12.4.17) takes the form,

$$\gamma_m(\tau_m, \tau_f) = \frac{x(\tau_f)\alpha_m(\tau_m, \tau_f)}{T_{mc}(\tau_m, \mathbf{v})} \tag{12.13.6}$$

for single males of type $\tau_m \in \Upsilon_m$.

Therefore, the multinomial expectations going into the function $N_{CF}(\tau_f, \tau_m, \mathbf{v})$ are:

$$x^* = x(\tau_f)\gamma_f(\tau_f, \tau_m) = \frac{x(\tau_f)y(\tau_m)\alpha_f(\tau_f, \tau_m)}{T_{fc}(\tau_f, \mathbf{v})} \tag{12.13.7}$$

for a single female of type τ_f, and

$$y^* = y(\tau_m)\gamma_m(\tau_m, \tau_f) = \frac{y(\tau_m)x(\tau_f)\alpha_m(\tau_m, \tau_f)}{T_{mc}(\tau_m, \mathbf{v})} \tag{12.13.8}$$

for a single male of type τ_m. One thus reaches the conclusion that the function $N_{CF}(\tau_f, \tau_m, \mathbf{v})$, in the abbreviated notation of Eqs. (12.13.7) and (12.13.8), has the form,

$$N_{CF}(\tau_f, \tau_m, \mathbf{v}) = \min(x^*, y^*)\ . \tag{12.13.9}$$

Working with this function for marital couple formation will be more complicated than that for extra-marital sexual contacts in Section 12.11, because it must be considered for all couple types $\varkappa = (\tau_f, \tau_m) \in \Upsilon_c$ rather than for just the cases where τ_f is a susceptible female type or τ_m is a susceptible male type. However, among the $m^2(n+1)^2$ couple types in the set Υ_c, there are only four cases to consider in deriving computational formulas for partial derivatives. These cases can be described as: $(\tau_f \in \Upsilon_{SF}, \tau_m \in \Upsilon_{SM})$, female and male susceptible; $(\tau_f \in \Upsilon_{SF}, \tau_m \in \Upsilon_{IM})$, female susceptible and male infective; $(\tau_f \in \Upsilon_{IF}, \tau_m \in \Upsilon_{SM})$, female infective and male susceptible; and $(\tau_f \in \Upsilon_{IF}, \tau_m \in \Upsilon_{IM})$, female and male infective.

As a first step to gaining insight into the forms of the partial derivative evaluated at a stationary vector $\widehat{\mathbf{v}}$, it will again be helpful to consider the approximation,

$$\eta_\theta\left(\frac{x}{y_1}, \frac{x}{y_2}\right) = \frac{x}{y_1}\left(\frac{2}{1 + \left(\frac{y_2}{y_1}\right)^\theta}\right)^{\frac{1}{\theta}} \tag{12.13.10}$$

to the min function for large $\theta > 0$ as in Eqs. (12.11.11) through (12.11.15). Thus, to apply this formulas let

$$x = x(\tau_f)y(\tau_m)\ , \tag{12.13.11}$$

$$y_1 = \frac{T_{fc}(\tau_f, \mathbf{v})}{\alpha_f(\tau_f, \tau_m)} \tag{12.13.12}$$

and

$$y_2 = \frac{T_{mc}(\tau_m, \mathbf{v})}{\alpha_m(\tau_m, \tau_f)}\ . \tag{12.13.13}$$

Then, to further simplify the notation, let

$$R_{fc}(\tau_f, \tau_m, \mathbf{v}) = \frac{y_2}{y_1} = \frac{\alpha_f(\tau_f, \tau_m)T_{mc}(\tau_m, \mathbf{v})}{\alpha_m(\tau_m, \tau_f)T_{fc}(\tau_f, \mathbf{v})} \tag{12.13.14}$$

and

$$g_{fc\theta}(\tau_f, \tau_m, \mathbf{v}) = \left(\frac{2}{1 + (R_{fc}(\tau_f, \tau_m, \mathbf{v}))^{\theta}}\right)^{\frac{1}{\theta}}\ . \tag{12.13.15}$$

With these definitions, the function $N_{CF}(\tau_f, \tau_m, \mathbf{v})$ in Eq. (12.13.9) may be expressed as:

$$N_{CF}(\tau_f, \tau_m, \mathbf{v}) = \frac{x(\tau_f)y(\tau_m)\alpha_f(\tau_f, \tau_m)}{T_{fc}(\tau_f, \mathbf{v})} g_{fc\theta}(\tau_f, \tau_m, \mathbf{v})\ . \tag{12.13.16}$$

A similar expression for this function could be derived by interchanging y_1 and y_2 in the above derivation.

The simplest formulas for partial derivatives of the function in Eq. (12.13.16) arise for the case $(\tau_f \in \Upsilon_{IF}, \tau_m \in \Upsilon_{IM})$ where both the female and male are infectives. For if a stationary population contains no infectives, then $\widehat{x}(\tau_f) = \widehat{y}(\tau_m) = 0$. By using the product rule for differentiation, it can be seen that all terms in a partial derivative of the function in Eq. (12.13.16) will contain either $\widehat{x}(\tau_f)$, $\widehat{y}(\tau_m)$, or both $\widehat{x}(\tau_f)$ and $\widehat{y}(\tau_m)$, when evaluated at a stationary vector $\widehat{\mathbf{v}}$. Therefore,

$$\frac{\partial N_{CF}(\tau_f, \tau_m, \widehat{\mathbf{v}})}{\partial x(\tau)} = 0 \tag{12.13.17}$$

for all single female types $\tau \in \Upsilon_f$. Similarly,

$$\frac{\partial N_{CF}(\tau_f, \tau_m, \widehat{\mathbf{v}})}{\partial y(\tau)} = 0 \tag{12.13.18}$$

for all single male types $\tau \in \Upsilon_m$.

Next consider the case $(\tau_f \in \Upsilon_{IF}, \tau_m \in \Upsilon_{SM})$ of a female infective and a male susceptible. From Eq. (12.13.16), it can be seen that for $\tau \neq \tau_f$ a partial derivative with respect to $x(\tau)$ evaluated at a stationary vector $\widehat{\mathbf{v}}$ will contain $\widehat{x}(\tau_f) = 0$ as a factor. Thus,

$$\frac{\partial N_{CF}(\tau_f, \tau_m, \widehat{\mathbf{v}})}{\partial x(\tau)} = 0 \tag{12.13.19}$$

for all $\tau \in \Upsilon_f$ such that $\tau \neq \tau_f$. But, for an infectious female type τ_f,

$$\frac{\partial N_{CF}(\tau_f, \tau_m, \widehat{\mathbf{v}})}{\partial x(\tau_f)} = \frac{\widehat{y}(\tau_m)\alpha_f(\tau_f, \tau_m)}{T_{fc}(\tau_f, \widehat{\mathbf{v}})} g_{fc\theta}(\tau_f, \tau_m, \widehat{\mathbf{v}}) . \tag{12.13.20}$$

Because the partial derivative of the function in Eq. (12.13.15) with respect to $y(\tau)$ for all $\tau \in \Upsilon_m$ evaluated at a stationary vector $\widehat{\mathbf{v}}$ will contain $\widehat{x}(\tau_f) = 0$ as a factor, it follows that:

$$\frac{\partial N_{CF}(\tau_f, \tau_m, \widehat{\mathbf{v}})}{\partial y(\tau)} = 0 \tag{12.13.21}$$

for all single male types $\tau \in \Upsilon_m$.

The case $(\tau_f \in \Upsilon_{SF}, \tau_m \in \Upsilon_{IM})$ of a female susceptible and a male infective has analogous formulas. In this case, because the partial derivative of the function in Eq. (12.13.16) with respect to $x(\tau)$ for all $\tau \in \Upsilon_f$ evaluated at a stationary vector $\widehat{\mathbf{v}}$ will contain $\widehat{y}(\tau_m) = 0$ as a factor, it follows that:

$$\frac{\partial N_{CF}(\tau_f, \tau_m, \widehat{\mathbf{v}})}{\partial x(\tau)} = 0 \tag{12.13.22}$$

for all single female types $\tau \in \Upsilon_f$. Moreover, for all $\tau \in \Upsilon_m$ such that $\tau \neq \tau_m$,

$$\frac{\partial N_{CF}(\tau_f, \tau_m, \widehat{\mathbf{v}})}{\partial y(\tau)} = 0 . \tag{12.13.23}$$

But, if $\tau = \tau_m$, then

$$\frac{\partial N_{CF}(\tau_f,\tau_m,\widehat{\mathbf{v}})}{\partial y(\tau_m)} = \frac{\widehat{x}(\tau_f)\alpha_f(\tau_f,\tau_m)}{T_{fc}(\tau_f,\widehat{\mathbf{v}})} g_{fc\theta}(\tau_f,\tau_m,\widehat{\mathbf{v}}) \ . \tag{12.13.24}$$

As in the one-sex partnership models described in Chapter 11, the case $(\tau_f \in \Upsilon_{SF}, \tau_m \in \Upsilon_{SM})$, in which both the female and male in a couple are susceptibles, leads to the most complex computational formulas for the partial derivatives in the Jacobian matrix for couple formation. At this point, it will be helpful in this case to consider alternative computational formulas to those just described so as to expedite the use of MAPLE. To this end write the function defined in Eqs. (12.13.15) and (12.13.16) in the alternative form,

$$N_{CF}(\tau_f,\tau_m,\mathbf{v}) = x(\tau_f)y(\tau_m)\alpha_f(\tau_f,\tau_m)\alpha_m(\tau_m,\tau_f)g_\theta^*(\tau_f,\tau_m,\mathbf{v}) \ , \tag{12.13.25}$$

where

$$g_\theta^*(\tau_f,\tau_m,\mathbf{v}) = \frac{1}{\alpha_m(\tau_m,\tau_f)T_{fc}(\tau_f,\mathbf{v})} g_{fc\theta}(\tau_f,\tau_m,\mathbf{v})$$

$$= \left(\frac{2}{(\alpha_m(\tau_m,\tau_f)T_{fc}(\tau_f,\mathbf{v}))^\theta + (\alpha_f(\tau_f,\tau_m)T_{mc}(\tau_m,\mathbf{v}))^\theta}\right)^{\frac{1}{\theta}} \ . \tag{12.13.26}$$

Then, there are four basic types of formulas for partial derivatives evaluated at a stationary vector $\widehat{\mathbf{v}}$.

One of these types arises by considering the variable $x(\tau_f)$ for a susceptible female type $\tau_f \in \Upsilon_{SF}$ who is a member of a couple of type (τ_f, τ_m). Then, it can be shown with the help of MAPLE that:

$$\frac{\partial N_{CF}(\tau_f,\tau_m,\widehat{\mathbf{v}})}{\partial x(\tau_f)} = \widehat{y}(\tau_m)\alpha_f(\tau_f,\tau_m)\alpha_m(\tau_m,\tau_f)g_\theta^*(\tau_f,\tau_m,\widehat{\mathbf{v}}) \times \frac{N_f(\tau_f,\tau_m,\widehat{\mathbf{v}})}{D_f(\tau_f,\tau_m,\widehat{\mathbf{v}})} \ , \tag{12.13.27}$$

where

$$N_f(\tau_f,\tau_m,\widehat{\mathbf{v}}) = (\alpha_m(\tau_m,\tau_f)T_{fc}(\tau_f,\widehat{\mathbf{v}}))^\theta T_{mc}(\tau_m,\widehat{\mathbf{v}})$$

$$+ (\alpha_f(\tau_f, \tau_m) T_{mc}(\tau_m, \widehat{\mathbf{v}}))^\theta \widehat{x}(\tau_f) \alpha_m(\tau_m, \tau_f) \tag{12.13.28}$$

and

$$D_f(\tau_f, \tau_m, \widehat{\mathbf{v}}) = ((\alpha_m(\tau_m, \tau_f) T_{fc}(\tau_f, \widehat{\mathbf{v}}))^\theta + (\alpha_f(\tau_f, \tau_m) T_{mc}(\tau_m, \widehat{\mathbf{v}}))^\theta)$$

$$\times T_{mc}(\tau_m, \widehat{\mathbf{v}}) . \tag{12.13.29}$$

Similarly, for a variable $y(\tau_m)$ for a susceptible male of type $\tau_m \in \Upsilon_{SM}$ who is a member of the couple type (τ_f, τ_m), it can be shown with the help of MAPLE that:

$$\frac{\partial N_{CF}(\tau_f, \tau_m, \widehat{\mathbf{v}})}{\partial y(\tau_m)} = \widehat{x}(\tau_f) \alpha_f(\tau_f, \tau_m) \alpha_m(\tau_m, \tau_f) g_\theta^*(\tau_f, \tau_m, \widehat{\mathbf{v}})$$

$$\times \frac{N_m(\tau_f, \tau_m, \widehat{\mathbf{v}})}{D_m(\tau_f, \tau_m, \widehat{\mathbf{v}})} , \tag{12.13.30}$$

where

$$N_m(\tau_f, \tau_m, \widehat{\mathbf{v}}) = (\alpha_f(\tau_f, \tau_m) T_{mc}(\tau_m, \widehat{\mathbf{v}}))^\theta T_{fc}(\tau_f, \widehat{\mathbf{v}})$$

$$+((\alpha_m(\tau_m, \tau_f) T_{fc}(\tau_f, \widehat{\mathbf{v}}))^\theta) \widehat{y}(\tau_m) \alpha_f(\tau_f, \tau_m) \tag{12.13.31}$$

and

$$D_m(\tau_f, \tau_m, \widehat{\mathbf{v}}) = ((\alpha_m(\tau_m, \tau_f) T_{fc}(\tau_f, \widehat{\mathbf{v}}))^\theta + (\alpha_f(\tau_f, \tau_m) T_{mc}(\tau_m, \widehat{\mathbf{v}}))^\theta)$$

$$\times T_{fc}(\tau_f, \widehat{\mathbf{v}}) . \tag{12.13.32}$$

A third type of formula arises when considering a female of type τ, $\tau \neq \tau_f$, who is not a member of the couple type (τ_f, τ_m). For this case, it can be shown with the help of MAPLE that:

$$\frac{\partial N_{CF}(\tau_f, \tau_m, \widehat{\mathbf{v}})}{\partial x(\tau)} = -\widehat{x}(\tau_f) \widehat{y}(\tau_m) \alpha_f(\tau_f, \tau_m) \alpha_m(\tau_m, \tau_f) g_\theta^*(\tau_f, \tau_m, \widehat{\mathbf{v}})$$

$$\times g_f(\tau_f, \tau_m, \widehat{\mathbf{v}}) \frac{\alpha_m(\tau_m, \tau)}{T_{mc}(\tau_m, \widehat{\mathbf{v}})} , \tag{12.13.33}$$

where

$$g_f(\tau_f, \tau_m, \widehat{\mathbf{v}}) = \frac{(\alpha_f(\tau_f, \tau_m) T_{mc}(\tau_m, \widehat{\mathbf{v}}))^\theta}{(\alpha_m(\tau_m, \tau_f) T_{fc}(\tau_f, \widehat{\mathbf{v}}))^\theta + (\alpha_f(\tau_f, \tau_m) T_{mc}(\tau_m, \widehat{\mathbf{v}}))^\theta} . \tag{12.13.34}$$

Finally, for a male of type τ, $\tau \neq \tau_m$, who is not a member of the couple type (τ_f, τ_m), it can be shown with the help of MAPLE that:

$$\begin{aligned} \frac{\partial N_{CF}(\tau_f, \tau_m, \widehat{\mathbf{v}})}{\partial y(\tau)} &= -\widehat{x}(\tau_f)\widehat{y}(\tau_m)\alpha_f(\tau_f, \tau_m)\alpha_m(\tau_m, \tau_f) g_\theta^*(\tau_f, \tau_m, \widehat{\mathbf{v}}) \\ &\quad \times g_m(\tau_f, \tau_m, \widehat{\mathbf{v}}) \frac{\alpha_f(\tau_f, \tau)}{T_{fc}(\tau_f, \widehat{\mathbf{v}})} , \end{aligned} \tag{12.13.35}$$

where

$$g_m(\tau_f, \tau_m, \widehat{\mathbf{v}}) = \frac{(\alpha_m(\tau_m, \tau_f) T_{fc}(\tau_f, \widehat{\mathbf{v}}))^\theta}{(\alpha_m(\tau_m, \tau_f) T_{fc}(\tau_f, \widehat{\mathbf{v}}))^\theta + (\alpha_f(\tau_f, \tau_m) T_{mc}(\tau_m, \widehat{\mathbf{v}}))^\theta} . \tag{12.13.36}$$

When numerically implementing formulas such as Eq. (12.13.36), it may be advisable to express such formulas in terms of ratios of the form in Eq. (12.11.14) to better cope with the potential problem of computer overflow for large values of θ.

Having set down formulas for the elements of the Jacobian matrix $\mathbf{J}_{CF}(\widehat{\mathbf{v}})$ for couple formation evaluated at a stationary vector $\widehat{\mathbf{v}}$, the next step is to provide an overview of the partitioned form of this matrix suitable for writing computer code. In terms of the notation in Eq. (12.10.12), observe that the sub-matrix whose rows are indexed by the set Υ_f of female types has the partitioned form,

$$\mathbf{J}_{FCF}(\widehat{\mathbf{v}}) = \left[\ \mathbf{J}_{FCF}(f, f, \widehat{\mathbf{v}}) \quad \mathbf{J}_{FCF}(f, m, \widehat{\mathbf{v}}) \quad \mathbf{0}_{m(n+1)\times m^2(n+1)^2}\ \right] , \tag{12.13.37}$$

where the rows and columns of $\mathbf{J}_{FCF}(f, f, \widehat{\mathbf{v}})$ are indexed by the set Υ_f, the rows and columns of $\mathbf{J}_{FCF}(f, m, \widehat{\mathbf{v}})$ are, respectively, indexed by the sets Υ_f and Υ_m, and $\mathbf{0}_{m(n+1)\times m^2(n+1)^2}$ is a $m(n+1) \times m^2(n+1)^2$ matrix of zeros. Recall that the latter matrix arises because the functions $N_{CF}(\tau_f, \tau_m, \mathbf{v})$ do not depend on the vector $\mathbf{v}_c$ for couples. Similarly, the sub-matrix whose rows are indexed by the set Υ_m of male types has the partitioned form,

$$\mathbf{J}_{MCF}(\widehat{\mathbf{v}}) = \left[\ \mathbf{J}_{MCF}(m, f, \widehat{\mathbf{v}}) \quad \mathbf{J}_{MCF}(m, m, \widehat{\mathbf{v}}) \quad \mathbf{0}_{m(n+1)\times m^2(n+1)^2}\ \right] . \tag{12.13.38}$$

Finally, the sub-matrix whose rows are indexed by the set Υ_c of couple types has the partitioned form

$$\mathbf{J}_{CCF}(\widehat{\mathbf{v}}) = \left[\ \mathbf{J}_{CCF}(c, f, \widehat{\mathbf{v}}) \quad \mathbf{J}_{CCF}(c, m, \widehat{\mathbf{v}}) \quad \mathbf{0}_{m^2(n+1)^2\times m^2(n+1)^2}\ \right] . \tag{12.13.39}$$

By way of illustrating the theory just developed in the remainder of this section, the elements the non-zero sub-matrices will be expressed in terms of the formulas for partial derivatives derived above for the simple case of $m = 1$ behavioral class with $n = 1$ stage of disease.

For this case, the two female types are $\tau_{f1} = (0)$, a susceptible, and $\tau_{f2} = (1)$, an infective, and the two male types, τ_{m1} and τ_{m2}, are defined similarly. Moreover, arranged in lexicographical order, the set of couple types Υ_c is:

$$\{\varkappa_1 = (\tau_{f1}, \tau_{m1}),\ \varkappa_2 = (\tau_{f1}, \tau_{m2}),\ \varkappa_3 = (\tau_{f2}, \tau_{m1}),\ \varkappa_4 = (\tau_{f2}, \tau_{m2})\} . \tag{12.13.40}$$

Because the formulas for the partial derivatives that make up the elements of the Jacobian matrix for couple formation are lengthy, it will be necessary to use an abbreviated notation when placing them in their appropriate locations in a matrix. For example, the derivative in Eqs. (12.13.27) through (12.13.29) will be denoted by $N(\tau_f, \tau_m)_{\tau_f}$; the other derivatives will be denoted similarly. With respect to the couple formation rate $\rho(\varkappa)$ in the differential equations of Eqs. (12.8.5) and (12.8.6), it will be assumed that for all couple types $\varkappa \in \Upsilon_c$ there is a positive constant ρ such that $\rho(\varkappa) = \rho$.

In this abbreviated notation, and from the above results on values of partial derivatives at a stationary vector $\widehat{\mathbf{v}}$, it can be seen that the 4×2 sub-matrix $\mathbf{J}_{CCF}(c, f, \widehat{\mathbf{v}})$ in Eq. (12.13.39) has the form,

$$\mathbf{J}_{CCF}(c, f, \widehat{\mathbf{v}}) = \begin{bmatrix} \rho N(\tau_{f1}, \tau_{m1})_{\tau_{f1}} & \rho N(\tau_{f1}, \tau_{m1})_{\tau_{f2}} \\ 0 & 0 \\ \rho N(\tau_{f2}, \tau_{m1})_{\tau_{f1}} & 0 \\ 0 & 0 \end{bmatrix} . \tag{12.13.41}$$

Similarly, the other 4×2 sub-matrix $\mathbf{J}_{CCF}(c, m, \widehat{\mathbf{v}})$ in Eq. (12.13.39) has the form,

$$\mathbf{J}_{CCF}(c, m, \widehat{\mathbf{v}}) = \begin{bmatrix} \rho N(\tau_{f1}, \tau_{m1})_{\tau_{m1}} & \rho N(\tau_{f1}, \tau_{m1})_{\tau_{m2}} \\ 0 & \rho N(\tau_{f1}, \tau_{m2})_{\tau_{m2}} \\ 0 & 0 \\ 0 & 0 \end{bmatrix}. \quad (12.13.42)$$

Examining Eq. (12.13.41), and from Eqs. (12.8.5) and (12.8.6), it can be seen that the 2×2 sub-matrix $\mathbf{J}_{FCF}(f, f, \widehat{\mathbf{v}})$ in Eq. (12.13.37), whose rows and columns are indexed by the set Υ_f of female types, has the form,

$$\mathbf{J}_{FCF}(f, f, \widehat{\mathbf{v}}) = \begin{bmatrix} -\rho N(\tau_{f1}, \tau_{m1})_{\tau_{f1}} & -\rho N(\tau_{f1}, \tau_{m1})_{\tau_{f2}} \\ -\rho N(\tau_{f2}, \tau_{m1})_{\tau_{f1}} & 0 \end{bmatrix}. \quad (12.13.43)$$

Similar observations with respect to Eq. (12.13.42) lead to the conclusion that the 2×2 sub-matrix $\mathbf{J}_{FCF}(f, m, \widehat{\mathbf{v}})$ in Eq. (12.13.37),whose rows and columns are, respectively, indexed by the sets Υ_f and Υ_m, has the form,

$$\mathbf{J}_{FCF}(f, m, \widehat{\mathbf{v}}) = \begin{bmatrix} J_{11} & J_{12} \\ 0 & 0 \end{bmatrix} \quad (12.13.44)$$

$J_{11} = -\rho N(\tau_{f1}, \tau_{m1})_{\tau_{m1}}$, $J_{12} = -\rho(N(\tau_{f1}, \tau_{m1})_{\tau_{m2}} + N(\tau_{f1}, \tau_{m2})_{\tau_{m2}})$.

Turning to the 2×2 sub-matrix $\mathbf{J}_{CCF}(c, f, \widehat{\mathbf{v}})$ in Eq. (12.13.39), whose rows and columns are, respectively, indexed by the sets Υ_m and Υ_f, it can be seen form Eq. (12.13.41) that:

$$\mathbf{J}_{CCF}(c, f, \widehat{\mathbf{v}}) = \begin{bmatrix} J_{11} & J_{12} \\ 0 & 0 \end{bmatrix} \quad (12.13.45)$$

$J_{11} = -\rho(N(\tau_{f1}, \tau_{m1})_{\tau_{f1}} + N(\tau_{f2}, \tau_{m1})_{\tau_{f1}})$, $J_{12} = -\rho N(\tau_{f1}, \tau_{m1})_{\tau_{f2}}$.

A similar inspection of Eq. (12.13.42) leads to the conclusion that the 2×2 sub-matrix $\mathbf{J}_{CCF}(c, c, \widehat{\mathbf{v}})$ in Eq. (12.13.39), whose rows and columns are indexed by the set Υ_m, has the form,

$$\mathbf{J}_{CCF}(c, c, \widehat{\mathbf{v}}) = \begin{bmatrix} -\rho N(\tau_{f1}, \tau_{m1})_{\tau_{m1}} & -\rho N(\tau_{f1}, \tau_{m1})_{\tau_{m2}} \\ 0 & -\rho N(\tau_{f1}, \tau_{m2})_{\tau_{m2}} \end{bmatrix}. \quad (12.13.46)$$

This completes the specification of the 6×6 Jacobian matrix $\mathbf{J}_{CF}(\widehat{\mathbf{v}})$ for couple formation in the simple case of $m = 1$ and $n = 1$.

12.14 Couple Formation for m ≥ 2 and n ≥ 2

The partitioned form of the Jacobian matrix for couple formation is presented in Eqs. (12.13.37) through (12.13.39), and as shown in Section 12.13, the elements of the sub-matrices in Eqs. (12.13.37) and (12.13.38) may be computed from the elements of the sub-matrices in Eq. (12.13.39). Therefore, when computing numerical versions of the Jacobian matrix for couple formation, it suffices to specify the elements of the sub-matrices $\mathbf{J}_{CCF}(c, f, \widehat{\mathbf{v}})$ and $\mathbf{J}_{CCF}(c, m, \widehat{\mathbf{v}})$, and then develop a procedure for computing the elements of the set of sub-matrices,

$$\{\mathbf{J}_{FCF}(f, f, \widehat{\mathbf{v}}), \mathbf{J}_{FCF}(f, m, \widehat{\mathbf{v}}), \mathbf{J}_{MCF}(m, f, \widehat{\mathbf{v}}), \mathbf{J}_{MCF}(m, m, \widehat{\mathbf{v}})\} \,. \tag{12.14.1}$$

As a starting point, this procedure will be illustrated for the case of $m = 1$ behavioral class and $n = 2$ stages of disease, and then an outline will follow, illustrating how the procedure may be generalized to cases such that $m \geq 2$ and $n \geq 2$.

For this case, the set Υ_f of female types contains the types $\tau_{f1} = (0)$, an infective, and $\tau_{f2} = (1)$ and $\tau_{f3} = (2)$, two infectious types. The three types of males, τ_{m1}, τ_{m2} and τ_{m3}, are defined similarly and constitute the set Υ_m of male types. For each fixed female type $\tau_f \in \Upsilon_f$, let

$$\Upsilon_c(\tau_f) = \{(\tau_f, \tau_m) \mid \tau_m \in \Upsilon_m\} \tag{12.14.2}$$

denote the indicated subset of couple types such that the female is of type τ_f. Then, the set Υ_c of couple types may be represented as the disjoint union:

$$\Upsilon_c = \bigcup_{\tau_f \in \Upsilon_f} \Upsilon_c(\tau_f) \,. \tag{12.14.3}$$

Let $\mathbf{J}_{CCF}(c, f, \tau_f)$ denote the sub-matrix of $\mathbf{J}_{CCF}(c, f, \widehat{\mathbf{v}})$ whose rows and columns are indexed, respectively, by the sets $\Upsilon_c(\tau_f)$ and Υ_f. Then, the sub-matrix $\mathbf{J}_{CCF}(c, f, \widehat{\mathbf{v}})$ may be represented in the partitioned form,

$$\mathbf{J}_{CCF}(c, f, \widehat{\mathbf{v}}) = \begin{bmatrix} \mathbf{J}_{CCF}(c, f, \tau_{f1}) \\ \mathbf{J}_{CCF}(c, f, \tau_{f2}) \\ \mathbf{J}_{CCF}(c, f, \tau_{f3}) \end{bmatrix} . \tag{12.14.4}$$

Similarly, the sub-matrix $\mathbf{J}_{CCF}(c, m, \widehat{\mathbf{v}})$ may be represented in the partitioned form,

$$\mathbf{J}_{CCF}(c, m, \widehat{\mathbf{v}}) = \begin{bmatrix} \mathbf{J}_{CCF}(c, m, \tau_{f1}) \\ \mathbf{J}_{CCF}(c, m, \tau_{f2}) \\ \mathbf{J}_{CCF}(c, m, \tau_{f3}) \end{bmatrix} , \tag{12.14.5}$$

where, for example, the rows of the sub-matrix $\mathbf{J}_{CCF}(c, m, \tau_{f1})$ are indexed by the set $\Upsilon_c(\tau_f)$ and the columns by the set Υ_m.

From an inspection of the general formulas for partial derivatives in Section 12.13, it can the seen that the 3×3 sub-matrix $\mathbf{J}_{CCF}(c, f, \tau_{f1})$ has the form,

$$\mathbf{J}_{CCF}(c, f, \tau_{f1}) = \begin{bmatrix} J_{11} & J_{12} & J_{13} \\ 0 & 0 & 0 \\ 0 & 0 & 0 \end{bmatrix} , \tag{12.14.6}$$

$J_{11} = \rho N(\tau_{f1}, \tau_{m1})_{\tau_{f1}}$, $J_{12} = \rho N(\tau_{f1}, \tau_{m1})_{\tau_{f2}}$, $J_{13} = \rho N(\tau_{f1}, \tau_{m1})_{\tau_{f3}}$, and the sub-matrix $\mathbf{J}_{CCF}(c, m, \tau_{f1})$ has the form

$$\mathbf{J}_{CCF}(c, m, \tau_{f1}) = \begin{bmatrix} J_{11} & J_{12} & J_{13} \\ 0 & J_{22} & 0 \\ 0 & 0 & J_{33} \end{bmatrix} . \tag{12.14.7}$$

$J_{11} = \rho N(\tau_{f1}, \tau_{m1})_{\tau_{m1}}$, $J_{12} = \rho N(\tau_{f1}, \tau_{m1})_{\tau_{m2}}$, $J_{13} = \rho N(\tau_{f1}, \tau_{m1})_{\tau_{m3}}$, $J_{22} = \rho N(\tau_{f1}, \tau_{m2})_{\tau_{m2}}$, $J_{33} = \rho N(\tau_{f1}, \tau_{m3})_{\tau_{m3}}$.

Furthermore, from an inspection of the results in Section 12.13, it can be seen that the sub-matrix $\mathbf{J}_{CCF}(c, f, \tau_{f2})$ has the form,

$$\mathbf{J}_{CCF}(c, f, \tau_{f2}) = \begin{bmatrix} 0 & \rho N(\tau_{f2}, \tau_{m1})_{\tau_{f2}} & 0 \\ 0 & 0 & 0 \\ 0 & 0 & 0 \end{bmatrix} , \tag{12.14.8}$$

and $\mathbf{J}_{CCF}(c, m, \tau_{f2}) = \mathbf{0}_{3\times3}$, a 3×3 zero matrix. Lastly, the sub-matrix $\mathbf{J}_{CCF}(c, f, \tau_{f3})$ has the form,

$$\mathbf{J}_{CCF}(c, f, \tau_{f3}) = \begin{bmatrix} 0 & 0 & \rho N(\tau_{f3}, \tau_{m1})_{\tau_{m3}} \\ 0 & 0 & 0 \\ 0 & 0 & 0 \end{bmatrix}, \tag{12.14.9}$$

and $\mathbf{J}_{CCF}(c, m, \tau_{f3}) = \mathbf{0}_{3\times3}$. It is clear that the patterns in the matrices displayed in Eq. (12.14.6) – (12.14.9) could easily be extended to cases such that $n \geq 3$.

The next step in describing the elements of the Jacobian matrix for couple formation is to set down a procedure for calculating the elements of the set of sub-matrices in Eq. (12.14.1) from the elements of the matrices in Eqs. (12.14.4) and (12.14.5). To this end, consider the elements in the first column of the 9×3 matrix $\mathbf{J}_{CCF}(c, f, \widehat{\mathbf{v}})$ in Eq. (12.14.4) and arrange them in a 3×3 matrix array denoted by:

$$\left[\rho N(\tau_f, \tau_m)_{\tau_{f1}} \mid \tau_f \in \Upsilon_f, \tau_m \in \Upsilon_c\right] . \tag{12.14.10}$$

The next step is to compute the row sums,

$$T_f(\tau_t)_{\tau_{f1}} = \sum_{\tau_m \in \Upsilon_m} \rho N(\tau_f, \tau_m)_{\tau_{f1}} \tag{12.14.11}$$

for $\tau_f \in \Upsilon_f$, and the column sums,

$$T_m(\tau_m)_{\tau_{f1}} = \sum_{\tau_f \in \Upsilon_f} \rho N(\tau_f, \tau_m)_{\tau_{f1}} \tag{12.14.12}$$

for $\tau_m \in \Upsilon_m$.

Then, the first column of the 3×3 sub-matrix $\mathbf{J}_{FCF}(f, f, \widehat{\mathbf{v}})$ is the 3×1 vector,

$$\begin{pmatrix} -T_f(\tau_{t1})_{\tau_{f1}} \\ -T_f(\tau_{t2})_{\tau_{f1}} \\ -T_f(\tau_{t3})_{\tau_{f1}} \end{pmatrix} . \tag{12.14.13}$$

It can also be seen that the first column of the 3×3 sub-matrix $\mathbf{J}_{MCF}(m, f, \widehat{\mathbf{v}})$ is:

$$\begin{pmatrix} -T_m(\tau_{m1})_{\tau_{f1}} \\ -T_m(\tau_{m2})_{\tau_{f1}} \\ -T_m(\tau_{m3})_{\tau_{f1}} \end{pmatrix} . \tag{12.14.14}$$

The first columns of the pair of sub-matrices $\mathbf{J}_{FCF}(c, m, \widehat{\mathbf{v}})$ and $\mathbf{J}_{MCF}(m, m, \widehat{\mathbf{v}})$ may be computed using a similar procedure. For these cases, arrange the elements of the first column of the 9×3 sub-matrix $\mathbf{J}_{CCF}(c, m, \widehat{\mathbf{v}})$ in Eq. (12.14.5) in a 3×3 matrix array,

$$[\rho N(\tau_f, \tau_m)_{\tau_{m1}} \mid \tau_f \in \Upsilon_f, \tau_m \in \Upsilon_c] \ . \tag{12.14.15}$$

Then, just as above, compute the row sums,

$$T_f(\tau_t)_{\tau_{m1}} = \sum_{\tau_m \in \Upsilon_m} \rho N(\tau_f, \tau_m)_{\tau_{m1}} \tag{12.14.16}$$

for $\tau_f \in \Upsilon_f$, and the column sums,

$$T_m(\tau_m)_{\tau_{m1}} = \sum_{\tau_f \in \Upsilon_f} \rho N(\tau_f, \tau_m)_{\tau_{m1}} \tag{12.14.17}$$

for $\tau_m \in \Upsilon_m$.

It then follows that the first column in the 3×3 sub-matrix $\mathbf{J}_{FCF}(f, m, \widehat{\mathbf{v}})$ is:

$$\begin{pmatrix} -T_f(\tau_{t1})_{\tau_{m1}} \\ -T_f(\tau_{t2})_{\tau_{m1}} \\ -T_f(\tau_{t3})_{\tau_{m1}} \end{pmatrix} . \tag{12.14.18}$$

Moreover, the first column in the 3×3 sub-matrix $\mathbf{J}_{MCF}(m, m, \widehat{\mathbf{v}})$ is:

$$\begin{pmatrix} -T_m(\tau_{m1})_{\tau_{m1}} \\ -T_m(\tau_{m2})_{\tau_{m1}} \\ -T_m(\tau_{m3})_{m_{f1}} \end{pmatrix} . \tag{12.14.19}$$

Clearly, from Eqs. (12.14.10) through (12.14.19), the procedure used to calculate the first columns of the set of sub-matrices in Eq. (12.14.1) could be extended to compute columns 2 and 3 in this set of matrices. It is also clear that the procedure just outlined could easily be extended to cases such that $n \geq 3$. As an exercise, it may be of interest to the reader to verify that the procedure just described would yield the matrices displayed in Eqs. (12.13.43) through (12.13.46) for case of $n = 1$ stage of disease.

To gain insight into the structure of the Jacobian matrix for couple formation for cases such that $m \geq 2$ behavioral classes and $n \geq 2$ stages of disease, it will suffice to consider the case of $m = 2$ and $n = 2$. For $j_1 = 1, 2$, let

$$\Upsilon_f(j_1) = \{(j_1, k_1) \mid k_1 = 0, 1, 2\} \tag{12.14.20}$$

denote the subset of three female types such that the female belongs to behavioral class j_1. The subsets of male types, $\Upsilon_m(1)$ and $\Upsilon_m(2)$, are defined similarly. Observe that, in this case, the sets Υ_f and Υ_m each contain 6 types.

As in Section 12.12, consider the subset of couple types where, for $\varkappa = (\tau_f = (j_1, k_1), \tau_m = (j_2, k_2))$,

$$A(j_1, j_2) = \{\varkappa = ((\tau_f, \tau_m) \mid k_1 = 0, 1, 2;\; k_2 = 0, 1, 2\} \tag{12.14.21}$$

is defined for each pair of behavioral classes (j_1, j_2), and the pairs (k_1, k_2) are arranged in lexicographical order. Equivalently, the set of 9 couple types $A(j_1, j_2)$ may also be represented in the form,

$$A(j_1, j_2) = \{\varkappa = ((\tau_f, \tau_m) \mid \tau_f \in \Upsilon_f(j_1);\; \tau_m \in \Upsilon_c(j_2)\}\ . \tag{12.14.22}$$

From this definition, it follows that the set Υ_c of 36 couple types may be represented as the disjoint union:

$$\Upsilon_c = \bigcup_{j_1=1}^{2} \bigcup_{j_2=1}^{2} A(j_1, j_2)\ . \tag{12.14.23}$$

As in Section 11.1, the disjoint sets in this union may be used to induce a useful partition of the matrices $\mathbf{J}_{CCF}(c, f, \widehat{\mathbf{v}})$ and $\mathbf{J}_{CCF}(c, m, \widehat{\mathbf{v}})$ in Eqs. (12.14.3) through (12.14.5). Thus, the matrix $\mathbf{J}_{CCF}(c, f, \widehat{\mathbf{v}})$ has the partitioned form,

$$\mathbf{J}_{CCF}(c, f, \widehat{\mathbf{v}}) = \begin{bmatrix} \mathbf{J}_{CCF}(c, f, 1, 1) \\ \mathbf{J}_{CCF}(c, f, 1, 2) \\ \mathbf{J}_{CCF}(c, f, 2, 1) \\ \mathbf{J}_{CCF}(c, f, 2, 2) \end{bmatrix}, \tag{12.14.24}$$

where, for example, the rows of the 9×6 sub-matrix $\mathbf{J}_{CCF}(c, f, 1, 1)$ are indexed by the set $A(1,1)$ of 9 couple types and the columns by the set Υ_f of 6 female types. Similarly, the matrix $\mathbf{J}_{CCF}(c, m, \widehat{\mathbf{v}})$ has the partitioned form,

$$\mathbf{J}_{CCF}(c, m, \widehat{\mathbf{v}}) = \begin{bmatrix} \mathbf{J}_{CCF}(c, m, 1, 1) \\ \mathbf{J}_{CCF}(c, m, 1, 2) \\ \mathbf{J}_{CCF}(c, m, 2, 1) \\ \mathbf{J}_{CCF}(c, m, 2, 2) \end{bmatrix}, \tag{12.14.25}$$

where, for example, the rows of the 9×6 sub-matrix $\mathbf{J}_{CCF}(c, m, 2, 2)$ are indexed by the set $A(2,2)$ of couple types and the columns by the set Υ_m of male types.

Each of the sub-matrices in Eqs. (12.14.24) and (12.14.25) may be further partitioned by fixing the disease state k_1 of the female member of a couple. Thus, for every triple (j_1, j_2, k_1), let

$$A(j_1, j_2, k_1) = \{\varkappa = (\tau_f, \tau_m) \mid k_2 = 0, 1, 2\} \tag{12.14.26}$$

denote the set of three couple types $\varkappa = (\tau_f = (j_1, k_1), \tau_m = (j_2, k_2))$ such that the three indices (j_1, j_2, k_1) are fixed but k_2 varies as indicated. Then, the sub-matrix $\mathbf{J}_{CCF}(c, f, 1, 1)$ in Eq. (12.14.24) may be represented in the partitioned form,

$$\mathbf{J}_{CCF}(c, f, 1, 1) = \begin{bmatrix} \mathbf{J}_{CCF}(c, f, 1, 1, 0) \\ \mathbf{J}_{CCF}(c, f, 1, 1, 1) \\ \mathbf{J}_{CCF}(c, f, 1, 1, 2) \end{bmatrix}. \tag{12.14.27}$$

In this matrix, the rows of the 3×6 sub-matrix $\mathbf{J}_{CCF}(c, f, 1, 1, 0)$ are indexed by the set $A(1,1,0)$ of couple types and set Υ_f of female types. Similar remarks hold for the other sub-matrices in Eq. (12.14.24).

Each sub-matrix in Eq. (12.14.25) may be partitioned in a manner similar to that in Eq. (12.14.27). The sub-matrix $\mathbf{J}_{CCF}(c, m, 2, 2)$, for example, has the partitioned form,

$$\mathbf{J}_{CCF}(c, m, 2, 2) = \begin{bmatrix} \mathbf{J}_{CCF}(c, m, 2, 2, 0) \\ \mathbf{J}_{CCF}(c, m, 2, 2, 1) \\ \mathbf{J}_{CCF}(c, m, 2, 2, 2) \end{bmatrix}. \tag{12.14.28}$$

The rows of the 3×6 sub-matrix $\mathbf{J}_{CCF}(c, m, 2, 2, 2)$ are indexed by the set $A(2, 2, 2)$ of couple types and the columns by the set Υ_m of male types. Furthermore, each of the sub-matrices in Eq. (12.14.25) may be partitioned in a manner similar to that in Eq. (12.14.28), but the details will be omitted.

As an aid to placing the partial derivatives in their correct locations in the Jacobian matrix, it will be helpful to further partition each sub-matrix $\mathbf{J}_{CCF}(c, f, j_1, j_2, k_1)$ into two sub-matrices whose columns are indexed by the sets $\Upsilon_f(1)$ and $\Upsilon_f(2)$ of female types belonging to behavioral class 1 and behavioral class 2, respectively. Thus,

$$\mathbf{J}_{CCF}(c, f, j_1, j_2, k_1) = \left[\ \mathbf{B}_{f1}(j_1, j_2, k_1) \quad \mathbf{B}_{f2}(j_1, j_2, k_1) \ \right] , \tag{12.14.29}$$

where the rows of the 3×3 matrices $\mathbf{B}_{f1}(j_1, j_2, k_1)$ and $\mathbf{B}_{f2}(j_1, j_2, k_1)$ are indexed by the set $A(j_1, j_2, k_1)$ of couple types and the columns are indexed, respectively by the sets $\Upsilon_f(1)$ and $\Upsilon_f(2)$ of the female types. The corresponding matrix $\mathbf{J}_{CCF}(c, m, j_1, j_2, k_1)$ of partial derivatives with respect to the variables in the vector for male types has the partitioned form,

$$\mathbf{J}_{CCF}(c, m, j_1, j_2, k_1) = \left[\ \mathbf{B}_{m1}(j_1, j_2, k_1) \quad \mathbf{B}_{m2}(j_1, j_2, k_1) \ \right] , \tag{12.14.30}$$

where the columns of the matrices $\mathbf{B}_{m1}(j_1, j_2, k_1)$ and $\mathbf{B}_{m2}(j_1, j_2, k_1)$ are indexed, respectively, by the sets $\Upsilon_m(1)$ and $\Upsilon_m(2)$ of male types.

As a further aid to correctly identifying partial derivatives, it will be helpful to explicitly denote each female type by its behavioral class and state with respect to disease. For example, a female of type (j_1, k_1) will be denoted by $\tau_{fk_1}(j_1)$, and similarly, a male of type (j_2, k_2) will be denoted by $\tau_{mk_2}(j_2)$. Rather than attempt to describe the sub-matrices in Eqs. (12.14.29) and (12.14.30) in a general notation, a procedure for constructing them will be illustrated by examples. As we shall see, the patterns displayed in Eqs. (12.14.6) through (12.14.9) can be generalized.

For example, in terms of the notation just introduced, the 3×3

matrix $\mathbf{B}_{f1}(1,1,0)$ has the form,

$$\mathbf{B}_{f1}(1,1,0)=\begin{bmatrix} F_{11} & F_{12} & F_{13} \\ 0 & 0 & 0 \\ 0 & 0 & 0 \end{bmatrix}, \tag{12.14.31}$$

for $F_{11} = \rho N(\tau_{f0}(1),\ \tau_{m0}(1))_{\tau_{f0}(1)}$, $F_{12} = \rho N(\tau_{f0}(1),\ \tau_{m0}(1))_{\tau_{f1}(1)}$, $F_{13} = \rho N(\tau_{f0}(1),\ \tau_{m0}(1))_{\tau_{f2}(1)}$, and the matrix $\mathbf{B}_{f2}(1,1,0)$ has the form,

$$\mathbf{B}_{f2}(1,1,0)=\begin{bmatrix} F_{11} & F_{12} & F_{13} \\ 0 & 0 & 0 \\ 0 & 0 & 0 \end{bmatrix}. \tag{12.14.32}$$

for $F_{11} = \rho N(\tau_{f0}(1),\ \tau_{m0}(1))_{\tau_{f0}(2)}$, $F_{12} = \rho N(\tau_{f0}(1),\ \tau_{m0}(1))_{\tau_{f1}(2)}$, $F_{13} = \rho N(\tau_{f0}(1),\ \tau_{m0}(1))_{\tau_{f2}(2)}$.

With regard to partial derivatives with respect to the elements of the vector for males, the sub-matrices in Eq. (12.14.30) have the forms,

$$\mathbf{B}_{m1}(1,1,0)=\begin{bmatrix} M_{11} & M_{12} & M_{13} \\ 0 & M_{22} & 0 \\ 0 & 0 & M_{33} \end{bmatrix}, \tag{12.14.33}$$

for $M_{11} = \rho N(\tau_{f0}(1),\ \tau_{m0}(1))_{\tau_{m0}(1)}$, $M_{12} = \rho N(\tau_{f0}(1),\ \tau_{m0}(1))_{\tau_{m1}(1)}$, $M_{13} = \rho N(\tau_{f0}(1),\ \tau_{m0}(1))_{\tau_{m2}(1)}$, with $M_{22} = \rho N(\tau_{f0}(1),\ \tau_{m1}(1))_{\tau_{m1}(1)}$, $M_{33} = \rho N(\tau_{f0}(1),\ \tau_{m2}(1))_{\tau_{m2}(1)}$; and

$$\mathbf{B}_{m2}(1,1,0)=\begin{bmatrix} M_{11} & M_{12} & M_{13} \\ 0 & 0 & 0 \\ 0 & 0 & 0 \end{bmatrix}. \tag{12.14.34}$$

for $M_{11} = \rho N(\tau_{f0}(1),\ \tau_{m0}(1))_{\tau_{m0}(1)}$, $M_{12} = \rho N(\tau_{f0}(1),\ \tau_{m0}(1))_{\tau_{m1}(1)}$, and $M_{13} = \rho N(\tau_{f0}(1),\ \tau_{m0}(1))_{\tau_{m2}(1)}$.

The next step is to display the matrices in Eqs. (12.14.31) through (12.14.34) for the case $k_1 = 1$. Thus, the only non-zero matrix in the set corresponding to those in Eqs. (12.14.31) through (12.14.34) has the form

$$\mathbf{B}_{f1}(1,1,1)=\begin{bmatrix} 0 & \rho N(\tau_{f1}(1),\tau_{m0}(1))_{\tau_{f1}(1)} & 0 \\ 0 & 0 & 0 \\ 0 & 0 & 0 \end{bmatrix}, \tag{12.14.35}$$

with $\mathbf{B}_{f2}(1,1,1) = \mathbf{B}_{m1}(1,1,1) = \mathbf{B}_{m2}(1,1,1) = \mathbf{0}_{3\times3}$. Similarly, for the case $k_1 = 2$,

$$\mathbf{B}_{f1}(1,1,2) = \begin{bmatrix} 0 & 0 & \rho N(\tau_{f2}(1), \tau_{m0}(1))_{\tau_{f2}(1)} \\ 0 & 0 & 0 \\ 0 & 0 & 0 \end{bmatrix}, \tag{12.14.36}$$

and $\mathbf{B}_{f2}(1,1,2) = \mathbf{B}_{m1}(1,1,2) = \mathbf{B}_{m2}(1,1,2) = \mathbf{0}_{3\times3}$. Observe the similarities of the patterns displayed in Eqs. (12.14.32) through (12.14.36) to those in Eqs. (12.14.6) through (12.14.9). To complete the description of the construction of the matrices $\mathbf{J}_{CCF}(c, f, \widehat{\mathbf{v}})$ and $\mathbf{J}_{CCF}(c, m, \widehat{\mathbf{v}})$ in Eqs. (12.14.24) and (12.14.25), variations of the procedure displayed in Eqs. (12.14.32) through (12.14.36) would need to be carried out on the remaining three pairs of behavioral classes $(1,2)$, $(2,1)$ and $(2,2)$, but the details will be left to the reader.

The last step in computing the elements of the Jacobian matrix for couple formation is that of computing the column vectors of the matrices in Eq. (12.14.1) from the columns of the matrices $\mathbf{J}_{CCF}(c, f, \widehat{\mathbf{v}})$ and $\mathbf{J}_{CCF}(c, m, \widehat{\mathbf{v}})$ in Eqs. (12.14.24) and (12.14.25). Although the details will be omitted, it suffices to say that an extension of the procedure outlined in Eqs. (12.14.10) through (12.14.19) could be used to compute the column vector of these matrices from those of $\mathbf{J}_{CCF}(c, f, \widehat{\mathbf{v}})$ and $\mathbf{J}_{CCF}(c, m, \widehat{\mathbf{v}})$. This completes the description of the procedure for computing the elements of the Jacobian matrix for couple formation.

12.15 Invasion Thresholds for m = n = 1

One of the simplest cases of the two-sex partnership models described in this section is that of $m = 1$ behavioral class and $n = 1$ stage of disease. For this case, there are two types of single females; namely, a susceptible and infected female denoted, respectively, by the symbols $\tau_{f1} = (0)$ and $\tau_{f2} = (1)$; the two types of single males, τ_{m1} and τ_{m2} are defined similarly. It also follows that in this simple case there are four types of couples, which may be denoted by the symbols $\varkappa_1 = (0,0)$, $\varkappa_2 = (0,1)$, $\varkappa_3 = (1,0)$, and $\varkappa_4 = (1,1)$. Because only relatively low dimensional arrays arise in Monte Carlo implementations of this model, it is well-suited to doing explorative computer experiments. Consequently, numerous computer experiments, designed to explore the behavior of the embedded deterministic model in relation to statistically summarized Monte Carlo realizations of the stochastic process, were carried out with the one-stage model.

In the early developmental stages of the stochastic two-sex stochastic partnership models under consideration, the only well-defined approach to finding threshold conditions for a particular assignment of parameter values was to use the branching process approximations studied in Chapters 8 and 9. Accordingly, the parameter assignments used in the experiment are presented in Table 12.15.1, and were chosen such that an epidemic would develop in a population according to the branching process approximation in Mode.[9]

Table 12.15.1. Parameter Assignments for the One-Stage Model.

Single Females: $(3996, 1)$
Single Males: $(3396, 1)$
Couples of Type $(0,0)$: 3204
$\lambda_f = \lambda_m = 1$
$q_{fem}(1) = q_{mem}(1) = 0.02$
$q_f(1) = q_m(1) = 0.11$
$\mu_{f0} = 1/720, \mu_{f1} = 1/60$
$\mu_{m0} = 1/660, \mu_{m1} = 1/60$
$\rho = 1/24, \delta = 1/24$
$\beta_{fem} = \beta_{mem} = 0.05$
$\beta_{fm} = \beta_{mm} = 0.05$

At a later date, following the development of software to compute eigenvalues of Jacobian matrices as outlined in previous sections of this chapter, it was also confirmed that the full 8×8 Jacobian matrix for a population containing infectives evaluated at a stationary vector for a population of susceptibles was unstable, which suggested that an epidemic would develop following the invasion of a few infective single females and males. As will be illustrated below, given the initial conditions and parameter assignments in Table 12.15.1, there is a positive probability that an epidemic would indeed develop in such a population, but, with some positive probability, it will also become extinct. It should be mentioned that the 8×8 **A**-matrix of embedded differential equations was also found to be stable, which suggested that the initial conditions would "wear off" in the sense of Eq. (10.7.17).

The first three rows of Table 12.15.1 were generated by finding the stationary vector of the embedded differential equations, following the numerical procedures outlined in Section 12.10. When rounded to the nearest integer, the stationary vector contained 3996 single females, 3396 single males, and 3204 couples as indicated in Table 12.15.1. It was assumed that the population of susceptibles was invaded by one infected individual of each sex. For simplicity, many of the parameter values for females and males were chosen as equal such as $q_f(1) = q_m(1) = 0.11$ for both females and males, with regard to marital sexual contacts. The rationale for choosing different probabilities of infection per sexual contact for marital and extra-marital contacts follows. For marital contacts, both partners may not take precautions to avoid infection because one partner may not know that the other is infected, but for extra-marital contacts, both females and males may take precautions to avoid infection. Though they seem high for HIV, for extra-marital contacts, the probabilities are in the range reported by Jacquez et al.[6]

For scale parameters in the latent exponential distributions, the reciprocals are the expected latent times spent in disease states in the absence of other competing risks. Hence, the basic death rate for susceptible females in the seventh row of Table 12.15.1 was assigned the value $\mu_{f0} = 1/720 = 1.3889 \times 10^{-3}$, corresponding to a life expectation of 720 months or 60 years. Similarly, the basic death rate for susceptible males was assigned the value $\mu_{m0} = 1/660$, corresponding to a life expectation of 660 months or $660/12 = 55$ years, since in many populations mortality rates for males are greater than those for females. The expectations assumed that females and males become sexually active in their late teens or early twenties. For both females and males, the incremental death rates for infected females and males in lines seven and eight of the table were chosen as $\mu_{f1} = \mu_{m1} = 1/60$ as determined by a latent expectation of 60 months or five years.

The parameters ρ and δ, governing couple formation and dissolution, were also interpreted as scale parameters in latent exponential distributions. For the experiments under consideration, values of these parameters were determined by $\rho = \delta = 1/24$, indicating that the expected waiting time among marital partners, as well as the expected duration of partnerships, was 24 months or two years. The rationale for choosing this value was that, according to the branching process approximation developed in Mode,[9] an epidemic would occur and spread in the population when the probabilities of infection per marital sexual contact were $q_f(1) = q_m(1) = 0.11$ as in line six of Table 12.5.1.

Finally, the parameters for the acceptance probabilities governing the choice of extra-marital and marital partnerships were chosen as $\beta_{fem} = \beta_{mem} = \beta_{fm} = \beta_{mm} = 0.05$, indicating that choices made in choosing sexual partners were "weakly" assortative. With respect to recruits, it was assumed that $\mu_f = \mu_m = 10$ so that, on average, 10 female and 10 male recruits entered the population per month. Furthermore, it was assumed that following the invasion of the initial infectives, none of the recruits were infective so that $\varphi_f(0) = \varphi_m(0) = 1$ and $\varphi_f(1) = \varphi_m(1) = 0$.

Apart from the initial numbers, which are larger than those used in a previous experiment, all parameter assignments in Table 12.15.1 are the same as those for experiment I reported in Sleeman and Mode.[12] At the time the experiments reported in that paper were run, however, the development of the software had progressed only to the point where the Min, Bar and Max trajectories could be computed from a sample of Monte Carlo realizations of the process. Moreover, the software contained no capability for estimating the probability that an epidemic becomes extinct by epoch from a sample Monte Carlo realizations of the process. Subsequently, the software was further developed not only to estimate the probability of extinction by epoch, but also to compute the trajectories of 25th, 50th and 75th quantiles from a Monte Carlo sample. As before, the software was also designed to include the Min, Bar and Max trajectories from a Monte Carlo sample as well as the Det trajectory as computed from the embedded deterministic model if so desired by an investigator.

As experimentation with the model progressed, it was realized that deeper insight into its behavior could be obtained if experiments of a rather long duration were conducted along with larger samples of Monte Carlo realizations. Consequently, unlike the results of the experiments reported in Sleeman and Mode,[12] which were based on 50 Monte Carlo realizations of the process each of 720 months or 60 years duration, the experiments reported in this chapter were based on 100 Monte Carlo realizations each of 1200 months or 100 years duration. Like all experiments reported in this book, the time unit was chosen as a month.

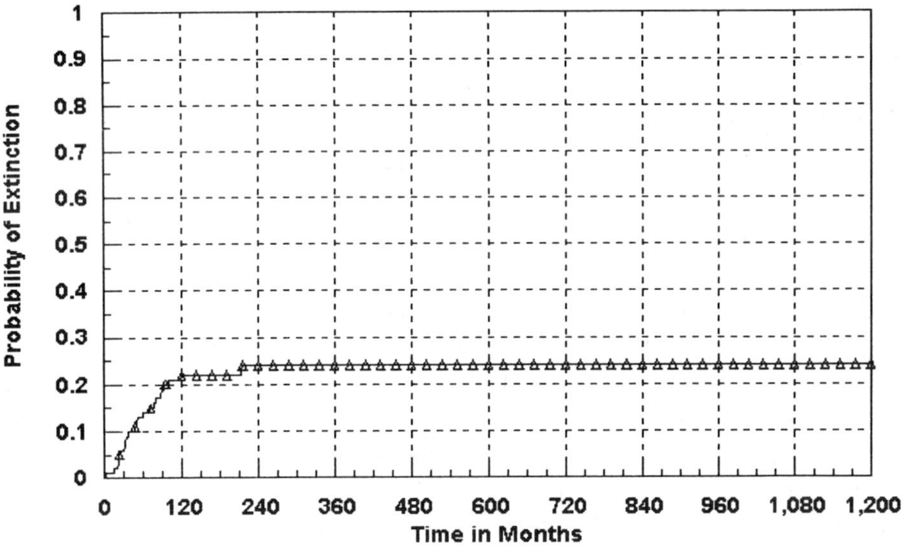

Figure 12.15.1. Probability Epidemic is Extinct by Epoch.

Estimates of the probability that an epidemic becomes extinct as a function of its duration expressed in epochs of one month are presented in Figure 12.15.1. As can be seen from this figure, the trajectory for the estimated probability of extinction converged to 0.24 at a point a little beyond about 200 months. Thus, given the initial conditions and parameter assignments in Table 12.15.1, the epidemic would eventually become extinct with an estimated probability of about 0.24.

The probability that an epidemic eventually becomes extinct is of basic importance in grasping the extent of the variability that may occur among the realizations of an epidemic governed by some stochastic process, but it is also of interest to gain insight into the extent of this variability among those realizations of the process in which an epidemic does become established in a population. In this connection, it is helpful to plot the trajectories of the 25th, 50th and 75th quantiles of a sample of Monte Carlo realizations of the process, which will be denoted by Q25, Q50 and Q75, respectively. Furthermore, to gain insight into the total extent of this variation, it will also be useful to include plots of the Min and Max trajectories. Finally, to get some idea of where the trajectory computed from the embedded deterministic model stands in relation those computed from a Monte Carlo sample, it will also be informative to include a plot of the Det trajectory. Plots of these trajectories for the number of infected females in couples by epoch are presented in Figure 12.15.2. Because the corresponding plots for males are similar given the initial conditions and parameters assignments under consideration, they will be omitted.

From an inspection of Figure 12.15.2, it is interesting to observe that for the first 30 years (360 months) of the projections, the position of the Det trajectory was between those of the Q75 and the Max trajectories. But, at the peak of the epidemic, which occurred somewhere in the interval 336 to 390 months, the Det trajectory was closer to the Max than to Q75. Thus, with respect to the peak of the epidemic and during the first 30 or so years of the projections, the Det trajectory seems to forecast the worst case scenario. Furthermore, a projection of an epidemic based on the embedded deteministic model would forecast that it would subside at a faster rate than actually occurred among the Monte Carlo realizations of the epidemic. For example, the Det trajectory did not come close to Q50 (the median trajectory of the Monte Carlo sample) until about 660 months into the projections. In the long run, however, the graphs in Figure 12.15.2 suggest that the Det trajectory converges to a value close to that of the Q75 trajectory, which suggests that, among 75% of the stochastic realizations of the process, fewer individuals would actually be infected than those predicted by forecasts based on the embedded deteministic model at any epoch. It should also be noted that at 1200 months (200 years) into the projections, the trajectories of Q25, Q50, Q75 and Det are quite close.

Another perspective from which to view the impact of an infectious disease on a population is that of the total population size. From this perspective, one would expect that the Min trajectory would represent the worst case of an epidemic in which there were many deaths due to disease; while the Max trajectory would represent those realizations in which there were fewer infected persons and, thus, fewer deaths due to disease. Figure 12.15.3 contains the graphs of the Min, Q25, Q50, Q75, Max and Det trajectories for the total size of the female population.

As can be seen from this figure, these trajectories did not diverge greatly until about 360 months into the projection, which indicates that the presence of infectives in the population had little impact on the size of the female population during this time period. Thereafter, however, these trajectories diverged, indicating that deaths from disease were having a significant impact on the population. During the time interval 360 to 720 months, the Det trajectory remained between the Min and Q25 trajectories, and tended to represent the worst case scenario of the epidemic. Thereafter, however, this trajectory occupied a place somewhere between the Q25 and Q50 trajectories, and tended to come closer to Q50. Like the examples presented in previous chapters, in this experiment there was a high level of stochasticity among realizations of the stochastic process with respect to the total size of the female population. Although it is not shown, the same set of trajectories for the total size of the male population exhibited a similar level of stochasticity.

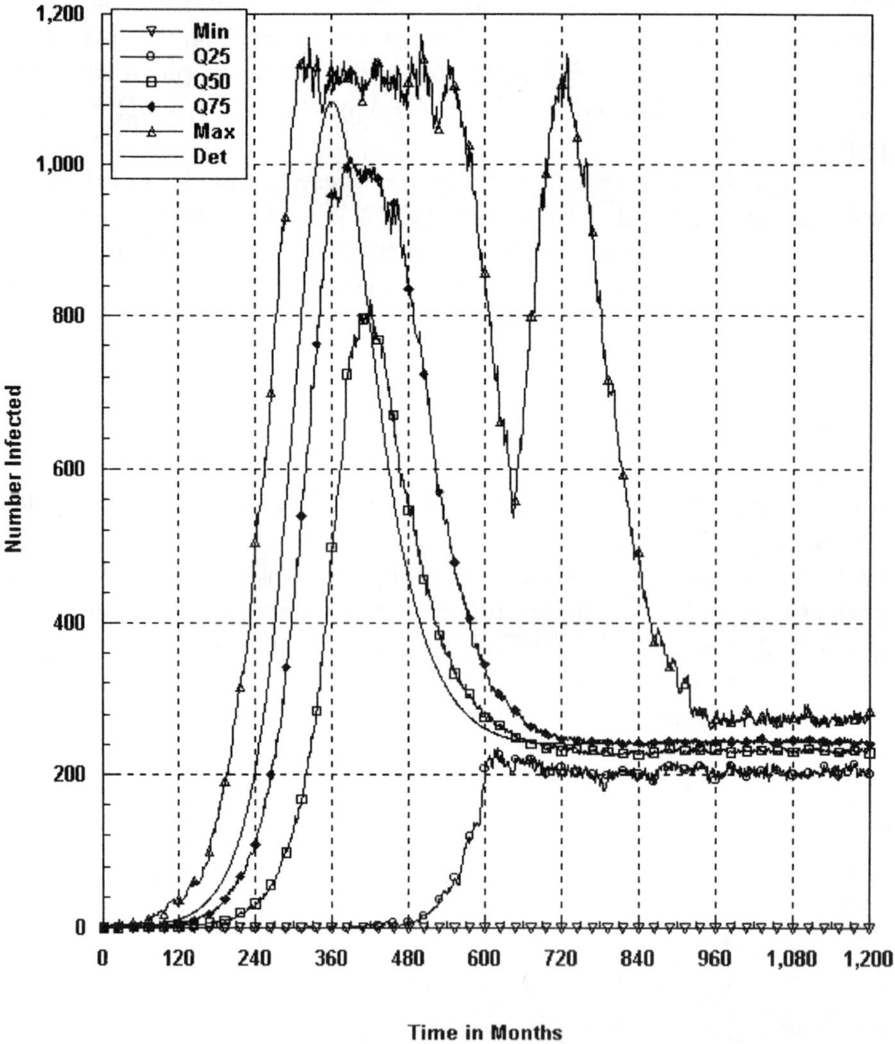

Figure 12.15.2. Number of Infected Females in Couples by Epoch.

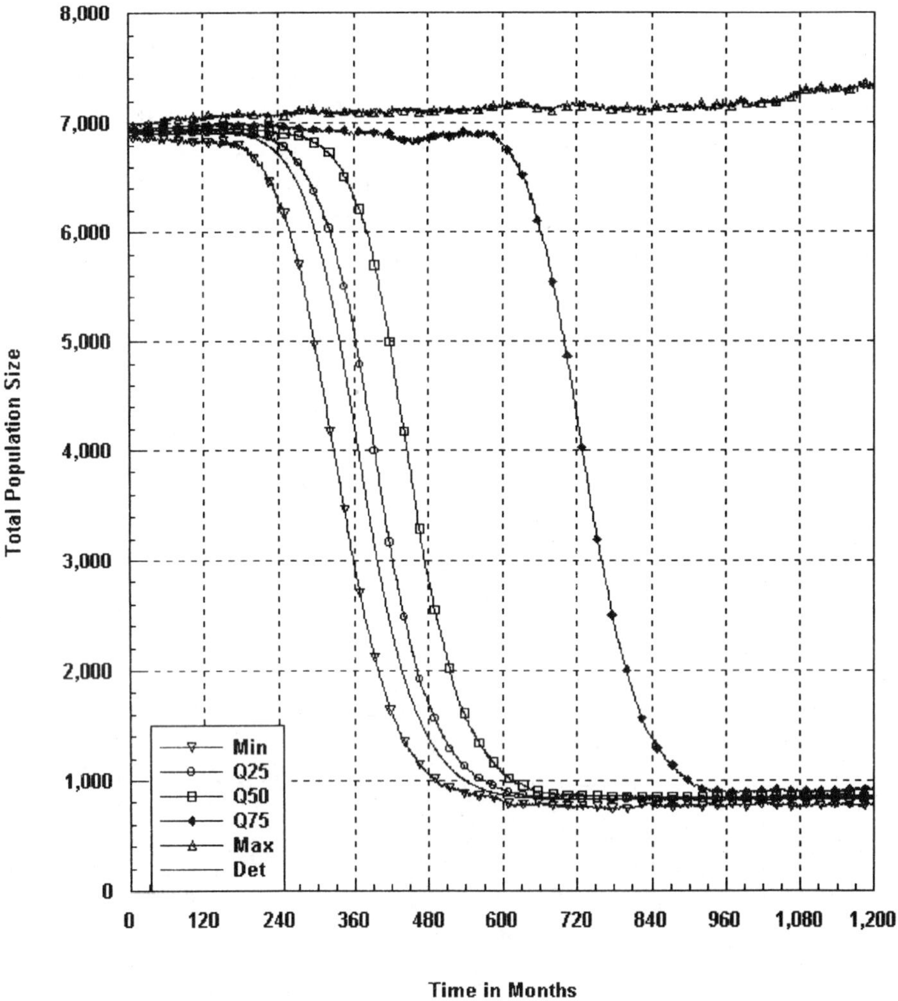

Figure 12.15.3. Total Population Size for Females by Epoch.

12.16 Four-Stage Model Applied to Epidemics of HIV/AIDS

It has been conjectured that the human immunodeficiency virus (HIV) may have been present in some populations for an unknown, but perhaps large number of decades, before it was recognized by the international community of scientists and laymen. The interesting book Grmek[5] may be consulted for an extensive discussion of whether acquired immune deficiency syndromes (AIDS) is an ancient disease. That several decades may elapse before the demographic impact of an infectious disease becomes apparent in a population seeded initially with one infective single female and male was illustrated in an experiment with the four-stage model reported in this section.

Table 12.16.1. Parameter Assignments for the Four-Stage Model.

Single Females: $(1378, 1, 0, 0, 0)$
Single Males: $(778, 1, 0, 0, 0)$
Couples of Type (0,0): 5822
$\lambda_f = \lambda_m = 0.25$
$q_{fem}(1) = q_{mem}(1) = 0.1$
$q_{fem}(2) = q_{mem}(2) = 0.05$
$q_{fem}(3) = q_{mem}(3) = 0.05$
$q_{fem}(4) = q_{mem}(4) = 0.1$
$q_f(j) = q_m(j) = q_{fem}(j) = q_{mem}(j),\ j = 1, 2, 3, 4$
$\mu_{f0} = 1/720, \mu_{f1} = 1/240$
$\mu_{f2} = \mu_{f3} = 1/240, \mu_{f4} = 1/23.8$
$\mu_{m0} = 1/660, \mu_{m1} = 1/180$
$\mu_{m2} = \mu_{m3} = 1/180, \mu_{m4} = 1/23.8$
$\rho = 1/12, \delta = 1/120$
$\beta_{fem} = \beta_{mem} = 0$
$\beta_{fm} = \beta_{mm} = 0$

The parameter assignments used in this experiment are presented in Table 12.16.1. According to the multitype branching process approximation in Mode,[10] an epidemic would develop in the population given these values of the parameters. Subsequent to the development of the software implementing the branching process approximations described in Chapters 8 and 9, software was also written to compute the eigenvalues of the 35×35 Jacobian matrix of the embedded differential equations evaluated at a stationary vector for a population containing only susceptibles evolving according the to parameter values in Table 12.16.1. It was found that this matrix was not stable, which also suggested that an epidemic would indeed develop in a population. As in other cases presented in Chapters 10 and 11, it was also found that the 35×35 **A**-matrix was stable so that as time increases the initial conditions "wear off".

The first two rows of the table contain the values of the stationary vector for the embedded differential equations rounded to the nearest integer. Observe that, by assumption, the initial population contained one infectious single female and male. As can be seen from the third row from the bottom of the table, in this experiment, durations of marital partnerships were long in the sense that the latent expectation for the duration of a marital partnership was $1/\delta = 120$ months or ten years, but the expected latent waiting time among marital partners was $1/\rho = 12$ months or one year. According to row 4 of the table, extra-marital sexual contacts occurred at a rate of about 3 per year or $\lambda_f = \lambda_m = 0.25$ per month. The values assumed for the probability of infection per extra-marital contact between a susceptible and infective are presented by stages of the disease in rows 5 through 8, and, for ease of presentation, it was assumed that these probabilities for marital contacts were the same as those for extra-marital contacts.

Assumed values for the death rate parameters for females and males are presented in rows 10 through 13. A person in stage 4 of the disease has a latent expectation of life span $1/\mu_{f4} = 1/\mu_{m4} = 23.8$ months. Finally, the parameter assignments in the last two rows of the table, $\beta_{fem} = \beta_{mem} = \beta_{fm} = \beta_{mm} = 0$, indicate that marital and extra-marital sexual partners were chosen at random with respect to stages of the disease. Not shown in the table are values of the γ-parameters for the durations of stay in stages 1, 2, and 3 of the disease for females and males. The values determined by $1/\gamma_f(1) = 1/\gamma_m(1) = 12$ months were based on some experimental results of Sleeman and Mode,[14,13] which suggested that the expected duration of stay in stage 1 of HIV disease may be longer than previously reported in the literature. The γ-values assigned for stages 2 and 3 of the disease were motivated by results reported by Longini et al.[7] and were determined by the equations $\gamma_f(2) = \gamma_m(2) = 1/52.62$ and $\gamma_f(3) = \gamma_m(3) = 1/62.89$. With respect to recruits, it was assumed that $\mu_f = \mu_m = 10$ so that, on average, 10 female and 10 male recruits entered the population per month. Furthermore, it was assumed that following the invasion of the initial infectives, none of the recruits were infective so that $\varphi_f(0) = \varphi_m(0) = 1$ and $\varphi_f(k) = \varphi_m(k) = 0$ for $k = 1, 2, 3, 4$.

It should be mentioned that parameter values presented Table 12.16.1 were also used in experiment II reported in Sleeman and Mode,[12] but with initial conditions differing from those given in the table, which were determined by finding the stationary vector of the embedded differential equations for the case of a population containing only susceptibles. Like those reported in Section 12.15, the software had been enhanced to statistically summarize the results of a sample of Monte Carlo realizations of the process. Included in these enhancements was a capability for calculating the probability that an epidemic becomes extinct as a function of the duration of the projections as well as a capability for computing quantile trajectories from a Monte Carlo sample. Finally, the experiment reported in Sleeman and Mode[12] used a Monte Carlo sample of size 50, whereas the sample size was raised to 100 for the experiments reported in this section, with the duration of each projection 1200 months or 100 years.

A graph of the estimated probability that an epidemic becomes extinct as a function of the duration of the projection by epoch is presented in Figure 12.16.1. As can be from this graph, by about 360 months into the projections, the population contained no infectives in 25 out of 100 Monte Carlo realizations of the process, indicating that the epidemic had become extinct. But, by the epoch of 1200 months, this number had increased to 27. Thus, given the initial conditions and parameter values in the table, an epidemic will eventually become extinct with an estimated probability of 0.27. In the figures presented below, attention will be focused on providing insights into what happened in the remaining 73 Monte Carlo realizations of the process in which the population contained at least one infective at 1200 months.

Unlike the graph presented in the previous section, where attention was focused on the female population, attention will be directed towards the male population in the following, but it should be mentioned that the corresponding graphs for the female population would be similar.

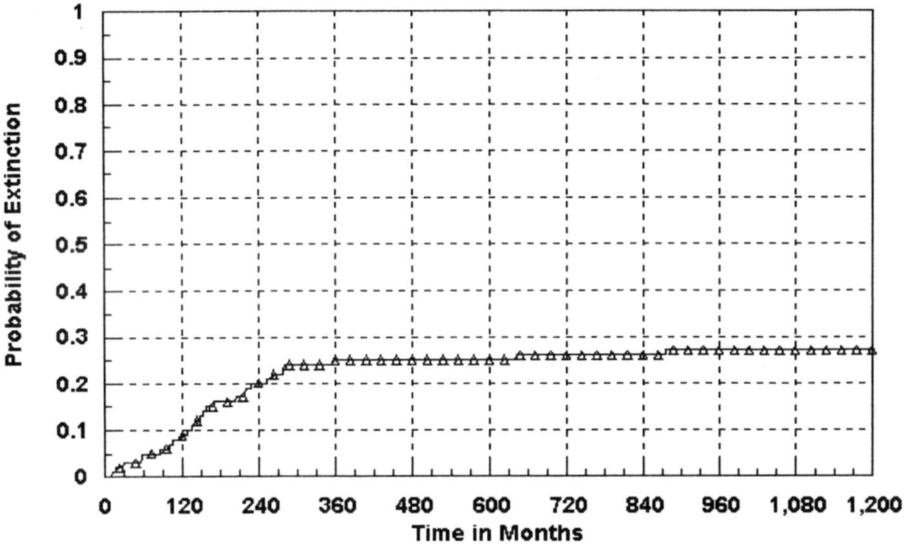

Figure 12.16.1. Probability Epidemic is Extinct by Epoch.

To provide some insight into the size of the epidemic within some component of the population, it is of interest to consider the cumulative numbers of infections that occurred following the introduction of initial infectives into the population. Graphs of the Min, Q25, Q50, Q75, Max and Det trajectories for the cumulative numbers of infected males in couples resulting from the invasion of the initial infectives are presented in Figure 12.16.2. As can be seen from these trajectories, among those realizations in which extinction did not occur, the development of the epidemic was slow; at 360 months into the projections, the Max trajectory stood at 81 but thereafter this trajectory rose at a more rapid rate and reached 8718 by 1200 months. In this experimental projection of an HIV/AIDS epidemic, the Det trajectory occupied a position between the Q75 and Max trajectories, but throughout these projections, this trajectory was closer to the Max than Q75. Just as with the experiments with the one-stage model presented in Section 12.15, the embedded deterministic model seems to reflect some of the worst case scenarios of the epidemic. It is also interesting to note that throughout the projections, the median trajectory Q50 occupied a position significantly lower than that of the Q75. For example, at epoch 1200 months, Q50 is equal to 2653 and Q75 is equal to 6765.

Another perspective from which to view the development of an epidemic within some component of the population is to consider the number of persons infected at any epoch in a projection. Graphs of the Min, Q25, Q50, Q75, Max and Det trajectories for the number of males in couples infected at any epoch are presented in Figure 12.16.3. These graphs are typical for that of a slowly-developing epidemic among those realizations of the process in which it did not become extinct. In a more rapidly-developing epidemic, one would expect to see these trajectories rise to a peak and then decline as an epidemic takes its toll on the population. However, there is little evidence of any decline in the number of infectives at some epoch until sometime after 1000 months into the projections in Figure 12.16.3. Evidently, if an investigator wished to observe more typical trajectories for the development of an epidemic, it appears necessary to continue the projections for another 100 years. That the Det trajectory lies somewhere between the trajectories Q75 and Max throughout most of the projections is consistent with the trajectories in Figure 12.16.2. This trajectory seems to represent some of the worst case scenarios among the possible realizations of an epidemic.

As in Section 12.15, it will be instructive to view the variability among realizations of an epidemic from the perspective of its impact on the size of some component of the population. Figure 12.16.4 contains graphs of the Min, Q25, Q50, Q75, Max and Det trajectories for the size of the male population. When compared with the graphs for the corresponding trajectories for the female population in Figure 12.15.3, it appears that the variability among the realizations of the process was somewhat less in these projections with the four-stage model than with the one-stage model of Section 12.15. By way of illustration, the initial size of the female population was 7201 and, at epoch 1200, the value of the Min trajectory was 780 in Figure 12.15.3. In terms of fractions, this number represents only $780/7201 \simeq 0.11$ of the initial population or a reduction in population size of about 89% among the worst case scenarios of the epidemic. On the other hand, the initial size of the male population was 6601 in Figure 12.16.4, and at epoch 1200, the value of the Min trajectory was 1909, which in fractional terms is about $1909/6601 = 0.29$ of the initial population or a reduction in population size of about 71% among the worst case scenarios of the epidemic. However, among the most benign cases of the epidemic, as represented by the Max trajectory in Figure 12.16.4, the value of Max at epoch 1200 (6716) is greater than the initial population size of 6601. Similarly, the values Max at epoch 1200 in Figure 12.15.3 was 7328, which was also greater than the initial value of 7201.

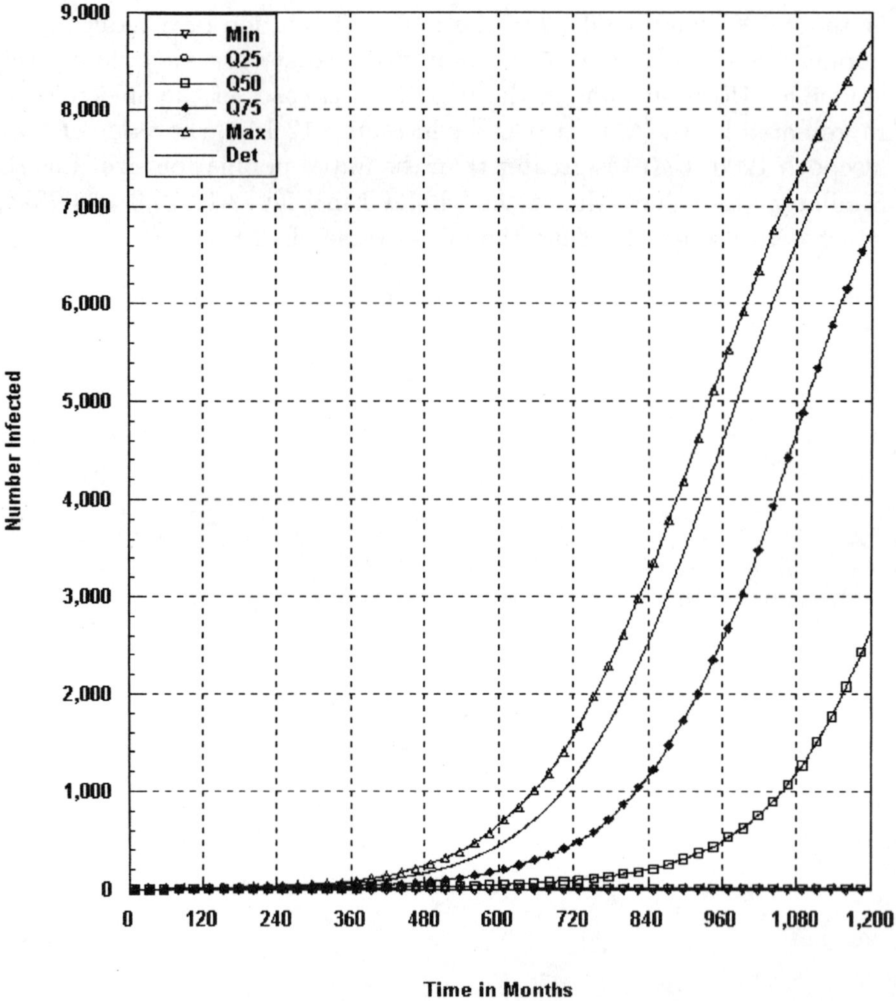

Figure 12.16.2. Cumulative Number of Infected Males in Couples.

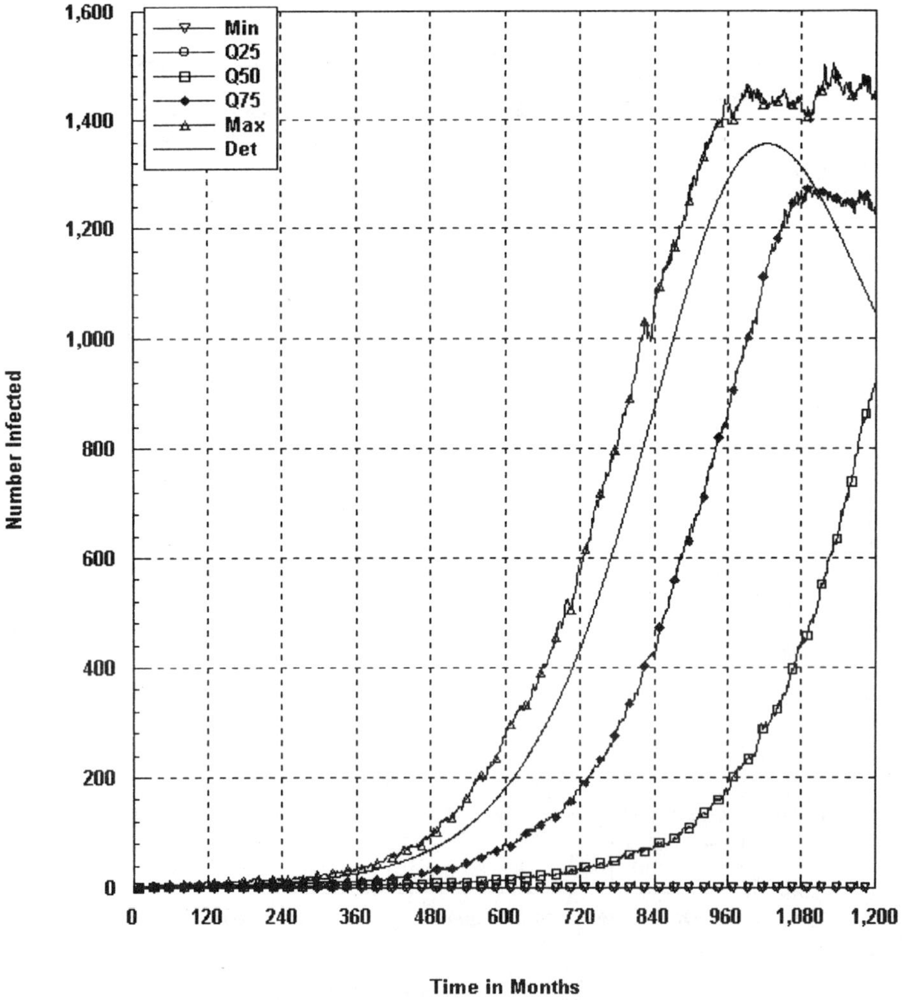

Figure 12.16.3. Number of Infected Males in Couples by Epoch.

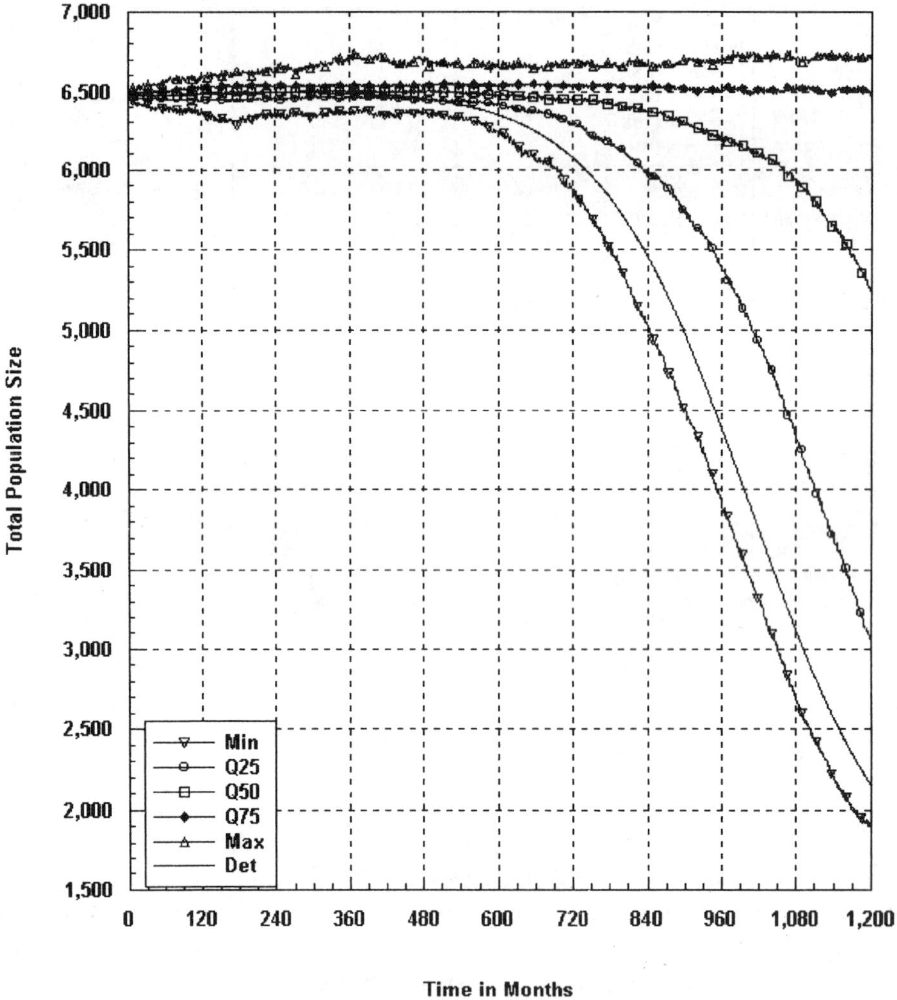

Figure 12.16.4. Total Population Size for Males by Epoch.

12.17 Highly Active Anti-Retroviral Therapy of HIV/AIDS

During recent years, a number of drugs, such as protease inhibitors, have been developed to treat people infected with HIV. Among the recent papers in the literature dealing with the impact of these drugs on patients infected with HIV are those of Buchbinder et al.,[2] Aboulafia[1] and Detels et al.[4] The treatment regimens administered to patients with HIV disease, which usually consists of combinations of drugs, are frequently referred to as highly active anti-retroviral therapy (HAART). In those patients who respond favorably to HAART, the effect is to reconstitute the immune system by reducing the viral load in their bodies, as measured by an increasing $CD4^+$ counts as opposed to decreasing counts in those patients who progressed to an AIDS-defining disease prior to the time anti-retroviral drugs were available. As the $CD4^+$ counts rise, a patient's immune system is better able to fight opportunistic infections that might otherwise be fatal. From the perspective of the models considered in this and other chapters, to accommodate those people who respond to HAART, the possibility that patients may move among stages of the disease needs to be taken into account, which may be accounted for in the structure of the 4×4 matrices $\boldsymbol{\Gamma}_f$ and $\boldsymbol{\Gamma}_m$ in the four-stage model under consideration (see Section 12.3 for details).

As in Section 12.16, it will be assumed for the sake of simplicity that the rates of transition among stages of disease are the same for females and males. And, to further simplify the presentation, it will be assumed that if γ_{fij} is the rate of transition from stage i to j, then the rate of transition from state j to i is γ_{fji}. Thus, if it is also supposed that the rates used in Section 12.16 continue to apply, then the matrix of latent risks for transitions among stages of HIV disease for females takes the form,

$$\boldsymbol{\Gamma}_f = \begin{bmatrix} 0 & 1/12 & 0 & 0 \\ 1/12 & 0 & 1/52.62 & 0 \\ 0 & 1/52.62 & 0 & 1/62.89 \\ 0 & 0 & 1/62.89 & 0 \end{bmatrix}. \tag{12.17.1}$$

From an inspection of this matrix, it can also be assumed that, during a small time interval, the only possible change in stage of disease is to a "neighboring" stage. This assumption seems reasonable, because one would not expect patients under HAART to respond instantaneously.

Another caveat to keep in mind, when interpreting the results of the computer experiments reported in this section, is that the rates in Eq. (12.17.1) are for a monthly time scale and are based on data for patients who progressed to an AIDS-defining disease without the benefit of anti-retroviral drugs. In reality, the reconstitution of the immune system under HAART may actually progress more rapidly than indicated by the reverse rates γ_{fji} in the matrix $\mathbf{\Gamma}_f$. However, given the present state of development of anti-retroviral drugs, HAART has not been observed to free a patient's body of HIV. In fact, HIV has returned to detectable levels in all patients for which HAART has been discontinued. Thus, the assumption implicit in the structure of the matrix $\mathbf{\Gamma}_f$, that no transition from a stage of disease to the disease-free state E_0 is possible, seems realistic.

To provide a basis for comparing the projections of epidemics for the experiments reported in this section with those reported in Section 12.16, a decision was made to use the initial conditions as well as the other values of parameters presented in Table 12.16.1 and elsewhere in that section. In other words, the computer input used for the experiments reported in this section differed from that used in Section 12.16 only with respect to the γ-parameters in the matrices $\mathbf{\Gamma}_f$ and $\mathbf{\Gamma}_m$. Moreover, as in Section 12.16, 100 Monte Carlo realizations of the process were computed with the length of each projection 1200 months or 100 years. One of the most noticeable effects of allowing transitions among stages of disease as determined by the matrix in Eq. (12.17.1) was that the estimated probability that an epidemic would eventually become extinct was 0.08 as compared to 0.27 in the experiments reported in Section 12.16. Evidently, with all other parameters and initial conditions held constant, the effect of allowing transitions among stages of disease was to increase the average length of the infectious period for each infective so that during their longer life spans an infectious person was at risk of infecting more susceptibles.

As in previous sections, the cumulative numbers of new infections were computed for various components of the population to gain some insight into the number of secondary cases produced by initial infectives. The Min, Q25, Q50, Q75, Max and Det trajectories of the cumulative number of infected males in couples are presented in Figure 12.17.1. When compared with the graphs of these trajectories presented in Figure 12.16.2, it can be seen that there were many more secondary infectives in the projections reported in this section than in Section 12.16. For example, in the worst cases of the epidemic as reflected by the Max trajectory at 1200 months, a cumulative total of 10904 males in couples had been infected as compared with 8718 cases in Figure 12.16.2. The differences between the Q25 trajectories in Figures 12.17.2 and 12.16.2 are even more striking. For example, at 1200 months in Figure 12.16.2, the value of the Q25 trajectory was only 8, due to an extinction probability of about 0.27; whereas that for the corresponding Q25 in Figure 12.17.1 was 8163, which reflects a lower probability of extinction.

From the perspective of administering health care to infected individuals, it is of interest to compute the number of persons infected in each component of the population by epoch (month) in a sample of Monte Carlo projections. Figure 12.17.2 contains the graphs of the Min, Q25, Q50, Q75, Max and Det trajectories of the number of infected males in couples by epoch. To gain some insights into the effects of allowing transitions among stages of disease, the graphs of these trajectories should be compared with those in Figure 12.16.3, especially for those realizations of the process in which the epidemic did not become extinct.

Unlike the projections summarized in Figure 12.16.3, where there was little evidence that the epidemic would peak until about 100 years into the projections, it appears from an inspection of the Q25, Q50 and Q75 trajectories in Figure 12.17.2 that the peak of the epidemic would be reached at some point in the time interval 900 to 1020 months or between 75 and 85 years. Interestingly, among the consequences of allowing transitions among stages of the disease is that an epidemic would develop at a slightly faster pace as compared to those cases in which disease stage transitions were allowed in one direction only (as in Section 12.16).

To complete the comparisons of the projections in this section with those presented in Section 12.16, Figure 12.17.3 contains the graphs of the Min, Q25, Q50, Q75, Max and Det trajectories for the total size of the male population. Comparing the graphs of these trajectories with those in Figure 12.16.4, an epidemic can have a greater impact on population size due to more deaths from disease when transitions among stages of disease are allowed rather than in one direction only. To illustrate the difference, it is of interest to compare the values of the Min, Q25, Q50, Q75 and Max trajectories for the two cases at 1200 months. When transitions disease stage transitions were allowed in only one direction as in Section 12.16, the values of these trajectories were Min 1909, Q25 3059, Q50 5234, Q75 6505 and Max 7716 (see Figure 12.16.4).

But, as can be seen from Figure 12.17.3, when transitions were allowed among stages, then these values were Min 1644, Q25 1851, Q50 2050, Q75 2613 and Max 6610. These comparisons among the two cases presented in Sections 12.16 and 12.17 illustrate that even though a disease can be treated effectively, these treatments may actually result in more people being infected unless measures are also taken to prevent infections. In conclusion, from an another inspection of the graphs of the Det trajectories in Figures 12.17.1, 12.17.2 and 12.17.3, it can be seen that if an investigator based his or her projections of an epidemic solely on the embedded deteministic model, there would be a tendency to project only the worst case scenario, as was the case for the projections presented in Section 12.16.

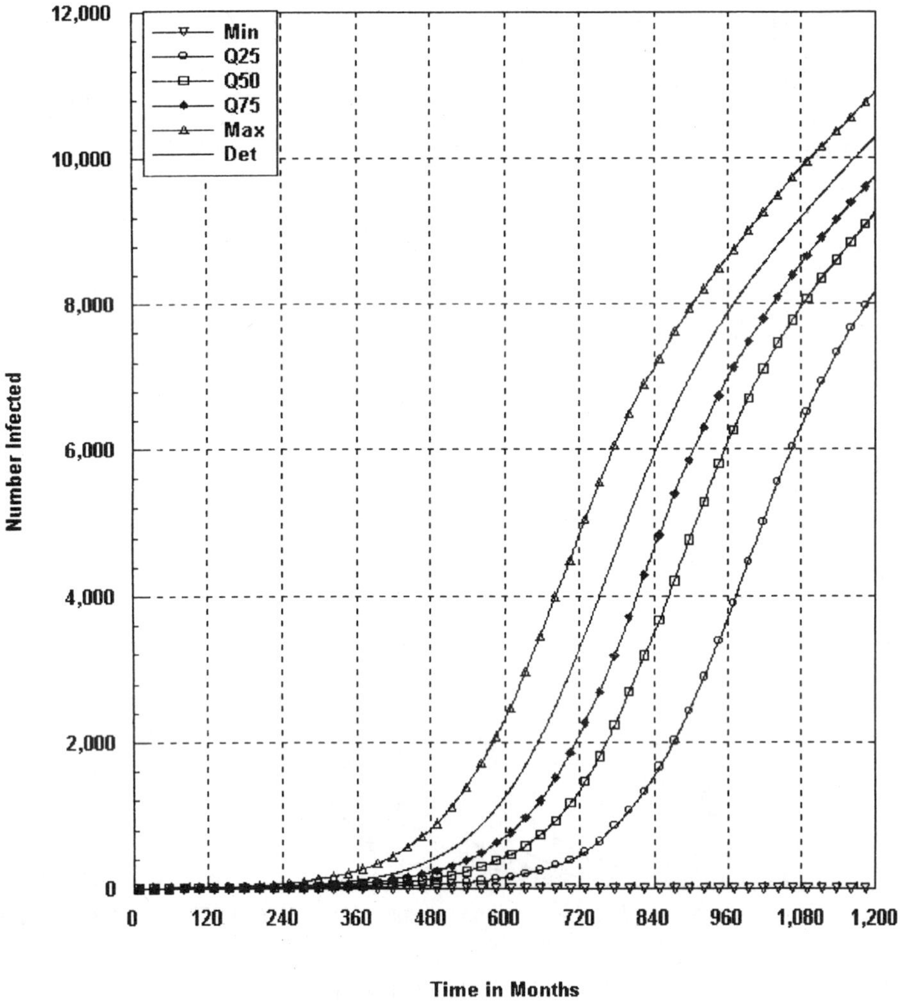

Figure 12.17.1. Cumulative Number of Infected Males in Couples.

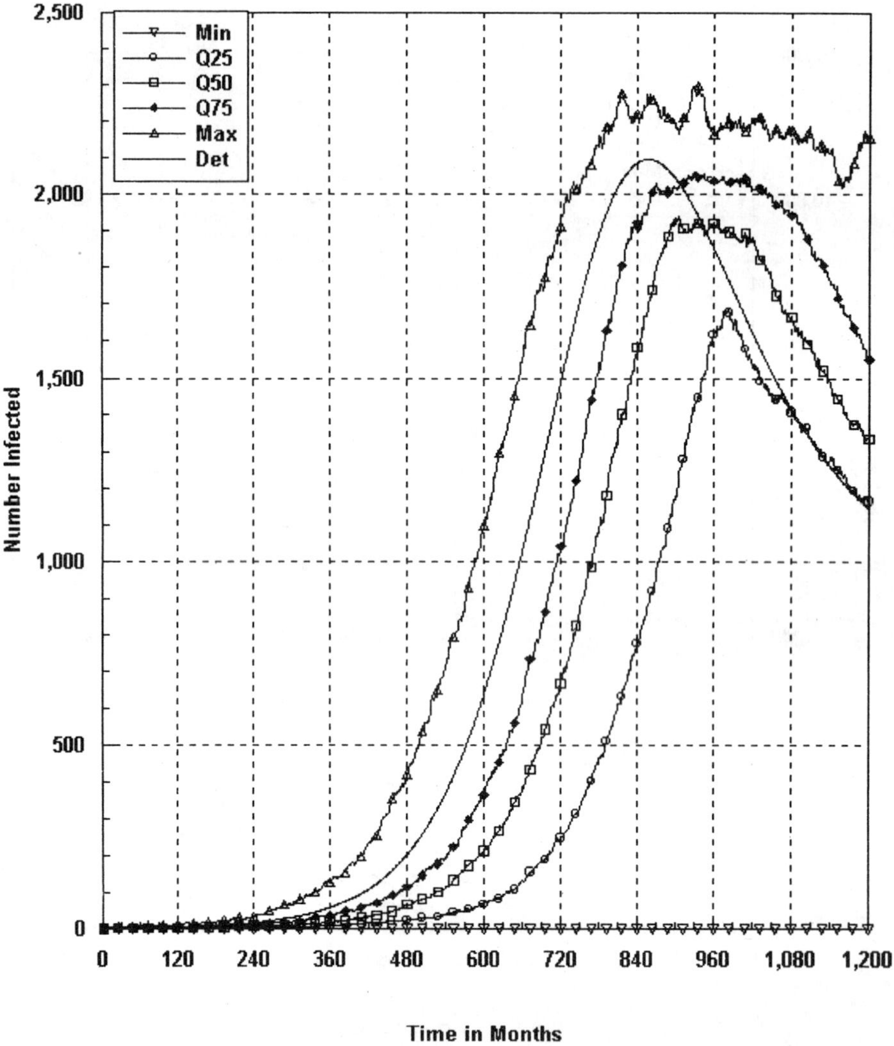

Figure 12.17.2. Number of Infected Males in Couples by Epoch.

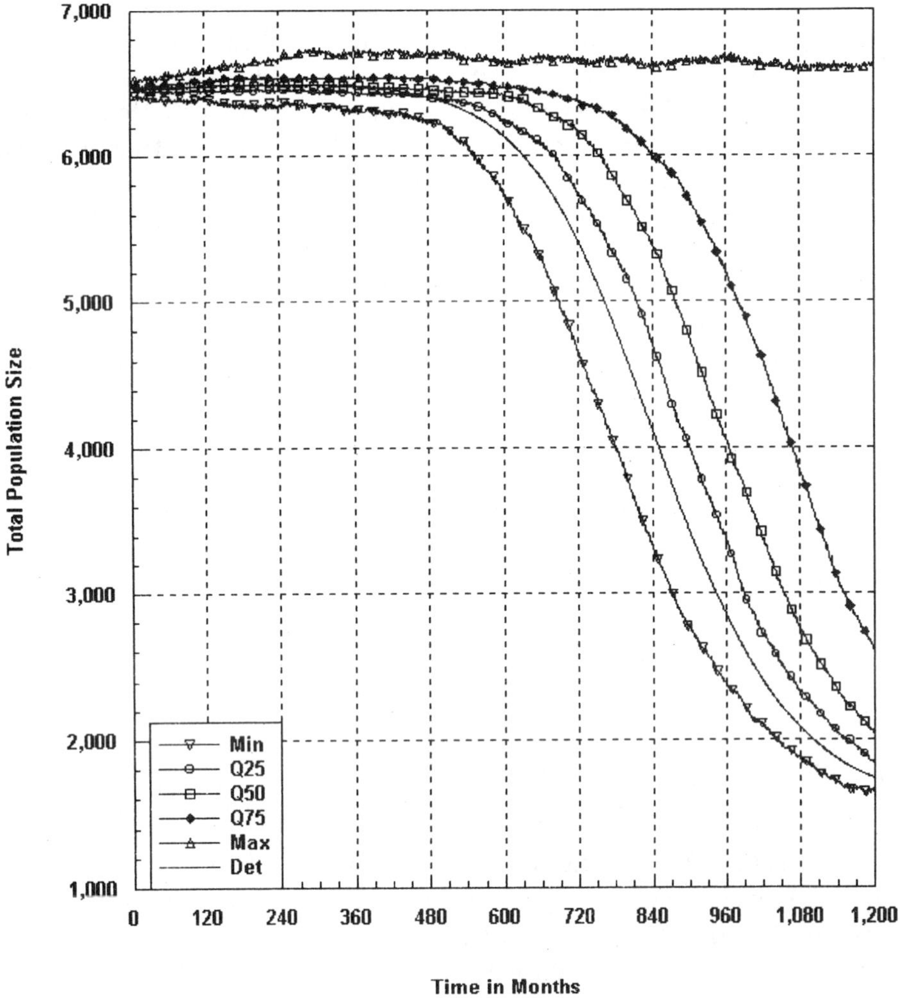

Figure 12.17.3. Total Population Size for Males by Epoch.

12.18 Epidemics of HIV/AIDS Among Senior Citizens

Infections of HIV among older heterosexual adults, which occur in some retirement communities, has been described by Whipple and Walsh[16] as the overlooked epidemic. Catina et al.[3] have documented risks of HIV transmission among the elderly; while Stall and Catina[15] have discussed risk behaviors for AIDS among late middle-aged and elderly Americans. Because HIV/AIDS epidemics among senior citizens in retirement communities is of concern to public health authorities, the computer input used to project HIV/AIDS epidemics in an elderly population will be described for a version of the two-sex model with $m = 2$ behavioral classes and $n = 1$ stage of disease in this section. Because persons of age 60 or more years may not live long enough to experience an incubation period of 15 or more years, a decision was made to use a $n = 1$ stage version of the model rather than a four-stage model as in Section 12.17.

Table 12.18.1. Parameters Affecting Risks of Infection.

$(\lambda_{f1}, \lambda_{f2}) = (0, 4)$
$(\lambda_{m1}, \lambda_{m2}) = (0, 4)$
$\boldsymbol{\eta}_f = (0, 1)$
$\boldsymbol{\eta}_m = (0, 1)$
$\gamma_{mc} = 8$
$\mathbf{p}_{fmar} = (0.98, 0.95)$
$\mathbf{p}_{fem} = (0.97, 0.94)$
$\mathbf{p}_{mmar} = (0.99, 0.97)$
$\mathbf{p}_{mem} = (0.98, 0.96)$

Table 12.18.1 contains the chosen values of the parameters affecting risks of being infected by either marital or extra-marital sexual contacts. In the first two rows, the expected numbers of extra-marital sexual partners per month are given for females and males. For example, the assignment $(\lambda_{f1}, \lambda_{f2}) = (0, 4)$ in the first row indicates that females in class 1 are monogamous in that the expected number of extra-marital sexual partners per month is $\lambda_{f1} = 0$; whereas, those in class 2 are highly active sexually in that they have an expected number of $\lambda_{f2} = 4$ extra-martial sexual partners per month. Identical remarks

apply to the parameter assignments $(\lambda_{m1}, \lambda_{m2}) = (0, 4)$ for males in the second row of Table 12.18.1. The vectors in the third and fourth rows represent the expected number of contacts per month per extra-martial sexual partner. For the case of the vector $\boldsymbol{\eta}_f = (0, 1)$, the value of $\eta_{f1} = 0$ is not meaningful from a substantive point of view because females in class 1 are monogamous, but some assigned value is required for the software to function properly. For females in class 2, the assignment $\eta_{f2} = 1$ indicates that highly active females have an expected number of $1 + \eta_{f2} = 2$ per extra-marital sexual partner per month. The same remark applies to the vector $\boldsymbol{\eta}_m = (0, 1)$ for males in the fourth row of Table 12.18.1. The parameter assignment $\gamma_{mc} = 8$ indicates that on average a marital couple has 8 sexual contacts per month.

It seems plausible to assume that a susceptible female has a higher probability of being infected per sexual contact with an infected male than that for a susceptible male when his female partner is infected. The rationale underlying this assumption is that a discharge of semen from an infected male into the vagina of a susceptible female may contain a higher concentration of infectious virus particles than a susceptible male may encounter on the vaginal walls of an infected female. The values in the vectors of escape probabilities in rows 6 through 9 of Table 12.18.1 have been chosen to reflect this assumption. For example, the vector $\mathbf{p}_{fmar} = (0.98, 0.95)$ of marital escape probabilities by behavioral class for females indicates that the probabilities that a susceptible female is infected $\mathbf{q}_{fmar} = \mathbf{1} - \mathbf{p}_{fmar} = (0.02, 0.05)$ per sexual contact with her infected male partner are higher than the corresponding probabilities for susceptible males $\mathbf{q}_{mmar} = \mathbf{1} - \mathbf{p}_{mmar} = (0.01, 0.03)$ (see rows 6 and 8 of Table 12.18.1). The same remarks apply to the vectors of escape probabilities $\mathbf{p}_{fem} = (0.97, 0.94)$ and $\mathbf{p}_{mem} = (0.98, 0.96)$ for extra-marital sexual contacts in rows 7 and 9 of Table 12.18.1.

Table 12.18.2. Parameters for Mortality, Marital Couple Formation-Dissolution, Extra-Marital Partnership Selection and Recruits.

$(\mu_{f0}, \mu_{f2}) = (1/240, 1/30)$
$(\mu_{m0}, \mu_{m2}) = (1/180, 1/30)$
$\beta_{fem1} = \beta_{fem2} = 1$
$\beta_{mem1} = \beta_{mem2} = 1$
$\beta_{f1} = \beta_{f2} = 1$
$\beta_{m1} = \beta_{m2} = 1$
$\rho = 1/12$
$\delta = 1/24$
$\mu_f = 5$
$\mu_m = 5$
$\varphi_f = (0.75, 0, 0.25, 0)$
$\varphi_m = (0.80, 0, 0.20, 0)$

The chosen values of the parameters for rates of mortality and rates of couple formation-dissolution as well as the values of β-parameters determining acceptance probabilities for selection of marital and extra-marital sexual partners and those of the parameters governing the entrance of female and male recruits into the population during any time interval are presented in Table 12.18.2. Note that it has been assumed that the age of female recruits entering the community is about 60 years. Thus, in row 1 of Table 12.18.2, the parameter assignments $(\mu_{f0}, \mu_{f1}) = (1/240, 1/30)$ indicate, by assumption, that the expectation of life remaining for a susceptible female recruit is $1/\mu_{f1} = 240$ months or 20 years, but after she is infected her latent expectation of life remaining is $1/\mu_{f2} = 30$ months or 2.5 years. According to the parameter assignments in row 2 of Table 12.18.2, the corresponding expectations of life for males are $1/\mu_{m1} = 180$ months or $180/12 = 15$ years and $1/\mu_{m2} = 30$ months or 2.5 years. Displayed in rows 3 and 4 of Table 12.18.2 are the values assigned to the β-parameters determining the acceptance probabilities for choices of extra-marital sexual partners for females and males, respectively. In rows 6 and 7 of Table 12.18.2 the corresponding values of the β-parameters for determining acceptance probabilities for choices of marital partners are displayed. If a reader is interested in the values of the acceptance probabilities determined by these parameter assignments, Eq. (11.16.1) may be consulted.

Rows 7 and 8 of Table 12.18.2 contain the assigned parameter values for the rates of couple formation and dissolution. Thus, according to row 7, the latent expected waiting time among marital partnerships is $1/\rho = 12$ months or one year, and expected duration of a marital partnership is $1/\delta = 24$ months or two years. The expected number of female and male recruits entering the community each month is $\mu_f = \mu_m = 5$ according to rows 9 and 10 of Table 12.18.2. Furthermore, according to the recruit probability vectors in rows 11 and 12 of Table 12.18.2, a female recruit is monogamous with probability 0.75 and the corresponding probability for males is 0.80. This assignment of probabilities was based on the plausible assumption that, on average, elderly females enjoy better health than elderly males, so that 80% of the males were assumed to be monogamous; while only 75% of the females were assumed to be monogamous. The monthly rates of transitions among the monogamous and highly sexually active behavioral classes were assumed to be low for both females and males as displayed by the rates in the matrices,

$$\boldsymbol{\Psi}_f = \boldsymbol{\Psi}_m = \begin{bmatrix} 0 & 1/1200 \\ 1/120 & 0 \end{bmatrix}. \tag{12.18.1}$$

It should be emphasized that, although the assigned values of the parameters just discussed are plausible, the values displayed above are actually hypothetical and should be viewed as part of an exercise in documenting the computer input used in an illustrative application of the model and software. For future applications of the model and software discussed in this section, it is recommended that an investigator search the voluminous HIV/AIDS literature for information pertaining to the parameters described above. In this connection, the use of the internet could greatly expedite the search for titles of relevant papers. Given assignments of parameters values such as those listed above, it is possible to calculate a stationary vector $\widehat{\mathbf{v}}$ of the embedded differential equations for the case where a population contains only susceptibles.

For the case of $m = 2$ behavioral classes and $n = 1$ stage of disease, the vector is 8×1 and has the partitioned form,

$$\widehat{\mathbf{v}} = \begin{pmatrix} \widehat{\mathbf{x}} \\ \widehat{\mathbf{y}} \\ \widehat{\mathbf{z}} \end{pmatrix}, \tag{12.18.2}$$

where

$$\widehat{\mathbf{x}} = \begin{pmatrix} \widehat{x}_1 \\ \widehat{x}_2 \end{pmatrix} \tag{12.18.3}$$

is a 2×1 vector of numbers of individuals in a stationary population for the two types of single females, $\widehat{\mathbf{y}}$ is a 2×1 similar vector for single males, and

$$\widehat{\mathbf{z}} = \begin{pmatrix} \widehat{z}_{11} \\ \widehat{z}_{12} \\ \widehat{z}_{21} \\ \widehat{z}_{22} \end{pmatrix} \tag{12.18.4}$$

is a 4×1 vector, whose elements are the numbers of couples of each type in the set of four couple types for the case a population contains only susceptibles.

By using a recursive numerical procedure similar to that described in Section 11.11, it can be shown that when this procedure was applied to the difference equation version of the embedded differential equations of this model and rounded to the nearest integer, the numerical values for the stationary vectors just described were:

$$\widehat{\mathbf{x}} = \begin{pmatrix} 572 \\ 75 \end{pmatrix}, \tag{12.18.5}$$

$$\widehat{\mathbf{y}} = \begin{pmatrix} 278 \\ 69 \end{pmatrix}, \tag{12.18.6}$$

$$\widehat{\mathbf{z}} = \begin{pmatrix} 432 \\ 27 \\ 71 \\ 23 \end{pmatrix}. \tag{12.18.7}$$

As an exercise, it is of interest to compare a theoretical estimate of the size of the female population at equilibrium with that determined by calculating the stationary vector. If the theory for the simpler one-sex and two-sex partnership models developed in Sections 11.11 and 12.10 hold for the two-sex model of this section, then a good guess for the size of the female population at equilibrium is the rate of female recruitment μ_f per unit time multiplied by $1/\mu_{f0}$, the expectation of life remaining after entering the population. For the parameter assignments used in this section, this value is $5 \times 240 = 1200$. But, according to the values in the vectors $\widehat{\mathbf{x}}$ and $\widehat{\mathbf{z}}$, the size of the female population size at equilibrium is:

$$572 + 75 + 432 + 27 + 71 + 23 = 1200 , \tag{12.18.8}$$

which matches the theoretical estimate exactly. For the case of males, the vectors $\widehat{\mathbf{y}}$ and $\widehat{\mathbf{z}}$ yield the value,

$$278 + 69 + 432 + 27 + 71 + 23 = 900 \tag{12.18.9}$$

for total population size at equilibrium. The theoretical number in this case is $\mu_m \times (1/\mu_{m0}) = 5 \times 180 = 900$, which again matches that in Eq. (12.18.9). These numerical results suggest that there is a theorem containing symbolic expressions for the theoretical sizes of the female and male populations at equilibrium, but it will left as an exercise for the reader to state and prove this theorem.

Just as in Section 11.16, it is of interest to test for the parameter assignments used in this section, whether the reduced 8×8 matrix $\mathbf{A}_S$ as well as the full 24×24 matrix $\mathbf{A}$ are stable to determine whether the initial conditions will wear off as $t \uparrow \infty$. For the set of parameter values under consideration, it was found that both these matrices were stable. Again, as a test of whether the software contains errors, it is also of interest to test whether the 8×8 Jacobian matrix,

$$\mathbf{J}_S(\widehat{\mathbf{v}}) = \mathbf{A}_S + \mathbf{J}_{CFS}(\widehat{\mathbf{v}}) \tag{12.18.10}$$

for the reduced system of differential equation is stable as expected when evaluated at the stationary vector $\widehat{\mathbf{v}}$.

If this matrix was not stable for the case where a population contains only susceptibles, then a software error would be suspected. It was found that for the parameter values under consideration this matrix was stable as expected, indicating that the software passed the test. A final step in finding an indicator as to whether an epidemic may develop when a few infectives are introduced into a population of susceptibles that has been evolving for a long period of time is to test the stability of the full 28×28 Jacobian matrix,

$$\mathbf{J}(\widehat{\mathbf{v}}) = \mathbf{A} + \mathbf{J}_{EM}(\widehat{\mathbf{v}}) + \mathbf{J}_{CF}(\widehat{\mathbf{v}}) \tag{12.18.11}$$

evaluated at the stationary vector $\widehat{\mathbf{v}}$. For the set of parameter values under consideration in this section, it was found that this matrix was not stable, suggesting that an epidemic may develop if a few infectives were introduced into a population of susceptibles. In the remaining sections of this chapter, the results of computer experiments designed to test the extent to which an HIV/AIDS epidemic may develop in a community of elderly females and males will be presented.

12.19 Invasions of Infectives for Elderly Heterosexuals

For the case of $m = 2$ behavioral classes and $n = 1$ stage of disease, there are four types of females and four types of males. For females, these types will be denoted by $\tau_{f1} = (1,0)$, $\tau_{f2} = (1,1)$, $\tau_{f3} = (2,0)$, and $\tau_{f4} = (2,1)$. The four types of males, τ_{m1}, τ_{m2}, τ_{m3}, and τ_{m4} are defined similarly. In this notation, sexually-active females and males are of types τ_{f4} and τ_{m4}, respectively. Table 12.19.1 contains descriptions of four invasion thresholds of infective and highly sexually-active single females and males into a community of elderly heterosexuals, which were used in computer experiments to compare the impact of each of these four thresholds of infectives, given the parameter values and initial numbers of susceptibles described in Section 12.18. It was also assumed that, following the invasions of the initial infectives, no infective recruits entered the population. Throughout all the experiments reported in this section, 100 Monte Carlo realizations of the process were computed for each invasion threshold and the length of each projection was 720 months or 60 years.

According the invasion threshold Initial 1, the initial population contained one infected highly sexually-active single male; whereas, in threshold Initial 2, it was assumed that the initial population contained one single female and one single male, who were both infected and highly sexually-active. In the invasion thresholds Initial 3 and Initial 4, the infectives in the initial population consisted of 2 and 10, respectively, of highly sexually-active individuals of each sex.

Table 12.19.1. Four Invasion Thresholds of Highly Sexually Active Single Females and Males for a Community of the Elderly.

Initial 1	$Y(0;\tau_{m4}) = 1$
Initial 2	$X(0;\tau_{f4}) = 1, Y(0;\tau_{m4}) = 1$
Initial 3	$X(0;\tau_{f4}) = 2, Y(0;\tau_{m4}) = 2$
Initial 4	$X(0;\tau_{f4}) = 10, Y(0;\tau_{m4}) = 10$

The graphs of the trajectories for each of these invasion thresholds for the probabilities of extinction by epoch in the set of four Monte Carlo projections with sample sizes of 100 are presented in Figure 12.19.1.

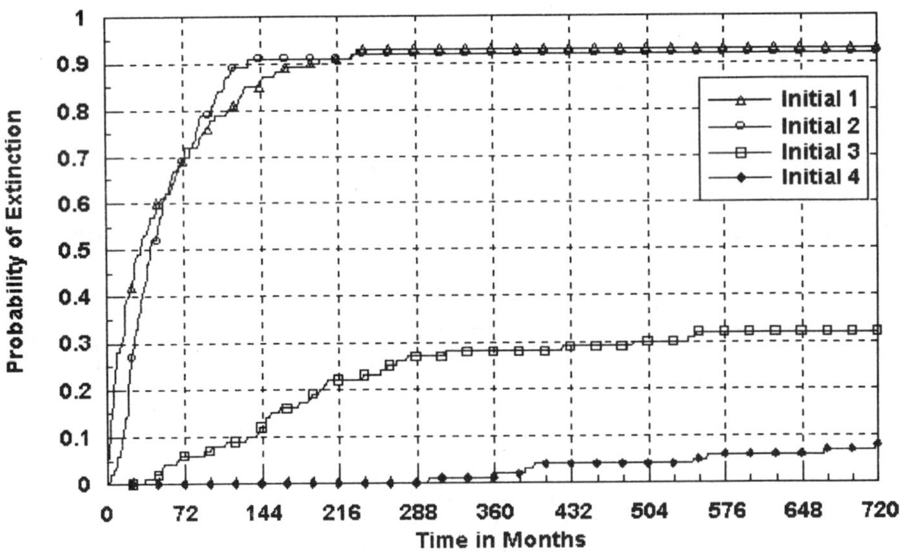

Figure 12.19.1. Probabilities of Extinction of the Epidemics by Epoch for Each of the Four Invasion Thresholds.

Inspecting these graphs, for invasion thresholds Initial 1 and Initial 2, the estimated probabilities of extinction of an epidemic within 60 years were high, i.e., 0.93 and 0.92, respectively. In both cases, convergence to these probabilities was rather rapid. But for Initial 3, the probability of extinction within 60 years, fell to 0.32, with convergence to this number being slower than for Initial 1 and 2. However, the probability of extinction of the epidemic within 60 years fell to 0.08 and convergence to this number appeared to be very slow for Initial 4. Thus, from these experiments one reaches the conclusion that with invasion thresholds of infectives in the neighborhood of either Initial 3 or Initial 4, there is a high probability that a major HIV/AIDS epidemic would be develop in the experimental community of elderly heterosexuals under consideration.

Even though the probability of extinction within 60 years may be high, as was the case for the invasion thresholds Initial 1 and Initial 2, rather severe epidemics may occur in some realizations of the process. On the other hand, when the probability of extinction is low, which was the case in the invasion threshold Initial 4, in some realizations of the process, relatively few individuals may be infected. To illustrate this variation among realizations of the process, the values of the Min, Q25, Q50, Q75, Max and Det trajectories at the epoch of 760 months for the cumulative numbers of infected monogamous females in couples are shown in Table 12.19.2.

Tables 12.19.2. Quantiles of Cumulative Numbers of Infected Monogamous Females in Couples at the Epoch of 720 Months.

Threshold	Initial 1	Initial 2	Initial 3	Initial 4
Min	0	0	0	79
Q25	0	0	15	279
Q50	0	0	276	302
Q75	1	1	304	322
Max	296	332	382	464
Det	345.04	349.77	370.64	380.17

From Table 12.19.2, it can be seen that the cumulative numbers of monogamous females that would be infected during a 60-year time span would be less than or equal to one for invasion thresholds Initial 1 and Initial 2 with an estimated probability of 0.75. However, according to the Max trajectory, as many as 296 and 332 females in this behavioral class would be infected with these invasion thresholds in the worst cases of the epidemic. With regard to invasion thresholds Initial 3 and Initial 4, note that the values of the median trajectory Q50 were 276 and 302, respectively. Thus, even though the probability of extinction of 0.32 within 60 years was considerably higher for Initial 3 than for Initial 4, the severity of the epidemic for Initial 3 would be nearly as great as that for Initial 4 with probability 0.5. As in the other examples of this chapter, the Det trajectory tends to overestimate the cumulative numbers of persons infected by the end of a projection.

The information in Table 12.19.2 provides some insight into the total numbers of persons that may be infected during a 60-year time span, but, from the point of view of providing health care for infected individuals, it is of interest to consider the numbers of persons infected at each epoch in a sample of projections. Figures 12.19.2 and 12.19.3 contain, respectively, the graphs of the Min, Q25, Q50, Q75, Max and Det trajectories for monogamous and highly sexually-active females in couples by epoch for the case of invasion threshold Initial 4. The corresponding graphs for males are presented in Figures 12.19.4 and 12.19.5. In terms of total population size of the community, relatively few infected persons may need care at any epoch. For, unlike the numbers presented in Table 12.19.2, the numbers of infected person displayed in these figures are in the low one and two digits, indicating that at any epoch there would be relatively few infected individuals who may need care. Is also interesting to note that, although the percentage of highly sexually-active individuals in the population at any time was in the range of about 15% to 25% of the total population, the numbers of infective individuals in this class exceeded the number of infectives in the monogamous class at some epochs, which was the majority of the population throughout the projections.

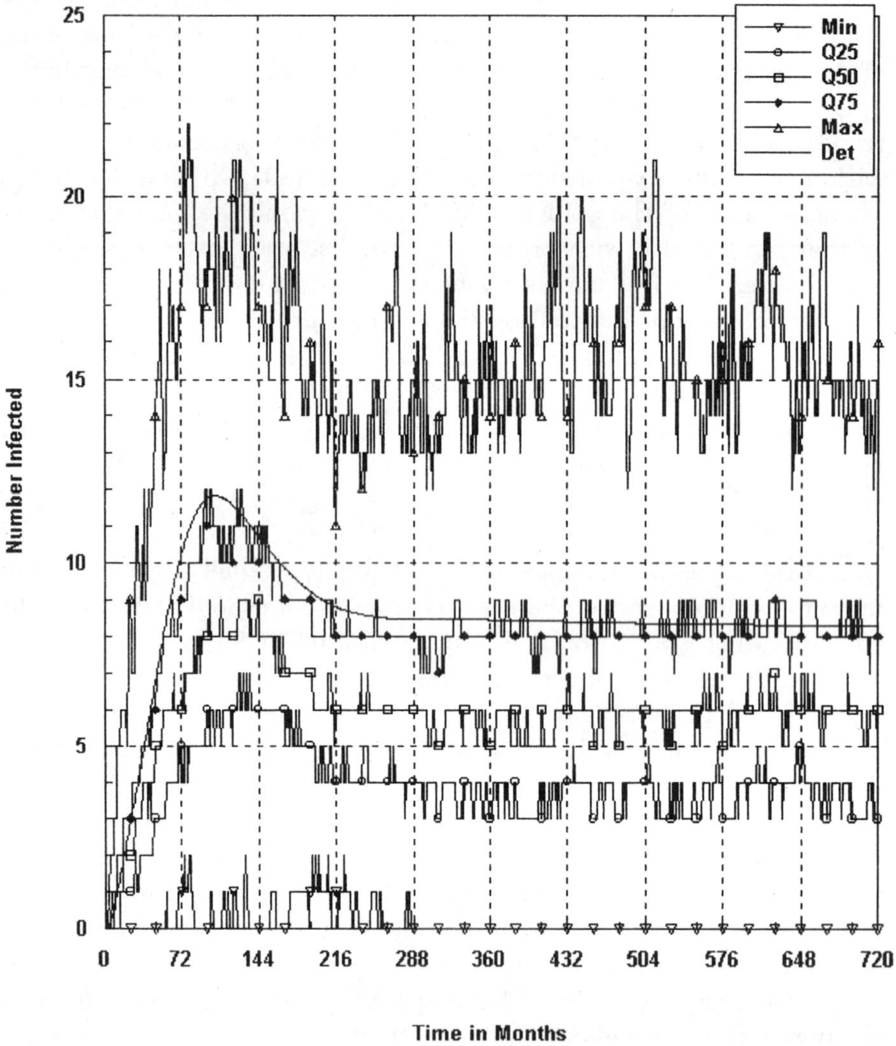

Figure 12.19.2. Number of Infected Monogamous Females in Couples by Epoch - Initial 4.

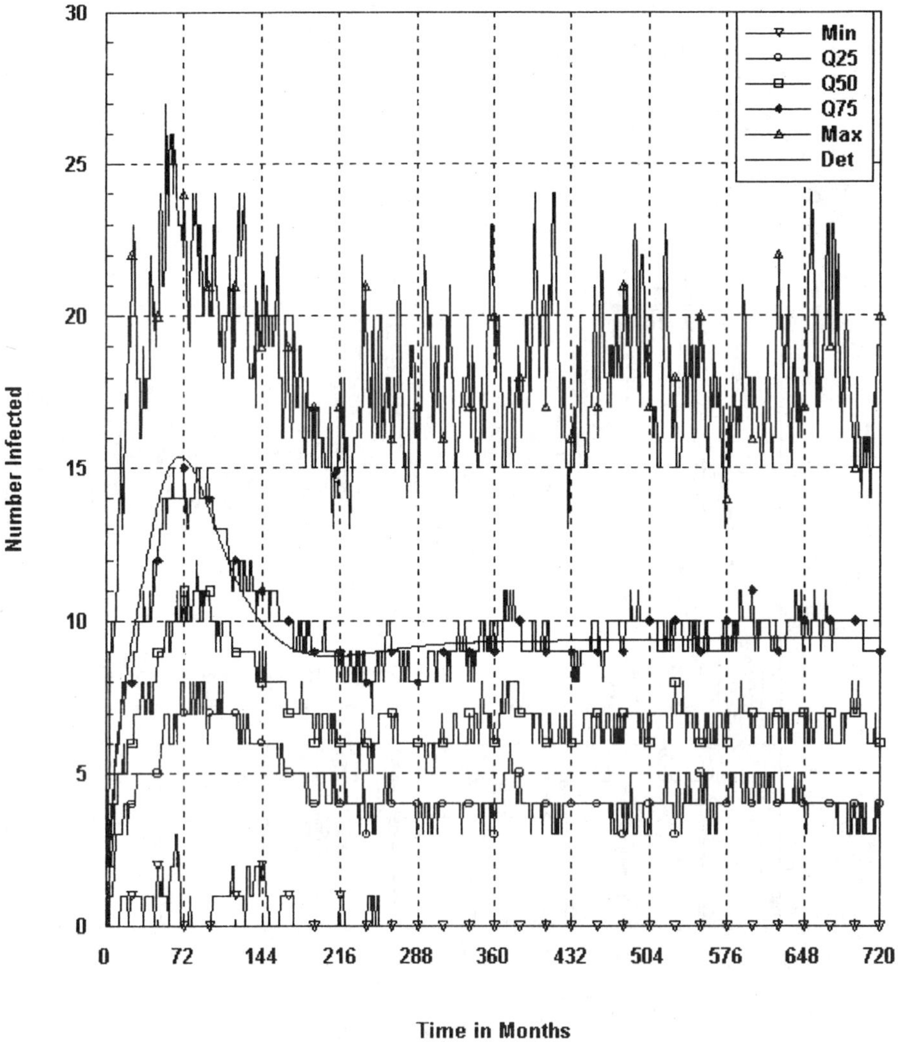

Figure 12.19.3. Number of Infected Highly Sexually Active Females in Couples by Epoch - Initial 4.

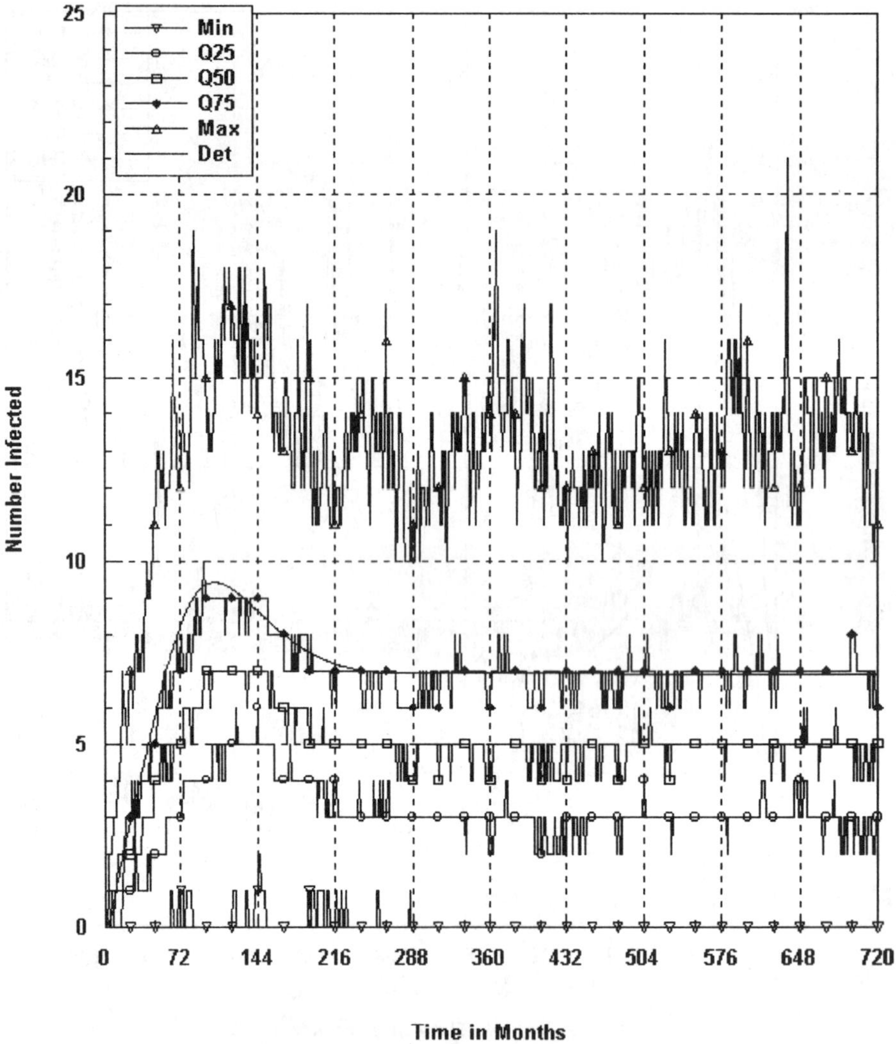

Figure 12.19.4. Number of Infected Monogamous Males in Couples by Epoch - Initial 4.

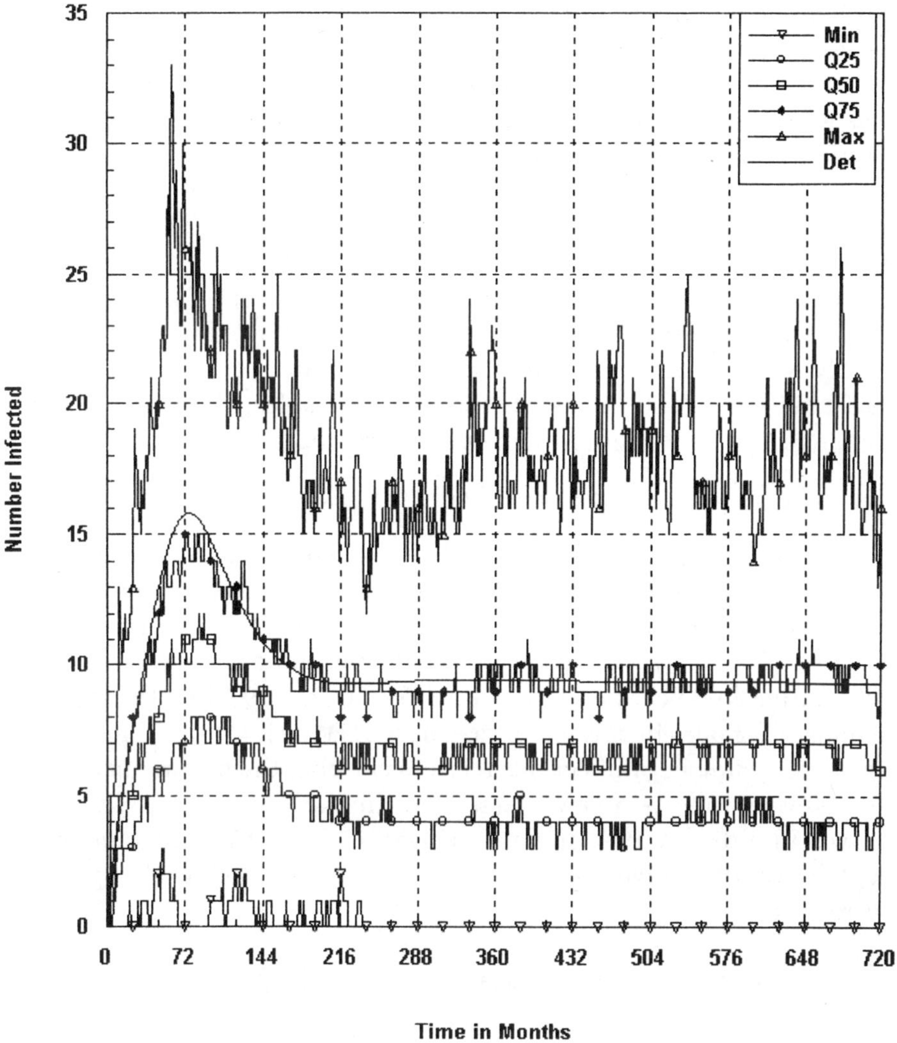

Figure 12.19.5. Number of Infected Highly Sexually Active Males in Couples by Epoch - Initial 4.

12.20 Recurrent Invasions of Infectious Recruits

The invasion thresholds considered in Section 12.19 may not be realistic for some communities of the elderly, because infectious recruits may enter the population with a positive probability during any time interval. In the computer experiments reported in this section, such a scenario was studied by supposing that all the parameter values described in Section 12.18 continued to be in force, the initial population contained no infectious individuals, but infectious recruits could enter the community with fixed probabilities during any time interval. The probability vectors for female and males recruits that were used in the experiments reported in this section are displayed in Table 12.20.1. Note that these vectors were derived from those in Table 12.18.2 by supposing that the highly sexually-active female and male recruits were infected with a probability of 1/100. Thus, for the case of females, the fourth element of the recruit vector $\boldsymbol{\varphi}_f$ was computed according to the formula

$$\varphi_{f4} = 0.25/100 = 0.0025 . \tag{12.20.1}$$

As in Section 12.19, 100 Monte Carlo realizations of the process were computed for 720 months or 60 years. According to the assigned values of the probabilities φ_{f4} and φ_{m4} in Table 12.120.1, the expected number of highly sexually-active female recruits entering the community during a 60-year period was $720 \times 5 \times 0.0025 = 9.0$ and the expected number for males in this class was $702 \times 5 \times 0.002 = 7.02$. Thus, on average, the number of infectious recruits entering the community during the 60-year time period was less than in the Initial 4 threshold displayed in Table 12.19.1, in which it was assumed that the numbers of highly sexually-active single females and males in the initial population were each 10.

Table 12.20.1. Probability Vectors for Female and Male Recruits.

Females	$\boldsymbol{\varphi}_f = (0.75, 0, 0.2475, 0.0025)$
Males	$\boldsymbol{\varphi}_m = (0.80, 0, 0.198, 0.002)$

Given the recruit probability vectors in Table 12.20.1, one would guess that at 720 months, in a sample of 100 Monte Carlo realizations of an epidemic, the community would contain no infectives in some number of these realizations. This was, in fact, the case, for in 21 out of a sample of 100 realizations. It is thus of interest to present some information on the variability among epidemics that developed in the remaining 79 realizations of the process. A useful way to view the variability in the sample of 100 realizations of the process is to display selected quantiles of the cumulative number of individuals infected within 60 years by behavioral class and sex. Displayed in Table 12.20.2 are selected quantiles and extreme values of the cumulative numbers of monogamous individuals in couples that were infected during the 60-year time span.

Table 12.20.2. Quantiles of Cumulative Numbers of Infected Monogamous Individuals in Couples at 720 Months.

Sex	Female	Male
Min	0	0
Q25	3	2
Q50	28	22
Q75	180	109
Max	303	200
Det	333.95	219.83

From Table 12.20.2, it can be seen that a "mild" epidemic would occur in the community in that only about 28 and 22 monogamous females and males, respectively, would be infected during the 60-year time span while they were members of a marital couple, with a probability of about 0.5. But, in the worst case of the epidemic, as represented by the upper extreme Max, as many as 303 females and 200 males in this classification may be infected in the 60-year time span. As in other sections, the values of the Det trajectory at 720 months exceeded those of the Max for both sexes.

Table 12.20.3 contains the quantiles and extreme values for the cumulative numbers of infected, highly sexually-active individuals in couples at 720 months. It is interesting to note that even though this high-risk behavioral class was only 15% to 25% of the population of couples, values of the summary statistics in Table 12.20.3 often exceed those in Table 12.20.2, indicating that a high-risk minority were, in some realizations of the process, contracting more infections than those in the majority lower-risk monogamous class.

Table 12.20.3. Quantiles of Cumulative Numbers of Infected Highly Sexually-Active Individuals in Couples at 720 Months.

Sex	Female	Male
Min	0	0
Q25	3	3
Q50	49	38
Q75	186	197
Max	326	353
Det	359.54	358.95

By definition, monogamous individuals have sexual contacts only with their martial partners, and thus no females or males were infected in the projections while they were members of the singles population. However, highly sexually-active females and males may experience sexual contacts while they are members of the singles population and thus may be infected.

Table 12.20.4. Quantiles of Cumulative Numbers of Infected Highly Sexually-Active Single Individuals at 720 Months.

Sex	Female	Male
Min	0	0
Q25	4	1
Q50	60	20
Q75	304	131
Max	566	246
Det	586.87	274.78

Displayed in Table 12.20.4 are the selected quantiles and extreme values for the cumulative numbers of infected, highly sexually-active individuals at 720 months while they were members of the singles population. As can be seen from these summary statistics, within a 60-year time span, substantial numbers of females and males may be infected while they are members of the singles population. Indeed, the numbers in this table are close to those in Tables 12.20.2 and 12.20.3. Curiously, in Tables 12.20.2 and 12.20.4, the values of Q75, Max and Det for males are considerably less than those for females, which may be a reflection of higher basic mortality rates and lower probabilities of infection per contact for males than for females.

Although the measures of variability displayed in the above tables, regarding the total size of an epidemic that may develop by behavioral class and sex during a 60-year time span, are of interest, it is perhaps of greater interest to graphically display measures of the variability in the numbers of persons infected at each epoch of a projection by behavioral class and sex. Figure 12.20.1 contains the graphs of the Q75, Max and Det trajectories for monogamous females and males in couples, depicting the numbers of persons infected at each epoch of the projections. As indicated in the figure, the graphs for females and males are in the upper panel and lower panels, respectively. Because the values of the Min, Q25 and Q50 trajectories were either small or zero throughout most of the projections, their graphs were not included. The corresponding graphs of the Q75, Max and Det trajectories of the numbers of infected highly sexually-active individuals in couples are displayed in Figure 12.20.2. From these graphs, it can be seen that at most epochs in the projections, the values of the Q75 trajectory were less than 10. Thus, at any epoch of the projections, 10 or fewer individuals would be infected among either monogenous or highly sexually-active females and males while they were members of couples, with a probability of about 0.75. But, among the worst cases of the epidemic, as indicated by the Max trajectory, the number of infected persons in couples would be in the range 10 to 20 for each sex and behavioral class after about 120 months or 10 years into the projections.

Although susceptible monogamous females and males cannot be infected while as members of the singles population, some single females and males in this class may be infected at any epoch in a projection due to infections acquired previously while they were members of couples. Figure 12.20.3 contains the graphs of the Q75, Max and Det trajectories of the numbers of monogamous single females and males at each epoch in the projections. Similarly, the graphs of the Q75, Max and Det trajectories for highly active single females and males are presented in Figure 12.20.4. Interestingly, according to these projections, the numbers of single females infected at any epoch were, for the most part, greater than those in couples in the most severe cases of the epidemic. For example, the Max trajectory for single monogamous females was in the range 20 to 30 at many epochs after about 120 months into the projections (see the upper panel in Figure 12.20.3); whereas, for highly sexually-active single females displayed in Figure 12.20.4, the Max trajectory was often in the range of 30 to 50 after about 120 months into the projections. The Max trajectory for single monogamous males was usually smaller, however, and was often in the range of 10 to 15 infected individuals after 120 months, which was close to that for infected males in couples. On the other hand, for highly sexually-active single males, the Max trajectory was often in the range of 20 to 30 infected individuals after 120 months into the projections.

These projections suggest that in the worst cases of HIV/AIDS epidemics in communities of the elderly, a majority of the infected females would belong to the singles population at any time. For the case of infected males at most epochs in the projections, the numbers of infected males among singles and couples would tend to be more equal. That a majority of infected females belonged to the singles population at most epochs in the projections considered in this section was attributable to two assumptions underlying the projections. One of these assumptions was that the probability of a susceptible female being infected per sexual contact with an infectious male was assumed to be higher than the corresponding probability for susceptible males. A second assumption was that, on average, females lived longer than males so that following the deaths of their male marital partners, they would return to the singles population.

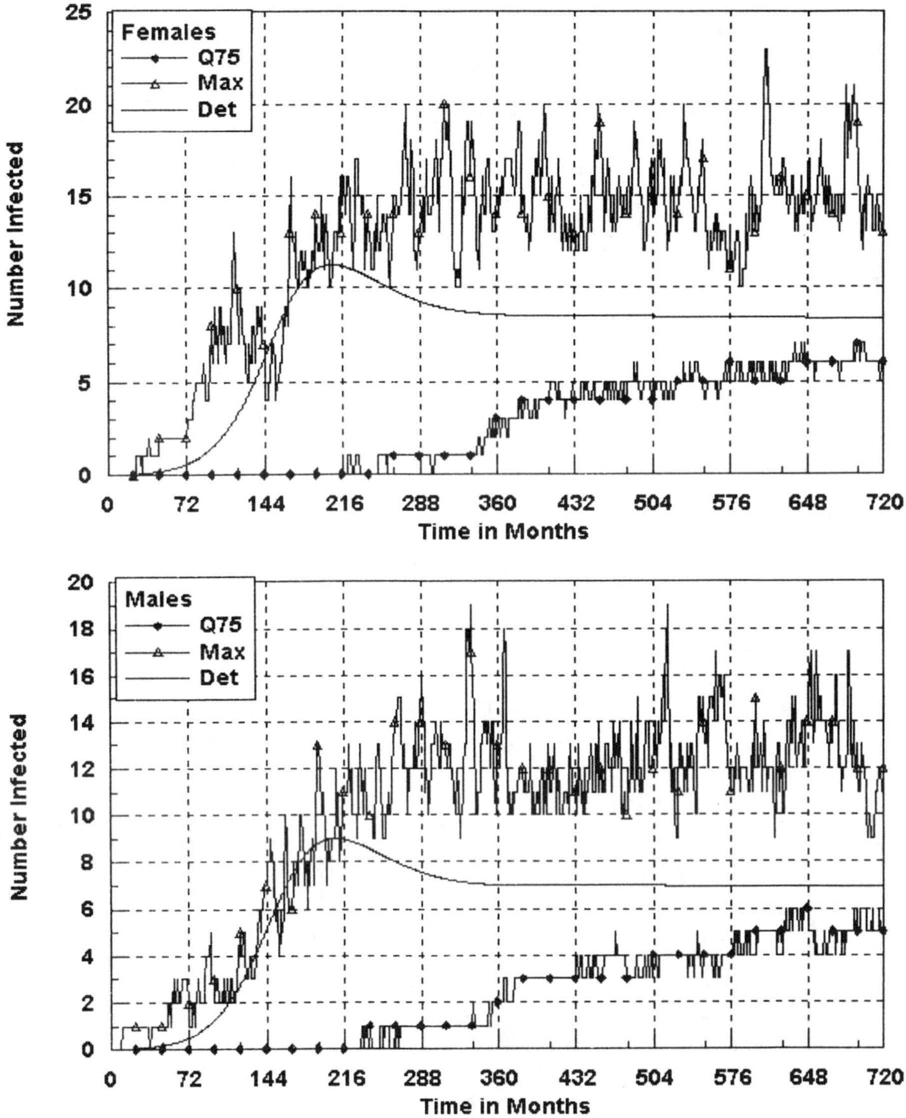

Figure 12.20.1. Quantiles of Numbers of Infected Monogamous Individuals in Couples by Epoch.

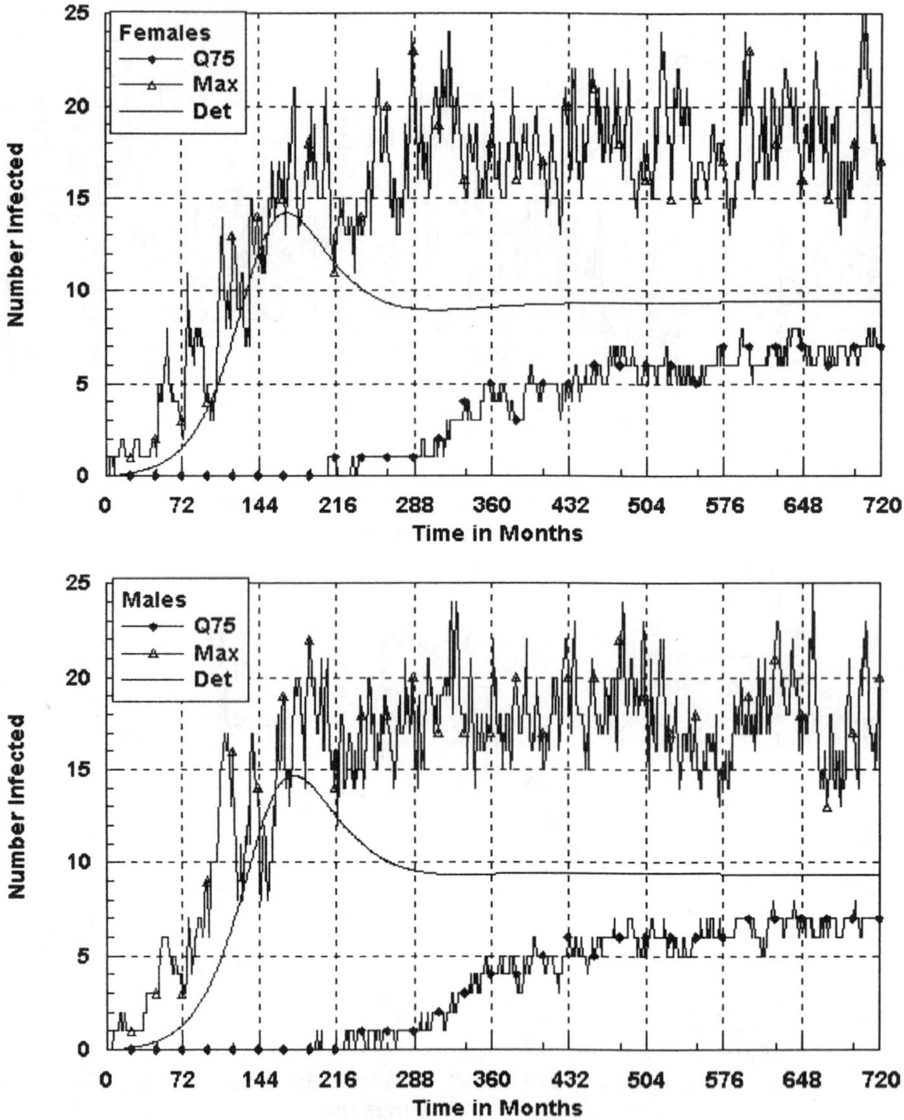

Figure 12.20.2. Quantiles of Numbers of Infected Highly Sexually Active Individuals in Couples by Epoch.

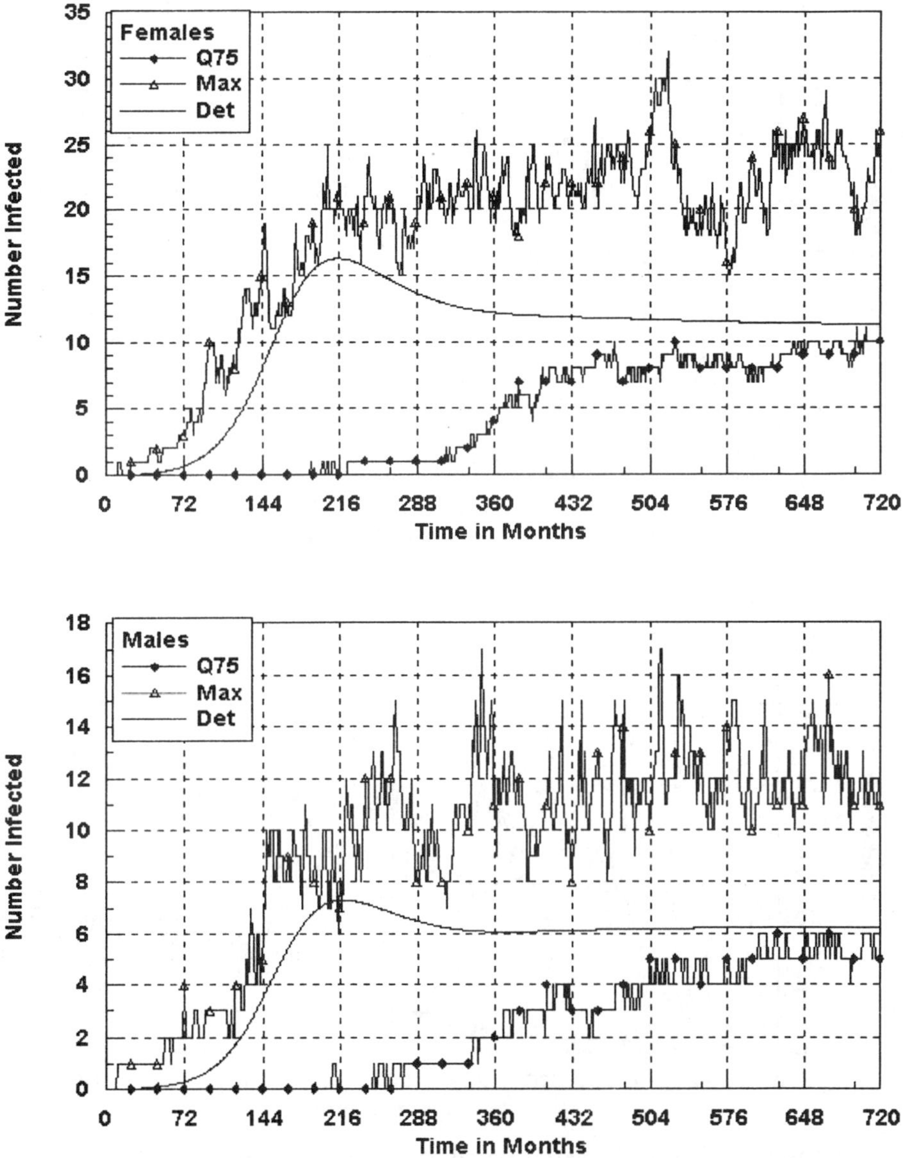

Figure 12.20.3. Quantiles of Numbers of Infected Monogamous Individuals in Singles Population by Epoch.

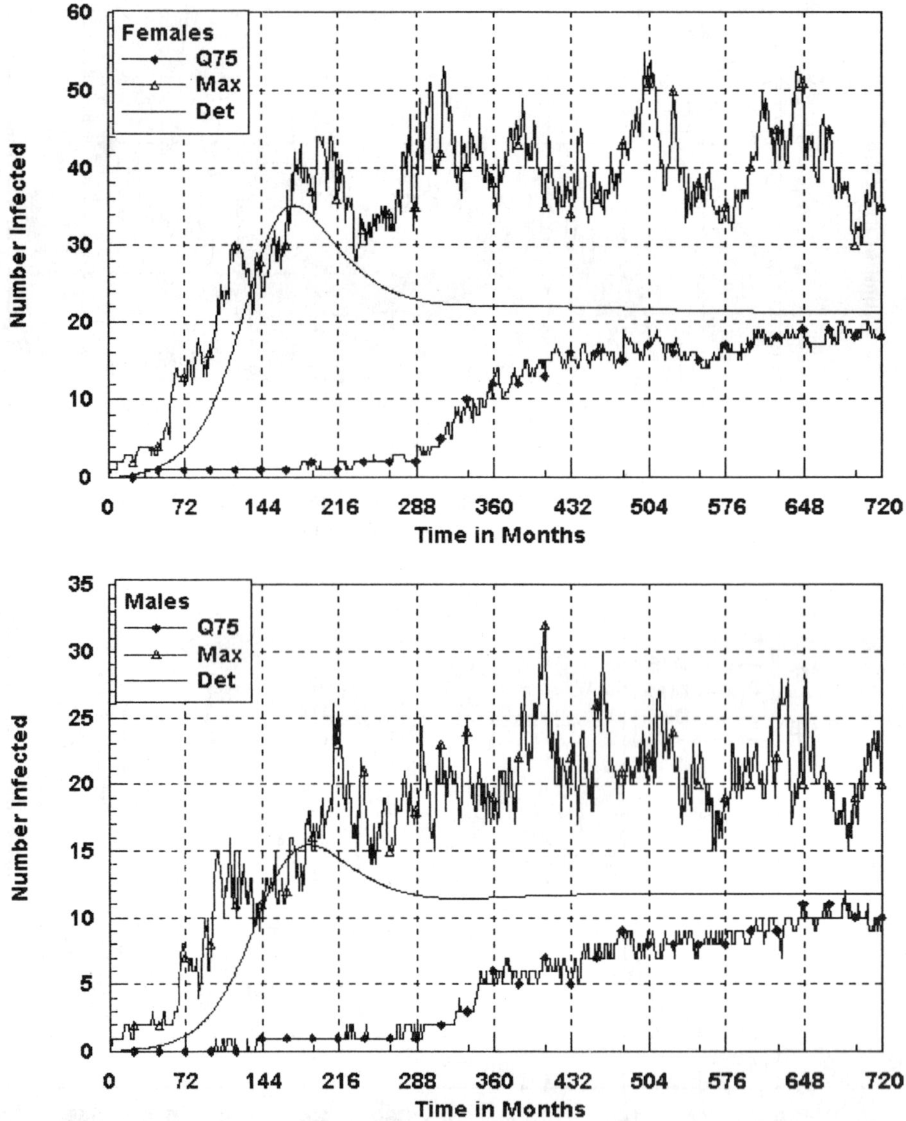

Figure 12.20.4. Quantiles of Numbers of Infected Highly Sexually Active Individuals in Singles Population by Epoch.

12.21 References

1. D. M. Aboulafia, Regression of Acquired Immunodeficient Syndrome-Related Pulmonary Kaposi's Sarcoma After Highly Active Antiretroviral Therapy, *Mayo Clinic Proceedings* **73:** 439-443, 1998.
2. S. P. Buchbinder, S. D. Holmberg, S. Scheer, G. Colfax, P. O'Maley and E. Vittinghoff, Combination Antiviral Therapy and Incidence of AIDS-Related Malignancies, *Journal of Acquired Immune Deficiency Syndromes and Human Retrovirology* **21:** S23-S26, Supplement 1, 1999.
3. J. A. Catina, H. Turner, et al. Older Americans and AIDS: Transmission Risks and Primary Research Needs, *The Gerontological Society of America* **29:** 373-381, 1989.
4. R. Detels, A. Munoz, G. McFarland, L. A. Kingsley, J. B. Margolick, J. Giorgi, L. K. Schrager and J. P. Phair, Effectiveness of Potent Antiviral Therapy on Time to AIDS and Death in Men with Known HIV Infection Duration, *Journal of the American Medical Association* **280:** 1497-1503, 1998.
5. M. D. Grmek with R. C. Maulitz and J. Duffin (translators), *History of AIDS - Emergence and Origin of a Modern Pandemic,* Princeton University Press, Princeton, New Jersey, 1990.
6. J. A. Jacquez, J. S. Koopman, C. P. Simon and I. M. Longini, Jr., Role of the Primary Infection in Epidemics of HIV Infection in Gay Cohorts, *Journal of Acquired Immune Deficiency Syndromes* **7:** 1169-1184, 1994.
7. I. M. Longini, Jr. et al., Modeling the Decline of CD4+ T-Lymphocyte Counts in HIV-Infected Individuals: A Markov Modeling Approach, *Journal of Acquired Immune Deficiency Syndromes* **4:** 1141-1147, 1991.
8. C. J. Mode, A Stochastic Model for the Development of an AIDS Epidemic in a Heterosexual Population, *Mathematical Biosciences* **107:** 491-520, 1991.
9. C. J. Mode, Threshold Parameters for a Simple Stochastic Partnership Model of Sexually Transmitted Diseases Formulated as a Two-Type CMJ-Process, *IMA Journal of Mathematics Applied in Medicine and Biology* **14:** 251-260, 1997.
10. C. J. Mode, Threshold Parameters for Stochastic Heterosexual Partnership Models of HIV/AIDS Formulated within Multitype CMJ-Processes, *Series in Mathematical Biology and Medicine* **6:** 383-405, O. Arino, D. Axelrod and M. Kimmel (eds.), *Advances in Mathematical Population Dynamics - Molecules, Cells and Man,* World Scientific Publishing Company, Singapore, New Jersey, London, Hong Kong,

1997.

11. C. J. Mode and C. K. Sleeman, A New Design of Stochastic Partnership Models for Epidemics of Sexually Transmitted Diseases with Stages, *Mathematical Biosciences* **156:** 95-122, 1999.

12. C. K. Sleeman and C. J. Mode, A Computer Exploration of Some Properties of Nonlinear Stochastic Partnership Models for Sexually Transmitted Diseases with Stages, *Mathematical Biosciences* **156:** 123-145, 1999.

13. C. K. Sleeman and C. J. Mode, On Fitting a Nonlinear Stochastic Model of a HIV/AIDS Epidemic to Public Health Data for the City of Philadelphia, *Series in Mathematical Biology and Medicine* **6:** 453-476, O. Arino, D. Axelrod and M. Kimmel (eds.), *Advances in Mathematical Population Dynamics - Molecules, Cells and Man,* World Scientific Publishing Company, Singapore, New Jersey, London, Hong Kong, 1997.

14. C. K. Sleeman and C. J. Mode, A Methodological Study on Fitting a Nonlinear Stochastic Model of the AIDS Epidemic in Philadelphia, *Mathematical and Computer Modelling* **26:** 33-51, 1997.

15. R. Stall and J. Catina, AIDS Risk Behaviors Among Late Middle-Aged and Elderly Americans, *Archives of Internal Medicine* **154:** 57-63, 1994.

16. B. Whipple and K. Walsh, The Overlooked Epidemic: HIV in Older Adults, *American Journal of Nursing* **96:** 23-28, 1996.

Chapter 13
AGE-DEPENDENT STOCHASTIC MODELS WITH PARTNERSHIPS

13.1 Introduction

When making decisions as to how to approach the construction of stochastic models accommodating the formation and dissolution of partnerships in human populations, it is natural to structure them based on some classification of individuals. For example, in the one-sex model considered in Chapter 11, individuals were classified by behavioral class and stage of disease, but in the two-sex model considered in Chapter 12, this classification was extended to include sex, behavioral class, and stage of disease. The objective of this chapter is to take initial steps towards extending this latter classification to include age. In computer simulation experiments, one is often interested in the evolution of an epidemic following the introduction of a few infectives into a population of susceptibles. As a first step toward reaching this objective, attention will be focused on a demographic component, i.e., a stochastic formulation that accommodates age as well as partnership formation and dissolution, but not the presence of infectious individuals. The second step will be to extend the formulation to include a component that accommodates infectives in the population.

At the outset, it should be mentioned that there is a rather extensive literature on demographic, age-dependent partnership models that belong to the deteministic paradigm. No attempt will be made to review this deteministic literature here, but the interested reader may consult a selected list of references contained in the recent paper by Martcheva.[5] Like much of the literature on deterministic age-dependent two-sex models, the formulation in this paper was based on a version of the McKendrick-von Foerster partial differential equations, and attention was focused on the existence of an eventual exponential equilibrium growth rate for an age-structured two-sex population.

However, as has been seen in the computer simulation experiments reported in Chapters 10-12, decades or even centuries may elapse before equilibrium is reached in the real world. Consequently, implementations of computer models with capabilities for accommodating transient behavior prior to reaching equilibrium are of fundamental importance in studying the evolution of epidemics. Indeed, as is often the case when studying evolutionary phenomena by computer intensive methods, the transient behavior of the model prior to reaching equilibrium, if it does exist, is often of more interest than its behavior following the attainment of equilibrium. It is, of course, recognized that in the deterministic literature there are a number of papers on the numerical integration of age-dependent partial differential equations belonging to the McKendrick-von Foerster class. Two recent contributions to this literature are the papers by Abia and Lopez-Marcos,[1] and Angulo and Lopez-Marcos.[2] But, because such numerical methods cannot accommodate the stochastic variability that is characteristic of most biological phenomena, they will not be considered in this chapter.

As the title of this chapter indicates, the primary focus of attention will be on the formulation and implementation of age-dependent stochastic models of sexually transmitted diseases in heterosexual populations with partnerships. In surveying the literature on mathematical models of epidemics, very few references on such age-dependent models can be found, particularly as they relate to the international HIV/AIDS epidemic. Among these rare references is the Ph.D. dissertation of Salsburg[14] on the formulation and implementation of a two-sex, age-dependent stochastic model designed to explore the evolution of an HIV/AIDS epidemic in a heterosexual population with three risk groups and behavioral classes for both females and males. Unlike the models described in Chapters 10-12, there were no provisions in the formulation for movement among behavioral classes which included females who were prostitutes, and males who repeatedly visited prostitutes.

There were two components in the model considered by Salsburg, whose implementation was predominantly an exercise in software engineering. At a higher level, there was an age-dependent demographic component, whose time unit of evolution was a year; then, at a lower level, there was an HIV/AIDS component, whose time unit of evolution was a month, for those individuals who were alive at the end of a year. This component, an extension of an earlier formulation (see Mode[7]), accommodated three risk groups for each sex. Such models, accommodating not only the age of an individual, but also behavioral classes and stages of disease, can give rise to high-dimensional arrays that are difficult to process, particularly when Monte Carlo realizations of the sample functions are computed. Consequently, only the embedded non-linear difference equations were implemented, because at that time, the desktop computers that were available had neither the memory nor the processor speed needed to carry out Monte Carlo simulation experiments within an acceptable period of time. Most of the scenarios studied by Salsburg[14] using the embedded non-linear difference equations assumed a small initial number of infected females and males. As has been illustrated by the examples in Chapters 10-12, if an investigator confines his or her attention to only the embedded deterministic model, the results can be quite misleading. The paper by Mode and Salsburg[13] may be consulted for some illustrative computer experiments using the embedded non-linear difference equations belonging to the demographic component of the model.

Subsequent to the completion of the work by Salsburg, the manufacturers of personal computers and the software industry made rapid progress in the development of desktop computers with respect to greater memory capacity, faster processor speed and improved user-friendliness. It thus became feasible to carry out Monte Carlo simulation experiments with two-sex HIV/AIDS models accommodating three behavioral classes for both sexes as reported in the Ph.D. thesis by Kamali.[4] Even though the desktop computers used by Kamali were more powerful than those used by Salsburg, they still lacked sufficient memory and the speed necessary to compute Monte Carlo realizations within an acceptable period of time for a stochastic model accommodating one-year age classes. Age was, therefore, not taken into account in the stochastic models considered by Kamali. Age classes could have been aggregated into five-year or even coarser aggregations so that the resultant arrays could be accommodated, but it was felt that the evolution of infections in a population might be obscured, since the status of individuals changed much more rapidly than the aging process. Moreover, it would certainly have complicated the numerical problems of dealing with two phenomena, the incidence of new infections and aging, that evolved on two different time scales. An example of a stochastic model of HIV infections in a homosexual population that accommodated not only a rather coarse aggregation of age classes, but also race is that of Tan and Xiang.[16]

An earlier non-published work by the authors addressed a non-age dependent stochastic model of an HIV/AIDS epidemic in a heterosexual population with one behavioral class. It was found that in projections of epidemics emanating from a few initial infective females and males, the trajectory of the embedded non-linear difference equations for the number of new infections in a population often departed significantly from the mean function calculated from a sample of Monte Carlo realizations of the process. Such departures were also observed in the computer experiments reported by Kamali with an extended form of the model that accommodated three behavioral classes for both sexes. In experiments with both the simple and more complex versions of the model, it was observed that such departures often depended significantly on the initial conditions chosen for a computer experiment. For example, if the initial conditions for a computer experiment were chosen as the state of the population following a long projection of 30 to 60 years, then this "irregular" behavior would tend to disappear in that the trajectory of the embedded deterministic model would be closer to that of the mean of a sample of Monte Carlo realizations of the process. As has been illustrated by the examples in Chapters 10-12, whether a stationary point consisting only of susceptibles in a population is stable or unstable for the embedded differential equations can be a useful indicator as to how trajectories of the stochastic model may behave.

When interpreting the results of computer experiments with a model, another question arises. To what extent has the design of the model influenced the observed results? For example, the design principles used in the models of Salsburg[14] and Kamali[4] differ from those discussed in Chapters 10-12 in that the concept of conditioning was used more frequently than that of competing risks. By way of illustrating these differences in design, consider the component of the model for the evolution of members of couples among stages of disease. In the designs used by Salsburg and Kamali, the probabilities for the evolution through the stages of disease by both members of a couple were conditioned on whether the partners did or did not separate during a time interval; whereas, in the designs set forth in Chapters 11 and 12, whether a couple separated during any time interval was only one of several competing risks in the matrix of latent risks governing the evolution of couples. Such design differences might appear inconsequential at first glance, but it can be shown by examples, which will not be presented here, that in some cases these differences can lead to quite different results. In numerical experiments, there might be differences with respect to the way the trajectory of the embedded deterministic model behaves in relation to a sample of Monte Carlo realizations of the process. As has been illustrated in Chapters 10-12, deterministic differential equations may be embedded in a stochastic model in a systematic way by judicious use of the concept of competing risks. The stability properties of these equations are useful indicators of how Monte Carlo realizations of a stochastic model may behave. Systematically applying design principles can be helpful not only in controlling errors during software development, but also in the comparison of the results of numerical experiments with different models. Consequently, the concept of competing risks will be used extensively in the design of the models in this chapter.

13.2 Parametric Models of Human Mortality

A question naturally arising is why study parametric models? Among the answers to this question is that one may use classical calculus and other mathematics to describe the model in a succinct form that may be communicated more easily among scientists than the encyclopedic numerical arrays commonly used in the study of human and animal mortality. As will be illustrated by examples, another advantage of parametric models is that their parameters often may be interpreted in meaningful biological and statistical terms. Furthermore, when a parametric model fits some data satisfactorily, then information may be moved among computers more easily than numerical forms of life tables when estimates of the parameters are available. The strategy used to develop a model for the entire life-span is to partition life-spans into three stages, infancy, mid-life and mature adulthood, and specify a latent risk function for each stage. To complete the model, a fourth latent risk function is added to accommodate accidents that may occur throughout life.

For many species of animals, infants are at high risk of death following hatching or birth, but as time passes the risk of death decreases. Therefore, the latent risk function for infant deaths will be assumed to have the exponential form,

$$\theta_0(x) = \alpha_0\beta_0 \exp\left[-\beta_0 x\right] \; , \tag{13.2.1}$$

where $x \geq 0$ and α_0 and β_0 are positive parameters. The integral of this latent risk function is:

$$H_0(x) = \int_0^x \theta_0(s)ds = \alpha_0\left(1 - \exp\left[-\beta_0 x\right]\right) \tag{13.2.2}$$

for $x \geq 0$, and, by definition, the latent survival function corresponding to this risk function is:

$$S_0(x) = \exp\left[-H_0(x)\right] \; . \tag{13.2.3}$$

In terms of this component of the model, the probability that an individual survives infancy is the limit,

$$\lim_{x\uparrow\infty} S_0(x) = S_0 = e^{-\alpha_0} \; . \tag{13.2.4}$$

Quite often an investigator will have some knowledge of the fraction S_0, which may be used to obtain an initial or trial estimate of α_0; namely $\alpha_0 = -\ln S_0$. Next observe that the term in parenthesis,

$$F_0(x) = 1 - \exp\left[-\beta_0 x\right] \tag{13.2.5}$$

in Eq. (13.2.2) is the distribution function of a random variable X_0 with expectation,

$$E[X_0] = \frac{1}{\beta_0} . \tag{13.2.6}$$

Thus, the parameter β_0 will determine the speed at which infant deaths occur. Small values of β_0 will correspond to longer infant survival times, while large values of β_0 will correspond to shorter survival times. Such ideas may be quantified by assigning trial values to $E[X_0]$ to find an estimate $\beta_0 = 1/E[X_0]$

Empirical risk functions for human mortality have been observed to have a mode somewhere between the ages of 20 and 35. For females, this mode may reflect risks due to childbearing, while for males this mode probably reflects more aggressiveness during these ages with the ensuing risk of death. These observations suggest the latent risk function for mid-life has the form,

$$\theta_1(x) = \alpha_1 f_1(x) , \tag{13.2.7}$$

where $f_1(x)$ is some probability density function with a mode that may be chosen for computational convenience. One such choice is the density for the log-normal distribution that has the formula,

$$f_1(x) = \frac{1}{\sqrt{2\pi}x\sigma} \exp\left[-\frac{1}{2}\left(\frac{\ln x - \mu}{\sigma}\right)^2\right] , \tag{13.2.8}$$

where $x > 0$, $\mu \in \mathbb{R}$ is a location parameter and $\sigma > 0$ is a scale parameter. One good reason for choosing the log-normal is that programs to numerically evaluate $\Phi(\cdot)$, the distribution function for a normal random variable with mean 0 and variance 1, are available in many software libraries. Moreover, it is easy to write programs to do these calculations.

For this density, the integral of the latent risk function takes the form,

$$H_1(x) = \int_0^x f_1(s)ds = \alpha_1 \Phi\left(\frac{\ln x - \mu}{\sigma}\right) , \tag{13.2.9}$$

where $\Phi(z)$ is the distribution function of a standard normal random variable. For this component of human mortality, the latent survival function is:

$$S_1(x) = \exp\left[-H_1(x)\right] \tag{13.2.10}$$

for $x > 0$. Unlike the infancy component of the model, in this case it is necessary to find trial values of three parameters α_1, μ and σ. Just as in the infancy component, the parameter α_1 may be determined from an estimate of the probability of surviving mid-life.

To connect the parameters μ and σ with more useful statistical interpretations, it can be shown that the mode of the log-normal density is:

$$m_1 = \exp\left[\mu - \sigma^2\right] . \tag{13.2.11}$$

And if X_1 is a log-normal random variable, then its expectation is:

$$E\left[X_1\right] = \mu_1 = \exp\left[\mu + \frac{\sigma^2}{2}\right] \tag{13.2.12}$$

Therefore, if some knowledge of m_1 is available, then by assigning a value of $\mu_1 > m_1$, the above equations may be solved for μ and σ. In fact, the solution is:

$$\sigma = \frac{1}{3}\sqrt{(6\ln\mu_1 - 6\ln m_1)}$$

$$\mu = \frac{1}{3}\ln m_1 + \frac{2}{3}\ln\mu_1 . \tag{13.2.13}$$

To accommodate accidents throughout the life-span, the latent risk function for this component will have the simple form $\theta_2(x) = \alpha_2$ for all $x \geq 0$, where α_2 is a positive constant. In this case, the integral of the risk function is:

$$H_2(x) = \int_0^x \theta_2(s)ds = \alpha_2 x \tag{13.2.14}$$

for $x \geq 0$. Therefore, for $x \geq 0$, the latent survival function has the simple form,

$$S_2(x) = \exp\left[-\alpha_2 x\right] . \tag{13.2.15}$$

A useful trial value of α_2, based on period studies of human mortality, is about 0.001. This component of the model is often referred to as the Makeham component.

A fourth two-parameter latent risk function, due to Gompertz circa the 19th century deals with risks of deaths at the older ages. Let α_3 and β_3 be positive parameters. Then, it will be assumed that for $x \geq 0$, the latent risk function $\theta_3(x)$ has the form,

$$\theta_3(x) = \alpha_3 \beta_3 \exp\left[\beta_3 x\right] . \tag{13.2.16}$$

Observe that, as it should, this risk function increases as age x of an individual increases, and by assumption, the risk of death increases exponentially with increasing age. The integral of this risk function has the form,

$$H_3(x) = \int_0^x \theta_3(s)ds = \alpha_3 \left(\exp\left[\beta_3 x\right] - 1\right) \tag{13.2.17}$$

for $x \geq 0$. Therefore, the latent survival function for this component is:

$$S_3(x) = \exp\left[-\alpha_3 \left(\exp\left[\beta_3 x\right] - 1\right)\right] \tag{13.2.18}$$

for $x \geq 0$. By applying a general, but standard formula, that a density is the risk function times the survival function, it can be seen that the probability density function of the Gompertz distribution has the form:

$$f_3(x) = \theta_3(x) S_3(x) = \alpha_3 \beta_3 \exp\left[\beta_3 x\right] \exp\left[-\alpha_3 \left(\exp\left[\beta_3 x\right] - 1\right)\right] \tag{13.2.19}$$

for $x \geq 0$. Although this distribution may be derived from intuitively appealing assumptions, it is more difficult to handle from a mathematical point of view than some other distributions that arise in probability and statistics. Nevertheless, because many advanced mathematical functions are now available in such software packages as MAPLE, MATHEMATICA and MATLAB to researchers, an outline of the mathematics used in analyzing the Gompertz distribution seems appropriate.

Because the parameters α_3 and β_3 do not have obvious statistical interpretations, such as an expectation or variance, it is difficult to assign tentative values to them. Quite often, however, there is some feeling about the modal age of death for those who survive to old age. Let m_3 denote the mode of the Gompertz distribution. Then, by using elementary calculus to find the maximum of the density $f_3(x)$, it can be shown that the equation,

$$\alpha_3 = \exp\left[-\beta_3 m_3\right] \tag{13.2.20}$$

supplies a connection between the parameters α_3, β_3 and m_3. In particular, if m_3 is assigned a value and β_3 is known, then α_3 is determined. But, to find a plausible value of β_3, more input is needed.

To this end, one may also have some idea about plausible values for σ_3, the standard deviation of the age of death among those who survive to old age. Thus, it would be helpful to express σ_3 in terms of the parameters of the Gompertz distribution. In this connection, it will be useful to consider the moment generating function of the Gompertz distribution, which is defined by,

$$M_3(s) = \int_0^\infty e^{sx} f_3(x)dx \tag{13.2.21}$$

for those values of s for which the integral converges. By using some advanced calculus, it can be shown that the moment generating function of the Gompertz distribution has the form,

$$M_3(s) = e^{\alpha_3}\left[\frac{\Gamma(\frac{s}{\beta_3}+1)}{\alpha_3^{\frac{s}{\beta_3}}} - \sum_{\nu=0}^{\infty}\frac{(-1)^{\nu}\alpha_3^{\upsilon+1}}{\nu!\left(\frac{s}{\beta_3}+\nu+1\right)}\right], \tag{13.2.22}$$

where $\Gamma(\cdot)$ is the famous gamma function and $s \in (-\epsilon, \infty)$ with $\epsilon > 0$ near zero. Recall that the gamma function is defined by the integral,

$$\Gamma(z) = \int_0^\infty x^{z-1}e^{-x}dx\ , \tag{13.2.23}$$

which converges for all $z > 0$. As is well-known, this function corresponds to the factorial function on the positive integers. In fact, if $z = n$, a positive integer, then $\Gamma(n) = (n-1)!$. In a word, this function fills the gaps among the integers, and, in particular, it can be shown that $\Gamma(\frac{1}{2}) = \sqrt{\pi}$.

If the random variable X_3 has a Gompertz distribution, then its expectation is:

$$E[X_3] = M_3^{(1)}(0) = \frac{dM_3(s)}{ds}\,|_{s=0} , \tag{13.2.24}$$

the second moment is:

$$E[X_3^2] = M_3^{(2)}(0) = \frac{d^2M_3(s)}{d^2s}\,|_{s=0} . \tag{13.2.25}$$

and the variance of the distribution is given by the well-known formula,

$$\sigma_3^2 = E[X_3^2] - (E[X_3])^2 . \tag{13.2.26}$$

After considerable analysis, it can be shown that the exact formula for the expectation is:

$$E[X_3] = e^{\alpha_3}\left[m_3 - \frac{C}{\beta_3} + \frac{1}{\beta_3}\sum_{\upsilon=0}^{\infty}\frac{(-1)^{\nu}\alpha_3^{\nu+1}}{\nu!(\nu+1)^2}\right] , \tag{13.2.27}$$

where $C \simeq 0.57721 \cdots$, is Euler's constant. Furthermore, the exact formula for the second moment is:

$$E[X_3^2] = e^{\alpha_3}\left[\left(m_3 - \frac{C}{\beta_3}\right)^2 + \frac{\pi^2}{\beta_3^2 6} - \frac{2}{\beta_3^2}\sum_{\upsilon=0}^{\infty}\frac{(-1)^{\nu}\alpha_3^{\nu+1}}{\nu!(\nu+1)^3}\right] . \tag{13.2.28}$$

The following two results:

$$\Gamma^{(1)}(1) = -C \tag{13.2.29}$$

and

$$\Gamma^{(2)}(1) = \frac{\pi^2}{6} + C^2 , \tag{13.2.30}$$

which were used in deriving the above formulas, are given in several books on special functions and advanced calculus.

When $\alpha_3 > 0$ is small, then $\exp[\alpha_3] \simeq 1$ and the above infinite series may be neglected. Thus, the approximations,

$$E[X_3] \simeq m_3 - \frac{C}{\beta_3} \tag{13.2.31}$$

and

$$E[X_3^2] \simeq \left(m_3 - \frac{C}{\beta_3}\right)^2 + \frac{\pi^2}{\beta_3^2 6} \tag{13.2.32}$$

hold for small α_3. Therefore, a formula for the approximate variance of the Gompertz distribution is:

$$\sigma_3^2 \simeq \frac{\pi^2}{\beta_3^2 6} \,. \tag{13.2.33}$$

Equivalently,

$$\beta_3 \simeq \frac{\pi}{\sigma_3\sqrt{6}} \tag{13.2.34}$$

is an approximate expression connecting the parameter β_3 with the standard deviation σ_3. This approximation is sometimes attributed to Siler.[15] However, if an investigator is working with MAPLE, MATHEMATICA, MATLAB or other software packages, programs may be written to compute the variance σ_3^2 more accurately, using the above infinite series. Thus, the accuracy of these approximations may be assessed. Among the classic books that contain information on the above mathematics are those of Artin[3] and Widder.[17]

As in the classical theory of competing risks, if it is assumed that the latent life-spans just described are independent, then the survival function for the entire life-span is:

$$S(x) = \prod_{\nu=0}^{3} S_\nu(x) \tag{13.2.36}$$

for $x \geq 0$. Observe that $S(0) = 1$. The risk function for the entire life-span is:

$$\theta(x) = \sum_{\nu=0}^{3} \theta_\nu(x) \,, \tag{13.2.37}$$

and the canonical formula for the probability density function of the entire life-span is:

$$f(x) = \theta(x)S(x) \ . \tag{13.2.38}$$

Given numerical values of the parameters, one could also compute the life table functions $p(x)$ and $q(x)$ according to the formulas,

$$p(x) = \frac{S(x)}{S(x-1)} \tag{13.2.39}$$

$$q(x) = 1 - p(x) = \frac{S(x-1) - S(x)}{S(x-1)} \tag{13.2.40}$$

for $x = 1, 2, \cdots, r$, the greatest age considered. By way of interpreting these conditional probabilities, observe that $p(x)$ is the conditional probability that an individual survives to age x, given that he was alive at age $x-1$. Thus, $q(x)$ is the conditional probability that an individual dies during the age interval $(x-1, x]$, given that he was alive at age x. From the point of view of statistical estimation, numerical values of the functions $q(x)$ obtained from widely-used life table methodology may be viewed as non-parametric estimates of the function $q(x)$ at some chosen ages $x = 1, 2, \cdots, r$. If $p(0)$ is defined as $p(0) = 1$, then the survival column of a life table is given by the function:

$$S(x) = \prod_{\nu=0}^{x} p(\nu) \tag{13.2.41}$$

at $x = 0, 1, 2, \cdots, r$ multiplied by some base number such as 100, 1000 or 100000.

Because females and males usually have different rates of mortality throughout all ages, different parameter values will need to be assigned to the two sexes in applying the model of mortality to heterosexual populations. Historically, changes in human mortality over time have been documented in many countries. To accommodate such changes, the eight parameters of the model may be constructed as functions of time. For examples of such time inhomogeneous laws of evolution in mortality, the interested reader may consult Mode et al.[10,9,11,12] Parametric models have also been used to incorporate heterogeneity and uncertainty into demographic projections (see Mode[6]).

13.3 Latent Risks for Susceptible Infants and Adolescents

As indicated in the introduction of this chapter, the first step in the development of an age-dependent demographic model accommodating such sexually transmitted diseases as HIV/AIDS, will be that of describing a formulation that does not accommodate infectives in a population. Just as in the mortality model described in the previous section, life cycle models for single females and males will be associated with stages of the life cycle. Consider, for example, a life cycle model component for single females prior to the time of sexual maturity when they become actively interested in finding partners. By definition, single females will leave this component of their life cycles when either they die, or enter the "marriage market", i.e., become sexually active or interested in finding potential sexual partners. One is thus led to consider a semi-Markovian type model with two absorbing states; namely, E_{11}-death and E_{12}-enters marriage market. To complete the description of the state space for this component, the transient state E_{20}-alive, indicating that an individual is alive, may be added.

The next step is to consider two latent risks functions, governing transitions from the transient state E_{20} to the absorbing states E_{11} and E_{12}. To simplify the exploration of ideas, it will be assumed that the laws of evolution of the process are time homogeneous. Let $\theta_{f1}(x)$ denote the latent risk of death for a female of age x at time t. Then, the probability that she dies during a small time interval $(t, t+h]$, i.e., undergoes the transition $E_{20} \rightarrow E_{11}$, is $\theta_{f1}(x)h + o(h)$. Similarly, for a female of age x at time t, let $\theta_{f2}(x)$ denote the latent risk governing entrance into the marriage market during a small time interval $(t, t+h]$. Then, the matrix of latent risks for infant and adolescent females has the simple form,

$$\mathbf{\Theta}_{f0}(x) = \begin{bmatrix} \theta_{f1}(x) & \theta_{f2}(x) & 0 \end{bmatrix}, \tag{13.3.1}$$

for females of age x. The matrix $\mathbf{\Theta}_{m0}(x)$ of latent risks for infant and adolescent males of age x is similar, and contains the latent risk functions $\theta_{m1}(x)$ and $\theta_{m2}(x)$. The next question that arises is: What parametric forms would be suitable for these risk functions?

A plausible form of the latent risk function $\theta_{f1}(x)$ would be the risk function in Eq. (13.3.1) plus a constant Makeham term to accommodate deaths due to accidents. Thus, for $x \geq 0$, the function $\theta_{f0}(x)$ could be chosen as,

$$\theta_{f1}(x) = \alpha_{f0}\beta_{f0}\exp\left[-\beta_{f0}x\right] + \alpha_{f2}\ , \tag{13.3.2}$$

where α_{f0} and β_{f0} are positive parameters for infant females, and a constant risk of accidental death for infant and adolescent females is given by $\alpha_{f2} > 0$. The corresponding risk function $\theta_{m1}(x)$ for males of age x could have the same functional form as that in Eq. (13.3.3), with parameters α_{m0}, β_{m0}, and α_{m2}.

In a population of adolescent females, let $\gamma_f > 0$ denote the minimum age at which they become interested in male sexual partners. Typically, this age would be in the interval 12 to 15 years. There is some empirical evidence (see Mode[8] chapter 4), that ages at first marriage in birth cohorts of females and males follow log-normal distributions with different parameter values for the two sexes. The age of first marriage and the minimum age for sexual activity γ_f for females may not be the same as that of first marriage, but it seems reasonable to assume that the shape of the distribution of the age of interest in sexual partners begins would be similar to that for first marriage ages. Thus, if X_f denotes a latent random variable for the age of first entrance into the marriage market, then it seems reasonable to assume that X_f has a log-normal distribution on the interval (γ_f, ∞) with distribution function,

$$\mathbb{P}\left[X_f \leq x\right] = \Phi\left(\frac{\ln(x - \gamma_f) - \mu_f}{\sigma_f}\right) \tag{13.3.3}$$

for $x > \gamma_f$. The parameters μ_f and σ_f could be chosen by following the procedure outlined in Eqs. (13.2.11) through (13.2.13), along with the knowledge that the mode of the distribution would be about 18 to 20 years, with the vast majority of females entering the marriage market before age 25.

It seems reasonable, therefore, to choose the functional form of the latent risk function $\theta_{f2}(x)$ as that for a log-normal distribution on the interval (γ_f, ∞) with parameters μ_f and $\sigma_f > 0$. For $x > 0$, let $f_1(x)$ denote the log-normal density in Eq. (13.2.8) with parameters μ_f and σ_f. Then, formally, for $x > \gamma_f$, this risk function would have the form,

$$\theta_{f2}(x) = \frac{f_1(x-\gamma_f)}{1-\Phi\left(\frac{\ln(x-\gamma_f)-\mu_f}{\sigma_f}\right)}, \tag{13.3.4}$$

and $\theta_{f2}(x) = 0$ for $0 \le x \le \gamma_f$. The latent risk function $\theta_{m2}(x)$ for males entering the marriage market could be defined as in Eq. (13.3.4) with parameters γ_m, μ_m and σ_m. An advantage of choosing functional forms for these risk functions as in Eq. (13.3.4) is that they can readily be computed for a given array of x-values using existing software packages.

Because the risk functions just defined apply only to infants and adolescents, it will be helpful to introduce succinct symbols for the component of the life cycle under consideration. For the case of females, let the symbol $\mathfrak{L}_{f0}$ denote this component and let the symbol $\mathfrak{L}_{m0}$ be defined similarly for males. Then, for females aged x in $\mathfrak{L}_{f0}$, the total risk function is:

$$\theta_f(x) = \theta_{f1}(x) + \theta_{f2}(x)\,. \tag{13.3.5}$$

Given that a female is born at time $t = 0$, the conditional probability that she is still in $\mathfrak{L}_{f0}$ at age $x > 0$ is:

$$S_f(x) = \exp\left[-\int_0^x \theta_f(s)ds\right]. \tag{13.3.6}$$

Therefore, given that a female is in $\mathfrak{L}_{f0}$ at time t, the conditional probability that she is still in $\mathfrak{L}_{f0}$ at age $x + h$ is:

$$\frac{S_f(x+h)}{S_f(x)} = \exp\left[-\int_x^{x+h} \theta_f(s)ds\right], \tag{13.3.7}$$

where $h > 0$.

For h sufficiently small, the integral may approximated by letting $\theta_f(s) = \theta_f(x)$ for all $x \le s \le x+h$. Then, by definition, given that a female in $\mathfrak{L}_{f0}$ is of age x at time t,

$$\pi_f(t, x; 0, 0) = \exp\left[-\theta_f(x)h\right] \tag{13.3.8}$$

is the conditional probability she is still in $\mathfrak{L}_{f0}$ at time $t+h$. Similarly, using a competing risk argument as initially outlined in Section 10.5, it can be shown that:

$$\pi_f(t,x,0,1) = (1 - \exp[-\theta_f(x)h]) \frac{\theta_{f1}(x)}{\theta_f(x)} \tag{13.3.9}$$

is the conditional probability this female dies, and

$$\pi_f(t,x;0,2) = (1 - \exp[-\theta_f(x)h]) \frac{\theta_{f2}(x)}{\theta_f(x)} \tag{13.3.10}$$

is the conditional probability that she enters the marriage market during $(t, t+h]$. A set of similar transition probabilities for males of age x in $\mathfrak{L}_{m0}$ at time t may also be calculated as in Eqs. (13.3.8) through (13.3.10), using the risk functions $\theta_{m1}(x)$ and $\theta_{m2}(x)$.

Many countries throughout the world collect data on human mortality and classify deaths by age at last birthday. From such classifications of data on mortality and estimates of the number of persons in an age group at some given time, it is possible to compute period life tables from which a times series of expectations of life at birth may be calculated for both females and males. As a general rule, expectations of life at birth for females often exceed those for males, and these expectations of life at birth for both sexes have increased over time in many countries during recent decades. Such empirical observations indicate that if investigators wish to project epidemics of HIV/AIDS (or other infectious diseases) over several decades, their models must accommodate latent risk functions that change in time. For infected persons, advances in drugs to treat the disease and also better nutrition may reduce their chances of death due to disease, which is another reason why models with time inhomogeneous laws of evolution need to be considered when projecting epidemics of infectious diseases over time periods involving several decades.

As suggested in Section 13.2, a useful approach to accommodating time inhomogeneous laws of evolution in a model whose latent risks depend on parameters is to devise schemes to let the parameters depend on time. For example, for the risk function in Eq. (13.3.2), the proportion of females that die in infancy is $\exp[-\alpha_{f0}]$. The larger the value of α_{f0}, the smaller the proportion of females who die in infancy. Thus, if expectations are such that infant mortality will decrease over the time period of the projection, the parameter α_{f0} could increase with time. With regard to medical intervention, small values of the parameters β_{f0} correspond to longer survival time of female infants. Therefore, if the expectation is that medical intervention will increase the survival times of infants, the parameter β_{f0} would decrease over time. Similar remarks hold for the parameters α_{m0} and β_{m0}, governing the survivability of infant males. Such ideas for constructing computer models with time inhomogeneous laws of evolution have been illustrated and implemented by Salsburg.[14]

Let $\theta_{f1}(t,x)$ and $\theta_{f2}(t,x)$ be latent risk functions for females in $\mathfrak{L}_{f0}$, which depend on t. Given some scheme for varying parameters in latent risks as functions of time, the transition probabilities in Eqs. (13.3.8) through (13.3.10) could be changed to accommodate such variation by using the risk functions $\theta_{f1}(t,x)$ and $\theta_{f2}(t,x)$ throughout the calculations in each epoch t of a projection. For example, let

$$S_h(N) = \{th \mid t = 0, 2, \cdots, N\} \tag{13.3.11}$$

denote the finite set of discrete time points over which an epidemic is to be projected, and let

$$A_{f0} = \{x \mid x = 0, 1, 2, \cdots, a_{f0}\} \tag{13.3.12}$$

denote the set of ages for females belonging to the $\mathfrak{L}_{f0}$ component of the life cycle. A similar set A_{m0} may be defined for males in $\mathfrak{L}_{m0}$ with a_{m0} as the greatest age. Typically, these ages would be expressed in years and each of the ages a_{f0} and a_{m0} could be in the interval $[18, 21]$. For every age $x \in A_{f0}$ and time point $t \in S_h(N)$, values of the risk functions $\theta_{f1}(t,x)$ and $\theta_{f2}(t,x)$ would need to be calculated and then substituted into the formulas in Eqs. (13.3.8) through (13.3.10) for the transition probabilities assigned to the intervals $(t, t+h]$. Similar remarks hold for the set of conditional probabilities,

$$\{\pi_m(t, x, 0, k) \mid k = 0, 1, 2\} \ , \tag{13.3.13}$$

governing transitions of males in $\mathfrak{L}_{m0}$ of age $x \in A_{m0}$ during a time interval $(t, t+h]$.

This section will be concluded with a brief overview of procedures for computing Monte Carlo realizations of the random functions describing the evolution of individuals in $\mathfrak{L}_{f0}$ and $\mathfrak{L}_{m0}$, along with a few remarks on the implementation of the age-dependent case. Let the random function $X(t, x)$ denote the number of females of age $x \in A_{f0}$ in $\mathfrak{L}_{f0}$ at time t. Among these individuals, let the random function $X_T(t+h, x, k)$ denote the number who undergo the transition $E_{20} \to E_{1k}$, $k = 1, 2$, during the time interval $(t, t+h]$. By definition, the random function $X_T(t+h, x, 0)$ denotes the number these individuals who do not undergo either of these transitions during $(t, t+h]$. As in previous chapters, let

$$\mathbf{X}_T(t+h.x) = (X_T(t+h, x, k) \mid k = 0, 1, 2) \tag{13.3.14}$$

and

$$\boldsymbol{\pi}_f(t, x) = (\pi_f(t, x; 0, k) \mid k = 0, 1, 2) \tag{13.3.15}$$

be vectors with the indicated elements.

Then, by assumption, given the random variable $X(t, x)$ at time t, the vector $\mathbf{X}_T(t+h.x)$ has a conditional multinomial distribution with index $X(t, x)$ and probability vector $\boldsymbol{\pi}_f(t, x)$. In symbols,

$$\mathbf{X}_T(t+h, x) \sim CMultinom\,(X(t, x), \boldsymbol{\pi}_f(t, x)) \ . \tag{13.3.16}$$

With regard to males in $\mathfrak{L}_{m0}$, let the random function $Y(t; x)$ denote the number of males of age $x \in A_{m0}$ at time t. As in Eqs. (13.3.14) and (13.3.15), one can define a random vector $\mathbf{Y}_T(t+h, x)$ and a vector $\boldsymbol{\pi}_f(t, x)$ of conditional probabilities such that $\mathbf{Y}_T(t+h, x)$ has a conditional multinomial distribution as in Eq. (13.3.16).

One of the practical problems that must be faced when implementing age-dependent models is that of processing large arrays. Ideally, if a computer has enough memory, then the ages of individuals could be calculated on the same time scale as that in the lattice $S_h(N)$ in Eq. (13.3.11). If this were the case, then the x in the random vector $\mathbf{X}_T(t+h, x)$ would be replaced the $x+h$, indicating that the age of each individual alive at time $t+h$ would advance by a time unit of length h. By way of illustration, if the time unit were a month, then the ages of all individuals would be expressed in terms of months. But, unfortunately, this practice could lead to such large arrays that processing them would not be feasible. One alternative would be to set all the parameters in the latent risk functions involving age to a yearly time scale. Then, for example, if a Monte Carlo projection were computed on a monthly time scale, then the age of all individuals of age x at the beginning of a 12 month time segment who were alive at the end of the segment could have their age advanced to $x+1$. Similar procedures have been implemented by Salsburg[14] to embed non-linear difference equations in a stochastic process.

13.4 Couple Formation in a Population of Susceptibles

By definition, females and males of age $x > a_{f0}$ and $y > a_{m0}$ will be eligible to be members of a couple. Let

$$A_{fm} = \{x \mid x > a_{f0}\} \tag{13.4.1}$$

denote the set of marriageable ages for females and define the set A_{mm} similarly for males. Females with marriageable ages $x \in A_{fm}$ will belong to stage $\mathfrak{L}_{fm}$ of the life cycle, and $\mathfrak{L}_{mm}$ will denote the corresponding stage for males. A couple will be said to be of type (x, y) if the female and male are, respectively, of ages x and y. Let

$$\Upsilon_c = A_{fm} \times A_{mm} = \{(x, y) \mid x > a_{f0},\ y > a_{m0}\} \tag{13.4.2}$$

denote the set of couple types.

Unlike the partnership models considered in Chapters 11 and 12, the set Υ_c will contain many more elements than those considered heretofore. For example, suppose the largest ages r_f and r_m of females and males considered in a projection are $r_f = r_m = 100$, where it is the case that $a_{f0} = a_{m0} = 18$ years of age. If the ages of all individuals were grouped into yearly age classes, there would be $100 - 18 = 82$ age groups for each sex, and the set Υ_c would contain $82 \times 82 = 6724$ elements. Restricting the formulation of the model to the deteminististic paradigm, any population projection requiring the recursive processing of 82×82 numerical arrays within a reasonable time span would be in the realm of practicality given the speed and memory of the desktop computers currently available.

However, when one considers transitions among types in the set Υ_c, due to the aging of individuals and other factors to be considered in a subsequent section, sparse arrays of latent risk functions with dimensions 6724×6724 would arise. Furthermore, even if the arrays were sparse and attention were confined to the deteministic paradigm, the recursive numerical processing that is required may be feasible. The problem of processing large arrays within a reasonable period of time arises in the replication of projections in Monte Carlo simulation experiments. If an investigator were to consider a more realistic stochastic formulation, then steps would have to be taken to reduce the dimensionality of the arrays.

One approach to reducing the dimensionality of the arrays to is observe that only a relatively small number of the couple types in the set Υ_c would actually be observed in a population at any time, because the ages of females and males in couples are positively correlated. To illustrate this observation geometrically, suppose the ages of females $x > a_{f0}$ form the x-axis and the ages of males $y > a_{m0}$ form the y-axis. Then, if plotted in the xy plane, the pairs of couple types (x, y) would cluster around the 45° line $y = x$ passing through the point (a_{f0}, a_{m0}). Some points would lie at considerable distances from this line, indicating that the ages of members of couples could differ by 10 or more years. But, in statistical enumerations of the ages of brides and grooms reported in many countries, the difference in ages would satisfy the inequality $0 \leq | x - y | \leq 5$ years in the vast majority of cases. If an investigator wishes to use such a restriction on the number of realized couple types, then number of elements in the set Υ_c would be greatly reduced in a computer implementation of the model, even if ages were grouped into yearly age classes. But, in the modelling of epidemics of sexually transmitted diseases, placing such restrictions on the number of couple types, or the types of sexual contacts, might result in omissions of a serious nature, particularly when extra-marital sexual contacts between persons of significantly different ages are taken into account.

The ideas outlined in Section 12.14 to formulate the model for couple formation may easily be extended to the age-dependent case. Let

$$\alpha_f(x,y) = \exp\left[-\beta_f \mid x - y \mid\right] \tag{13.4.3}$$

denote the conditional probability that a single female in $\mathfrak{L}_{mf}$ of age $x \in A_{fm}$ finds a single male of age $y \in A_{mm}$ acceptable as a potential marriage partner, where β_f is a parameter such that $\beta_f \geq 0$. Similarly, let $\alpha_m(y,x)$ denote the conditional probability, depending on a parameter $\beta_m \geq 0$, that a single male in $\mathfrak{L}_{mm}$ of age $y \in A_{mm}$ finds a single female of age $x \in A_{fm}$ acceptable as a potential marriage partner. Unlike the acceptance probabilities considered in Chapters 10, 11 and 12, ages of individuals provide a "ready made" quantification of the variables x and y in Eq. (13.4.3).

Let the random function $X(t;x)$ denote the number of single females of age x in $\mathfrak{L}_{fm}$ at time t. Then, at time t the total number of single females in the population at time t is:

$$X(t;\cdot) = \sum_{x \in A_{fm}} X(t;x) > 0 \tag{13.4.4}$$

and

$$U_f(t;x) = \frac{X(t;x)}{X(t;\cdot)} \tag{13.4.5}$$

is the frequency of single females of age $x \in A_{fm}$ at time t. Similarly, let the random function $Y(y;t)$ denote the number of single males of age $y \in A_{mm}$ in the population at time t, and let $Y(t;\cdot) > 0$ denote the total number of single males in stage $\mathfrak{L}_{mm}$ at time t. Then, the frequency $U_m(t;y)$ of single males of age $y \in A_{mm}$ in the population at time t can be defined as in Eq. (13.4.5).

By following the procedures of Section 12.4, an application of Bayes' formula yields the expression:

$$\gamma_f(t;x,y) = \frac{U_m(t;y)\alpha_f(x,y)}{\sum_{\nu \in A_{mm}} U_m(t;\nu)\alpha_f(x,\nu)} \tag{13.4.6}$$

for the conditional probability that a single female of age $x \in A_{fm}$ has contact with a potential single male marriage partner of age $y \in A_{mm}$ during the time interval $(t, t+h]$. By using the same argument, it can be shown that the corresponding conditional probability that a single male of age $y \in A_{mm}$ has contact with a potential single female marriage partner of age $x \in A_{fn}$ during the time interval $(t, t+h]$ has the form,

$$\gamma_m(t; y, x) = \frac{U_f(t; x)\alpha_m(y, x)}{\sum_{\nu \in A_{fm}} U_f(t; \nu)\alpha_m(y, \nu)} . \tag{13.4.7}$$

Let

$$\mathbf{\Gamma}_f(t; x) = (\gamma_f(t; x, y) \mid y \in A_{mm}) \tag{13.4.8}$$

denote a vector of contact probabilities for single females who are of age $x \in A_{fm}$ at time t, and let $\mathbf{\Gamma}_m(t; y)$ denote a similar vector of contact probabilities for single males of age $y \in A_{mm}$ at time t.

Given $X(t; x)$ single females of age $x \in A_{fm}$ at time t, let the random function $Z_f(t; x, y)$ represent the number single males of age $y \in A_{mm}$ selected as potential marriage partners during the time interval $(t, t+h]$. Similarly, among the $Y(t; y)$ single males of age $y \in A_{mm}$ at time t, let the random function $Z_m(t; y, x)$ denote the number of single females of age $x \in A_{fm}$ selected as potential marriage partners during this time interval. Furthermore, for single females of age x, let

$$\mathbf{Z}_f(t; x) = (Z_f(t; x, y) \mid y \in A_{mm}) \tag{13.4.9}$$

denote a random vector with elements $Z_f(t; x, y)$; define a similar random vector $\mathbf{Z}_m(t; y)$ with elements $Z_m(t; y, x)$ for single males of age $y \in A_{mm}$ at time t. Given $X(t; x)$, the random vector $\mathbf{Z}_f(t; x)$ has a conditional multinomial distribution with index $X(t; x)$ and probability vector $\mathbf{\Gamma}_f(t; x)$ for every single female of age $x \in A_{fm}$ at time t by assumption. In symbols,

$$\mathbf{Z}_f(t; x) \sim CMultinom\left(X(t; x), \mathbf{\Gamma}_f(t; x)\right) . \tag{13.4.10}$$

Similarly, by assumption, for single males of age $y \in A_{mm}$ at time t,

$$\mathbf{Z}_f(t; x) \sim CMultinom\left(Y(t; y), \mathbf{\Gamma}_m(t; y)\right) . \tag{13.4.11}$$

As in Section 12.4, let the random function $N_{CF}(t; x, y)$ denote the potential number of couples of type $(x, y) \in \Upsilon_c$ that may be formed during the time interval $(t, t+h]$, and let the random function

$Z_{CF}(t;x,y)$ denote the actual number of couples of this type that may be formed during this time interval. Then, $N_{CF}(t;x,y)$ will chosen as

$$N_{CF}(t;x,y) = \min\{Z_f(t;x,y), Z_m(t;y,x)\} \ . \tag{13.4.12}$$

To determine the random function $Z_{CF}(t;x,y)$, let $\rho(x,y)$ denote the rate of couple formation during any time interval. Then, during any time interval $(t, t+h]$,

$$q_{CF}(x,y;h) = 1 - \exp\left[-\rho(x,y)h\right] \tag{13.4.13}$$

is the conditional probability that a couple of type (x,y) is formed during the time interval $(t, t+h]$. Finally, it will be assumed that $Z_{CF}(t;x,y)$ has as conditional binomial distribution with index $N_{CF}(t;x,y)$ and probability $q_{CF}(x,y;h)$. In symbols,

$$Z_{CF}(t;x,y) \sim CBinom\left(N_{CF}(t;x,y), q_{CF}(x,y;h)\right) \ . \tag{13.4.14}$$

From the algorithms just outlined, it can be seen that the random function $N_{CF}(t;x,y)$ in Eq. (13.4.12) satisfies equalities and inequalities similar to those in Eqs. (12.4.8) through (12.4.10) with probability one for all t, x and y. Recall that these constraints must hold when one considers the potential number of couples of any type that may be formed during any time interval $(t, t+h]$.

13.5 Births in a Population of Susceptibles

A demographic property of a population not explicitly taken into account in all the models considered in the previous chapters, is that during any time interval, births may be added to the population. Actually, whenever a model accommodates recruits entering the population during any time interval, as was the case with those presented in Chapters 10, 11 and 12, births occurring a decade or more prior to a point in time may be taken into account implicitly by supposing recruits are teenage individuals becoming sexually active. Nevertheless, in epidemics that may persist in a population over many generations, such as HIV/AIDS, it is of considerable interest to formulate stochastic models that accommodate births, for it is known that HIV and other viruses may be transmitted from infected mothers to their infants in utero. It should be mentioned that there already exists a rather extensive literature on stochastic models of human reproduction (see, for example, Mode[8] and the references contained therein). But, these models are rather complex. They were formulated to take into account many aspects of human reproduction, such as the use of contraceptives, which would be useful in evaluating the impact of family planning programs. However, due to this level of complexity, such models would be unsuitable as components of epidemic models. Consequently, in this section, a simpler approach to constructing stochastic models accommodating the flow of births into a population will be presented.

Let $a_L < a_U$ denote, respectively, the lower and upper ages of child bearing for human females. When age is expressed in years, then typically $a_L \in (15, 20]$ and $a_U \in (50, 55]$. Next consider the partition,

$$a_L = x_1 < x_2 < \cdots < x_k < x_{k+1} = a_U \tag{13.5.1}$$

of the interval $(a_L, a_U]$ of child bearing ages. A concept that is widely used in demography is that of the gross fertility rate, which will be denoted by μ_{GTF}. To interpret this number, suppose it was possible to observe over time the number of live births each woman in birth cohorts experienced throughout the age interval $(a_L, a_U]$, given that she is still alive at age a_U. Then, μ_{GTF} would be the expected number of live births per women in this cohort. Now, with respect to the partition in Eq. (13.5.1), let $b(x)$ denote some probability density function $b(x_i)$ such that:

$$\sum_{i=1}^{k} b(x_i) = 1 \, . \tag{13.5.2}$$

In the demographic literature, this density is sometimes referred to as the distribution of age of child bearing. In the simplified stochastic model of human reproduction to be presented in this section, the number $b(x_i)\mu_{GTF}$ will be interpreted as follows: Given that a women is of age x_i at time t, $b(x_i)\mu_{GTF}$ is the expected number of live births experienced during the time interval $(t, t+h]$.

One approach to computing the density of age of child bearing is to consider a random variable V with range $[0, 1]$ with a beta type density:

$$f(v) = \frac{\Gamma(\alpha+\beta)}{\Gamma(\alpha)\Gamma(\beta)} v^{\alpha-1}(1-v)^{\beta-1} \tag{13.5.3}$$

defined for $v \in (0,1)$, where $\alpha > 0$ and $\beta > 0$ are parameters. Then, define the random variable,

$$X = a_L + (a_U - a_L)V \,, \tag{13.5.4}$$

which maps the interval $[0,1]$ onto the interval $[a_L, a_U]$. Observe that the inverse map

$$V = \frac{X - a_L}{a_U - a_L} \tag{13.5.5}$$

maps the interval $[x_i, x_{i+1}]$ onto the interval

$$\left[y_i = \frac{x_i - a_L}{a_U - a_L},\ y_{i+1} = \frac{x_{i+1} - a_L}{a_U - a_L} \right] \tag{13.5.6}$$

in $[0,1]$. By definition,

$$\begin{aligned} b(x_i) &= P\left[x_i < X \le x_{i+1}\right] \\ &= P\left[y_i < V \le y_{i+1}\right] \\ &= \int_{y_i}^{y_{i+1}} f(v)dv \end{aligned} \tag{13.5.7}$$

for $i = 1, 2, \cdots, k$. Given estimates of the parameters α and β and the availability of such software packages as MAPLE or MATLAB on a desktop computer, the density function in Eq. (13.5.7) could easily be computed. Salsburg[14] provides an example in which the parameters α and β were estimated by non-linear least squares from demographic data. The choice of the beta density in Eq. (13.5.3) is, of course, arbitrary; moreover, other choices of parametric densities could be equally convenient and useful.

For a typical female of age x in the child bearing ages, let $\xi(x)$ be a random variable with range $n = 0, 1, 2, \cdots$, denoting the number of live births she experiences during a time interval $(t, t+h]$. It will be assumed that $\xi(x)$ has Poisson distribution with parameter $b(x)\mu_{GTF}$. To fix ideas, suppose all live births may be attributed to females in couples, and let the random function $Z(t;x,y)$ denote the number of type (x,y)-couples in the population at time t. Then, the random function,

$$X_c(t;x) = \sum_y Z(t;x,y) \tag{13.5.8}$$

represents the number of females in couples at time t who may experience lives births during the time interval $(t, t+h]$. As in previous chapters, let $\mathfrak{B}(t)$ stand for the evolution of the process up to time t. Given $\mathfrak{B}(t)$, let $\xi_i(x)$, $i = 1, 2, \cdots$, denote a sequence conditionally independent and identically distributed random variables whose common distribution is that of $\xi(x)$. Then, for females in couples of age x at time t, the total number of live births experienced during the time interval $(t, t+h]$ is given by the random function,

$$B(t;x) = \sum_{i=1}^{X_c(t;x)} \xi_i(x)\,, \tag{13.5.9}$$

where, by definition, if $X_c(t;x) = 0$, then $B(t;x) = 0$.

As is well-known, given $\mathfrak{B}(t)$, it can be shown that the random function $B(t;x)$ has a conditional Poisson distribution with parameter $X_c(t;x)b(x)\mu_{GTF}$. When the child bearing ages are partitioned as in Eq. (13.5.1), then, in Monte Carlo simulation experiments, the total number of births added to the population during the time interval $(t, t+h]$ is given by the random function,

$$B(t) = \sum_{i=1}^{k} B(t;x_i) \tag{13.5.10}$$

with conditional expectation,

$$E\left[B(t) \mid \mathfrak{B}(t)\right] = \sum_{i=1}^{k} X_c(t;x_i)b(x_i)\mu_{GTF}\,. \tag{13.5.11}$$

Moreover, if it is assumed that the summands in Eq. (13.5.10) are conditionally independent given $\mathfrak{B}(t)$, then it follows that the random function $B(t)$ in Eq. (13.5.10) has a Poisson distribution with parameter Eq. (13.5.11).

Whenever two sexes are distinguished in a population, live births will classified as either a girl or a boy. Let p_g and p_b denote, respectively, a live birth is a girl or boy, where $p_g + p_b = 1$. Then, because given $\mathfrak{B}(t)$, the random function $B(t)$ has a conditional Poisson distribution, it can be shown that there are two conditionally independent Poisson distributed random functions $B_g(t)$ and $B_b(t)$ such that:

$$B(t) = B_g(t) + B_b(t) \ . \tag{13.5.12}$$

Furthermore, it can be shown that $B_g(t)$ and $B_b(t)$ have parameters,

$$\lambda_f(t) = p_g E\left[B(t) \mid \mathfrak{B}(t)\right]$$

$$\lambda_m(t) = p_b E\left[B(t) \mid \mathfrak{B}(t)\right] \tag{13.5.13}$$

respectively.

In some Monte Carlo simulation experiments, the parameters $\lambda_f(t)$ and $\lambda_m(t)$ may be sufficiently small so that realizations of the random functions $B_g(t)$ and $B_b(t)$ may be computed, using an algorithm designed to compute realizations directly from a Poisson distribution. In some cases, however, these parameters may be so large that a central limit theorem may be applied. For, let $X \sim N(\mu, \sigma^2)$ symbolize that a random variable X has a normal distribution with expectation μ and variance σ^2, and let $Y \cong X$ symbolize that the distribution of a random variable Y is approximately that of X. Then, if $\lambda_f(t)$ is large,

$$B_g(t) \cong X_g \sim N(\lambda_f(t), \lambda_f(t)) \ , \tag{13.5.14}$$

and similar result holds for the random function $B_b(t)$. Let Z denote a standard random variable such that $Z \sim N(0,1)$. A realization of the random variable X_g may then be computed according to the formula:

$$X_g = \lambda_f(t) + Z\sqrt{\lambda_f(t)} \ . \tag{13.5.15}$$

It is easy to write code or use existing software packages to compute values of a standard normal random variable Z that are approximately independently and identically distributed. Hence, realizations of the random variable X_g for girls, and the corresponding X_b for boys, may be computed efficiently, because in each epoch in a Monte Carlo projection, only two realizations of a random variable $Z \sim N(0,1)$ need to be computed.

However, realizations of the random variable in Eq. (13.5.15) will not, in general, be non-negative integers, which are required in Monte Carlo simulation experiments. Thus, it becomes necessary to adjust the random variables X_g and X_b. Let $[x]$ denote the greatest integer in a real number x. Then, realizations of the random function $B_g(t)$ will be computed using the formula:

$$B_g(t) = \max(0, [X_g]) . \tag{13.5.16}$$

When $\lambda_f(t)$ is sufficiently large, this formula would be justified because negative values of X_g would occur with a negligibly small probability. Similar remarks hold for computing realizations of the random function $B_b(t)$ for boys.

Although illegitimate births have not been explicitly discussed, the above formulas could easily be extended to include single females in the child bearing ages at each epoch of a projection. Another way in which the formulation presented in this section may be extended is that of allowing for time inhomogeneity in the birth process. For example, by inspecting historical data in many countries of the world, it can be seen that the gross fertility rate has declined over time. One approach to taking such time inhomogeneity into account is to suppose the gross fertility rate $\mu_{GFR}(t)$ is a decreasing function of t. Then, by way of simplification, if it is assumed that the density of age of child bearing $b(x)$ does not change over time, then the fertility rate for women of age x in couples at time t would be $b(x)\mu_{GFR}(t)$. Moreover, under the assumptions outlined above, all formulas of this section would continue to apply.

13.6 Latent Risks with Infectives

As illustrated in Section 13.3, whenever the ages of individuals are accommodated in a model, matrices of latent risks for life cycle models of either singles or couples can become very large Thus, as in Section 13.3, for the case of single members of a population, attention will be confined to sub-matrices of latent risks for each age and with $n = 1$ stage of disease. For example, consider a single female of age $x \leq a_{f0}$ in the infant and youth component of a population prior to entrance into the marriage market. Prior to becoming sexually active, females in this age class cannot be infected by sexual contacts, but, if a mother is infected with HIV, then with some positive probability she will transmit the virus to her infant prior to or during the birth process. Although the birth process described in Section 13.5 does not take this possibility into account, it could easily be extended to taking into account infected mothers passing infections to their infants. One is thus led to consider the following state space, with three absorbing states and two transient states, for the life cycle model for these individuals. Let the absorbing states E_{11} and E_{12} denote, respectively, that a death can be attributed to a cause other than disease and to disease, and let E_{13} denote an absorbing state, indicating entrance into the marriage market. The two transient states of the life cycle model will be denoted by E_{20} and E_{21} and represent, respectively, a susceptible and infected person.

Given these definitions of states, suppose the rows of the matrix of latent risks are indexed by the two transient states and the columns are indexed by the set of five states. Then, the 2×5 matrix $\mathbf{\Theta}_{f0}(x)$ of latent risks for females of age $x \leq a_{f0}$ has the form,

$$\mathbf{\Theta}_{f0}(x) = \begin{bmatrix} \theta_{f1}(x) & 0 & \theta_{f3}(x) & 0 & 0 \\ \theta_{f1}(x) & \theta_{f2}(x) & \theta_{f3}(x) & \theta_{f0}(x) & 0 \end{bmatrix}. \tag{13.6.1}$$

By way of explanation, because the first row of this matrix is indexed by the susceptible state E_{20}, the only risks of transitions from this state are death from a cause other than disease, $E_{20} \to E_{11}$, with risk function $\theta_{f1}(x)$, and entrance into the marriage market, $E_{20} \to E_{13}$, with risk function $\theta_{f3}(x)$. Note that the transition, $E_{20} \to E_{21}$, indicating a susceptible female of age x is infected, has a zero risk, because prior to becoming sexually active there is no risk of contracting a sexually transmitted disease.

The second row of the matrix contains those risk functions for transitions out of the state E_{21}, representing an infected individual. For an infected person, the transition $E_{21} \to E_{12}$, indicates death from a cause other than disease. Thus, the risk function $\theta_{f2}(x)$ has been added to the second row of the matrix, governing transitions from the transient state E_{21} to the set of absorbing states. The risk function $\theta_{f0}(x)$ is that for the transition $E_{21} \to E_{20}$, indicating that an infected person has been cleared of an infection. For the case of HIV, this risk function may be positive, because it has been observed that an infant born to a mother infected with HIV may test positive, but subsequently his or her body may be cleared of the virus. For most ages such that $0 < x \leq a_{f0}$, the risk $\theta_{f0}(x)$ would be zero, because so far no treatment regimen has been observed to completely clear a body of HIV. It is clear that the 2×5 matrix of latent risks $\boldsymbol{\Theta}_{m0}(y)$ for males with ages $0 \leq y \leq a_{m0}$ would have the same structure as that in Eq. (13.6.1).

Before proceeding to describe matrices of latent risk for singles in the marriageable ages, it is appropriate to make some remarks about the functional forms of the risk functions in Eq. (13.6.1). The functional form of the risk function $\theta_{f1}(x)$ could be chosen as in Eq. (13.3.2) and that for $\theta_{f3}(x)$ could be chosen as in Eq. (13.3.4). Having made these choices for the risk functions $\theta_{f1}(x)$ and $\theta_{f3}(x)$, there remains the task of choosing the risk functions $\theta_{f2}(x)$ and $\theta_{f0}(x)$ in the second row of $\boldsymbol{\Theta}_{f0}(x)$. As in previous chapters, the simplest choice for the function $\theta_{f2}(x)$ is to assume there is a positive constant μ_{f1} such that:

$$\theta_{f2}(x) = \mu_{f1} \tag{13.6.2}$$

for all $0 \leq x \leq a_{f0}$. Similarly, for the case of infected females in this age class, suppose there is a positive constant μ_{f20} such that:

$$\theta_{f0}(0) = \mu_{f20} \, , \tag{13.6.3}$$

but $\theta_{f0}(x) = 0$ for all $0 < x \leq a_{f0}$. Only infants in the early states of life may be cleared of HIV in this specification of the risk functions; for other ages in this class it is not possible to clear a body of the virus.

For single females of marriageable age $x > a_{f0}$, there is no need to include a risk function for entrance into the marriage market. It suffices to consider a set of two absorbing states E_{11} and E_{12}, representing causes of death as defined above. To complete the definition of the state space for the life cycle model for single females in these ages, the set of transient states will again consist of the two states E_{20} and

E_{21}, as previously defined. Then, for a single female of age $x > a_{f0}$, the 2×4 matrix $\boldsymbol{\Theta}_{fm}(x)$ of latent risks has the form,

$$\boldsymbol{\Theta}_{fm}(x) = \begin{bmatrix} \theta_{fm1}(x) & 0 & 0 & \theta_{fm02}(x) \\ \theta_{fm1}(x) & \theta_{fm2}(x) & 0 & 0 \end{bmatrix} . \tag{13.6.4}$$

The latent risk function $\theta_{fm1}(x)$ is that for death due to causes other than disease and is the sum of three components defined in Section 13.2. Thus,

$$\theta_{fm1}(x) = \frac{\alpha_{f1}}{\sqrt{2\pi} x \sigma_f} \exp\left[-\frac{1}{2} \left(\frac{\ln x - \mu_f}{\sigma_f} \right)^2 \right]$$

$$+ \alpha_{f2} + \alpha_{f3}\beta_{f3} \exp\left[\beta_{f3} x\right] . \tag{13.6.5}$$

As can be seen, the first component is that for the accident hump somewhere between the ages of 20 and 35 and consists of a log-normal density, weighted by the factor $\alpha_{f1} > 0$ such that $\exp[-\alpha_{f1}]$ is the fraction of females surviving past age 35. The parameters μ_f and σ_f pertain to females and may be calculated as in Eqs. (13.2.11) through (13.2.13). The second component is $\alpha_{f2} > 0$, the Makeham term for accidents throughout the whole of life, and the third term is the Gompertz risk function for risk of death at the older ages, depending on positive parameters α_f and β_f specific to females. As in Eq. (13.6.2), it will be assumed that the risk of death due to disease, $\theta_{fm2}(x) = \mu_{f1} > 0$, is constant for all $x > a_{f1}$.

Finally, the risk function $\theta_{fm02}(x)$ is that for the transition $E_{20} \to E_{21}$, indicting that a susceptible single female of age x at some time t has been infected during the time interval $(t, t+h]$. No attempt will be made in this section to derive a formula for this risk function. By consulting Section 12.5, it can be seen that similar techniques could be used to derive a formula for the risk function $\theta_{fm02}(x)$. More precisely, this function should be written as $\theta_{fm02}(t; x)$ to emphasize that it would depend on the sample functions of the process at time t. When specifying the matrices of latent risks in Eqs. (13.6.1) and (13.6.4), care should be taken that the parameters in all risk functions are expressed in terms of the same time unit such as a month or year.

The next task to be considered in this section is that of defining the state space and matrix of latent risks for the life cycle model for a couple of type (x, y) with ages $x > a_{f0}$ and $y > a_{m0}$. For this component of the system, the set of absorbing states will contain five elements. Let E_{DIS} denote the event of couple dissolution by either separation or divorce; let E_{f11} and E_{f12} denote, respectively, a female death from a cause other than disease or a death due disease; the absorbing states E_{m11} and E_{m12} are defined similarly for male deaths. The set of transient states will contain four elements denoted by $(0,0)$, $(0,1)$, $(1,0)$ and $(1,1)$. As in Chapter 12, the symbol $(0,0)$ indicates that both the female and male of a couple are susceptible; the symbol $(0,1)$ indicates that the female is susceptible, but the males is infected; and the two remaining symbols, $(1,0)$ and $(1,1)$, are interpreted similarly. For singles, the rows of the matrix of latent risks for couple evolution will be indexed by the set of transient states and the columns of the entire state space. Thus, the matrix of latent risks for couples is 4×9, and for each couple type (x, y) and time t, it may represented in the partitioned form,

$$\boldsymbol{\Theta}_c(t; x, y) = [\boldsymbol{\Theta}_{c1}(t; x, y), \boldsymbol{\Theta}_{c2}(t; x, y)] \ , \tag{13.6.6}$$

where $\boldsymbol{\Theta}_{c1}(t; x, y)$ is a 4×5 matrix of risks governing transitions from the set of transient states to the set of absorbing states, and $\boldsymbol{\Theta}_{c2}(t; x, y)$ is a 4×4 matrix governing transitions among the transient states.

With with respect to risks of death, the latent risks described above for females and males may again be used in the matrix $\boldsymbol{\Theta}_{c1}(t; x, y)$, but to complete the specification of this matrix, risks for couple dissolution need to be included. Thus, for each couple type (x, y) and time t, this matrix will have the form,

$$\boldsymbol{\Theta}_{c1}(t; x, y) = \begin{bmatrix} \delta & \theta_{fm1}(x) & 0 & \theta_{mm1}(y) & 0 \\ \delta & \theta_{fm1}(x) & 0 & \theta_{mm1}(y) & \theta_{mm2}(y) \\ \delta & \theta_{fm1}(x) & \theta_{fm2}(x) & \theta_{mm1}(y) & 0 \\ \delta & \theta_{fm1}(x) & \theta_{fm2}(x) & \theta_{mm1}(y) & \theta_{mm2}(y) \end{bmatrix} . \tag{13.6.7}$$

In this matrix, δ is the risk of couple dissolution per unit time, the risk function $\theta_{fm1}(x)$ for females of age x is defined as in Eq. (13.6.5), and $\theta_{fm2}(x) = \mu_{f1}$ is a positive constant for all $x > a_{f0}$. The risk functions $\theta_{mm1}(y)$ and $\theta_{mm2}(y)$ are defined similarly for males of age y, but with parameters specific to males. It should be mentioned that the assumption of a constant risk δ for couple dissolution is a bit unrealistic. It has been observed empirically that the longer a couple stays together, the less the risk of their dissolution due to separation or divorce. Thus, δ should be a decreasing function of z, the duration of marriage. But the inclusion of this variable would greatly increase the number of couple types to be considered since a couple type (x, y, z) would contain three variables. It should be mentioned that Kamali[4] worked with a model accommodating the variable z, but the design of the system differed from that under consideration in that matrices of competing latent risks were not used.

With regard to transitions among transient states in the life cycle model for couples, the 4×4 matrix of latent risks for a couple of type (x, y) at time t takes the form,

$$\boldsymbol{\Theta}_{c2}(t; x, y) = \begin{bmatrix} 0 & \theta_{mm02}(t; y) & \theta_{fm02}(t; x) & 0 \\ 0 & 0 & 0 & \theta_{fm012}(t; x) \\ 0 & 0 & 0 & \theta_{mm102}(t; y) \\ 0 & 0 & 0 & 0 \end{bmatrix}. \tag{13.6.8}$$

The risk function $\theta_{mm02}(t; y)$ is that for the transition $(0,0) \to (0,1)$, indicating that the male member of a couple of age y at time t was infected during the time $(t, t+h]$ by extra-marital sexual contacts; the risk function $\theta_{fm02}(t; x)$ is similarly defined for the transition $(0,0) \to (1,0)$, indicating that a susceptible female of age x at time t was infected during the time interval $(t, t+h]$ by extra-marital sexual contacts. Note that the risk function $\theta_{fm012}(t; x)$ is for the transition $(0,1) \to (1,1)$, indicating that a susceptible female was infected during the time interval $(t, t+h]$ by either marital or extra-marital sexual contacts. Finally, the risk function $\theta_{mm102}(t; y)$ is for the transition $(1,0) \to (1,1)$ and has a similar interpretation for susceptible males. Although the details will be omitted, explicit formulas for these risk functions could be derived using the ideas set forth in Section 12.5.

In closing this brief overview of a procedure for the formulation of stochastic models of epidemics in the age-dependent case when infectives are included in a population, it is appropriate to make few remarks as to how the model of Chapter 12 may be extended to accommodate age. The first of these remarks concerns transitions from one age class to another. Although some ideas for handling these transitions have been discussed in the closing paragraph of Section 13.3, such transitions have been omitted in this section, because they would depend on the scheme used to group ages. For example, if ages were grouped into intervals of length one year and the time unit for sexual contacts was one month, then ages would be held constant for 12 time units, and at the end of the 12th unit, the ages of all live individuals would be advanced one year. Similar remarks hold if age intervals were grouped in two years. Because the aging process is slow compared to progression of some infectious diseases, it would seem reasonable to hold the risk functions constant on age intervals of lengths one or two years. However, if one used age intervals of length five years, as is often the case in practice, then there might be some question as to whether the risk functions should be held constant for the five-year interval, particularly at the older ages when rates of aging increase rather rapidly.

On the other hand, it may be feasible to use age classes of varying length, depending on the risks of death that vary according to age. For example, during the first five years of life, as well for ages 70 or greater, it would seem reasonable to use a finer grouping of ages, such as one or two years, to reflect greater changes in the risks of death. But, for ages 5 to 70, age groupings of three to five years may be appropriate, because the risks of death change more slowly in these ages. It is clear that after a decision has been made as to which classification of ages is to be used in a computer implementation, the ideas of chain multinomial distributions developed in Chapter 12 could be used to compute Monte Carlo realizations of the process on some discrete time lattice with an equal spacing $h > 0$ of points; moreover, the techniques used to embed non-linear differences equations in the stochastic process on this lattice could also be extended to age-dependent models discussed in this chapter. If a finite number of age classes remain fixed so that they may be accommodated in finitely many types of individuals, then, as in Chapters 10, 11, and 12, by letting $h \downarrow 0$ in the non-linear difference equations, it can be shown that a large system of ordinary differential equations would arise, which in principle could be used to get a handle on threshold conditions. However, if age were viewed as a continuous variable, then as $h \downarrow 0$, one is lead to the conjecture that a system of partial differential equations would arise, but the derivation of such equations will be left as a future research exercise.

13.7 References

1. L. M. Abia and J. C. Lopez-Marcos, On the Numerical Integration of Non-Local Terms for Age-Structured Population Equations, *Mathematical Biosciences* **157:** 147-168, 1999.
2. O. Angulo and J. C. Lopez-Marcos, Numerical Schemes for Size-Structured Population Equations, *Mathematical Biosciences* **157:** 169-188, 1999.
3. E. Artin, *The Gamma Function,* New York, Chicago, San Francisco, Toronto, London, Holt, Rinehart and Winston, 1964.
4. R. Kamali, *A Methodological Investigation of an AIDS Epidemic in a Heterosexual Population through Extra-Marital Sexual Contacts,* Ph. D. Thesis, Drexel University Library, Philadelphia Pennsylvania, 1996.
5. M. Martcheva, Exponential Growth in Age-Structured Two-Sex Populations, *Mathematical Biosciences* **157***:* 1-22, 1999.
6. C. J. Mode, On Statistically Assessing Critical Population Size of an Endangered Species in a Random Environment, *IMA Journal of Mathematics Applied in Medicine and Biology* **5**: 147-166, 1988.
7. C. J. Mode, A Stochastic Model for the Development of an AIDS Epidemic in a Heterosexual Population, *Mathematical Biosciences* **107:** 491-520, 1991.
8. C. J. Mode, *Stochastic Processes in Demography and Their Computer Implementation,* Springer-Verlag, Berlin, Heidelberg, New York, Tokyo, 1985.
9. C. J. Mode and M. E. Jacobson, On Estimating Critical Population Size of an Endangered Species, *Mathematical Biosciences* **85**: 185-209, 1987.
10. C. J. Mode and M. E. Jacobson, A Study of the Impact of Environmental Stochasticity on Extinction Probabilities by Monte Carlo Integration, *Mathematical Biosciences* **83**: 105-125, 1987.
11. C. J. Mode, G. T. Pickens and D. C. Ewbank, Demographic Heterogeneity and Uncertainty in Population Projections, *IMA Journal of Mathematics Applied in Medicine and Biology* **4**: 223-236, 1987.

12. C. J. Mode and T. Root, Projecting Age-Structured Populations in a Random Environment, *Mathematical Biosciences* **88**: 223-245, 1988.

13. C. J. Mode and M. A. Salsburg, On the Formulation and Computer Implementation of an Age-Dependent Two-Sex Demographic Model, *Mathematical Biosciences* **118:** 211-240, 1993.

14. M. A. Salsburg, *The Formulation and Implementation of a Stochastic Model that Explores HIV Infection,* Ph.D. Thesis, Drexel University Library, Philadelphia, Pennsylvania, 1992.

15. W. A. Siler, Competing-Risk Model for Animal Mortality, *Ecology* **60:** 750-759, 1979.

16. W. Y. Tan and Z. Xiang, A Stochastic Model for the HIV Epidemic and Effects of Age and Race on the HIV Infection in Homosexual Populations, *Series in Mathematical Biology and Medicine* **6:** 425-451, O. Arino, D. Axelrod and M. Kimmel (eds.), *Advances in Mathematical Population Dynamics - Molecules, Cells and Man,* World Scientific Publishing Company, Singapore, New Jersey, London, Hong Kong, 1997.

17. D. Widder, *Advanced Calculus*, New York, Prentice Hall, 1947.

Chapter 14
EPILOGUE - FUTURE RESEARCH DIRECTIONS

14.1 Modeling Mutations in Disease Causing Agents

A feature common to all the stochastic structures presented in Chapters 10, 11 and 12, as well as the initial steps toward a formulation of age dependent models presented in Chapter 13, is that of modeling various aspects of human behavior that can play decisive roles as to whether an epidemic of a sexually transmitted disease develops, following the introduction of infectives into a population of susceptibles. Among the aspects of human behavior considered were the expected number of either marital or extra-marital sexual contacts per unit time, probabilities of infection per contact, and choices of partners as modeled in contact structures expressed in terms of acceptance probabilities. Further work directed at refining these formulations and developing the necessary software seems warranted, but there is also a need for research in other directions. Apart from a few computer exercises in Chapters 10, 11 and 12, where mutational events were simulated by supposing that during any time interval an infectious recruit entered a population of susceptibles with small probability, no attention was given to mutations occurring in a disease-causing agent that the recruits were supposed to carry. It is known, however, that mutations play a basic role in the evolution of disease-causing agents, and attempts to control epidemics often center around developing strategies to cope with new mutations that have occurred in a disease-causing organism.

A question that naturally arises, therefore, is how should one approach the modeling of mutations in disease-causing agents? Mutations are unpredictable and are thus stochastic in nature. Hence, the development of stochastic models will certainly be among the more fruitful routes to pursue as was first demonstrated by Fisher,[1] who used a branching process in his study of the survival of a mutant gene. But, at this point time, the precise routes such modeling efforts may take are not clear, although it seems worthwhile to speculate on some of the possibilities. If, for example, mutations are approached at the gene level, then for those disease-causing agents whose genomes are relatively simple, developing a stochastic model with a state space $\mathfrak{S}$ that encompasses a rather large set of possible mutations and interactions among them may be feasible, particularly if computer intensive methods were used. According to the interesting and informative book by Oldstone,[3] some disease-causing viruses are examples of organisms with relatively few genes. For, it has been reported that each of the viruses causing measles, yellow fever, poliomyelitis and Lassa fever, as well as the Ebola virus, Hantavirus and HIV, have fewer than 10 genes.

By way of illustrating some ideas in selecting state spaces, suppose the genome of an organism has 10 loci with two alleles at each locus. Then, the total number of genotypes would be $2^{10} = 1024$; if there were 3 alleles at each locus, then $3^{10} = 59049$ genotypes would be possible. A set of genotypes, either realized or potential, could be selected as a state space. On the other hand, if the interaction of genes is the primary focus of attention, then it may be of interest to consider combinations of genes as elements of a state space. For example, if it is of interest to ascertain the number of ways a set of genes may interact, then one is led to consider combinations of genes taken 2 at a time, 3 at a time, and so on. For the case of n genes, the total number of combinations taking at least 2 at a time is:

$$\sum_{k=2}^{n} \binom{n}{k} = 2^n - n - 1 . \tag{14.1.1}$$

For the case of $n = 10$ genes, this number is $2^{10} - 10 - 1 = 1013$. Because it is now possible to represent state spaces $\mathfrak{S}$, containing 1024, 59049 or 1013 elements on many personal computers, working with state spaces of these sizes is becoming increasingly feasible for many investigators with limited budgets.

Evidently, combinations of "new" mutant genes with others in the pathogen seem to interact with genes in the host in such a way that a mutant version of the pathogen is able to evade the defenses of the host's immune system that was formerly resistant to the pathogen. Two questions that naturally arise are what is the nature of this interaction and how may it be studied. In this connection, in a recent news article by Marshall,[2] some interesting results that offer hope in answering these questions were reported for two disease-causing organisms. Briefly, microarrays of DNA, containing thousand of human genes, are now becoming increasingly available to investigators, making it possible to test interactions of human genes with those of a pathogen. In an experiment with two strains of the Ebola virus, which were not harmful to humans, researches at the US Army Medical Research Institute in Frederick, Maryland, compared the gene expression profiles of normal human leukocytes with those infected with the virus. These experiments suggest that the genes in one strain of the virus induced genes in the host to produce immune-system regulators called cyctokines and chemokines, as well as inhibitors of a cell death process called apoptosis. According to investigators, these results suggest how the deadly Zaire strain of the virus spreads so rapidly in an infected individual. Further information on the Ebola virus may be found in Oldstone.[3] British researchers, using related techniques and working with a microarray of DNA from the bacterium *Mycobacterium tuberculosis* that causes tuberculosis (TB), suggested that the pathogen competes with the host for iron and induces a dormancy response that may help TB evade immune attack.

Because microarrays of DNA may be produced at relatively low cost, it seems plausible that in future many researchers will be conducting experiments similar to those mentioned above in which interactions of genes in the pathogen and host will be studied. As time passes, it seems likely that such studies will lead to the construction of large data bases, which upon analysis will not only suggest ways to develop therapeutic measures to control or eliminate mutant forms of a pathogen after it invades a host, but may also may provide information on sets of mutant genes in terms of changes in the molecular structures differentiating them. Changes in molecular structures may in turn be viewed mathematically as some types of transformations among the elements of a state space consisting of genes or perhaps combinations of genes that constitute the genome of a pathogen. The genomes of more pathogens will be sequenced, and as the data becomes available from these efforts and from the types of experiments discussed above, it may be possible to formulate the structure of the genome of a pathogen mathematically in terms of a well-defined state space with transformations connecting existing or potential elements of this space expressed in terms of transition probabilities with unknown parameters. Moreover, using such data, it should be possible to estimate the unknown parameters and develop a stochastic framework that would aid in assigning predictive probabilities of which mutations or transformations are most likely to occur in the future.

In summary, it seems unlikely that it will be possible to eliminate most existing pathogens or to predict with certainty which new pathogens may arise in the future as a result of an evolutionary process whose details are not, as yet, well understood. But, with the ongoing development of technology that aids in the study of mutational phenomena at the molecular level, there are very good reasons to believe that the details of this evolutionary process will be further illuminated and aid in man's quest to respond more quickly and effectively with measures to combat the detrimental effects of mutational changes in existing pathogens or the emergence of new ones. As in the past, however, variation and uncertainty, which are characteristic of all biological systems, will be an intrinsic part of these evolutionary processes, and the need to come to grips with this variation and uncertainty in predicting mutational changes in pathogens at the level of practical applications will stimulate the development of new stochastic models and computer intensive methods, whose structures can, at present, be only dimly perceived. In closing, it should be mentioned in that there already exists some literature on mathematical models dealing with mutational changes that have occurred in at the cellular level in man in connection with cancer and other studies. For readers interested in such topics, one point of entry into this literature is the recent deterministic paper by Polanski, Kimmel and Swierniak,[4] and the references cited therein.

14.2 References

1. R. A. Fisher, *The General Theory of Natural Selection,* New York, Dover, 1958.

2. E. Marshall, Do-It-Yourself Gene Watching, *Science* **286:** 444-447, 1999.

3. M. B. A. Oldstone, *Viruses, Plagues, and History,* New York, Oxford, Oxford University Press, 1998.

4. A. Polanski, M. Kimmel and A. Swierniak, Qualitative Analysis of the Infinite Dimensional Model of Evolution of Drug Resistance, *Series in Mathematical Biology and Medicine* **6:** 595-612, O. Arino, D. Axelrod and M. Kimmel (eds.), *Advances in Mathematical Population Dynamics - Molecules, Cells and Man,* World Scientific Publishing Company, Singapore, New Jersey, London, Hong Kong, 1997.

AUTHOR INDEX

SUBJECT INDEX